Intraoperative Mapping of Cognitive Networks

Emmanuel Mandonnet • Guillaume Herbet
Editors

Intraoperative Mapping of Cognitive Networks

Which Tasks for Which Locations

Springer

Editors
Emmanuel Mandonnet
Department of Neurosurgery
Lariboisière Hospital
Paris Brain Institute (ICM)
and Paris University
Paris
France

Guillaume Herbet
Department of Neurosurgery
Gui de Chauliac Hospital, Montpellier
& Institute of Functional Genomics
University of Montpellier, INSERM, CNRS
Montpellier
France

ISBN 978-3-030-75070-1 ISBN 978-3-030-75071-8 (eBook)
https://doi.org/10.1007/978-3-030-75071-8

This Springer imprint is published by the registered company Springer Nature Switzerland AG
The registered company address is: Gewerbestrasse 11, 6330 Cham, Switzerland

Foreword

With the exception of a few seminal works by pioneers in surgical brain mapping, such as Wilder Penfield and George Ojemann, the link between neurosurgery and basic neuroscience remained weak for about a century. The reinforcement of interactions across technical and conceptual advances in the understanding of dynamic processes underpinning neural functions, and clinical implications in brain-damaged patients, especially in those who need cerebral surgery, is now a reality. Remarkably, the emerging field of connectomics, which resulted in the elaboration of original models in cognitive neuroscience based upon intercommunications between distributed neural networks, and challenging the obsolete localizationist framework yet still entrenched in the neurosurgical and neurological communities, opened new avenues to explore neuroplastic mechanisms. Indeed, predicting potentials and limitations of neural redeployment at the individual level is very valuable to preserve an optimal quality of life in patients who will undergo brain surgery. Besides epilepsy, such an ambitious aim is particularly critical in neurooncology, since the life expectancy significantly increased in brain tumor patients in the past two decades, mainly due to early and extensive surgical resections.

To this end, beyond the contribution of perioperative noninvasive functional neuroimaging, intra-surgical awake mapping by means of direct cortical and axonal electrostimulation, able to transitorily and repeatedly disrupt specific functional systems as well as their interplay, and combined with real-time behavioral monitoring, allows structural-functional correlations throughout the surgical act. The ultimate aim is to decipher the individual connectome and to tailor the resection according to the functional circuitry, most of the time already reorganized due to the prior tumor progression, in order to find the best compromise between the oncological and neurological aspects. In this connectome-based approach, awake surgery should be considered in a systematic way regardless of the tumor location. Therefore, an optimal selection of tasks to be administrated during the cognitive monitoring is of utmost importance, to optimize the extent of resection and thus survival while minimizing the functional risk. Importantly, such a selection must be based not only on the relationships between the tumor and the surrounding cortico-subcortical neural circuits but also on the definition of a personalized quality of life by the patient him/herself, taking into consideration his/her wishes as well as his/her environment.

Making the link between patients' expectations, neural foundations of behavior, and surgical planning implies first to revisit the traditional rigid and reductionist model of brain organization which prevailed for too long, and which commonly led to a simplistic view in clinical practice, that is, to propose a battery of tasks according to the lobar cortical localization of a cerebral lesion. This is the reason why a textbook on intraoperative mapping of cognitive networks was desperately needed. Led by the editors, Emmanuel Mandonnet and Guillaume Herbet, this collective body of work will serve as a comprehensive book for all multidisciplinary neurosurgical teams with a flexible and individualized perspective of brain surgery. In fact, what makes this volume so unusual is its translational approach bringing together experts in various fields, including not only neurosurgeons but also neuropsychologists, speech therapists, neurologists, neuroanatomists, neurophysiologists, and neuroscientists. The philosophical positions the authors have taken in rethinking the neural bases sustaining functional networks, with a progression from unimodal segregated systems (as vision) to more integrated complex systems and their dynamic interactions in a meta-networking perspective (as creativity), as well as the implication for neurosurgical management are quite unique and innovative, to say the least.

The book is organized in a logical and informative fashion, starting with chapters covering the neurobiology of sensorimotor and visuospatial functions and the application of such knowledge to select and administrate adapted tasks into the operating theater. I particularly like the way in which movement was redefined, that is, beyond the output pyramidal system that should be preserved to avoid postoperative hemiparesis in classical neurosurgery (usually performed under general anesthesia), as an interplay between networks mediating movement execution and movement control, making possible a mapping and monitoring of complex skills (as bimanual coordination) in awake patients who expressed their desire to preserve a perfect conation. The second part of the textbook is dedicated to various aspects of oral and written language, which still represents for the vast majority of neurosurgeons the optimal (or even the sole) indication of awake mapping. Yet, as demonstrated in the next chapters, higher-order cognitive functions have also to be considered, whatever the hemisphere involved by the lesion, including in the right side wrongly claimed as "nondominant" in the older literature. Besides nonverbal semantics and executive functions, an important issue is the introduction of tasks capable of providing during surgery insights into the theory of mind, which is critical for interpersonal relationships: this breakthrough goes beyond the classical view of a damaged brain taken in isolation, disconnected from its social environment. Another original concept is the multitasking throughout the resection, increasing the cognitive demand by playing with the inter-system communication without extending the duration of surgery, so taking account of the practical constraints in the operating room, especially the risk of patient tiredness. Finally, future prospects are discussed, paving the way for monitoring more integrated aspects of human being, such as personality, creative behavior, and intuition. These high-order considerations raise *in fine* indirectly the problem of the onco-functional balance, since the price to pay to optimize intraoperative mapping could be to interrupt prematurely the resection: such medico-surgical as well as philosophical discussion needs to take place in a systematic manner with the patient and his/her family before each surgery, to select tasks "à la carte."

Modern neurosurgery should play a pivotal role in developing the synapse between, on one hand fundamental neuroscience, by designing on the basis of factual observations new models of dynamic spatiotemporal integration within and across neural circuits underpinning constant plastic reconfiguration, and on the other hand clinical applications, by using such an instability of the connectome to increase survival of brain-damaged patients while preserving their conation, cognition, emotion, and adapted behavior—in order to give them the opportunity to make their own choices regarding long-term projects. I have no doubt that this comprehensive and unique textbook edited by Dr. Mandonnet, Dr. Herbet, and their colleagues will serve this purpose with considerable distinction. I applaud them for bringing everything known about this complicated subject, so far poorly explored, within the confines of one textbook, which will be the definitive source on this topic. This volume is a major contribution that will be significant in the history not only of neurosurgery and cerebral mapping but also of clinical neurology and neurosciences. This is a must-read for anyone in the field—and beyond!

Hugues Duffau
Department of Neurosurgery
Gui de Chauliac hospital
Montpellier University Medical Center
Institute of Functional Genomics
University of Montpellier, INSERM U1191
Montpellier
France

Preface

In the first half of the twentieth century, Wilder Penfield was the first neurosurgeon to use, in a systematic way, cortical electrostimulation in awake patients with the aim of mapping functional areas surrounding an epileptogenic focus to be removed. In the years 1940–1950, together with his student Theodore Rasmussen, who was both neurosurgeon and neurologist, they depicted with great accuracy not only the well-known homunculus describing the topographical organization of the different parts of the body within the pre- and post-central sensorimotor areas but also other sensory areas such as auditory or visual cortex. They further provided a detailed mapping of associative temporal areas, the stimulation of which triggered complex cognitive phenomenon, like experiencing vivid memories. Later on, Penfield collaborated with neuropsychologists Donald Hebb and Brenda Milner, and they introduced in the mapping procedure several cognitive tasks like picture naming, writing, and reading [1]: the modern intraoperative cognitive monitoring was born.

Following this line of clinical practice for epilepsy surgery, the neurosurgeon George Ojemann and the neuropsychologist Catherine Mateer further introduced new behavioral tasks, in an attempt to evaluate and preserve, in addition to naming, syntax and verbal working memory [2]. Moreover, Ojemann envisioned that brain tumor patients should also benefit from applying the principles of intraoperative brain mapping with electrical stimulation under awake conditions. In the early 1990s, he guided the first steps in the field of two of his young fellows, Mitch Berger and Hugues Duffau. Together, they completely renewed the field of surgical neuro-oncology: Mitch Berger clearly demonstrated the survival benefit of maximizing the resection [3], while Hugues Duffau pushed further the potentialities of functional preservation. Indeed, he extended the mapping to the white matter pathways [4] and he introduced, in collaboration with neuropsychologists, new cognitive tasks, such as the line bisection paradigm [5]. Almost 30 years later, awake surgery for brain tumors has considerably spread over the world and is firmly considered as the most reliable tool to guide the neurosurgeon in a maximally safe resection.

What is meant by safe resection? The answer to this important question greatly evolved over time. At first, preserving motor and language functions was the main objective. Hence, in addition to the detection of stimulation-induced movements, picture naming was, and still is, the essential task to be monitored throughout the resection. But then, it became apparent that clinical and neuropsychological postoperative examinations revealed that sparing areas responsive at picture naming task did not prevent deterioration in other language and cognitive functions, such as reading, writing, speaking spontaneously, spatial awareness, mentalizing, attention, cognitive flexibility, inhibition, emotion recognition, and so on. In particular, Herbet and Duffau demonstrated the importance of mapping the right hemisphere [6], a tumor location for which many teams previously did not consider awake surgery. Following their pioneering work, different teams around the world started to introduce new tasks in order to monitor a variety of cognitive functions, with the good intention to improve overall cognitive outcome. However, because there is always the possibility that such tasks are introduced for addressing some purely scientific questions rather than for the direct benefit of patients [7], some rules should be kept in mind when choosing to use a new task intraoperatively.

First, the necessity to preserve a specific function should be thoroughly discussed with the patient during the preoperative interview. The goal is to define with the patient which cognitive profile would allow him to enjoy his life. This cognitive profiling differs for a musician, an engineer, a school teacher, or a building worker. From this starting point, a set of tasks tapping into the cognitive functions to be preserved could be selected. This is something neurosurgeons are not well trained for. The help of neuropsychologists is already essential here and, in fact, our brief historical review clearly highlights that a successful awake surgery relies on the smooth collaboration within a neurosurgeon/neuropsychologist pair.

The next step is to select, according to the location of the tumor, a limited number of tasks aimed to map the different neurocognitive networks invaded by or close to the tumor. This is an incredibly big challenge, because there are no simple structure-function mappings in the cognitive domain. The reasons for this are multiple and beyond the scope of this introduction, but we can briefly mention the three major ones:

- Efficient cognitive functioning results from the synchronized interaction of several spatially distant but connected areas.
- Such network-level organization exhibits an important interindividual variability.
- Network resilience to injury also greatly varies between individuals, as patients are unequal regarding neuroplastic potentialities.

As the aim of this book is to give an extensive overview of our current state of knowledge regarding this crucial question, these three points will be repeatedly addressed in the course of the chapters. But here again, the dialog with the neuropsychologist is also essential: any deficit evidenced in the preoperative evaluation should act as a strong warning that the corresponding function is at risk and that it should be monitored intraoperatively. Noninvasive preoperative functional mapping (task-based and resting state fMRI, tractography, MEG, TMS, …) has also an important role to play, as it provides a means to partly account for interindividual variability. The most striking example is given by the preoperative identification of uncommon reversed lateralization of verbal and visuo-spatial hemispheres, an essential information to integrate in the selection of intraoperative tasks [8].

Ultimately, there still remain many unclear points, and it is our hope that the reading of our book will motivate new neurosurgeon/neuropsychologist pairs to shed some light on some of those, through a retrospective in-depth analysis of the data collected during their experience in perioperative mapping of cognitive networks.

Paris, France — Emmanuel Mandonnet
Montpellier, France — Guillaume Herbet

References

1. Penfield W, Roberts L. Speech and brain mechanisms [Internet]. Princeton University Press, Princeton. 1959 [cited 2021 Jan 16]. Available from: https://press.princeton.edu/books/hardcover/9780691642635/speech-and-brain-mechanisms
2. Ojemann G, Mateer C. Human language cortex: localization of memory, syntax, and sequential motor-phoneme identification systems. Science. 1979;205(4413):1401–3.
3. Berger MS, Deliganis AV, Dobbins J, Keles GE. The effect of extent of resection on recurrence in patients with low grade cerebral hemisphere gliomas. Cancer. 1994;74(6):1784–91.
4. Duffau H, Capelle L, Sichez N, Denvil D, Lopes M, Sichez J-P, et al. Intraoperative mapping of the subcortical language pathways using direct stimulations. An anatomo-functional study. Brain.2002;125(Pt 1):199–214.
5. Thiebaut de Schotten M, Urbanski M, Duffau H, Volle E, Lévy R, Dubois B, et al. Direct evidence for a parietal-frontal pathway subserving spatial awareness in humans. Science. 2005;309(5744):2226–8.
6. Herbet G, Duffau H. Revisiting the functional anatomy of the human brain: toward a meta-networking theory of cerebral functions. Physiol Rev. 2020;100(3):1181–228.
7. Mandonnet E, Herbet G, Duffau H. Letter: Introducing new tasks for intraoperative mapping in awake glioma surgery: clearing the line between patient care and scientific research. Neurosurgery. 2020;86(2):E256–7.
8. Mandonnet E, Mellerio C, Barberis M, Poisson I, Jansma JM, Rutten G-J. When right is on the left (and vice versa): a case series of glioma patients with reversed lateralization of cognitive functions. J Neurol Surg A Cent Eur Neurosurg. 2020;81(2):138–46.

Contents

Part I

Sensorimotor and Visuo-Spatial Functions

Motor Control

1

Lorenzo Bello, Christian F. Freyschlag, and Fabien Rech

1.1 Neural Basis of Motor Control

Surgical mapping and tumor removal require a good understanding of the cortical and subcortical organization of the motor control network. To this end, we will review here the main components which might be considered during surgery.

The primary motor cortex (M1), classically considered as the core of the motor system, is located on the lateral and medial face of the precentral gyrus and is constituted by Brodmann area 4 [1], containing pyramidal cells, from which emerge the "pyramidal" tract. This fascicle is going through the posterior limb of the internal capsule, decussates (for 80–85% of the fibers [2]) in the brainstem, and finally projects in the spinal cord, where it has the main control on the motoneuron of the IX couch of Rexed [3]. It presents a broad somatotopy [4], with region dedicated to the face and upper limb located laterally and region dedicated to the lower limb located medially. However, this classical view of the Penfieldian homunculus needs to be nuanced because there are many overlapping (up to four parts of the body) on the precentral gyrus [5]. In fact, the functional organization of the primary motor cortex is likely more oriented toward the goal of action and the precentral gyrus should be analyzed in terms of ethological action map rather than somatotopic map [6].

L. Bello
Neurosurgical Oncology Unit, Department of Oncology and Hemato-Oncology, Università degli Studi di Milano, Milan, Italy
e-mail: lorenzo.bello@unimi.it

C. F. Freyschlag
Department of Neurosurgery, Medical University of Innsbruck, Innsbruck, Austria
e-mail: christian.freyschlag@i-med.ac.at

F. Rech (✉)
Service de Neurochirurgie, Université de Lorraine, CHRU-Nancy, Nancy, France

Université de Lorraine, CNRS, CRAN, Nancy, France
e-mail: f.rech@chru-nancy.fr

E. Mandonnet, G. Herbet (eds.), *Intraoperative Mapping of Cognitive Networks*,
https://doi.org/10.1007/978-3-030-75071-8_1

Immediately anterior to the precentral gyrus are located the dorsal (PMd) and ventral (PMv) premotor cortex, corresponding to Brodmann area 6. Both regions show strong connections with the supplementary motor area (SMA), M1, the spinal cord, and the superior (PMd) and inferior (PMv) parietal lobule [7, 8] in the framework of a large frontoparietal network. The PMd extends over the superior and middle frontal gyrus. The rostral PMd is involved in executive function, attention, and working memory whereas caudal PMd could be more dedicated to movement preparation and execution [9]. The PMd seems to be involved in decisional process during movement selection based on arbitrary clues [10, 11] and codes the conditional probability of a movement based on the body position to preselect the optimal motor program [12] probably thanks to dense connections with the superior parietal lobule through the superior longitudinal fascicle branch I (SLF I) [13]. fMRI studies reported a more complex functional segregation of the PMd, especially between working memory, attention, motricity of hand, eye movement, and action [14, 15].

The PMv is located on the ventral part of the precentral gyrus. By virtue of its connection to the inferior parietal lobule via the SLF III [13], its role is to adapt the hand shape to the object to favor the grasp contrary to the PMd which is involved in reaching [11]. Functional imaging studies suggest that the PMv is at least divided in two subregions activated, respectively, during spatial location (dorsal part of the PMv) and grasping observation (ventral part of the PMv). It is then one crucial component of the mirror neuron network [16]. Left PMv has also been identified as a crucial part of the speech network [17].

PMd and PMv over the precentral gyrus play a role in motor control as direct stimulations can elicit movement arrest emphasizing the role of such areas in motor control [18] (Figs. 1.1, 1.2, and 1.3). Recent studies based on direct electrical stimulation (DES) suggest that the precentral gyrus can be divided in several parts as proposed by neuroimaging studies (Fig. 1.4) [19]. Interestingly, three of these subareas are responsible of identical clinical responses during DES, thus excluding a simple somatotopic distribution of the network involved in motor control and reinforcing the hypothesis of ethological organization. Moreover, both hand movement and speech can be disturbed during single electrostimulation over both PMv and PMd, pleading in favor of a complex organization and interactions between the language and the motor networks at this level [20].

The SMA is located on the medial face of the brain on Brodmann area 6. It is classically divided into a rostral preSMA and a caudal SMAproper [21] although the cellular organization plead more for a continuum without sharp borders [22]. The SMA is connected to the alpha motor neuron of the spinal cord, the inferior frontal gyrus (IFG), PMd, PMv, M1, and superior (SPL) and inferior (IPL) parietal lobules [7, 23, 24]. Patterns of connections between the preSMA and the SMA proper are slightly different. PreSMA has connections with cognitive areas whereas SMA proper has only connections with motor and premotor area [24]. A somatotopic organization has been identified into the SMAproper with, rostrally to caudally, language in the dominant hemisphere, then face, upper limb, and finally lower limb area [25]. PreSMA is involved in internally generated movement [26] and the complex preSMA/SMAproper is involved in complex sequences of movements as

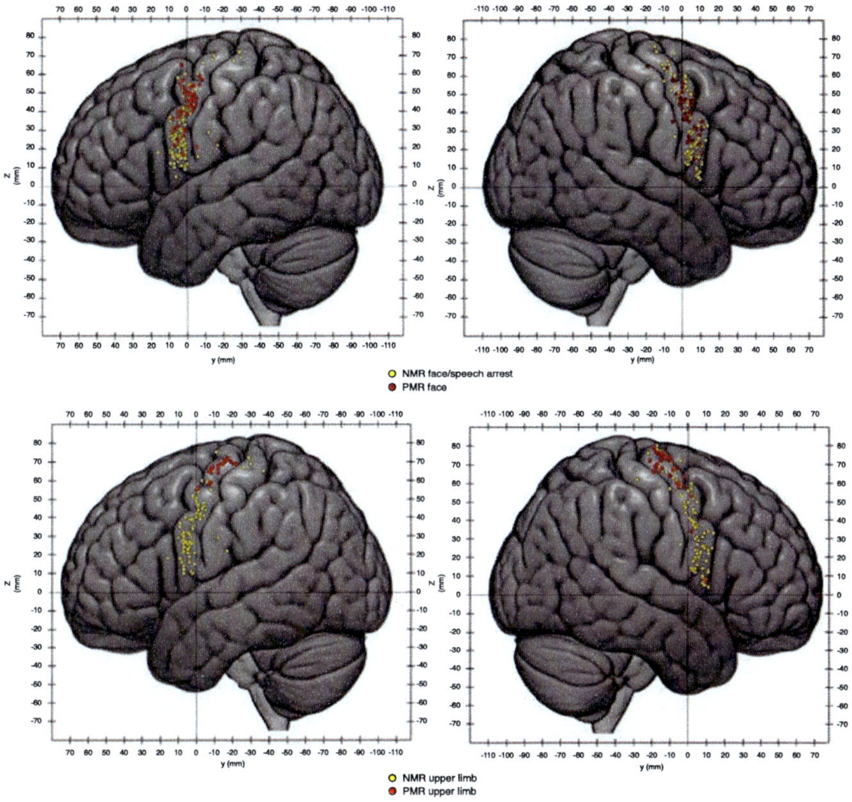

Fig. 1.1 Overlap between negative motor (NMR) and positive motor (PMR) responses. Yellow dots = NMRs; red dots = PMRs. Top = face & speech; bottom = upper limb. The coordinates correspond to the MNI reference space (with permission of [19])

well as in temporal sequencing [27, 28], bimanual coordination [29], learning [30], task switching [31], and inhibition [24]. Given the putative numerous roles of the SMA, it has been suggested it is working through action-condition associations where motor behaviors are selected thanks to rules depending on conditions and requiring inhibition to select the appropriate sequences. Learning would then consist in creating the optimal action-condition associations. Under this view, the SMA should be considered as a whole and a continuum linking cognitive areas to motor ones thanks to action-condition associations [24]. These hypotheses tend to be confirmed by electrostimulation procedures which, despite a broad somatotopy, failed to identify sharpened borders into the SMA [32].

The SMA is connected with the IFG and the ventral part of the precentral gyrus through the frontal aslant tract (FAT). DES of the left and right FAT can induce speech arrest and surgery to the contact of the left FAT is followed by spontaneous speech disorders, confirming the role of this network in the speech initiation and

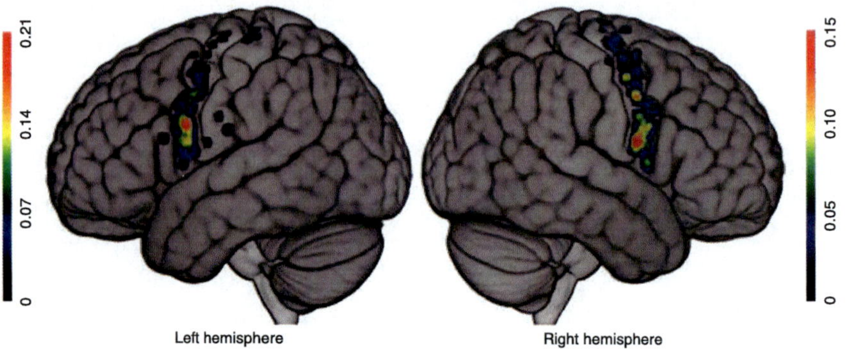

Fig. 1.2 Probabilistic map of face/speech arrest negative motor responses for each hemisphere. The color bar indicates the probability. Scales were adjusted for each hemisphere, to highlight differences inside the precentral gyrus (with permission of [19])

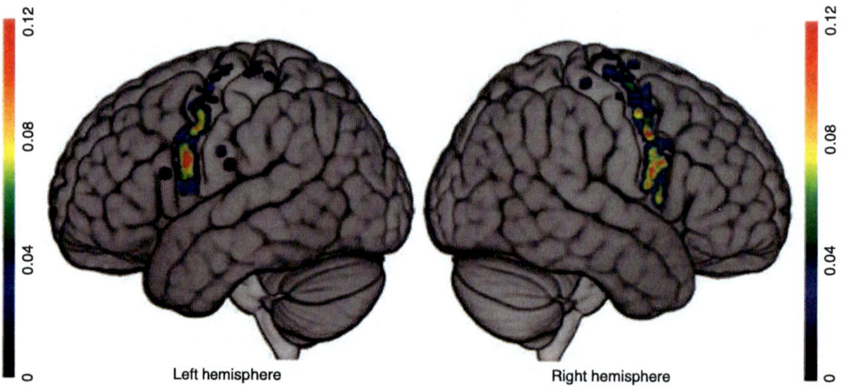

Fig. 1.3 Probabilistic map of upper limb negative motor responses for each hemisphere. The color bar indicates the probability. Scales were adjusted for each hemisphere, to highlight differences inside the precentral gyrus (with permission of [19])

verbal fluency in the left hemisphere [33, 34]. SMA, PMd, and PMv are connected to the caudate nucleus through the frontal-striatal tract (FST). DES of the FST elicits movement arrest of the contralateral upper and lower limb, but also of bimanual movement and a reduction in verbal fluency (observed at the contact of the left FST) [33]. A somatotopic organization of the fibers subserving motor control has also been identified thanks to DES. Indeed, it is possible to disturb the ongoing movement (by inducing usually a movement arrest without loss of tone or consciousness—a so-called negative motor response [18]) of the lower limb posteriorly, medially, and superiorly, very close to the SMAproper (Fig. 1.5d) while site eliciting movement arrest of the upper limb is located more laterally, ventrally, and anteriorly (Fig. 1.5b). Between those sites are found site eliciting bilateral upper limbs arrest during a unilateral single DES (Fig. 1.5c). Finally, sites eliciting

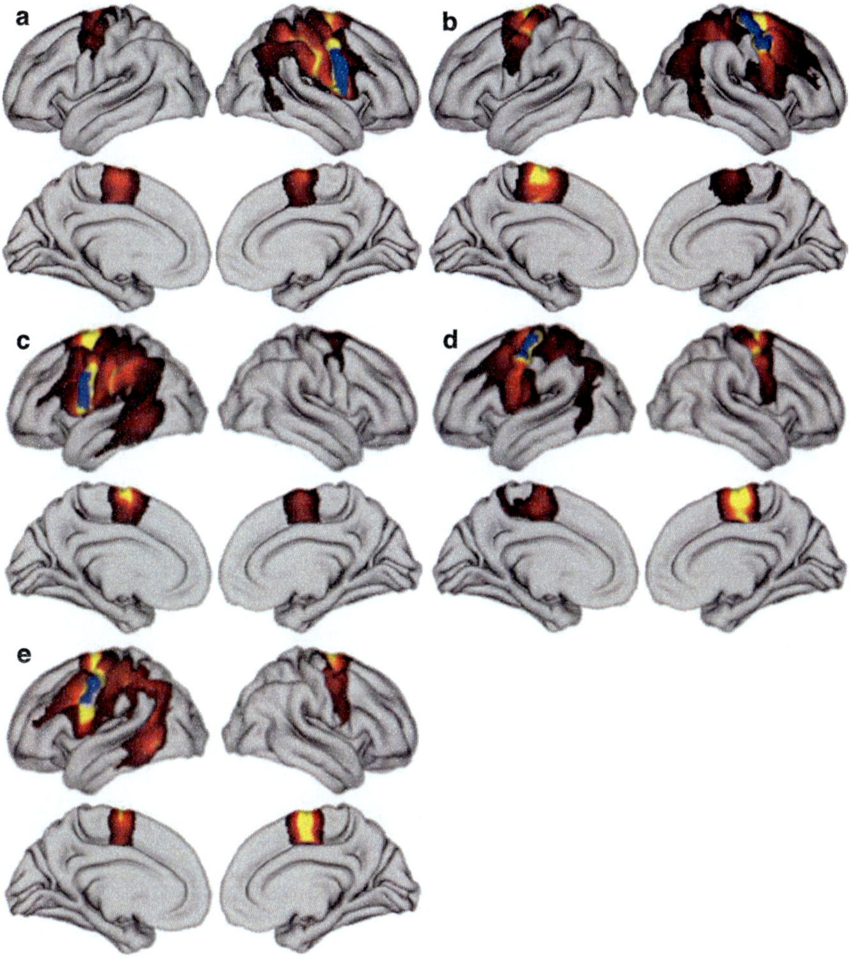

Fig. 1.4 Clusters of negative motor responses involving speech and upper limb (in blue). Each figure (**a**–**e**) represents the ispi- and contralateral connections on the lateral and medial faces of the hemispheres. Area connected structurally to the cluster with a probability superior to 95% are shown in red-yellow gradient. It is then possible to see how each cluster shares common connected area and conversely how cortical area is connected to several clusters. (**c**–**e**) Show three clusters over the precentral gyrus. The central cluster (**e**) includes connections of both dorsal and ventral clusters (**c**, **d**). Data about clusters are coming from Rech et al. (2019) (with permission of [20])

movement arrest of the face or speech are located the most anteriorly, laterally, and ventrally (Fig. 1.5a) [35, 36]. Despite an apparent dispersion of those sites, they are always located in a somatotopic manner at the individual level. The distribution of each kind of sites shows the orientation of the fibers subserving motor control, going from the premotor area to the head of the caudate nucleus and corresponding

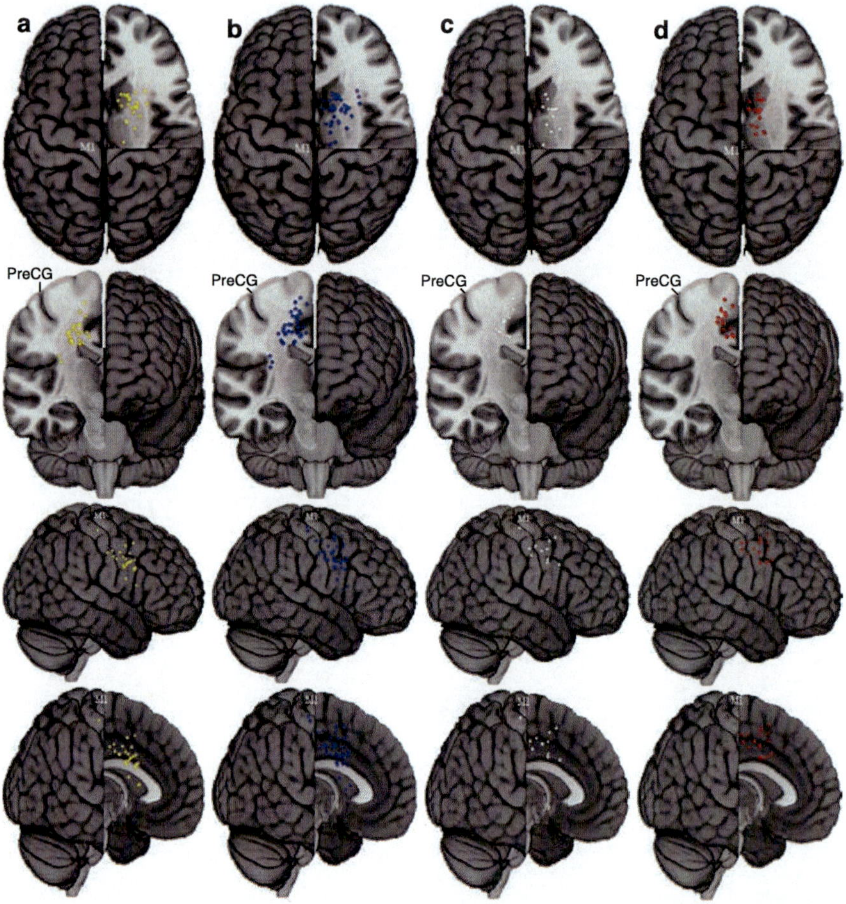

Fig. 1.5 Repartition of sites eliciting negative motor responses (NMR) according to the kind of NMRs observed. All sites have been reported on a single side for a better visual appreciation. Each dot corresponds to a site of NMR (n = 18 patients). Axial, coronal, and sagittal views (with and without ipsilateral brain) are shown on each row. Each column corresponds to a single kind of NMRs. First column (**a**) with yellow dots: face/speech. NMR. Second column (**b**) with blue dots: contralateral upper limb NMR. Third column (**c**) with white dots: bilateral NMR. Fourth column (**d**) with red dots: lower limb NMR. Spatial distribution between each kind of NMR can, therefore, be analyzed for each plane (with permission of [35])

to the FST. As the FAT is slightly more anterior and lateral than the FST, sites of speech arrest/face are more likely due to FAT stimulation [33].

Such area as PMd, PMv, SMA, and M1 are strongly connected through U-fibers [37]. Association fibers such as the SLF I, II, and III connect the SPL, intraparietal sulcus (IPS), and IPL to the PMd and PMv and play a role in motor control as revealed by subcortical DES in the parietal lobe which can inhibit or accelerate contralateral body parts or both hands [38]. Interestingly, cortical terminations of each fascicle are overlapping and highlight the middle part of the precentral gyrus where numerous projections seem to converge, even from the arcuate fascicle (Figs. 1.4e and 1.6) [39, 40]. This region has been recently considered as an important hub for motor awareness as stimulation makes the patient unconscious of a DES-related motor arrest [41]. Conversely, each subpart of the precentral gyrus shares frontal and parietal connections with other subparts (Figs. 1.4 and 1.6).

Such findings, and especially those revealed by DES, are in favor of a complex functional organization of cortical areas and tend to confirm that terms like PMd, PMV, SMAproper, and preSMA are too restrictive to apprehend the complexity of motor functions. At a subcortical level, the complex organization of the white

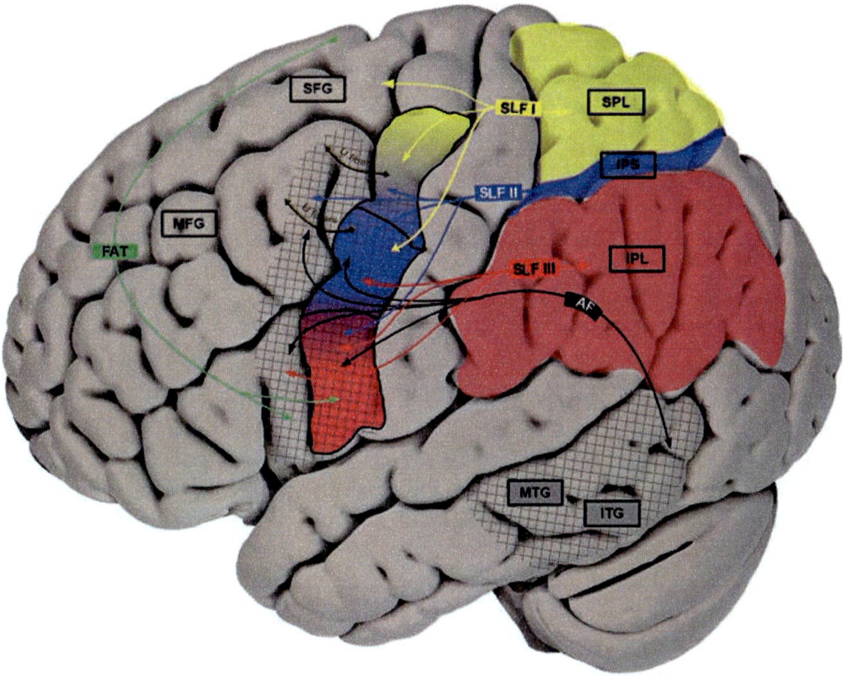

Fig. 1.6 Networks involving motor control and cortical connections. Clusters of negative motor responses are identified by black solid line over the preCG. Colors of the clusters correspond to the parietal origin of fibers. A gradient inside the preCG appears and is consecutive to a dorsoventral progressive modification of the connectivity, from the SLF I (yellow), the SLF II (blue), and finally the SLF III (red). Cortical terminations of the AF are also shown with black crossed lines up to the lower part of the dorsal cluster. The frontoparietal stream and its dorsoventral organization and overlapping are visible and allow to understand the segregation inside the precentral gyrus as well as the complex connectivity of the precentral gyrus with the frontal and the parietal lobe. *SFG* superior frontal gyrus, *MFG* middle frontal gyrus, *SPL* superior parietal lobule, *IPS* intraparietal sulcus, *IPL* inferior parietal lobule, *MTG* middle temporal gyrus, *ITG* inferior temporal gyrus, *SLF* superior longitudinal fasciculus, *IFOF* inferior fronto-occipital fasciculus, *AF* arcuate fasciculus, *FAT* frontal aslant tract (adapted with permission of [20])

matter under the precentral gyrus has been well described [37] but exploring this region with DES remains difficult as the surgical approach to the precentral gyrus is limited anteriorly by fibers of the FST and the FAT and posteriorly by somesthetic fibers.

1.2 Review About Evidence of Long-Term Deficits in Patients Who Did Not Benefit from Intraoperative Monitoring of Motor Control

Avoidance of motor deficits is probably one of the most relevant concerns in brain tumor surgery, above all when tumor involves primary motor cortex and its descending fibers. Such a concern is in fact based on evidence showing that resection of tumors located within M1 or near the corticospinal tract can produce postoperative motor deficits from 2% up to 30% of patients [42–46]. Although in most of the cases, when an EMG/MEPs monitoring is used, such deficits are not permanent and tend to recover during the first 3 months, developing new protocols to shorten this transient period of deficits and limit their functional impact remains an important surgical concern. Importantly, recent retrospective analysis [46] of patients operated for glioma located to approximately 2 cm from the precentral and postcentral sulcus demonstrated that despite the intraoperative neurophysiological mapping routinely used in brain tumor resection appears to be a good tool to preserve basic motor functions (i.e., the general ability to move arms and/or hands), difficulties in programming and execution of complex action or fine movements are often reported postoperatively by patients. Crucially such subtle difficulties can negatively affect the patients' quality of life [47]. Taken together these data suggest that the standard approach, although efficient in most tumors involving M1 originating fibers, may have important limitations. When used in case of tumors involving the premotor or the parietal areas, the preservation of M1 and its originating fibers may be not enough to preserve motor function. This is due to the role of non-primary motor areas in performing and adapting movement to the action's goal and to the relevance of the subcortical neural network connecting these cortical areas as previously described. Therefore, while M1 and its descending fibers are identified by DES without the need of patient's collaboration, structures involved in higher level of motor programming and movement control (PMd, PMv, and SMA) can be mapped only while the patient is performing an ongoing motor task, in awake conditions.

1.3 Review About Knowledge Gained from Lesion-Symptom Mapping

While the effect of M1 lesion in producing severe paralysis or complete paresis has been clear for almost a century, the role of non-primary motor cortices in high-level motor programming has been described more recently. Specifically, lesion mapping studies of apraxia, i.e., the inability to perform voluntary complex movement induced by neurological lesions in the absence of primary sensory or motor disorders, suggest the involvement of parietal and frontal regions (PMd, PMv, and SMA) [48–55]. Notably the two main classifications of apraxia, namely ideomotor apraxia (inability to imitate gesture of a model) and ideational apraxia (inability to perform pantomime without visual model), were disentangled in human through lesion-symptom mapping suggesting that areas specifically related to posterior IPS and SPL were more strongly associated with imitation. Conversely, pantomime deficits were associated with regions such as the supramarginal gyrus, the middle temporal gyrus, and the extreme capsule [56]. Together with these studies mainly pointing at a distributed cortical network, recently growing evidence has also highlighted the fundamental role of the white matter fibers connecting the abovementioned regions [57]. Specifically, the connections between the inferior parietal regions and the premotor cortex seem to play a crucial role. In monkeys and humans, this circuit was recently defined as the "lateral grasping network," and demonstrated to be specifically active during hand movement in light and in darkness, pointing to its crucial role in hand tool manipulation even in a haptically driven context [58–60].

1.4 Review of the Different Tasks Newly Designed to Monitor Motor Control Intraoperatively

Standard motor monitoring using continuous MEPs/EMG recording is nowadays a mandatory and highly efficient protocol for the identification of motor sites in patients with tumors in descending motor pathways [44, 61, 62]. However, as mentioned before, when tumors are located at "distant" location from the central sulcus, yet involving relevant sensorimotor network areas (premotor or parietal regions), the standard approach requires the addition of supplemental higher order motor tasks in awake conditions. To date two main cognitive-motor tasks are routinely applied to monitor sensory motor integration and praxis. The simplest is to ask the patients to continually perform a repetitive voluntary movement of the upper limb (flexion-extension of the harm or finger-to-thumb task), and to observe the interferences generated by DES during the task performance [35, 63, 64]. This identifies all cortical and subcortical sites producing a modulation (i.e., an acceleration, slowdown, or interruption) of the ongoing movement. A second, recently developed task is the hand-manipulation-task (hMT) [46]. The patient is asked to perform a rotational movement on a tool shaped like a screwdriver. Although both approaches are similar, the latter requires a higher level of dexterity and haptic not visually guided interaction with an object, introducing in the motor task the investigation of the sensory-motor integration, a crucial component of motor control [65]. From a surgical viewpoint, specific patterns of interference on task execution (both behavioral and EMG) were associated with different parieto-frontal positive areas, providing surgeons with a highly specific tool to navigate within the praxis network: the M1 block is characterized by tonic muscle activation, the S1 by clonic twitches and release of the object, and the SMG and vPM by the arrest of movement without muscle activation. Moreover, the stimulation of the dorsomedial sectors of the premotor cortex induced a slow deceleration of the movement and a loss of rhythmicity in the hand–object interaction [46].

1.5 Review of Studies Evidencing a Functional Improvement in Series of Patients Operated on With Versus Without Motor Control Monitoring

Cortical and subcortical brain mapping under awake or asleep conditions remain the gold standard of functional guided brain tumor resection. The authors are not aware of any study published that compared in a randomized fashion brain mapping to no functional guidance at all. However, there are centers that do not rely on mapping techniques during the resection of a potentially eloquent brain tumor.

Magill et al. [44] analyzed 49 patients undergoing resections of tumors located primarily within the motor cortex. Awake craniotomy was performed in 65% of cases using standard neurophysiological monitoring and active hand/limb movement, while 35% were done under general anesthesia. The mean extent of resection was 91%. New or permanent postoperative motor deficits occurred in 20 patients. Of the permanent deficits, 14 were mild, 4 were moderate, and 2 were severe (3.8% of cases). A matched case-control study by Gerritsen et al. [66] compared awake brain mapping with no surgical adjunct technologies. Not only the extent of resection was significantly increased under awake and mapping conditions (94.9% vs. 70.3%), but the rate of postoperative complications was generally lower in the awake mapping group. In their large series of insular gliomas, Simon et al. [67] described their experience in a cohort of 94 consecutive patients. Their protocol of resection comprised a microsurgical (mostly transsylvian) approach with electrophysiological monitoring (MEP) resulting in a 13% rate of permanent hemiparesis. These results confirm that monitoring the primary motor pathway with MEPs technique is not enough to avoid permanent motor deficit.

Martino et al. [64] reported a series study with 21 patients operated under awake procedure for removal of frontal tumors located in the superior frontal gyrus. The motor mapping procedure required the patients to perform different motor tasks (fingers-to-thumb opposition and bimanual alternate flexion and extension of the two hands). In the immediate postoperative period, 12 out of 21 showed a limb motor worsening, while at 3–6 months after surgery only 4 patients showed worsened performances compared with preoperative phase. Interestingly, only cortical mapping was used to find motor control disturbances and subcortical mapping was only used to monitor the pyramidal pathway explaining probably the rate of permanent deficit even if patients were operated awake (as subcortical fibers subserving motor control were removed (Fig. 1.5)). Using a similar approach, Gabarrós et al. [63] studied 15 patients with tumors infiltrating the premotor cortex. All patients were operated under awake conditions. While primary motor cortex was identified with DES, the SMA was mapped asking the patients to perform a classical contralateral finger opposition motor task. At 6 months follow-up, five patients showed permanent deficits interfering with daily life activities. These results confirm that assessing movement during surgery improves results but shows also that a cortical mapping of active motor function is not sufficient to prevent permanent deficit.

Finally, in a study of low-grade glioma invading the SFG, it has been shown that preservation of the motor control fibers during an active motor task in awake surgery leads to no permanent deficit whereas identification and resection of such fibers for oncological purposes up to the pyramidal pathway lead to a SMA syndrome and to permanent deficit in bimanual coordination and motor control [68]. In a recent study authors investigated the efficacy of a novel task requiring hand–tool interaction (hMT) by comparing the incidence of postoperative ideomotor apraxia (immediate and 1 month after surgery) between patients undergoing the standard motor mapping with ($n = 79$) and without ($n = 41$) the hMT [46]. Crucially, the task dramatically reduced the incidence of postoperative ideomotor apraxia (global incidence 2.5% when the task was used in comparison with 50% when it was not applied) and the need of postoperative rehabilitation. These results finally confirm that preservation of cortical and subcortical structure involved in motor control is crucial to prevent permanent motor deficit in motor and premotor regions.

Illustrative Case (Fig. 1.7)

30-year-old woman presenting a tumor of the superior frontal gyrus evoking a low-grade glioma and revealed by seizure (a–d: pre- and postoperative MRI T2 FLAIR sequences). Decision to proceed to a tumor resection under awake condition to map language as well as motor control networks. e: results of the cortical mapping with 1 and 2: contraction of the upper limb, 3: contraction of the face and motor seizure of the face, 4: speech arrest, 5 slowdown of the speech and upper limb and motor arrest of the hand (negative motor response), 6 semantic paraphasia. (f) Results of the subcortical mapping with 8 corresponding to movement arrest of the upper limb and acceleration of the counting very close to the midline. Retractor shows the ventricle, which is widely opened, exposing the head of the caudate nucleus (smooth and white above the retractor). g–j: tumor cavity (blue) overlapped on a brain MNI 152 template with white matter fascicles coming from Rojkova's atlas [69]. FAT (red) and FST (green) are shown. FAT is more anterior than FST, explaining why it is usually a limit posteriorly and laterally during resection (at the level of the tip of the retractor usually). In this case, it is interesting to note that tag 8 corresponds likely to both termination of the FAT and FST because the protocol consisted in asking the patient to count and move, in order to detect for disturbance in motor control of the speech and upper limb.

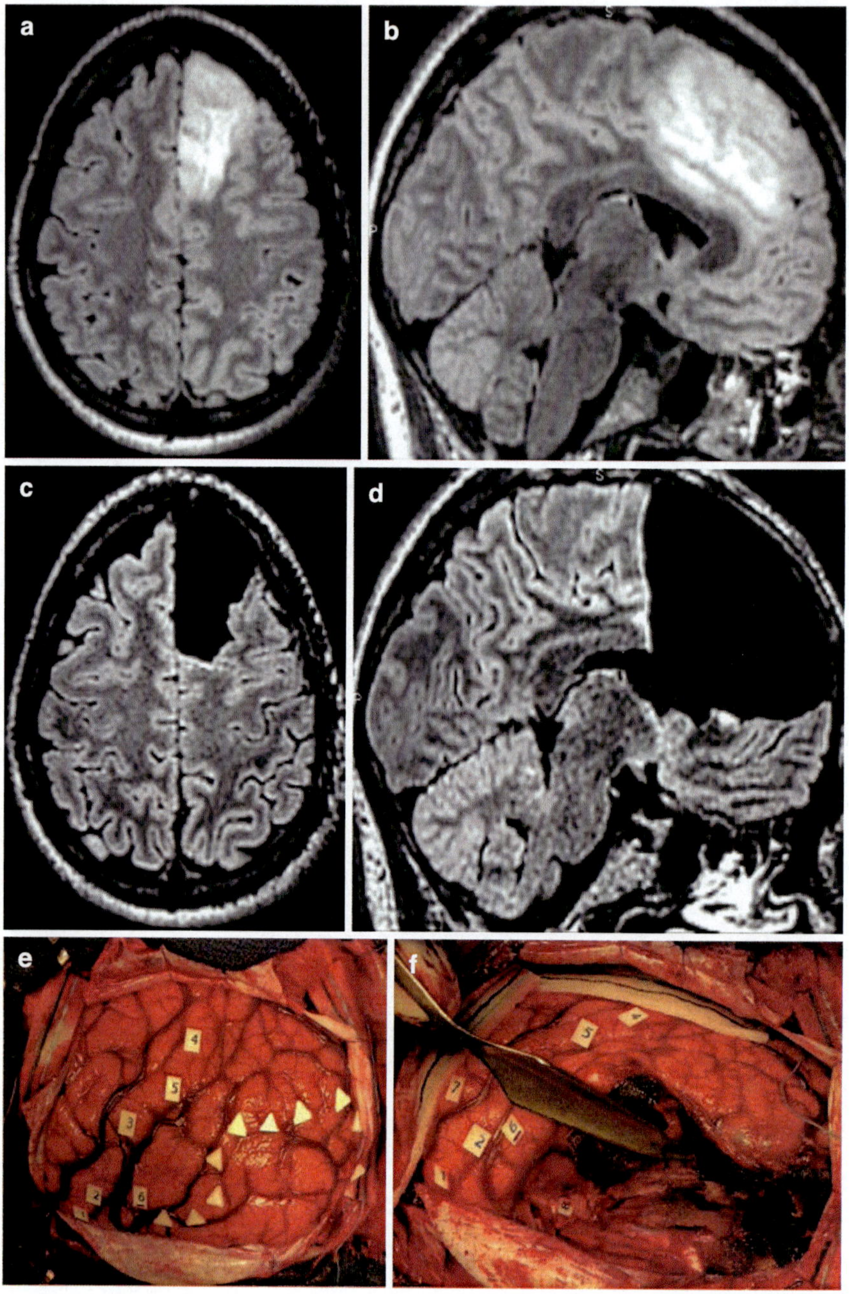

Fig. 1.7 Illustrative case

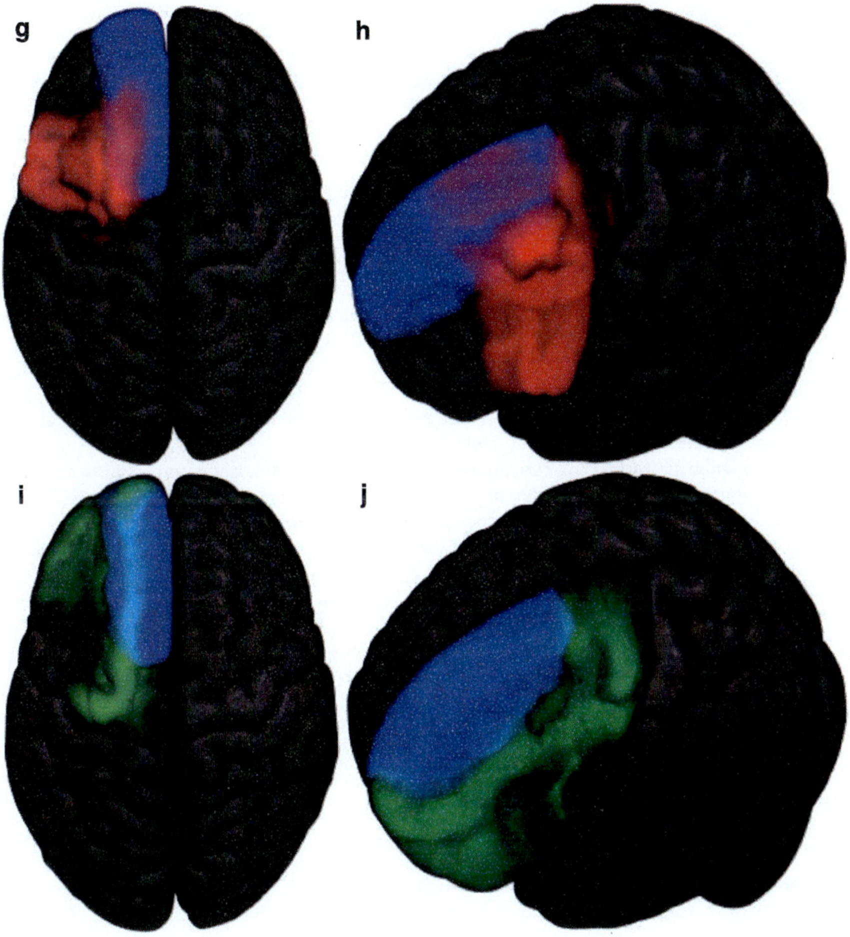

Fig. 1.7 (continued)

1.6 Conclusion

Taken together these data suggest that MEPs/EMG motor monitoring, mainly performed in asleep conditions, can be effectively complemented with active (awake condition) motor tasks (complex movement or interaction with tools) for resection of tumor located in premotor and parietal regions. It also shows that cortical and subcortical mapping of motor control are mandatory to preserve the motor control network and avoid permanent deficit. Such approach can help the neurosurgeon not only to preserve basic motor function but also higher order motor skills with a significant improvement of quality of life.

References

1. Brodmann K. Vergleichende Lokalisationslehre der Grosshirnrinde in ihren Prinzipien dargestellt auf Grund des Zellenbaues. Barth. 1909.
2. Lacroix S, Havton LA, McKay H, Yang H, Brant A, Roberts J, Tuszynski MH. Bilateral corticospinal projections arise from each motor cortex in the macaque monkey: a quantitative study. J Comp Neurol. 2004;473:147–61.
3. Bortoff GA, Strick PL. Corticospinal terminations in two new-world primates: further evidence that corticomotoneuronal connections provide part of the neural substrate for manual dexterity. J Neurosci. 1993;13:5105–18.
4. Penfield W, Boldrey E. Somatic motor and sensory representation in the cerebral cortex of man as studied by electrical stimulation. Brain. 1937;60(389):1937.
5. Catani M. A little man of some importance. Brain. 2017;140:3055–61.
6. Graziano MSA. Ethological action maps: a paradigm shift for the motor cortex. Trends Cogn Sci. 2016;20:121–32.
7. Dum RP. Frontal lobe inputs to the digit representations of the motor areas on the lateral surface of the hemisphere. J Neurosci. 2005;25:1375–86.
8. He SQ, Dum RP, Strick PL. Topographic organization of corticospinal projections from the frontal lobe: motor areas on the lateral surface of the hemisphere. J Neurosci. 1993;13:952–80.
9. Picard N, Strick PL. Imaging the premotor areas. Curr Opin Neurobiol. 2001;11:663–72.
10. Chouinard PA, Paus T. The primary motor and premotor areas of the human cerebral cortex. Neuroscientist. 2006;12:143–52.
11. Hoshi E, Tanji J. Distinctions between dorsal and ventral premotor areas: anatomical connectivity and functional properties. Curr Opin Neurobiol. 2007;17:234–42.
12. Glaser JI, Perich MG, Ramkumar P, Miller LE, Kording KP. Population coding of conditional probability distributions in dorsal premotor cortex. Nat Commun. 2018;9:1788. https://doi.org/10.1038/s41467-018-04062-6.
13. Makris N, Kennedy DN, McInerney S, Sorensen AG, Wang R, Caviness VS, Pandya DN. Segmentation of subcomponents within the superior longitudinal fascicle in humans: a quantitative, in vivo, DT-MRI study. Cereb Cortex. 2005;15:854–69.
14. Genon S, Li H, Fan L, et al. The right dorsal premotor mosaic: organization, functions, and connectivity. Cereb Cortex. 2017;27(3):2095–110. https://doi.org/10.1093/cercor/bhw065.
15. Schubotz RI, Anwander A, Knösche TR, von Cramon DY, Tittgemeyer M. Anatomical and functional parcellation of the human lateral premotor cortex. NeuroImage. 2010;50:396–408.
16. Rizzolatti G, Sinigaglia C. The mirror mechanism: a basic principle of brain function. Nat Rev Neurosci. 2016;17:757–65.
17. van Geemen K, Herbet G, Moritz-Gasser S, Duffau H. Limited plastic potential of the left ventral premotor cortex in speech articulation: evidence from intraoperative awake mapping in glioma patients. Hum Brain Mapp. 2014;35:1587–96.
18. Lüders H, Lesser RP, Morris HH, Dinner DS. Negative motor responses elicited by stimulation of the human cortex. In: Wolf P, Dam M, Janz D, editors. Advances in epileptology. New York: Raven Press; 1987. p. 229–31.
19. Rech F, Herbet G, Gaudeau Y, Mézières S, Moureau J-M, Moritz-Gasser S, Duffau H. A probabilistic map of negative motor areas of the upper limb and face: a brain stimulation study. Brain. 2019;142(4):952–65. https://doi.org/10.1093/brain/awz021.
20. Rech F, Wassermann D, Duffau H. New insights into the neural foundations mediating movement/language interactions gained from intrasurgical direct electrostimulations. Brain Cogn. 2020;142:105583.
21. Picard N, Strick PL. Motor areas of the medial wall: a review of their location and functional activation. Cereb Cortex. 1996;6:342–53.
22. Geyer S, Matelli M, Luppino G, Zilles K. Functional neuroanatomy of the primate isocortical motor system. Anat Embryol. 2000;202:443–74.

23. Dum RP, Strick PL. Spinal cord terminations of the medial wall motor areas in macaque monkeys. J Neurosci. 1996;16:6513–25.
24. Nachev P, Kennard C, Husain M. Functional role of the supplementary and pre-supplementary motor areas. Nat Rev Neurosci. 2008;9:856–69.
25. Fontaine D, Capelle L, Duffau H. Somatotopy of the supplementary motor area: evidence from correlation of the extent of surgical resection with the clinical patterns of deficit. Neurosurgery. 2002;50:297–305.
26. Cunnington R, Windischberger C, Deecke L, Moser E. The preparation and execution of self-initiated and externally-triggered movement: a study of event-related fMRI. NeuroImage. 2002;15:373–85.
27. Gerloff C, Corwell B, Chen R, Hallett M, Cohen LG. Stimulation over the human supplementary motor area interferes with the organization of future elements in complex motor sequences. Brain. 1997;120:1587–602.
28. Shima K, Tanji J. Neuronal activity in the supplementary and presupplementary motor areas for temporal organization of multiple movements. J Neurophysiol. 2000;84:2148–60.
29. Gerloff C, Andres FG. Bimanual coordination and interhemispheric interaction. Acta Psychol. 2002;110:161–86.
30. Nakamura K, Sakai K, Hikosaka O. Effects of local inactivation of monkey medial frontal cortex in learning of sequential procedures. J Neurophysiol. 1999;82:1063–8.
31. Rushworth MFS, Hadland KA, Paus T, Sipila PK. Role of the human medial frontal cortex in task switching: a combined fMRI and TMS study. J Neurophysiol. 2002;87:2577–92.
32. Trevisi G, Eickhoff SB, Chowdhury F, Jha A, Rodionov R, Nowell M, Miserocchi A, McEvoy AW, Nachev P, Diehl B. Probabilistic electrical stimulation mapping of human medial frontal cortex. Cortex. 2018;109:336–46. https://doi.org/10.1016/j.cortex.2018.06.015.
33. Kinoshita M, de Champfleur NM, Deverdun J, Moritz-Gasser S, Herbet G, Duffau H. Role of fronto-striatal tract and frontal aslant tract in movement and speech: an axonal mapping study. Brain Struct Funct. 2015;220:3399–412.
34. Dragoy O, Zyryanov A, Bronov O, et al. Functional linguistic specificity of the left frontal aslant tract for spontaneous speech fluency: evidence from intraoperative language mapping. Brain Lang. 2020;208:104836.
35. Rech F, Herbet G, Moritz-Gasser S, Duffau H. Somatotopic organization of the white matter tracts underpinning motor control in humans: an electrical stimulation study. Brain Struct Funct. 2016;221(7):3743–53.
36. Rech F, Herbet G, Moritz-Gasser S, Duffau H. Disruption of bimanual movement by unilateral subcortical electrostimulation. Hum Brain Mapp. 2014;35:3439–45.
37. Catani M, Dell'Acqua F, Vergani F, Malik F, Hodge H, Roy P, Valabregue R, Thiebaut de Schotten M. Short frontal lobe connections of the human brain. Cortex. 2012;48:273–91.
38. Almairac F, Herbet G, Moritz-Gasser S, Duffau H. Parietal network underlying movement control: disturbances during subcortical electrostimulation. Neurosurg Rev. 2014;37:513–6; discussion 516–7.
39. Fernández-Miranda JC, Wang Y, Pathak S, Stefaneau L, Verstynen T, Yeh F-C. Asymmetry, connectivity, and segmentation of the arcuate fascicle in the human brain. Brain Struct Funct. 2015;220:1665–80.
40. Parlatini V, Radua J, Dell'Acqua F, Leslie A, Simmons A, Murphy DG, Catani M, Thiebaut de Schotten M. Functional segregation and integration within fronto-parietal networks. NeuroImage. 2017;146:367–75.
41. Fornia L, Puglisi G, Leonetti A, Bello L, Berti A, Cerri G, Garbarini F. Direct electrical stimulation of the premotor cortex shuts down awareness of voluntary actions. Nat Commun. 2020;11:705.
42. Keles GE, Lundin DA, Lamborn KR, Chang EF, Ojemann G, Berger MS. Intraoperative subcortical stimulation mapping for hemispherical perirolandic gliomas located within or adjacent to the descending motor pathways: evaluation of morbidity and assessment of functional outcome in 294 patients. J Neurosurg. 2004;100:369–75.

43. Luther N, Kondziolka D, Kano H, Mousavi SH, Flickinger JC, Lunsford LD. Motor function after stereotactic radiosurgery for brain metastases in the region of the motor cortex. J Neurosurg. 2013;119:683–8.
44. Magill ST, Han SJ, Li J, Berger MS. Resection of primary motor cortex tumors: feasibility and surgical outcomes. J Neurosurg. 2018;129:961–72.
45. Obermueller T, Schaeffner M, Gerhardt J, Meyer B, Ringel F, Krieg SM. Risks of postoperative paresis in motor eloquently and non-eloquently located brain metastases. BMC Cancer. 2014;14:21.
46. Rossi M, Fornia L, Puglisi G, et al. Assessment of the praxis circuit in glioma surgery to reduce the incidence of postoperative and long-term apraxia: a new intraoperative test. J Neurosurg. 2018;130:17–27.
47. Hanna-Pladdy B, Heilman KM, Foundas AL. Ecological implications of ideomotor apraxia: evidence from physical activities of daily living. Neurology. 2003;60:487–90.
48. Buxbaum LJ, Randerath J. Limb apraxia and the left parietal lobe. Handb Clin Neurol. 2018;151:349–63.
49. Buxbaum LJ, Shapiro AD, Coslett HB. Critical brain regions for tool-related and imitative actions: a componential analysis. Brain. 2014;137:1971–85.
50. De Renzi E, Faglioni P, Lodesani M, Vecchi A. Performance of left brain-damaged patients on imitation of single movements and motor sequences. Frontal and parietal-injured patients compared. Cortex. 1983;19:333–43.
51. Geschwind N. The apraxias: neural mechanisms of disorders of learned movement. Am Sci. 1975;63:188–95.
52. Goldenberg G, Hermsdörfer J, Glindemann R, Rorden C, Karnath H-O. Pantomime of tool use depends on integrity of left inferior frontal cortex. Cereb Cortex (New York, NY: 1991). 2007;17:2769–76.
53. Varney NR, Damasio H. Locus of lesion in impaired pantomime recognition. Cortex. 1987;23:699–703.
54. Watson RT, Fleet WS, Gonzalez-Rothi L, Heilman KM. Apraxia and the supplementary motor area. Arch Neurol. 1986;43:787–92.
55. Weiss PH, Ubben SD, Kaesberg S, Kalbe E, Kessler J, Liebig T, Fink GR. Where language meets meaningful action: a combined behavior and lesion analysis of aphasia and apraxia. Brain Struct Funct. 2016;221:563–76.
56. Hoeren M, Kümmerer D, Bormann T, Beume L, Ludwig VM, Vry M-S, Mader I, Rijntjes M, Kaller CP, Weiller C. Neural bases of imitation and pantomime in acute stroke patients: distinct streams for praxis. Brain. 2014;137:2796–810.
57. Sperber C, Wiesen D, Goldenberg G, Karnath H-O. A network underlying human higher-order motor control: insights from machine learning-based lesion-behaviour mapping in apraxia of pantomime. Cortex. 2019;121:308–21.
58. Binkofski F, Buccino G, Posse S, Seitz RJ, Rizzolatti G, Freund H. A fronto-parietal circuit for object manipulation in man: evidence from an fMRI-study. Eur J Neurosci. 1999;11:3276–86.
59. Borra E, Gerbella M, Rozzi S, Luppino G. The macaque lateral grasping network: a neural substrate for generating purposeful hand actions. Neurosci Biobehav Rev. 2017;75:65–90.
60. Nelissen K, Vanduffel W. Grasping-related functional magnetic resonance imaging brain responses in the macaque monkey. J Neurosci. 2011;31:8220–9.
61. Rossi M, Conti Nibali M, Viganò L, et al. Resection of tumors within the primary motor cortex using high-frequency stimulation: oncological and functional efficiency of this versatile approach based on clinical conditions. J Neurosurg. 2019:1–13.
62. Szelényi A, Bello L, Duffau H, Fava E, Feigl GC, Galanda M, Neuloh G, Signorelli F, Sala F. Intraoperative electrical stimulation in awake craniotomy: methodological aspects of current practice. Neurosurg Focus. 2010;28:7.
63. Gabarrós A, Martino J, Juncadella M, et al. [Intraoperative identification of the supplementary motor area in neurooncological surgery]. Neurocirugia (Asturias, Spain). 2011;22:123–32.
64. Martino J, Gabarrós A, Deus J, Juncadella M, Acebes JJ, Torres A, Pujol J. Intrasurgical mapping of complex motor function in the superior frontal gyrus. Neuroscience. 2011;179:131–42.

65. Glencross DJ, Piek JP (eds) Motor control and sensory motor integration: issues and directions. Elsevier, Amsterdam; New York. 1995.
66. Gerritsen JKW, Viëtor CL, Rizopoulos D, Schouten JW, Klimek M, Dirven CMF, Vincent AJ-PE. Awake craniotomy versus craniotomy under general anesthesia without surgery adjuncts for supratentorial glioblastoma in eloquent areas: a retrospective matched case-control study. Acta Neurochir. 2019;161:307–15.
67. Simon M, Neuloh G, von Lehe M, Meyer B, Schramm J. Insular gliomas: the case for surgical management. J Neurosurg. 2009;110:685–95.
68. Rech F, Duffau H, Pinelli C, Masson A, Roublot P, Billy-Jacques A, Brissart H, Civit T. Intraoperative identification of the negative motor network during awake surgery to prevent deficit following brain resection in premotor regions. Neurochirurgie. 2017;63:235–42.
69. Rojkova K, Volle E, Urbanski M, Humbert F, Dell'Acqua F, Thiebaut de Schotten M. Atlasing the frontal lobe connections and their variability due to age and education: a spherical deconvolution tractography study. Brain Struct Funct. 2016;221:1751–66.

Vision

2

Philippe Menei, Anne Clavreul, Morgane Casanova, David Colle, and Henry Colle

2.1 Introduction

At the first glance, mapping of the vision seems to be an easy task! In reality, it is as challenging as for the most complex cognitive functions. This is due to the very wide domain covered by the word "vision." Vision is the perception of the surrounding environment using light in the visible spectrum reflected by the objects in the environment. The spatial array of the environment available to perception is called the visual field (VF). Visual perception is different from visual acuity, which refers to how clearly a person sees.

The major difficulty in visual perception is that what people see is not simply a translation of retinal stimuli. Indeed, vision initiates several cognitive intricate functions, difficult to dissociate in the everyday life. Among them:

- The neural mechanisms underlying stereo vision, motion perception, and color vision.

P. Menei
Department of Neurosurgery, Teaching Hospital, Angers, France

CRCINA, UMR 1232 INSERM/CNRS, Angers, France

Department of Neurosurgery, University of Angers, CHU Angers, CRCINA, Angers, France
e-mail: phmenei@chu-angers.fr

A. Clavreul
Department of Neurosurgery, University of Angers, CHU Angers, CRCINA, Angers, France
e-mail: anne.clavreul@univ-angers.fr

M. Casanova
Rennes Institute of Electronics and Telecommunications, FAST Team (Facial Analysis Synthesis and Tracking) UMR CNRS, Centrale Supélec, Rennes, France

D. Colle · H. Colle (✉)
Department of Neurosurgery, St Lucas General Hospital, Ghent, Belgium
e-mail: Henry.Colle@AZSTLUCAS.BE

E. Mandonnet, G. Herbet (eds.), *Intraoperative Mapping of Cognitive Networks*,
https://doi.org/10.1007/978-3-030-75071-8_2

- Visual cognition, often associated with high-level vision and top-down visual processing, allowing constructing visual entities by collecting perceived parts into coherent wholes, determining which parts belong together [1].
- Visuospatial cognition referring to the ability to identify, integrate, and analyze space and visual form, details, structure in more than one dimension. All of these are essential for visuospatial skills and visuospatial working memory.
- Object, face, emotion and word recognition, reading [2–5].
- Visual attention embracing many aspects, including spatial attention which allows to selectively process visual information through prioritization of an area within the visual field, but also object-based attention and social attention [6].
- The social vision belonging to social cognition, strongly itself linked to the previous described attention and visuospatial cognition. Vision plays a critical role in the development and maintenance of social exchange. The human visual system is particularly attuned at processing social cues, allowing "reading" others' mental and emotional states and making snap judgments about their characters and dispositions. The gaze plays a major role in all these processes.

The mapping of these last cognitive functions is specifically discussed in other chapters of this book (see Chaps. 4 and 18). The present one will be focused on a primary aspect of the vision, the VF, but necessarily, other complex visual functions will be addressed.

2.2 Neuroanatomy of the Visual System

The anatomy and physiology of the neural visual system are complex, though more and more understood [7]. The neural visual system is constituted by the photoreceptive cells in the retina, also known as the rods and cones, which detect the photons of light and respond by producing neural impulses. The cones which are specialized for maximum visual acuity are centered in a retinal area called fovea. The fovea is employed for accurate vision in a small region in the center of the VF. Common wisdom holds that, vision outside the fovea is severely impoverished. We know now that peripheral vision can provide useful information, peripheral acuity, and color vision. Nevertheless, color perception is best in the fovea and declines in the periphery. Sensitivity to red-green color variations declines more steeply toward the periphery than sensitivity to luminance or blue-yellow colors [8]. Extensive work in the past years has shown that observers can perform many recognition tasks with short presentation times that preclude multiple fixations. This includes object recognition, scene perception, recognition of social actions and face, and emotion perception [9, 10].

The retinal signals are transmitted by the optic nerve. The optic nerves from both eyes meet and cross at the optic chiasm. At this point the information coming from both eyes is combined and then splits according to the VF. The corresponding halves of the field of view (right and left) are sent to the left and right halves of the brain, respectively, to be processed (Fig. 2.1).

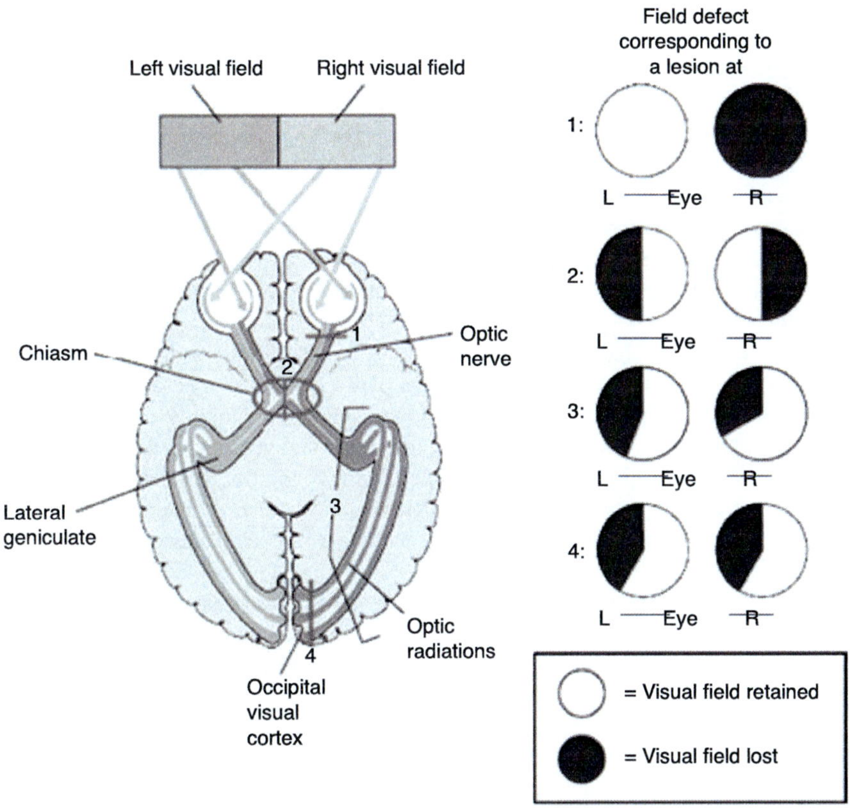

Fig. 2.1 Anatomy of the visual system and visual field defect function of the lesion site

From optic chiasm, information from the right visual field travel in the left optic tract, those from the left visual field travels in the right optic tract.

Each optic tract terminates in a sensory relay nucleus in the thalamus of the brain: the lateral geniculate nucleus (LGN). In fact, the LGN is not just a simple relay station but it is also a center for processing. It receives reciprocal input from the cortical and subcortical layers and reciprocal innervation from the visual cortex.

The neurons of the LGN then relay the visual information to the cortex through a pathway of white matter fibers: the optic radiations (OR). There is one such tract on each side of the brain, each one including an upper and a lower division. Depending on the level of a transection, a specific visual field defect will appear (Fig. 2.1).

The right side of primary visual cortex deals with the left half of the VF of both eyes, and similarly for the left brain. A small region in the center of the field of view, the foveal vision, is processed redundantly by both halves of the brain.

The LGN sends signals to primary visual cortex, also called V1 or striate cortex. It creates a bottom-up saliency map of the visual field to guide attention or eye gaze to salient visual locations.

From this primary visual cortex, visual information is secondarily processed in the visual association cortex also called extrastriate cortex, which include the cortical area V2, V3, V4, and V5/MT [11]. As visual information passes forward through the visual hierarchy, the complexity of the neural representations increases. Whereas a V1 neuron may respond selectively to a line segment of a particular orientation, neurons in the lateral occipital complex respond selectively to complete object, and neurons in visual association cortex may respond selectively to human faces, or to a particular object.

Recent descriptions of visual association cortex describe a division into two functional pathways, a ventral and a dorsal pathway. This conjecture is known as the dual streams hypothesis [12]. The dorsal stream, commonly referred as the "where" pathway, is involved in spatial attention. The ventral stream, commonly referred as the "what" pathway, is involved in the recognition, identification, and categorization of visual stimuli. However, there is still much debate about the degree of specialization within these two pathways, since they are in fact heavily interconnected.

Lesion of primary visual cortex, as OR, leads to a contralateral homonymous hemianopia or quadrantanopia. Bilateral lesions can cause complete cortical blindness and can sometimes be accompanied by a condition called Anton-Babinski syndrome, which is when a patient is blind but denies having any visual deficit.

In the area called the sagittal stratum which connects the occipital lobe to the rest of the brain, OR are anatomically close to other white matter fascicles [13–16]. These fascicles are particularly close at the level of the atrium of the lateral ventricle, where they are ordered from the surface to the ependyma: U fibers, arcuate/superior longitudinal fascicle complex, vertical occipital fascicle, middle and inferior longitudinal fascicles, inferior fronto-occipital fascicle, optic radiations, and tapetum fibers [17–19].

In the dominant hemisphere (usually left), all these white matter pathways participate to verbal language and reading; in the minor hemisphere, they participate to attentional functions and visuospatial and social cognition.

2.3 What Does Really Mean Mapping the Vision?

Diffusion tensor imaging (DTI)-based tractography of white matter tracts as well as visual functional MRI can be combined with intraoperative navigation and displayed on neuronavigation. This approach can provide useful information regarding the surgical strategy but is limited in the context of brain tumor as peri-tumoral edema is known to alter the visualization of the white matter tracts on diffusion tractography [20–22]. The OR, as all white matter fascicles, lack consistent anatomical landmark, especially in tumor surgery, where a mass effect and displacement of white matter structures is common. So mapping the vision should be a physiological and functional exploration. During awake brain surgery, the anatomical structures physiologically explored are the OR and the visual cortex.

Direct electrical stimulation (DES) of OR leads to "positive" and "negative" "phenomena." The reason for the appearance to a symptom or another is not clearly understood (intensity, site of the DES). The negative symptoms are interpreted as a disturbance of the visual processing, resulting in a scotoma. The positive are interpreted as antero- or retrograde stimulation of neurons resulting in phosphenes in the corresponding contralateral visual field [23, 24]. It has been postulated that the warning of phosphene-evoked stimulation to alert the surgeon of an imminent anatomical disruption of the OR might not be sensitive enough. Indeed, it is possible that phosphenes are triggered only when the stimulation site is already within the OR, thus leading to a visual deficit. However, this limitation might be compensated by increasing the stimulation intensity, thus securing a margin between the resection and the OR (see Fig. 2.2). In fact, complexity of elicited visual phenomena increases in a postero-anterior axis and can be categorized into simple (e.g., flashing lights), intermediate (simple geometrical shapes), and complex forms or visual distortion [25, 26]. It has been described that the left occipital cortex would have a substantially lower sensitivity for stimulation and would lack complex shapes compared with the visually dominant right occipital lobe during extraoperative stimulation

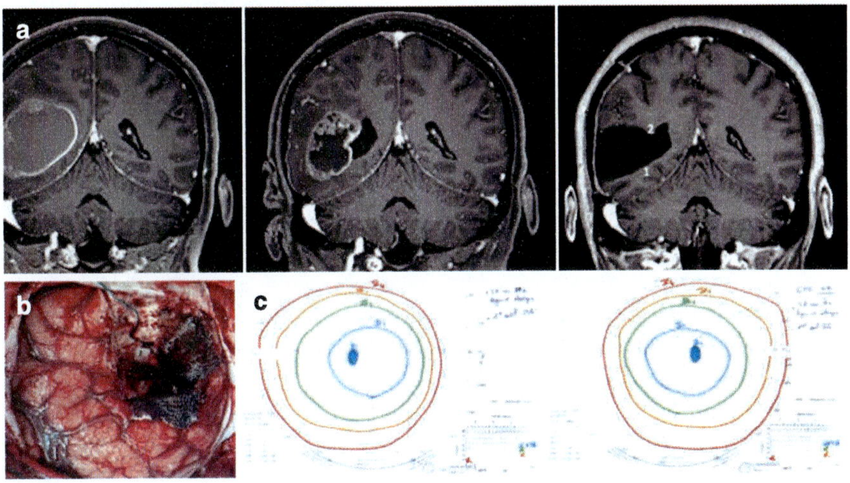

Fig. 2.2 (a) Coronal slices of T1 gado in a patient-case with a brain metastasis. Left: at diagnosis. Patient had a complete hemianopia. Middle: Just after puncture of the cyst. Right: 1 month after complete resection under awake conditions with visual field testing according to the quadrants picture naming procedure. Numbers 1 and 2 correspond to tags 1 and 2 of the figure (b). (b) Intraoperative photography. When stimulating tag 2 at 3 mA, the patient was unable to name the picture in the left lower quadrant, as image recognition was disturbed by phosphenes. When stimulating tag 1 at 3 mA, the patient reported phosphenes in the left upper quadrant. The tumor had entered the ventricle in between tag 1 and 2, splitting the upper and lower half of the optic radiations in two separate parts. (c) Postoperative Goldman perimetry 1 month after awake resection, demonstrating a quasi-normal visual field

using depth electrodes [25]. But in the condition of an awake surgery it should be reminded that the majority of the primary cortex is buried in the calcarine fissure and thus is inaccessible for stimulation.

Negative phenomenon might be related to DES of the white matter fascicles connecting the visual cortex to other networks (as inferior longitudinal fasciculus and inferior-fronto-occipital fasciculus), leading to a large variety of symptoms, in the domain of attention (unilateral neglect), reading (alexia), object recognition (visual agnosia), face recognition (prosopagnosia), emotion recognition, empathy, and theory of mind.

2.4 Why to Map the Visual Field?

The VF is a major compound of vision and there is an obvious clinical interest in mapping it. VF defect is a postoperative handicap, which has been largely underestimated by neurosurgeons. While functional disability is minimal with a superior quadrantanopia, permanent hemianopia is a significant handicap that impairs daily life activities, particularly the ability to drive a motor vehicle or to read [27, 28].

The normal monocular human visual field extends to approximately 60° nasally from the vertical meridian in each eye, to 107° temporally, and approximately 70° above and 80 below the horizontal meridian.

VF is currently assessed by manual or automated perimeters and it is a time-consuming process (Fig. 2.3). The monocular visual field is measured by perimetry. This may be kinetic, where spots of light are shown on the white interior of a half sphere and slowly moved inward until the observer sees them (Goldman perimeter), or static, where the light spots are flashed at varying intensities at fixed locations in the sphere until detected by the subject. Commonly used perimeters are the automated Humphrey Field Analyzer, the Heidelberg Edge Perimeter, or the Oculus. The binocular VF can be measured by merging results from monocular fields or by using a Binocular Humphrey Esterman VF test (EVFT) (Carl Zeiss Meditec). Binocular visual field testing programs are readily available in various automated perimeters.

Concerning the stimulus, five different sizes are defined by Roman numerals I through V. Each stimulus covers a fourfold greater area, ranging from 0.25 mm^2 for a size I stimulus to 64 mm^2 for a size V stimulus. The light sensitivity threshold is expressed in decibel, calibrated on the most intense perimetric stimulus that the device can display, and not in luminance unit.

It is important to know that results between different perimeters are similar, but not identical. That is mainly due to the differences in the hardware used and the luminosity of the devices [29]. As the available luminosity and luminosity steps of one device approaches the other, the results become more comparable, if both perimeters are running the same algorithm. Moreover, visual field testing is a subjective examination. Testing the same eye/patient twice in the same day using the same machine does not produce identical results.

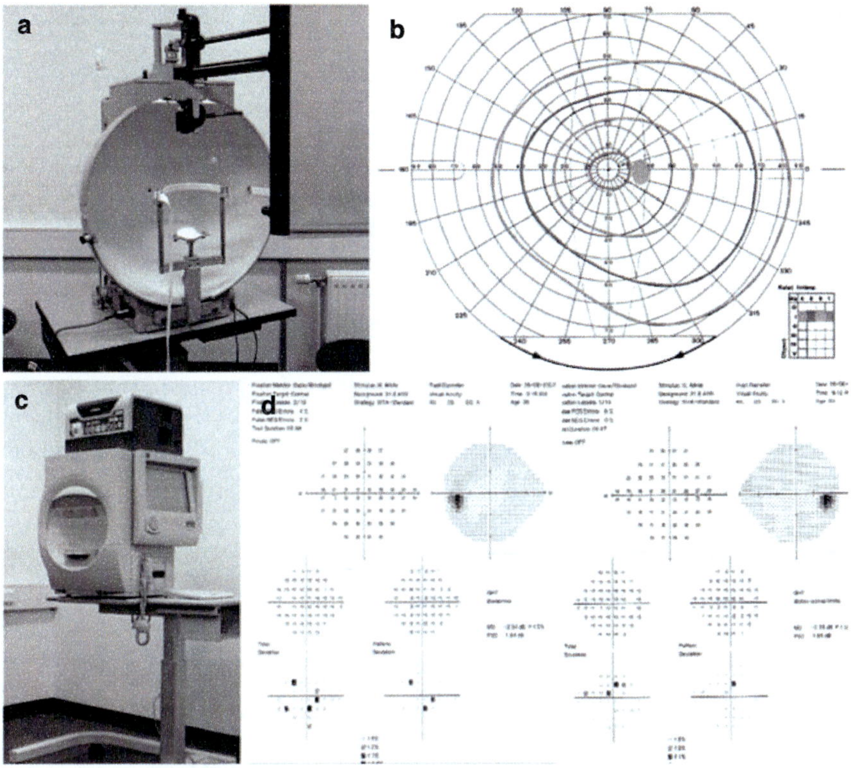

Fig. 2.3 VF testing: (**a**) Godman perimeter (**b**) and monocular VF result, right eye, (**c**) automated perimeter (**d**) monocular VF result, right and left eye

For a driving license, most of the European country regulations are based on EU Directive 2009/113/EC that requires a horizontal visual field at least 50° left and right from the vertical meridian in each eye and 120° horizontally in total, and 20° above and below the horizontal meridian (European Commission Official Journal of the European Union 2009/112/EC; Ammend Commission Directive Annex III, 52:223–227. Done at Brussels, 25 August 2009). No description of which visual field test to be used has been included in the European Commission's regulations. These criteria may vary depending on the country legislation. However, the functional scoring system developed by Esterman is the current gold standard for testing binocular visual fields and is used by many national driving authorities.

Mapping of more elaborate aspect of vision as reading, spatial attention, and face and emotion recognition has to be discussed depending on the patient and the lesion location [30].

2.5 When to Map the VF?

As for all brain mapping programming, two elements must be taken into account.

The first one is the patient, more specifically his medical history (e.g., ophthalmologic status), his profession, and his hobbies. The visual status of the patient and whether or to what extent a postoperative visual field deficit is acceptable should be a pivotal discussion between the patient and surgeon prior to surgery.

The prognosis is important also. Even if a hemianopia is a significant handicap, it has to be balanced with the oncological benefit of a large resection. The situation would be dramatically different for an epilepsy surgery [31–33].

Finally, the localization of the lesion is a major point. This is particularly an issue in anterior temporal lobe resection, which is an efficient treatment for refractory temporal lobe epilepsy [34, 35]. Surgical damage to Meyer loop, the most anterior part of the optic radiation, results in a visual field deficit in between 48 and 100% of patients. Resection of tumors in the posterior temporal lobe or adjacent to the atrium may be also associated with an injury to the OR, resulting in postoperative VF deficits.

2.6 Cortical Visual Evoked Potential

Several reports have suggested that cortical visual evoked potentials (VEPs) can be reliably recorded intraoperatively and that they may predict postoperative visual function.

Several reports showed that intraoperative monitoring of the visual cortex is feasible under general anesthesia, using visual evoked potential with subdural electrodes and photic stimulation through closed eyelids with a strobe light [36–38].

The method can be performed during awake craniotomy also. In this situation, direct cortical visual evoked potential (VEP) recording, subcortical recordings from the OR, and subcortical stimulation of the OR can be combined to assess visual function and proximity of the lesion to the OR [39].

Other reports have highlighted the limitations and questioned the reliability of intraoperative VEP monitoring, suggesting that there was no correlation between intraoperative VEP changes and VF outcome [40, 41]. Indeed, the presence of a robust cortical VEP at baseline in visually compromised patients is of concern and brings into question the value of this technique. One possible explanation of this phenomenon is that the VEPs generated by the intact contralateral visual cortex can mask the presumed VEP waveform deficiencies generated by the ipsilateral visual system.

Intraoperative electrophysiological monitoring of the visual pathways is feasible under general and local anesthesia. However, it could be postulated that VEP recordings are not reliable for warning the surgeon about an imminent anatomical disruption of the OR.

2.7 Review of the Different Tools and Tasks Designed to Monitor Visual Field and Other Vision Functions

The different approaches and tools described in this chapter are mainly developed to explore the VF, but new tools targeting the more cognitive aspects of vision are under development and will be shortly discussed.

VF evaluation can be done *by confrontation*, when the examiner, linguist or psychologist, moves his fingers in the four corners of the VF, in a concentric way, as during a classical neurological examination. However, this method lacks accuracy and reproducibility, and is frequently hard to execute in the patient's and examiner's position; only rough data can be collected and comparison between successive evaluations is difficult. Specific tools have been then evaluated: dish, screen, and virtual reality headset.

2.7.1 DISH/Large Perimetry Chart Experience

In this approach, close to the Goldman test, the patient focused on a target on a large screen or board 3 ft away in the center of his VF. There are few publications, and to date two clinical cases have been reported.

Nguyen et al. described for the occipital cortex mapping in one patient, in sitting position, the use of a combined static and kinetic perimetry, with a standard flashing checkerboard task for each eye [42]. The necessity of a sitting position and the cumbersome of the system are real limitations.

More recently, Joswing et al. reported an illustrative case of their well-established practice for awake perimetry testing for surgery epilepsy using a visual board [43, 44]. The patient is installed in lateral decubitus position with a large perimetry chart on a stand turned to 90° placed in front of him. The patient is provided with a laser pointer, and, in response to ongoing electrocortical stimulation of several visual cortical areas, has to point exactly toward the perimetry chart to acknowledge any positive or negative changes in his vision.

The examiner moved an object toward the target, and the patient signaled when they saw it in their periphery.

2.7.2 Screen Experience

Since during awake cortico-subcortical mapping the tasks usually are presented on a laptop or tablet screen, the use of this tool seems obvious. The screen has to be presented at a constant distance, perpendicular to and nearby the patient's face, that should nevertheless always remain observable (evaluation of facial movements, emotion, possibility of seizures, avoidance of claustrophobia,...).

Currently, when a standard 15″ screen is used (diagonal 39.6 cm, horizontal 34.5 cm, vertical 19.4 cm), it is placed at 20–25 cm from the nasion, so the horizontal screen length equals the double of the distance screen/eye, offering a lateral angle of 50° (Fig. 2.4).

2.7.2.1 Picture Naming in Quadrants (Montpellier Experience)

Another approach has been proposed by Duffau et al.: it consists in presenting two images situated diagonally on a screen divided into four quadrants [45, 46]. This task has been proposed for lesion involving the sagittal stratum in either hemisphere. As language tracts and optic radiations are very close within the temporo-occipito-parietal junction, a stimulation of the language pathways would result in naming disturbances for the two diagonally placed pictures, whereas misnaming for only one of the two pictures would be rather linked to a visual disturbance. In the study of Gras-Combe et al., this procedure allowed to avoid full hemianopia in 13 out of the 14 patients, demonstrating its utility. Figure 2.2 provides an illustrative case with full preservation of left VF in a patient with a right temporal metastasis. Optic radiation were mapped intraoperatively by means of picture naming in quadrants.

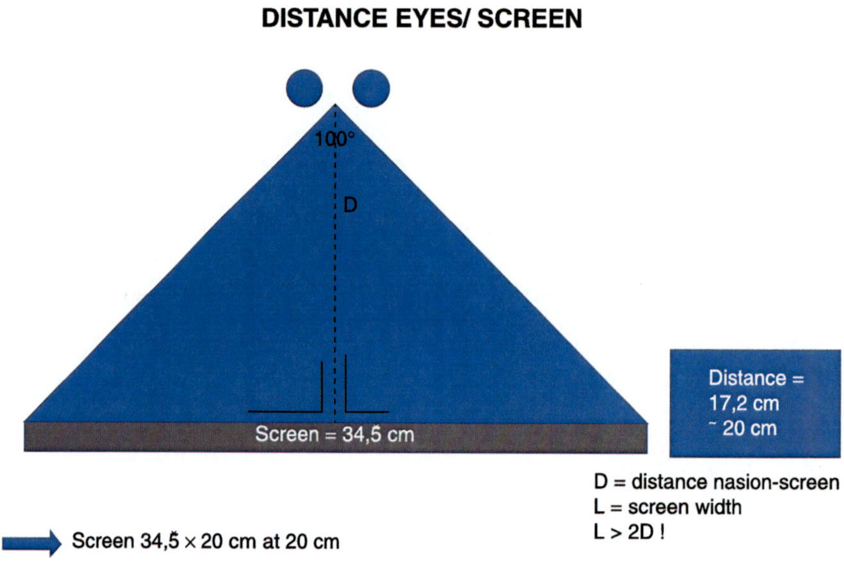

Fig. 2.4 Scheme of relative distance between eyes and screen, depending on screen's width, to obtain a lateral angle of 50° × 2

2.7.2.2 Colored Dots Visual Field Testing (Gent Experience)

Since 2012, we have developed at the Saint-Lucas General Hospital Gent a combination of simple visual field testing, preferably with evaluation of extinction (with avoidance of eye movements).

When a reference point is placed at the center of the presented screen, and the patient fixes it, only coarse shapes and colors can be recognized out of the central view, so we avoided presenting objects or complex figures, since this induces involuntary eye movements (saccades), biasing the proper visual field evaluation.

During VF testing, the patient has to fix a central point (e.g., star, differentiating it from dots), while points appear at the periphery, either in a single quadrant or in opposed quadrants, to allow evaluation of extinction.

As background, a black display is preferable (Fig. 2.5a), to enhance the contrast with the presented colors; moreover, most glioma operations are performed in an obscured room (use of microscope, 5 ALA,…), where a bright background can be disturbing.

The procedure as used in classical perimetry is subjective: the patient's answer—to see or not to see the dot (yes or no)—cannot be verified; on the contrary, when the patient mentions a color, the response can be controlled (correct or not): this makes the testing very reliable without loss of time. Another advantage of the use of colors

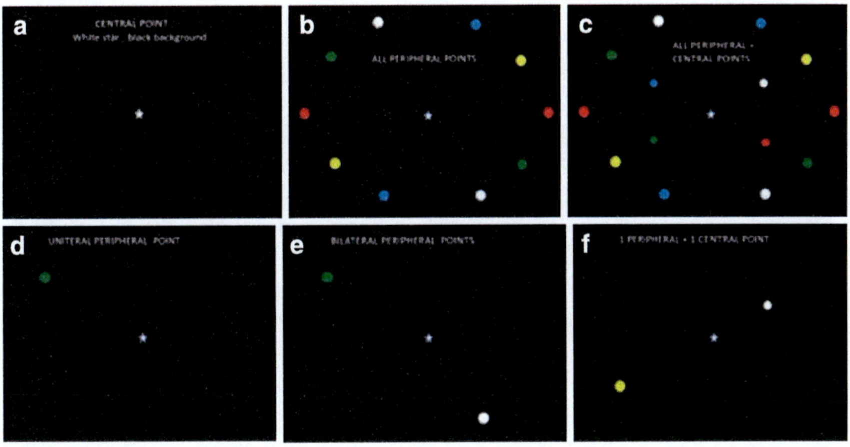

Fig. 2.5 Presentation of colored points at peripheral and central locations, uni- or bilateral, and central star to be fixed, on a dark background. (**a**) Central white star, on black background. (**b**) All 10 peripheral points. (**c**) All 10 peripheral + 4 central points. (**d**) 1 Peripheral point. (**e**) 2 points, both peripheral. (**f**) 2 points, 1 peripheral, 1 central

(except in color-blind people where the test has to be adapted in function of their deficit) is that recognition is very fast, easy for the patient, and even usable in illiterate patients; moreover, it is valuable in tired patients, and easy to verify.

Either flashing light points, moving or colored points or combinations can be proposed to the patient. In our opinion, to evaluate correctness of the answer, colored dots are preferable, after exclusion of color blindness. Moreover, description of colors (e.g., "red and blue") is faster and more reliable than description of the quadrant (e.g., "right inferior and left superior").

Colors are displayed as follows (Fig. 2.5b).

Beside the 10 points displayed clockwise at the periphery (10 mm), 4 more points can be presented more centrally in the 4 angles (8 mm), providing some evaluation in case of *there is already some degree of* visual field deficit (Fig. 2.5c).

Either one point can be displayed at one side, or 2 points, one in each hemi-field; in case of 1 testing point, it is preferably located hetero-laterally to the lesion (Fig. 2.5d). To make the test more sensitive, we use 2 points presented in both peripheral hemi-fields (Fig. 2.5e), or 1 peripheral and 1 central (Fig. 2.5f). The occurrence of an extinction phenomenon (the ipsilesional stimulus impedes the perception of the contralesional stimulus) could detect earlier a VF deficit; nevertheless, it should be pointed out that the extinction phenomena is classically described in unilateral neglect meaning that the 2 points test explore vision and attention at the same time, as in ecological conditions.

When projected on a Goldman perimetry, the dots are in the normal I3 isoptere, and correspond to a VF retained as standard for quality of life: Superior: 20°, Lateral: 50°, Inferior: 20, Medial: 10° (see Fig. 2.6a, b).

The task can be implemented by asking the patient to click on the point on the touch screen; so combined analysis of visual field and movement is obtained.

Of course, the color visual field test has to be evaluated and trained preoperatively in regard to classical visual field evaluation with Goldman perimeter.

In our approach, the color visual field test is alternated with the G.E.N. Task, which provides global multimodal testing, integrating the visual field evaluation with other-language and non-language-functions. Since the optic radiations are located in the vicinity of inferior fronto-occipital, inferior longitudinal, and arcuate fascicles, these tracts could be lesioned at the same time, and hence evaluated together within one task; this can be obtained with the G.E.N.T. (see Chap. 19), where besides visual field, auditory, reading, naming, nonverbal semantics, and syntax can be evaluated simultaneously by asking the patient to make a short sentence with a written subject or verb and four drawn objects (Fig. 2.7).

This task is presented on the same screen at the same distance to the eyes, so immediate and easy switching from one to the other kind of testing is possible without any screen manipulation, avoiding loss of time. However, as for the picture naming in quadrants, there is a risk that the patient makes a saccade as a mean to compensate the stimulation-induced visual field deficit, resulting in a risk of false negative.

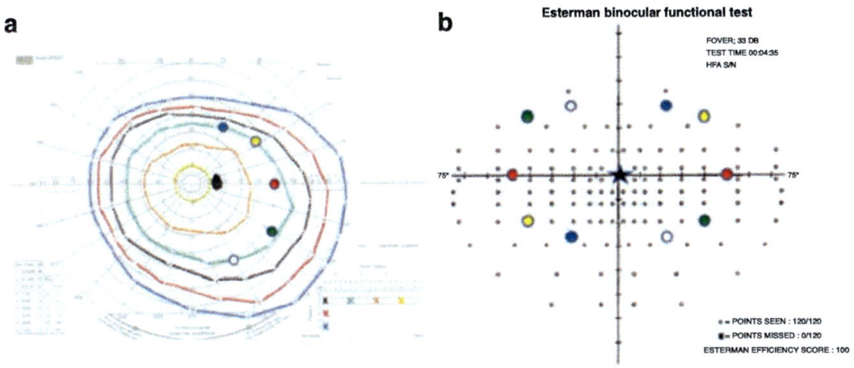

Fig. 2.6 (**a**) Projection of peripheral colored dots on Goldmann perimeter (monocular). (**b**) Projection of peripheral colored dots on Esterman Test (binocular)

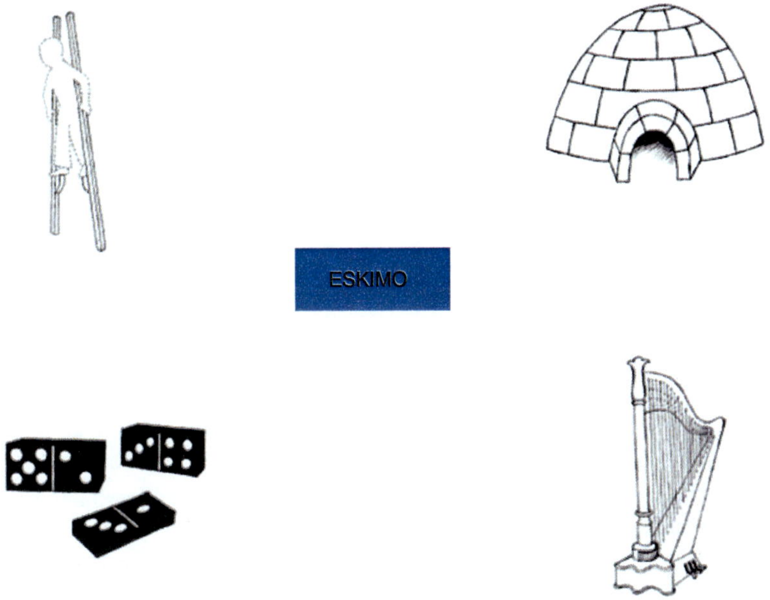

Fig. 2.7 One trial of the GENTask. The patient is asked to produce a short sentence like "The Eskimo lives in an igloo"

2.7.3 Virtual Reality Headset (Angers Experience)

VF evaluation with a virtual reality headset (VRH) has been already described, but none to date has yet studied the capabilities offered by these systems in the identification of functional brain areas and implementation of tests of cognitive and visual functions in patients during awake cranial surgery [47–49]. Indeed, the developed headsets and software were oriented for bedside evaluation, and to detect and quantify VF defect in ophthalmologic pathology such as glaucoma.

An adapted procedure for VF testing in the condition of an awake surgery needed to be developed.

In 2017, we started in Angers to develop this procedure with an Oculus DK1 VRH (Oculus, Menlo Park, California), which has a binocular visual field of 80°. The developed software was based on Esterman test that is officially used to assess visual field defects for driving license authorization according to the European recommendations. In order to be compatible with the VRH, the Esterman test had to be modified.

The mean difficulties dealing with VR technology is the rapidity of progress and the constant release of new more performing and affordable VRH. We then adapted our software to the Oculus DK2 which has a binocular visual field of 90°. Our modified Esterman test in its latest version explored the 45° around the central visual axis of a binocular visual field, which does not meet all the French criteria on driving licenses, but can detect important visual defects that may impair the quality of life.

In the operative room, while the neurosurgeon performs direct cortical or subcortical electrostimulation, the orthoptist provides luminous stimuli on the control screen. The patient gives an oral answer to the examiner according to whether or not he sees the luminous stimulus (Fig. 2.8).

Our goal was to assess the efficiency of the VRH in detecting visual defects, rather than comparing two bedsides visual field assessment techniques. Nevertheless, we compared our test with an automated perimetry and comparison showed that 90% of the patients with a VF defect were well classified with our approach.

The proof of concept of this approach was done for a 66-year-old male, right-handed, blind in his right eye due to a history of ischemic optic neuropathy, who had surgery for a left parieto-temporal malignant glioma [50].

We then adapted our software to another VRH model: the Samsung Gear VR combined with a Samsung S7 smartphone (visual field 96°).

Presently, we are using the HTC Vive (visual field 110°) [51]. The major advance was to combine the VRH HTC Vive with an eye-tracking device (Tobii Pro SDK) able to track the full HTC Vive field of view and to perform a pupil measurement.

The first VF test was piloted by an orthoptist, enhancing accuracy, but weighting down the procedure. We developed another version, easier to pilot, exploring a VF of 80° with six possible red dots on a black background (Fig. 2.9). Indeed, the maximum visual field attainable in the virtual reality headset, taking into account its mechanical characteristics, is 110°. However, if we keep the foam to maximize the user comfort and if we do not impose to press the headset against the face as much as possible, then the visual field is around 90°.

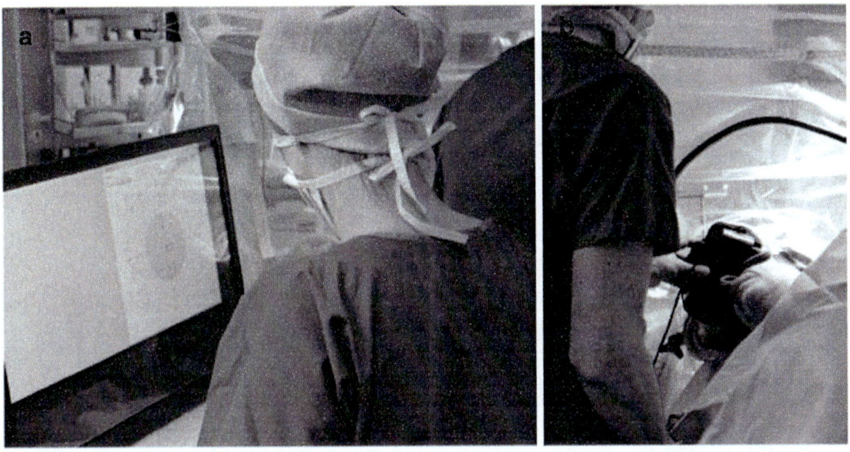

Fig. 2.8 Modified Esterman test. (**a**) View of the screen piloted by the orthoptist. Left: the gray area represents what the patient is seeing. Each stimulus appears as a white dot on a gray background, while the patient has to stare the central yellow dot; Right: modified Esterman test grid, allowing the orthoptist to select the part of the visual field to be tested and one of the 20 pre-settled points; (**b**) patient wearing the virtual reality headset

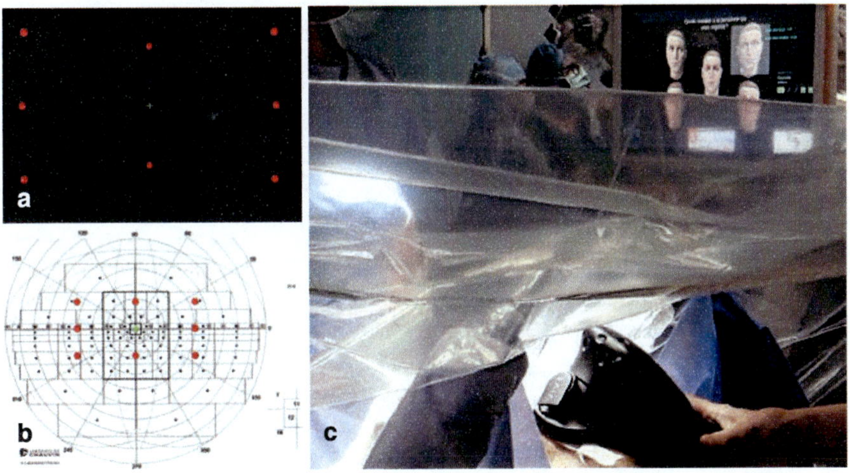

Fig. 2.9 VF testing with the VRH HTC vive. (**a**) What the patient sees, the eight possible dots are presented, (**b**) the same dots projected on an Esterman grid; (**c**) perioperative view, with exploration of social vision using interactive avatars. The screen shows what the patient is seeing in the VRH, his gaze is represented as a green spot

According to our experience, the phosphenes elicited by DES are more distinct in patients wearing a VRH with a dark background. What the patient sees in the VRH is projected on one of the neuronavigation system's screen. Thanks to the eye tracking, the patient gaze can be followed online on the screen, materialized as a green point (Fig. 2.9). This gives an essential control of the patient gaze, and warrants that the patient was really fixing the central dot during the VF testing, without eye saccades. Moreover, once the task has been completed, gaze layout can be displayed on the screen as lines, heat map, or statistics, combined if necessary with pupillometry data, which is particularly helpful during testing of a complex aspect of vision (Fig. 2.10).

Now, a prospective study is ongoing comparing with all the described limitations, our VF test to an automatized perimetry (TRIAL.GOV **NCT04288505**). In the future, technical features of Virtual Reality Headset are going to be improved, and it will probably soon be possible to explore a wider visual field in these devices.

Parallelly, we are exploring more cognitive aspects of the vision, such as attention and visuospatial and social cognition. Indeed, there are several interactions between awareness, spatial attention, and vision of affectively and socially significant items or faces [52, 53].

VR offers tools for creating realistic simulations of social situation. Eye-tracking sensor technology can determine the patient's level of attention, to where and to

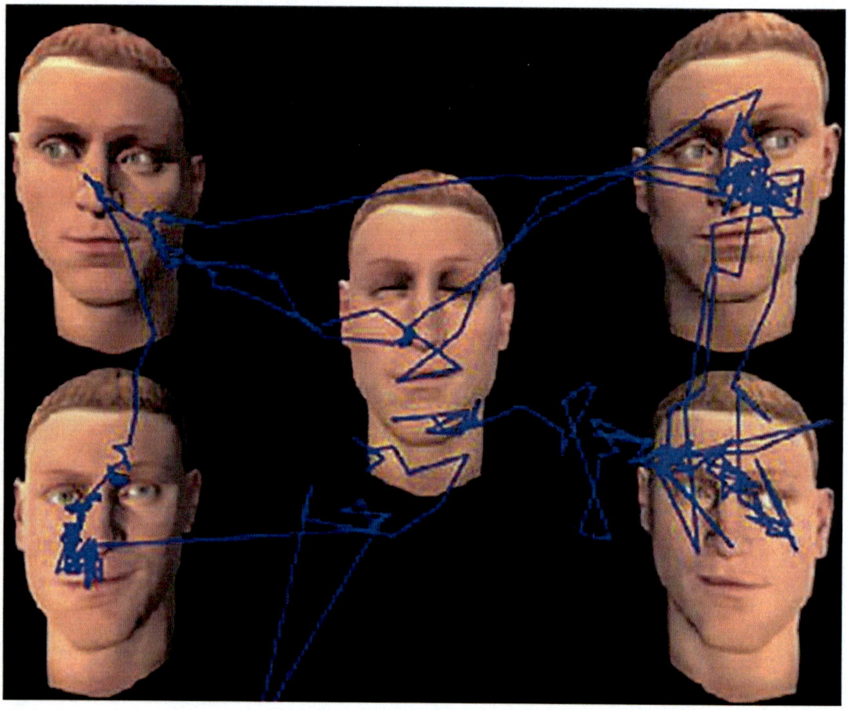

Fig. 2.10 The eye-tracking recording (blue line) after a social vision task. The patient is asked to search for the avatar trying to make visual contact. Once the avatar looking at the patient is identified and visual contact is established for a period of 0.6 s, the avatar expresses a dynamic facial emotion. The patient is asked to describe the avatar's emotion or to describe his feelings about the desire to communicate or engage in social contact expressed by the avatar

what the patient is focusing his attention, as well as his pupillometry. Interactivity is another interesting aspect of VR. Eye-tracking technology provides a whole new way to interact with VR content. For example, eye-tracking data of participants can be used for real-time control of a virtual character's attention or facial emotion (Figs. 2.9 and 2.10).

We demonstrated the safety of this approach with VRH during a brain mapping procedure [54]. We are now developing VR interactive tasks, using avatars and more recently actors, allowing to explore with a VRH combined with eye tracking, during a brain mapping procedure, the VF, the attentional processes, and theory of mind (Fig. 2.10) [55].

2.8 Conclusion

Different approaches have been developed to explore the VF during an awake surgery, and many groups use them already in routine. However, the value of intraoperative mapping of the visual pathways during resection of tumors adjacent to the OR is still unclear. That could be explained by several points.

First, to test the reliability of all these perioperative VF testing, they would have to be compared with bedside binocular automated perimetry. Nevertheless, as mentioned above, the results between different perimeters are not identical and VF testing is a subjective examination. The variability is significant, and that makes the comparison between a perioperative perimetry test and an automated perimetry quite difficult.

Secondly, a larger number of comparable patients and a randomized trial are needed to establish the benefit of VF mapping in terms of eligibility to drive, or more globally on quality of life.

The VF is an important compound of the vision, but does not represent itself the whole complex cognitive process of the vision. Vision and language are intimately processed in the dominant hemisphere. On the other hand, attention, visuospatial cognition, and social vision are interconnected also in the "minor hemisphere" (see Chaps. 4 and 18). Attentional or visual cognition defects can be more disabling than a VF defect, leading to the necessity to develop more comprehensive approaches to map the "vision," and to test the patients before and after the surgery.

References

1. Vernon D. Visual cognition. In: Ikeuchi K, editor. Computer vision: a reference guide. Boston: Springer US; 2014. p. 860–2.
2. Adolphs R. Recognizing emotion from facial expressions: psychological and neurological mechanisms. Behav Cogn Neurosci Rev. 2002;1:21–62.
3. Carreiras M, Armstrong BC, Perea M, Frost R. The what, when, where, and how of visual word recognition. Trends Cogn Sci. 2014;18:90–8.
4. Freiwald WA. The neural mechanisms of face processing: cells, areas, networks, and models. Curr Opin Neurobiol. 2020;60:184–91.

5. Riesenhuber M, Poggio T. Neural mechanisms of object recognition. Curr Opin Neurobiol. 2002;12:162–8.
6. Harris LR, Jenkin M. Vision and attention. In: Jenkin M, Harris L, editors. Vision and attention. New York: Springer; 2001. p. 1–17.
7. Prasad S, Galetta SL. Anatomy and physiology of the afferent visual system. Handb Clin Neurol. 2011;102:3–19.
8. Hansen T, Pracejus L, Gegenfurtner KR. Color perception in the intermediate periphery of the visual field. J Vis. 2009;9:26.1–12.
9. Fademrecht L, Bülthoff I, de la Rosa S. Action recognition in the visual periphery. J Vis. 2016;16:33.
10. Rosenholtz R. Capabilities and limitations of peripheral vision. Annu Rev Vis Sci. 2016;2:437–57.
11. Huff T, Mahabadi N, Tadi P. Neuroanatomy, visual cortex. In: StatPearls. Treasure Island: StatPearls Publishing; 2020.
12. Mishkin M, Ungerleider LG. Contribution of striate inputs to the visuospatial functions of parieto-preoccipital cortex in monkeys. Behav Brain Res. 1982;6:57–77.
13. Di Carlo DT, Benedetto N, Duffau H, Cagnazzo F, Weiss A, Castagna M, Cosottini M, Perrini P. Microsurgical anatomy of the sagittal stratum. Acta Neurochir (Wien). 2019;161:2319–27.
14. Jitsuishi T, Hirono S, Yamamoto T, Kitajo K, Iwadate Y, Yamaguchi A. White matter dissection and structural connectivity of the human vertical occipital fasciculus to link vision-associated brain cortex. Sci Rep. 2020;10:820.
15. Rokem A, Takemura H, Bock AS, Scherf KS, Behrmann M, Wandell BA, Fine I, Bridge H, Pestilli F. The visual white matter: the application of diffusion MRI and fiber tractography to vision science. J Vis. 2017;17:4.
16. Takemura H, Pestilli F, Weiner KS, Keliris GA, Landi SM, Sliwa J, Ye FQ, Barnett MA, Leopold DA, Freiwald WA, et al. Occipital white matter tracts in human and macaque. Cereb Cortex. 2017;27:3346–59.
17. Capilla-Guasch P, Quilis-Quesada V, Regin-Neto M, Holanda VM, González-Darder JM, de Oliveira E. White matter relationships examined by transillumination technique using a lateral transcortical parietal approach to the atrium: three-dimensional images and surgical considerations. World Neurosurg. 2019;132:e783–94.
18. Koutsarnakis C, Kalyvas AV, Komaitis S, Liakos F, Skandalakis GP, Anagnostopoulos C, Stranjalis G. Defining the relationship of the optic radiation to the roof and floor of the ventricular atrium: a focused microanatomical study. J Neurosurg. 2019;130:1728–39.
19. Peltier J, Nicot B, Baroncini M, Zunon-Kipré Y, Haidara A, Havet E, Foulon P, Page C, Lejeune J-P, Le Gars D. Anatomie de la substance blanche périventriculaire. Neurochirurgie. 2011;57:151–5.
20. Roux FE, Ibarrola D, Lotterie JA, Chollet F, Berry I. Perimetric visual field and functional MRI correlation: implications for image-guided surgery in occipital brain tumours. J Neurol Neurosurg Psychiatry. 2001;71:505–14.
21. Shinoura N, Suzuki Y, Yamada R, Tabei Y, Saito K, Yagi K. Relationships between brain tumor and optic tract or calcarine fissure are involved in visual field deficits after surgery for brain tumor. Acta Neurochir (Wien). 2010;152:637–42.
22. Winston GP, Daga P, White MJ, Micallef C, Miserocchi A, Mancini L, Modat M, Stretton J, Sidhu MK, Symms MR, et al. Preventing visual field deficits from neurosurgery. Neurology. 2014;83:604–11.
23. Dobelle WH, Mladejovsky MG. Phosphenes produced by electrical stimulation of human occipital cortex, and their application to the development of a prosthesis for the blind. J Physiol. 1974;243:553–76.
24. Šteňo A, Hollý V, Fabian M, Kuniak M, Timárová G, Šteňo J. Direct electrical stimulation of the optic radiation in patients with covered eyes. Neurosurg Rev. 2014;37:527–33.
25. Jonas J, Frismand S, Vignal J-P, Colnat-Coulbois S, Koessler L, Vespignani H, Rossion B, Maillard L. Right hemispheric dominance of visual phenomena evoked by intracerebral

stimulation of the human visual cortex: Right Hemispheric Dominance of Visual Phenomena. Hum Brain Mapp. 2014;35:3360–71.
26. Lee HW, Hong SB, Seo DW, Tae WS, Hong SC. Mapping of functional organization in human visual cortex: electrical cortical stimulation. Neurology. 2000;54:849–54.
27. Bowers AR. Driving with homonymous visual field loss: a review of the literature. Clin Exp Optom. 2016;99:402–18.
28. Zihl J. Visual scanning behavior in patients with homonymous hemianopia. Neuropsychologia. 1995;33:287–303.
29. Manji H, Plant GT. Epilepsy surgery, visual fields, and driving: a study of the visual field criteria for driving in patients after temporal lobe epilepsy surgery with a comparison of Goldmann and Esterman perimetry. J Neurol Neurosurg Psychiatry. 2000;68:80–2.
30. Chan-Seng E, Moritz-Gasser S, Duffau H. Awake mapping for low-grade gliomas involving the left sagittal stratum: anatomofunctional and surgical considerations. J Neurosurg. 2014;120:1069–77.
31. Blume WT, Whiting SE, Girvin JP. Epilepsy surgery in the posterior cortex. Ann Neurol. 1991;29:638–45.
32. Salanova V, Andermann F, Olivier A, Rasmussen T, Quesney LF. Occipital lobe epilepsy: electroclinical manifestations, electrocorticography, cortical stimulation and outcome in 42 patients treated between 1930 and 1991. Surgery of occipital lobe epilepsy. Brain J Neurol. 1992;115(Pt 6):1655–80.
33. Yang P-F, Jia Y-Z, Lin Q, Mei Z, Chen Z-Q, Zheng Z-Y, Zhang H-J, Pei J-S, Tian J, Zhong Z-H. Intractable occipital lobe epilepsy: clinical characteristics, surgical treatment, and a systematic review of the literature. Acta Neurochir (Wien). 2015;157:63–75.
34. Ebeling U, Reulen HJ. Neurosurgical topography of the optic radiation in the temporal lobe. Acta Neurochir (Wien). 1988;92:29–36.
35. Sincoff EH, Tan Y, Abdulrauf SI. White matter fiber dissection of the optic radiations of the temporal lobe and implications for surgical approaches to the temporal horn. J Neurosurg. 2004;101:739–46.
36. Curatolo JM, Macdonell RA, Berkovic SF, Fabinyi GC. Intraoperative monitoring to preserve central visual fields during occipital corticectomy for epilepsy. J Clin Neurosci. 2000;7:234–7.
37. Kamada K, Todo T, Morita A, Masutani Y, Aoki S, Ino K, Kawai K, Kirino T. Functional monitoring for visual pathway using real-time visual evoked potentials and optic-radiation tractography. Neurosurgery. 2005;57:121–7; discussion 121–7.
38. Ota T, Kawai K, Kamada K, Kin T, Saito N. Intraoperative monitoring of cortically recorded visual response for posterior visual pathway. J Neurosurg. 2010;112:285–94.
39. Shahar T, Korn A, Barkay G, Biron T, Hadanny A, Gazit T, Nossek E, Ekstein M, Kesler A, Ram Z. Elaborate mapping of the posterior visual pathway in awake craniotomy. J Neurosurg. 2018;128:1503–11.
40. Cedzich C, Schramm J, Fahlbusch R. Are flash-evoked visual potentials useful for intraoperative monitoring of visual pathway function? Neurosurgery. 1987;21:709–15.
41. Raudzens PA. Intraoperative monitoring of evoked potentials. Ann N Y Acad Sci. 1982;388:308–26.
42. Nguyen HS, Sundaram SV, Mosier KM, Cohen-Gadol AA. A method to map the visual cortex during an awake craniotomy. J Neurosurg. 2011;114:922–6.
43. Girvin JP. Operative techniques in epilepsy. Cham: Springer International Publishing; 2015.
44. Joswig H, Girvin JP, Blume WT, Burneo JG, Steven DA. Awake perimetry testing for occipital epilepsy surgery. J Neurosurg. 2018;129:1195–9.
45. Duffau H, Velut S, Mitchell M-C, Gatignol P, Capelle L. Intra-operative mapping of the subcortical visual pathways using direct electrical stimulations. Acta Neurochir (Wien). 2004;146:265–9; discussion 269–70.
46. Gras-Combe G, Moritz-Gasser S, Herbet G, Duffau H. Intraoperative subcortical electrical mapping of optic radiations in awake surgery for glioma involving visual pathways. J Neurosurg. 2012;117:466–73.

47. Kimura T, Matsumoto C, Nomoto H. Comparison of head-mounted perimeter (imo®) and Humphrey Field Analyzer. Clin Ophthalmol Auckl N Z. 2019;13:501–13.
48. Tsapakis S, Papaconstantinou D, Diagourtas A, Droutsas K, Andreanos K, Moschos MM, Brouzas D. Visual field examination method using virtual reality glasses compared with the Humphrey perimeter. Clin Ophthalmol Auckl N Z. 2017;11:1431–43.
49. Wroblewski D, Francis BA, Sadun A, Vakili G, Chopra V. Testing of visual field with virtual reality goggles in manual and visual grasp modes. Biomed Res Int. 2014;2014:206082.
50. Mazerand E, Le Renard M, Hue S, Lemée J-M, Klinger E, Menei P. Intraoperative subcortical electrical mapping of the optic tract in awake surgery using a virtual reality headset. World Neurosurg. 2017;97:424–30.
51. Casanova M, Clavreul A, Soulard G, Delion M, Aubin G, Ter Minassian A, Seguier R, Menei P. Immersive virtual reality and ocular tracking for brain mapping during awake surgery: prospective evaluation study. J Med Internet Res. 2021;23(3):e24373.
52. Bernard F, Lemée J-M, Ter Minassian A, Menei P. Right hemisphere cognitive functions: from clinical and anatomic bases to brain mapping during awake craniotomy part I: clinical and functional anatomy. World Neurosurg. 2018a;118:348–59.
53. Lemée J-M, Bernard F, Ter Minassian A, Menei P. Right hemisphere cognitive functions: from clinical and anatomical bases to brain mapping during awake craniotomy. Part II: neuropsychological tasks and brain mapping. World Neurosurg. 2018;118:360–7.
54. Delion M, Klinger E, Bernard F, Aubin G, Minassian AT, Menei P. Immersing patients in a virtual reality environment for brain mapping during awake surgery: safety study. World Neurosurg. 2020;134:e937–43.
55. Bernard F, Lemée J-M, Aubin G, Ter Minassian A, Menei P. Using a virtual reality social network during awake craniotomy to map social cognition: prospective trial. J Med Internet Res. 2018b;20:e10332.

3 Frontal Eye Fields

Guillaume Herbet

3.1 Anatomy and Connectivity of FEFs

3.1.1 Physiological Definition and Brief Historical Background

The frontal eye field is defined physiologically as a restrict area of the primate's posterior prefrontal cortex whose low-intensity electrostimulation is associated with involuntary ocular movements [1, 2]. Such observation go back far into the past; indeed, David Ferrier [3] was the first to report that, in some animals (including monkeys), stimulating an area situated in the posterior half of the superior and middle frontal cortex caused head and eye movements to the opposite side as well as dilatation of pupils in some cases. Since that time, the finding of a frontal ocular area has been widely replicated, first in lower and higher primates (e.g., [4, 5]) and then in humans in the context of neurosurgery. On the latter point, Foerster [6, 7] found conjugate horizontal deviation of the eyes to the opposite side, and sometimes upward deviation, in response to stimulation of the posteriormost portion of the middle frontal gyrus. Likewise, Penfield and collaborators [8, 9] not only confirmed that applying stimulation on the posterior part of the dorsolateral prefrontal cortex (caudal part of the mid-lateral area according to the authors) caused "adversive movements" of the eyes toward and upward the hemisphere contralateral to the stimulation, but also reported that epileptic discharges in areas situated in or in the vicinity of the ocular frontal areas replicated some of the clinical observations evoked during stimulation, including eye movements [10]. Penfield and associates also identified eye-related areas in other frontal structures, including the precentral gyrus [9].

G. Herbet (✉)
Department of Neurosurgery, Gui de Chauliac Hospital, Montpellier & Institute of Functional Genomics, University of Montpellier, INSERM, CNRS, Montpellier, France
e-mail: guillaume.herbet@igf.cnrs.fr

E. Mandonnet, G. Herbet (eds.), *Intraoperative Mapping of Cognitive Networks*,
https://doi.org/10.1007/978-3-030-75071-8_3

3.1.2 Localization of the FEFs

As reviewed by Vernet et al. [11], the precise location of the FEF is variable across species (i.e., nonhuman primates versus humans) and depends on both the technique used to locate it (i.e., electrostimulation, PET, fMRI, TMS) and the behavior paradigm employed to trigger its neural activity. In the unanesthetized monkey, the FEF has been typically found in the anterior bank of the pre-arcuate sulcus around the posterior end of the sulcus principalis, using either electrostimulation procedure (e.g., [12–14]) or electrophysiological recordings in concert with oculomotor behavior tasks (e.g., [15, 16]). In humans, the exact location of the FEF slightly diverges across studies. Neuromodulation studies in patients implanted with subdural electrodes for epilepsy surgery identified the FEF "*in front of or at the level of the motor representation* [of the hand]" [17], or "*at the posterior end of the middle frontal gyrus immediately anterior to the precentral gyrus and in proximity to the superior frontal sulcus*" [18]. Electrostimulation studies conducted with "awake" patients in the context of low-grade glioma surgery confirmed the FEF as located in the posteriormost part of the middle frontal gyrus in front of the primary motor cortex, just below the intersection of the precentral sulcus and the superior frontal sulcus [19, 20]. It is worthing of note, however, that electrostimulation procedure has potential shortcomings in its ability to identify the FEF as it cannot interfere with the neurons situated in the adjacent sulci at low-intensity threshold, explaining why neuroimaging studies provide different results (see below). Moreover, the functional definition of the FEFs is intrinsically linked to observation of ocular movements in response to stimulation, though other visuo-motor activities are able to activate the FEFs. However, because neurosurgery is a clinical situation and not an experimental one, such visuo-motor tasks are routinely not included in the intra-operative protocol to spot the FEF.

As briefly mentioned above, neuroimaging literature mainly based on positron emission tomography (PET) and functional magnetic resonance imaging (fMRI) has provided a more complete picture of the possible location of the FEFs, with the advantage of using a wide range of behavior tasks able to fire it, including without being exhaustive self-paced, externally paced, imagined, visually guided, and memory-guided saccades (for a detailed review, see [11, 21, 22]). In a meta-analysis of available PET datasets, Paus [22] found a consistent location of the FEF very close to the precentral sulcus with however a great deal of across-study variability along a medial-to-lateral axis possibly due to the type of visuo-motor tasks employed. In the review of Amiez and Petrides [12] based on fMRI literature, the FEF was reportedly located in the depth of the precentral gyrus at the intersection with the superior frontal sulcus. However, in individual studies, the FEF was occasionally found in the anteriormost part of precentral gyrus [23], or at least extending in this region [24]. Other fMRI works have suggested an inferior to superior functional subdivision of the FEF [25–27], possibly corresponding to reflexive and volitional demands, respectively [21]. In brief, neuroimaging literature mainly localizes the FEF in the precentral sulcus close to the superior frontal sulcus with however some variabilities that may reflect either task requirements or differences in the statistical approach used to process neuroimaging data. Alternatively, the across-study variability in the precise localization of the FEF may be explained by the considerable interindividual variability in sulcal anatomy notably regarding its shape, size, and location [28].

3.1.3 Connectivity of FEFs

The frontal eye fields are at the heart of a complex and very distributed sensorimotor network supporting the planning, execution, and regulation of saccadic eye movements. This neural circuitry has been the target of numerous reviews; the aim here is to provide a general overview of what it is currently known without going into too much details. Besides, we have to keep in mind that much of it is accepted about the anatomical connectivity of the FEFs is derived from either autoradiographic or electrophysiological recording techniques performed in nonhuman primates. Generally, experimental evidence suggests that the FEFs exert a directed influence on the oculomotor system through four main subcortical, descending pathways [29], all of which have been reviewed by Squire et al. [30] as follows (Fig. 3.1). The first that projects to the deep layer of the ipsilateral colliculus has a direct influence on all aspects of saccade-related activity [31]. The second projects to the ipsilateral basal ganglia with a relay in the striatum. The third projects to the cerebellum via the pontine nuclei. The fourth projects to mesencephalic and pontine nuclei that form what is called the saccade generator circuit. Besides, the FEFs are closely connected

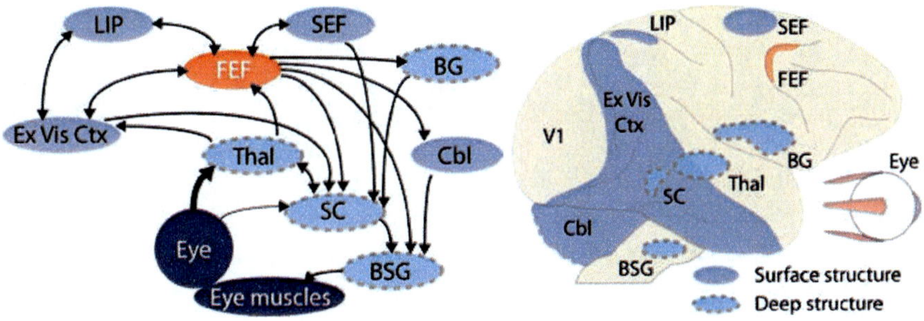

Fig. 3.1 The connectivity and anatomical locations of the frontal eye field (FEF) and other structures within the visual and oculomotor systems of the rhesus macaque monkey brain. **Left panel**, diagram of the connectivity of the FEF (orange) with other visual and oculomotor structures. Some connections that do not directly involve the FEF are omitted. **Right panel**, locations of the brain regions pictured in the left panel shown in the lateral view of the monkey brain. In both panels, surface structures other than the FEF are colored darker blue. Deep structures are illustrated as lighter blue and with a dashed outline. **Abbreviations**: *BG* basal ganglia, *BSG* brainstem saccade generator, *Cbl* cerebellum, *Ex Vis Ctx* extrastriate visual cortex, *LIP* lateral intraparietal area, *SC* superior colliculus, *SEF* supplementary eye field, *Thal* thalamus, *V1* primary visual cortex. From Ryan Fox Squire et al. [30] Frontal eye field. Scholarpedia, 7(10):5341, revision #13743. This figure is licensed under the Creative Commons Attribution 3.0: http://www.scholarpedia.org/article/Frontal_eye_field

to a number of fronto-cortical regions also involved in saccadic eye movements, an anatomo-functional organization which seems to be well preserved between monkeys and humans [12]. This includes the supplementary eye field and the cingulate eye field. In humans, the former is located in the superior frontal gyrus, rostral to the supplementary motor area, whereas the latter lodges within the cingulate sulcus [12, 29]. The FEFs have also bi-directional connections with different areas of the visual system in both the ventral (inferior-temporal cortex) and the dorsal (postero-parietal) stream, as revealed by tracer studies in monkey [32–34]. A recent resting-state functional connectivity study, performed in monkey and humans concurrently, not only confirmed the results from autoradiographic studies, but also indicated that the functional connectivity of the FEF is globally preserved across the two species. More specifically, the FEF was coupled in humans with multiple frontal areas (including the supplementary eye field, the cingulate eye field, the dorsolateral prefrontal cortex, and an area around the inferior frontal sulcus), posterior parietal areas (especially the inferior parietal lobule, the intraparietal sulcus and the precuneal cortex), and temporo-occipital areas (especially within and around the lateral occipitotemporal sulcus) [35]. Taken as a whole, current literature demonstrates that the FEF is intimately connected, functionally and structurally, with both the oculomotor and the visual systems.

3.2 Putative Functions of the FEF

3.2.1 Ocular-Motor Behaviors

As evoked above, it is widely accepted that the FEF is strongly involved in the network supporting planning, generation, and control of saccades as it interfaces with a wide range of cortical or subcortical areas known to participate in such ocular-motor activities. The results from fMRI studies indeed showed that numerous behavior tasks, manipulating the reflexive, voluntary, or predictive aspect of saccadic activity, are able to trigger functional activity of the FEFs (for a review, [11]). However, fMRI is not designed to draw causal anatomo-functional interferences. Therefore, patients' performances are of major interest to better define the functional involvement of a given area. Lesion studies, mainly dealing with stroke patients, reportedly described oculomotor deficits following partial or major insult to the FEF. Lesions affect either the reflexive or the voluntary aspect of saccadic movements, with however a greater impact on intentional saccades [11]. These disturbances generally manifest by increased latencies in the ipsi- or/and contralesional visual fields, irrespective to the behavior paradigms used. In a study using a comprehensive assessment of oculomotor behaviors, it was shown that the FEF has an important role in the disengagement from central fixation, the control of contralateral saccades, saccade prediction and the control of smooth pursuit and optokinetic nystagmus in the ipsilesional hemisphere [36]. Another example is that FEF damage can induce difficulties in performing vertical saccades during visual exploration [37]. Today, most of what has been found in patients has been replicated using another technique allowing causal anatomo-functional correlations in neurologically healthy participants, namely transcranial magnetic stimulation (TMS). These studies, reviewed by Vernet et al. [11], generally showed that TMS impulses induce longer latencies mainly of contralesional or bilateral saccades in the context of reflexive or voluntary saccades. They also indicated that TMS can interfere with saccade execution in anti-saccade or memory-guided behavioral paradigms.

3.2.2 Saliency Map and Saccade Target Selection

Rapid saccadic eye movement is needed to orient gaze toward items of interest in an often complex and fast-changing visual environment. Currently, it is believed that the FEF may participate in generating a salience map that gauges and selects the most salient or conspicuous aspects of the visual scene for further foveal processing. This process of "saccade target selection" is guided by both bottom-up, perceptual aspect of visual items and top-down knowledge (i.e., goals or expectations) of the individual [38]. As a matter of fact, pharmaceutical inactivation of the FEF in monkeys can lead to a target-selection deficit [39], as for the superior colliculus [40]. In a visual search paradigm, this deficit manifests by a greater proportion or erroneous saccades toward visual distractors while the capacity of performing saccades toward visual targets is preserved in the absence of such distractors.

3.2.3 Visuospatial Attention and Awareness

By virtue of its connections in visual associative areas [34], the FEF is increasingly thought as a visual area itself, at the interface between the oculomotor system and the network maintaining aspects of visuospatial attention. In this regard, it is interesting to highlight that, in the monkey brain, fMRI studies have suggested a functional compartmentalization of the FEF into a lateral and medial sector that might be involved in, respectively, short and ample saccades [41]. Consistent with the supposed behavior role of short and ample saccades during the vision of natural or dynamics environments (i.e., short saccades allow precise identification of object features in the service of grasping and manipulation whereas larger saccades are associated with reaching and trunk movements), it was shown that ventral FEF was functionally coupled with areas of the ventral stream involved in object processing and manipulation while dorsal FEF synchronized with areas of the dorsal stream. This shows how involved is the FEF, though differentially, in visually guided behaviors—at least in monkeys. This functional division of the FEF seems to agree with tracer studies showing that the ventral and the dorsal FEF have a dissimilar pattern of anatomical connectivity. For example, the work by Schall et al. [34] in monkeys indicated that the ventral FEF (equivalent to lateral) hosts projections from the foveal representation in retinotopically organized areas and from areas that represent the central vision in the inferotemporal cortex whereas the medial FEF (equivalent to dorsal) received projections from the peripheral representation in retinotopically organized areas and from areas involved in peripheral vision. This connectivity, both functional and structural, in the visual system has led to the hypothesis whereby the FEF might be cognitively penetrated and thus might play a role in the control of visual attention, independently of its role in saccadic movements. This hypothesis has been at least partially validated in lesional studies performed in the monkey, as unilateral lesions of the FEF did cause inattention to stimuli on the opposite side of the visual field in various studies (e.g., [42–44]). This observation agrees with studies showing that pharmaceutical inactivation of FEF causes an increase of reaction times to detect contralateral targets in visual search paradigms in the absence of saccades, suggesting that FEF does contribute to attention shifts and perception (e.g., [45]). This role has been further supported by observation that low-intensity stimulation of the FEF, adjusted for hindering the overt production of saccadic movements, can transitorily improve the deployment of covert attention [46].

In humans, the FEF has currently a central position in the most authoritative anatomo-functional models of attention. For example, in the model by Corbetta and Shulman [47] mainly based on fMRI and lesional literature, the FEF together with the intraparietal sulcus—forming the so-called dorsal attention system—is critical for controlling the top-down aspect of attention, while the ventral system composed of the temporoparietal junction and the inferior frontal gyrus is rather involved in detecting and shifting attention toward unexpected stimuli. Interestingly enough, the FEF especially in the right hemisphere is thought to be an area allowing functional exchanges between the two attention systems [48] as it is also modulated by stimuli-driven reorienting of attention [49]. The possible coupling between attention and saccades was evidenced in a quantitative meta-analysis of fMRI datasets where functional maps of, respectively, attention shifts and saccadic eye movements widely overlapped, notably in the FEF [50].

Neuropsychological studies in humans confirmed the role of the FEF, especially in the right hemisphere, in visuospatial attention, as its damage is associated with spatial neglect. For example, Thiebaut de Schotten et al. [51] assessed the cortical and white matter correlates of spatial neglect based on the behavioral performances of stroke patients. Among the range of analyses performed, an overlay subtraction analysis was achieved between patients with neglect versus patients without neglect. The results revealed that patients with neglect were more frequently lesioned in the frontoparietal network, including but not uniquely the right FEF. On a different but interconnected matter, fMRI and TMS studies have suggested a role of the left FEF in the modulation of conscious visual perception possibly through the system of attention reorienting [52, 53].

3.3 Intraoperative Mapping of the FEF in "Awake" Surgery for Diffuse Low-Grade Glioma

To the best of our knowledge, there are only two studies describing the clinical manifestations associated with electrostimulation of the FEF in the context of glioma surgery. In the first one, direct electrostimulation along with electro-oculography recordings was performed in a 34-year woman operated on for a glioma invading the right frontal cortex including the FEF [19]. Before the surgical procedure, a functional MRI was achieved in an attempt to identify the network of areas involved in saccadic movements, in particular the FEF. A simple oculomotor task that consisted in performing self-paced symmetric horizontal saccades was used as functional localizer. As expected, the task triggered functional activations in the supplementary eye field, in the intraparietal sulcus, and in the left FEF (located in the precentral gyrus, at the intersection with the superior frontal sulcus according the figure provided). The lack of significant activation in the ipsilesional FEF was interpreted as due to the lesional infiltration of the structure even if an activation was revealed when using less conservative statistical threshold. In the operating theater, electrostimulation was applied on the cerebral cortex while the patient was engaged in two concurrent behavioral scenarios. In the first condition, the patient was simply asked to visually fix on a target placed in front of her eyes. In the alternative condition (a saccade task similar to that used in MRI scanner), the patient was asked to perform continuously horizontal saccades. In the first condition, four sites located in the most anterior part of the precentral gyrus, behind the lateral half of the middle frontal gyrus, caused conjugate contraversive eye movements when stimulated at low current intensity (1.8 mA in average). Ocular metrics suggested not saccadic, but smooth pursuit ocular deviations. In the second one, suppression of saccades was provoked four times at one site (a site identical to condition one) (Fig. 3.2).

In the second study, six glioma patients in whom ocular deviations were evoked in the frontal cortex were included [20] (Fig. 3.3). Importantly, sites associated with ocular deviations could be situated in the frontal white matter as well. At the cortical level, ocular deviations were evoked by interfering with an area located in front of the primary motor cortex of the face within the posterior part of the middle frontal gyrus, just below the intersection of the precentral gyrus and the superior frontal sulcus. This anatomical situation corresponds to what is generally observed in electrostimulation studies conducted with tumor [19] or epileptic patients [18, 54]. Interestingly, while the majority of sites were associated with horizontal ocular deviations, a conjugate upward deviation was elicited in one patient (in addition to a horizontal one), an observation that has been already reported, albeit rarely, in the previous medical literature (e.g., [7, 8, 55]). As hypothesized by Kaiboriboon et al. [56], this kind of results suggest that the FEF might be topologically severed into two subareas along a rostral-to-caudal axis. At the subcortical level, three sites associated with horizontal deviations were identified in the white matter underneath the cortical FEF, in particular in fibers running under the posterior half of the middle frontal gyrus. Vertical deviations were not induced possibly because the fibers emanating from the caudal FEF were not stimulated. As diffusion tractography was not

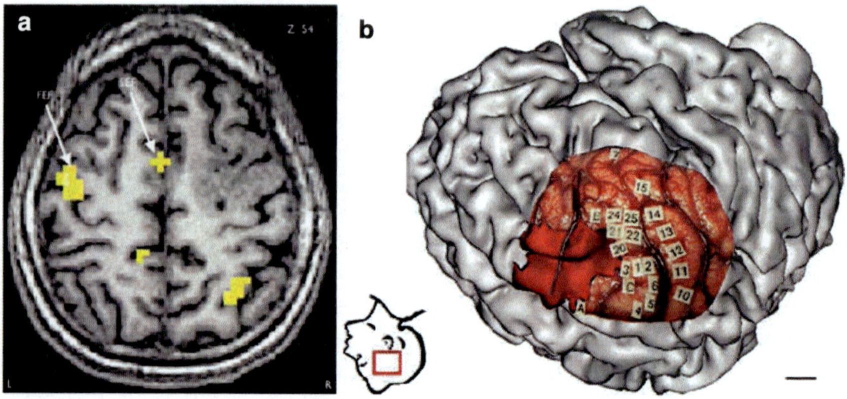

Fig. 3.2 Location of the FEF in a study combining preoperative activation fMRI and direct electrostimulation in a single glioma patient. (**a**) Preoperative fMRI showing left FEF, supplementary eye field, and parietal activation, induced by a self-paced horizontal saccade task. *R* right, *L* left. (**b**) Intraoperative picture overlaid onto the three-dimensional reconstruction of the patient's brain. Electrostimulation of the regions labeled 20, 21, 22, and 24 elicited contraversive smooth eye movements whereas the area corresponding to the label 21 elicited both smooth eye movements and saccade suppression. Bar represents 1 cm in length (with permissions from WOLTERS KLUWER HEALTH, INC)

used in this study and because a vast number of association and projection tracts run in the white matter deep in the middle frontal gyrus, it was not possible to identify which fibers formed the oculomotor tract. However, in view of the fronto-striatal tract's projections in both the FEF and the striatum (a nucleus known to participate in oculomotor behaviors, see above) [57], it is likely that the oculomotor tract might in fact be part of this projection tract.

All-in-all, although brain stimulation studies conducted with glioma patients are at the very least rare, they not only confirmed the location of the FEF in the posteriormost part of the middle frontal gyrus, around the junction between the precentral and the superior frontal sulci, but also identified for the first time the white matter connections that might be involved in eye control.

3.4 Functional Consequences of FEF Surgical Removal

To our knowledge, there are currently no reports assessing the functional consequences of surgical removal of the FEF in the particular context of glioma neurosurgery.[1] However, as the anatomo-functional organization of the FEF seems

[1] Note that Bourdillon et al. [56] reported the case of an 11-year old woman in whom a surgical resection of the right FEF was performed due to the presence of a cavernoma that caused epileptic discharge (during seizure, the patient experienced tonic eye deviation toward the opposite side). According the authors, no neurological impairments were observed after surgery but we do not know the way the patient was assessed.

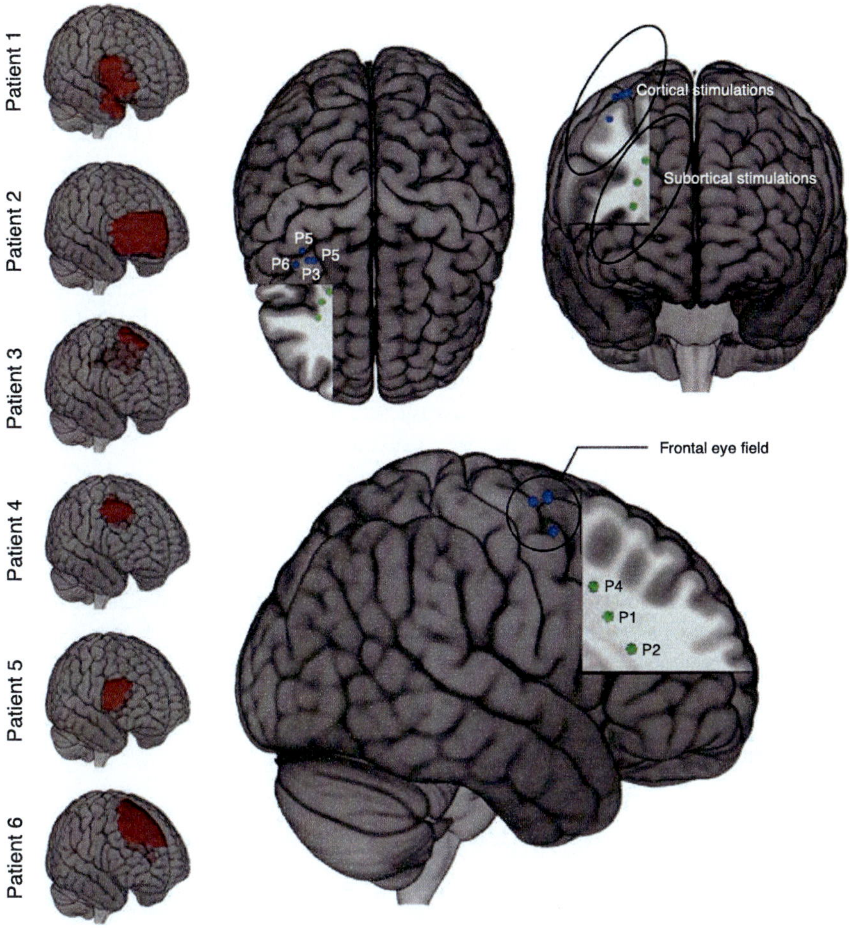

Fig. 3.3 Cortical and subcortical topography of sites associated with oculomotor deviations as revealed by electrostimulation mapping in diffuse low-grade patients (with permissions from Springer)

phylogenetically well preserved between humans and monkeys [12], the results from ablation studies conducted with the latter are in our opinion particularly relevant—even if, of course, the pathophysiological bases of the resulting deficits are not exactly the same (i.e., acute lesion in monkey versus graded lesion in humans).

3.4.1 On Ocular Behaviors

Historically, Ferrier and Yeo [59] were the first to perform ablations of the FEF in macaque and dog-faced monkeys. They observed that unilateral lesioning of this structure caused a deviation of both the head and the eyes toward the ipsilesional side. However, contrary to bilateral lesions for which the impairment was permanent, the deviations dissipated in the next days. Soon after, Sherrington [60] found that the removal of the cerebral region anterior to the motor cortex provoked conjugate horizontal of the eyes on the opposite side. Since that time, the effect of ablating the FEF on ocular behaviors has been repeatedly reported. For example, Schiller [61] demonstrated that both unilateral and bilateral FEF lesions produced only temporary deficits in eye movements. Lynch [62] found that surgical removal of both FEF induced a dramatic impairment of visual pursuit in a behavior task consisting of visually tracking a moving target, while the monkey's ability to produce accurate saccades was only slightly impaired. Schiller and Chou [63] showed that FEF ablation produced major and permanent deficits on tasks in which monkeys were trained to make saccadic eye movements toward targets presented at various temporal asynchronies, suggesting a major role of this structure in temporal ordering and processing speed for visually guided saccadic eye movement generation. Keating [64] confirmed that FEF ablation had a dramatic effect on visual predictive and nonpredictive pursuit. Interestingly, this effect disappeared 1–3 weeks after surgical removal in case of unilateral lesions, but reappeared after lesioning of the other in the contralateral hemisphere.

As mentioned above, the effects of FEF surgical removal in humans have not been the target of specific reports. As a consequence, the few lesion studies conducted with patients presenting with ischemic stroke affecting the FEF are interesting to consider. From these studies [36, 65–68], reviewed and criticized by Vernet et al. [11], the general picture is that FEF lesions mainly affect voluntary saccadic movements, less reflexive ones.

3.4.2 On Visuospatial Attention

It is known that FEF removal in monkeys provokes clinical manifestations very close to those observed in humans in case of unilateral spatial neglect. Welch and Stuteville [44] observed that lesioning a small area located in the depth of the posterior part of the superior limb of the arcuate sulcus (approximating the location of the FEF) caused unilateral neglect. Likewise, surgical lesion of the arcuate gyrus, at the caudal part of the principalis sulcus, induced nonsensory neglect (related to a defect of intentional behavior) in a study by Watson et al. [69], a conclusion that was reached by Valenstein et al. [43] based on the behavioral performances of monkeys following ablation of the arcuate sulcus. Watson confirmed that the ablation of the arcuate gyrus is associated postoperatively with neglect, but that the induced neglect is more severe when the lesion is accompanied with a corpus callosum disconnection [70].

To close this part of the chapter, it appears that surgical removal of the FEF in monkeys does induce abnormal oculomotor behaviors and impaired visuospatial processing, but the disturbances are more acute and long-lasting in the event of bilateral damage or when the corpus callosum is additionally lesioned. In our own clinical experience, the surgical removal of the FEF (which is very rare) or of its neighboring structures (which is frequent given the strong incidence of diffuse low-grade gliomas in the superior frontal gyrus) almost systematically induces a spatial neglect, albeit transitory, characterized by an inability to voluntary explore the contralesional visual field. From a neuropsychological standpoint, patients with such type of neglect fail to complete a cancellation task but perform well on a line bisection task contrary to patients with a parietal neglect who fail on both tasks (Fig. 3.4). These dissociable components of spatial neglect have already been outlined in a former study conducted with stroke patients, the results of which have prompted the authors to propose that neglect is a polymorph syndrome (see Chap. 4 and [71]).

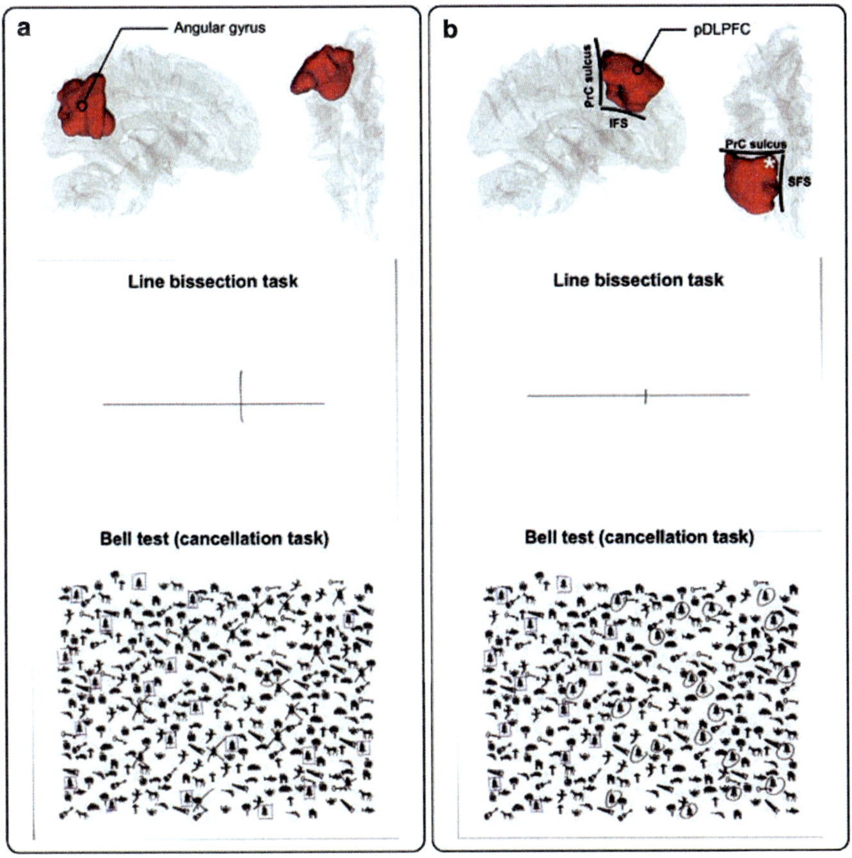

Fig. 3.4 Neglect signs following a surgical resection in (**a**) the right inferior parietal lobule (angular gyrus) or (**b**) affecting at least partially the right FEF (posterior dorsolateral prefrontal cortex resection with the precentral sulcus and the superior frontal sulcus as posterior and superior limits, respectively). In the latter case, only the cancellation task is affected whereas in the former both tasks are affected. Note that bells which are encircled in blue are items omitted by the patients. The right FEF is indicated by a white star. *pDLPFC* posterior dorsolateral prefrontal cortex, *IFS* inferior frontal sulcus, *PrC* precentral, *SFS* superior frontal sulcus

3.5 Perspectives

3.5.1 Why Searching for FEF Oculomotor Responses? Surgical Considerations

Beyond the goal of avoiding long-lasting, and possibly highly debilitating impairments on visually guided behaviors, functional identification of the cortical FEF is very useful in finding the latero-posterior limits of resections concerning the posteriormost part of the superior frontal gyrus including the supplementary motor area as well as the supero-posterior limits of resections targeting the posterior part of the dorsolateral cortex. Likewise, identification of the oculomotor white matter pathway, likely forming a dedicated strata of the fronto-striatal tract [20], is one of the functional limits when operating in the deep matter of the dorsolateral prefrontal cortex. Of course, because the white matter of the dorsolateral cortex is an area where crosses at least four imposing white matter connectivities (i.e., fronto-striatal tract, frontal asltant tract, inferior fronto-occipital fasciculus, and superior longitudinal fasciculus branch II), other tasks are usually employed to map the white matter fibers surrounding the pathway projecting in the FEF, such as a mentalizing task in the right hemisphere ([72, 73]; see Chap. 18), a non-verbal semantic association task in both cerebral hemispheres ([74, 75]; see Chap. 15), or a motor task to map the negative motor network ([76–78]; see Chap. 1).

3.5.2 Should We Use Other Behavioral Tasks to Map the FEF and Its Underlying White Matter Connectivity?

In connection with the latter section, specific studies assessing neuropsychologically the behavioral consequences of FEF removal in humans are, to the best our knowledge, inexistent. Consequently, in the context of glioma surgery, it is unknown whether resection of the FEF as well as its neighboring and interconnected structures can lead to permanent and disabling impairments, in the left or the right hemisphere. Stated another way, although patients do not seem to present with chronic impairments, we currently do not know the exact neuroplasticity potential of this frontal area, contrary to nearest regions such as the supplementary motor area [79]. To provide insight into this important clinical matter, it would be especially relevant to plan a longitudinal study aimed at assessing the functional counterparts of FEF removal on oculomotor behaviors and spatial awareness and more generally on neuropsychological functions—before, immediately after, and a while after surgery. The results of this kind of well-controlled studies will allow to decide whether or not additional behavioral paradigms are needed to identify and spare subregions of the FEF not associated with ocular movements. At the present time, the FEF is indeed identified as such when ocular deviations, horizontal or more rarely vertical, are provoked. It is not beyond the bounds of possibility that other tasks may be considered, as visuospatial tasks gauging the voluntary component of visual attention, beyond the line bisection task which is useless because of its inability to capture the process of directed visuo-attentional exploration. In this respect, I am aware that some medical centers usually employed a cancellation task implemented in a touchscreen environment to assess this aspect of visuospatial attention at the whole-brain level [80]. However, once again, if patients recover spontaneously, it seems inappropriate to use such tasks at the risk of interfering with the onco-functional balance [81]. For example, in Charras et al. [82], 20 patients with a right diffuse low-grade glioma were assessed with a range of visuospatial attention tasks (including four cancellation tasks) the day before, 4 days after, and 3 months after surgery. Although half of the patients presented with visuospatial deficits, including exploratory deficits on the contralesional side, immediately after surgery, all of them fully recovered 3 months after surgery. However, no patients had a tumor around the FEF in this study, so the issue remains.

3.6 Conclusion

The FEF is a complex area interfacing between the oculomotor and the spatial attention systems. Until now, the FEF (and recently its underlying connectivity) was identified by observation of horizontal and sometimes vertical ocular deviations during direct electrostimulation. Although this mapping seems sufficient to avoid permanent deficits in the execution and regulation of oculomotor behaviors, it remains that there is no available evidence that patients did recover completely, especially with regard to higher level processes such as attention orienting, visual search, and awareness. It is thus advocated to mount studies, ideally longitudinally designed, to assess in a fine-grained manner the behavior performances of patients with a tumor damaging the FEF or areas situated in its vicinity. In the event of lasting and disabling impairments, then new tasks should be considered.

References

1. Crosby EC, Henderson JW. The mammalian midbrain and isthmus regions. Part II. Fiber connections of the superior colliculus. B. Pathways concerned in automatic eye movements. J Comp Neurol. 1948;88(1):53–91.
2. Smith WK. The frontal eye fields. The precentral motor cortex. 1949. p. 314–6.
3. Ferrier D. On the localisation of the functions of the brain. Br Med J. 1874;2(729):766.
4. Leyton AS, Sherrington CS. Observations on the excitable cortex of the chimpanzee, orang-utan, and gorilla. Q J Exp Physiol Transl Integr. 1917;11(2):135–222.
5. Vogt C. Zur Kenntnis der electrich erregbaren Hirnrinden-Gebiete bei den Saugetieren. J Psychol Neurol. 1907;8:277–456.
6. Foerster O. The cerebral cortex in man. Lancet. 1931;2:309–12.
7. Foerster O. The motor cortex in man in the light of Hughlings Jackson's doctrines. Brain. 1936;59(2):135–59.
8. Penfield W, Boldrey E. Somatic motor and sensory representation in the cerebral cortex of man as studied by electrical stimulation. Brain. 1937;60(4):389–443.
9. Rasmussen T, Penfield W. The human sensorimotor cortex as studied by electrical stimulation. In: Federation proceedings. 1947. p. 184.

10. Penfield W, Erickson TC. Epilepsy and cerebral localization. Publisher: Clarles C. Thomas 1941.
11. Vernet M, Quentin R, Chanes L, Mitsumasu A, Valero-Cabré A. Frontal eye field, where art thou? Anatomy, function, and non-invasive manipulation of frontal regions involved in eye movements and associated cognitive operations. Front Integr Neurosci. 2014;8:66.
12. Amiez C, Petrides M. Anatomical organization of the eye fields in the human and non-human primate frontal cortex. Prog Neurobiol. 2009;89(2):220–30.
13. Bruce CJ, Goldberg ME. Primate frontal eye fields. I. Single neurons discharging before saccades. J Neurophysiol. 1985;53(3):603–35.
14. Robinson DA, Fuchs AF. Eye movements evoked by stimulation of frontal eye fields. J Neurophysiol. 1969;32(5):637–48.
15. Bizzi E. Discharge of frontal eye field neurons during saccadic and following eye movements in unanesthetized monkeys. Exp Brain Res. 1968;6(1):69–80.
16. Bruce CJ, Goldberg ME, Bushnell MC, Stanton GB. Primate frontal eye fields. II. Physiological and anatomical correlates of electrically evoked eye movements. J Neurophysiol. 1985;54(3):714–34.
17. Godoy J, Lüders H, Dinner DS, Morris HH, Wyllie E. Versive eye movements elicited by cortical stimulation of the human brain. Neurology. 1990;40(2):296.
18. Blanke O, Spinelli L, Thut G, Michel CM, Perrig S, Landis T, et al. Location of the human frontal eye field as defined by electrical cortical stimulation: anatomical, functional and electrophysiological characteristics. Neuroreport. 2000;11(9):1907–13.
19. Milea D, Lehericy S, Rivaud-Pechoux S, Duffau H, Lobel E, Capelle L, et al. Antisaccade deficit after anterior cingulate cortex resection. Neuroreport. 2003;14(2):283–7.
20. Montemurro N, Herbet G, Duffau H. Right cortical and axonal structures eliciting ocular deviation during electrical stimulation mapping in awake patients. Brain Topogr. 2016;29(4):561–71.
21. McDowell JE, Dyckman KA, Austin BP, Clementz BA. Neurophysiology and neuroanatomy of reflexive and volitional saccades: evidence from studies of humans. Brain Cogn. 2008;68(3):255–70.
22. Paus T. Location and function of the human frontal eye-field: a selective review. Neuropsychologia. 1996;34(6):475–83.
23. Darby DG, Nobre AC, Thangaraj V, Edelman R, Mesulam M-M, Warach S. Cortical activation in the human brain during lateral saccades using EPISTAR functional magnetic resonance imaging. NeuroImage. 1996;3(1):53–62.
24. Petit L, Clark VP, Ingeholm J, Haxby JV. Dissociation of saccade-related and pursuit-related activation in human frontal eye fields as revealed by fMRI. J Neurophysiol. 1997;77(6):3386–90.
25. Berman RA, Colby CL, Genovese CR, Voyvodic JT, Luna B, Thulborn KR, et al. Cortical networks subserving pursuit and saccadic eye movements in humans: an FMRI study. Hum Brain Mapp. 1999;8(4):209–25.
26. Luna B, Thulborn KR, Strojwas MH, McCurtain BJ, Berman RA, Genovese CR, et al. Dorsal cortical regions subserving visually guided saccades in humans: an fMRI study. Cereb Cortex (New York, NY: 1991). 1998;8(1):40–7.
27. Perry RJ, Zeki S. The neurology of saccades and covert shifts in spatial attention: an event-related fMRI study. Brain. 2000;123(11):2273–88.
28. Petit L, Pouget P. The comparative anatomy of frontal eye fields in primates. Cortex. 2019;118:51–64.
29. Schall JD. Visuomotor functions in the frontal lobe. Annu Rev Vis Sci. 2015;1:469–98.
30. Squire RF, Steinmetz NA, Moore T. Frontal eye field. Scholarpedia. 2012;7(10):5341.
31. Helminski JO, Segraves MA. Macaque frontal eye field input to saccade-related neurons in the superior colliculus. J Neurophysiol. 2003;90(2):1046–62.
32. Barbas H, Mesulam M-M. Organization of afferent input to subdivisions of area 8 in the rhesus monkey. J Comp Neurol. 1981;200(3):407–31.
33. Huerta MF, Krubitzer LA, Kaas JH. Frontal eye field as defined by intracortical microstimulation in squirrel monkeys, owl monkeys, and macaque monkeys II. Cortical connections. J Comp Neurol. 1987;265(3):332–61.

34. Schall JD, Morel A, King DJ, Bullier J. Topography of visual cortex connections with frontal eye field in macaque: convergence and segregation of processing streams. J Neurosci. 1995;15(6):4464–87.
35. Hutchison RM, Gallivan JP, Culham JC, Gati JS, Menon RS, Everling S. Functional connectivity of the frontal eye fields in humans and macaque monkeys investigated with resting-state fMRI. J Neurophysiol. 2012;107(9):2463–74.
36. Rivaud S, Müri RM, Gaymard B, Vermersch AI, Pierrot-Deseilligny C. Eye movement disorders after frontal eye field lesions in humans. Exp Brain Res. 1994;102(1):110–20.
37. Pflugshaupt T, Nyffeler T, von Wartburg R, Hess CW, Müri RM. Loss of exploratory vertical saccades after unilateral frontal eye field damage. J Neurol Neurosurg Psychiatry. 2008;79(4):474–7.
38. Thompson KG, Bichot NP. A visual salience map in the primate frontal eye field. Prog Brain Res. 2005;147:249–62.
39. McPeek RM, Keller EL. The effects of reversible inactivation of Frontal Eye Field and Superior Colliculus on saccade target selection. J Vis. 2003;3(9):694.
40. Schiller PH, Sandell JH, Maunsell JH. The effect of frontal eye field and superior colliculus lesions on saccadic latencies in the rhesus monkey. Journal of neurophysiology. 1987;57(4):1033–49.
41. Babapoor-Farrokhran S, Hutchison RM, Gati JS, Menon RS, Everling S. Functional connectivity patterns of medial and lateral macaque frontal eye fields reveal distinct visuomotor networks. J Neurophysiol. 2013;109(10):2560–70.
42. Kennard MA. Alterations in response to visual stimuli following lesions of frontal lobe in monkeys. Arch Neurol Psychiatry. 1939;41(6):1153–65.
43. Valenstein E, Watson RT, Van Den Abell T, Carter R, Heilman KM. Response time in monkeys with unilateral neglect. Arch Neurol. 1987;44(5):517–20.
44. Welch K, Stuteville P. Experimental production of unilateral neglect in monkeys. Brain. 1958;81(3):341–7.
45. Wardak C, Ben Hamed S, Olivier E, Duhamel J-R. Differential effects of parietal and frontal inactivations on reaction times distributions in a visual search task. Front Integr Neurosci. 2012;6:39.
46. Moore T, Fallah M. Microstimulation of the frontal eye field and its effects on covert spatial attention. J Neurophysiol. 2004;91(1):152–62.
47. Corbetta M, Shulman GL. Control of goal-directed and stimulus-driven attention in the brain. Nat Rev Neurosci. 2002;3(3):201–15.
48. Vossel S, Geng JJ, Fink GR. Dorsal and ventral attention systems: distinct neural circuits but collaborative roles. Neuroscientist. 2014;20(2):150–9.
49. Corbetta M, Patel G, Shulman GL. The reorienting system of the human brain: from environment to theory of mind. Neuron. 2008;58(3):306–24.
50. Grosbras M-H, Laird AR, Paus T. Cortical regions involved in eye movements, shifts of attention, and gaze perception. Human brain mapping. 2005;25(1):140–54.
51. Thiebaut de Schotten M, Tomaiuolo F, Aiello M, Merola S, Silvetti M, Lecce F, et al. Damage to white matter pathways in subacute and chronic spatial neglect: a group study and 2 single-case studies with complete virtual "in vivo" tractography dissection. Cereb Cortex. 2014;24(3):691–706.
52. Chica AB, Paz-Alonso PM, Valero-Cabré A, Bartolomeo P. Neural bases of the interactions between spatial attention and conscious perception. Cereb Cortex. 2013;23(6):1269–79.
53. Chica AB, Valero-Cabré A, Paz-Alonso PM, Bartolomeo P. Causal contributions of the left frontal eye field to conscious perception. Cereb Cortex. 2014;24(3):745–53.
54. Thurtell MJ, Mohamed A, Lüders HO, Leigh RJ. Evidence for three-dimensional cortical control of gaze from epileptic patients. Journal of Neurology, Neurosurgery & Psychiatry. 2009;80(6):683–5.
55. Kaiboriboon K, Lüders HO, Hamaneh M, Turnbull J, Lhatoo SD. EEG source imaging in epilepsy—practicalities and pitfalls. Nat Rev Neurol. 2012a;8(9):498.

56. Kaiboriboon K, Lüders HO, Miller JP, Leigh RJ. Upward gaze and head deviation with frontal eye field stimulation. Epileptic Disord. 2012b;14(1):64–8.
57. Leh SE, Ptito A, Chakravarty MM, Strafella AP. Fronto-striatal connections in the human brain: a probabilistic diffusion tractography study. Neurosci Lett. 2007;419(2):113–8.
58. Bourdillon P, Guénot M, Beuriat P-A, Ostrowsky-Coste K. The frontal eye field. Neurology. 2018;91(4):e398–9.
59. Ferrier D, Yeo GF. XIX. A record of experiments on the effects of lesion of different regions of the cerebral hemispheres. Philos Trans R S Lond. 1884;175:479–564.
60. Sherrington CS. Further experimental note on the correlation of action of antagonistic muscles. Br Med J. 1893;1(1693):1218.
61. Schiller PH, True SD, Conway JL. Deficits in eye movements following frontal eye-field and superior colliculus ablations. Journal of neurophysiology. 1980;44(6):1175–89.
62. Lynch JC. Frontal eye field lesions in monkeys disrupt visual pursuit. Exp Brain Res. 1987;68(2):437–41.
63. Schiller PH, Chou IH. The effects of frontal eye field and dorsomedial frontal cortex lesions on visually guided eye movements. Nat Neurosci. 1998;1(3):248–53.
64. Keating EG. Frontal eye field lesions impair predictive and visually-guided pursuit eye movements. Exp Brain Res. 1991;86(2):311–23.
65. Gaymard B, Ploner CJ, Rivaud-Pechoux S, Pierrot-Deseilligny C. The frontal eye field is involved in spatial short-term memory but not in reflexive saccade inhibition. Exp Brain Res. 1999;129(2):288–301.
66. Guitton D, Buchtel HA, Douglas RM. Frontal lobe lesions in man cause difficulties in suppressing reflexive glances and in generating goal-directed saccades. Exp Brain Res. 1985;58(3):455–72.
67. Henik A, Rafal R, Rhodes D. Endogenously generated and visually guided saccades after lesions of the human frontal eye fields. J Cogn Neurosci. 1994;6(4):400–11.
68. Pierrot-Deseilligny CH, Rivaud S, Gaymard B, Agid Y. Cortical control of reflexive visually-guided saccades. Brain. 1991;114(3):1473–85.
69. Watson RT, Miller BD, Heilman KM. Nonsensory neglect. Ann Neurol. 1978;3(6):505–8.
70. Watson RT, Valenstein E, Day AL, Heilman KM. The effect of corpus callosum lesions on unilateral neglect in monkeys. Neurology. 1984;34(6):812.
71. Binder J, Marshall R, Lazar R, Benjamin J, Mohr JP. Distinct syndromes of hemineglect. Arch Neurol. 1992;49(11):1187–94.
72. Herbet G, Lafargue G, Moritz-Gasser S, Bonnetblanc F, Duffau H. Interfering with the neural activity of mirror-related frontal areas impairs mentalistic inferences. Brain Struct Funct. 2015;220(4):2159–69.
73. Yordanova YN, Duffau H, Herbet G. Neural pathways subserving face-based mentalizing. Brain Struct Funct. 2017;222(7):3087–105.
74. Herbet G, Moritz-Gasser S, Duffau H. Direct evidence for the contributive role of the right inferior fronto-occipital fasciculus in non-verbal semantic cognition. Brain Struct Funct. 2017;222(4):1597–610.
75. Moritz-Gasser S, Herbet G, Duffau H. Mapping the connectivity underlying multimodal (verbal and non-verbal) semantic processing: a brain electrostimulation study. Neuropsychologia. 2013;51(10):1814–22.
76. Kinoshita M, de Champfleur NM, Deverdun J, Moritz-Gasser S, Herbet G, Duffau H. Role of fronto-striatal tract and frontal aslant tract in movement and speech: an axonal mapping study. Brain Struct Funct. 2015;220(6):3399–412.
77. Rech F, Herbet G, Gaudeau Y, Mézières S, Moureau J-M, Moritz-Gasser S, et al. A probabilistic map of negative motor areas of the upper limb and face: a brain stimulation study. Brain. 2019;142(4):952–65.
78. Rech F, Herbet G, Moritz-Gasser S, Duffau H. Somatotopic organization of the white matter tracts underpinning motor control in humans: an electrical stimulation study. Brain Struct Funct. 2016;221(7):3743–53.

79. Herbet G, Maheu M, Costi E, Lafargue G, Duffau H. Mapping neuroplastic potential in brain-damaged patients. Brain. 2016;139(3):829–44.
80. Conner AK, Glenn C, Burks JD, McCoy T, Bonney PA, Chema AA, et al. The use of the target cancellation task to identify eloquent visuospatial regions in awake craniotomies. Cureus. 2016;8(11):e883.
81. Mandonnet E, Herbet G, Duffau H. Introducing new tasks for intraoperative mapping in awake glioma surgery: clearing the line between patient care and scientific research. Neurosurgery. 2020;86(2):E256–7.
82. Charras P, Herbet G, Deverdun J, De Champfleur NM, Duffau H, Bartolomeo P, et al. Functional reorganization of the attentional networks in low-grade glioma patients: a longitudinal study. Cortex. 2015;63:27–41.

Spatial Cognition

4

Paolo Bartolomeo and Emmanuel Mandonnet

4.1 Introduction

During a walk, you want to cross a trafficked boulevard. You stop at a pedestrian crossing and watch the traffic light while waiting for the green pedestrian sign, while the cars are passing by. As soon as the green arrives, the cars stop and you start to cross, but at the last moment an unruly cyclist cuts you off: you narrowly avoid him. Your attention processes have allowed you to manage this situation in the best possible way, by selecting important information (voluntary attention on the traffic light) in order to maintain a finalized behavior (crossing the street) despite distractions. However, attention also allowed you to react quickly and appropriately to an unforeseen and potentially dangerous event (automatic attention captured by the cyclist).

4.2 Networks of Attention in the Brain

During the last decades, neuroimaging studies have provided extensive information on the neural implementation of spatial attention [1, 2]. Thanks to this work, we now know that there is no single region in the brain that manages attentional

P. Bartolomeo (✉)
Sorbonne Université, Inserm U 1127, CNRS UMR 7225, Paris Brain Institute, ICM, Hôpital de la Pitié-Salpêtrière, Paris, France
e-mail: paolo.bartolomeo@icm-institute.org

E. Mandonnet
Sorbonne Université, Inserm U 1127, CNRS UMR 7225, Paris Brain Institute, ICM, Hôpital de la Pitié-Salpêtrière, Paris, France

Department of Neurosurgery, Lariboisière Hospital, Paris Brain Institute (ICM) and Université de Paris, Paris, France
e-mail: emmanuel.mandonnet@aphp.fr

E. Mandonnet, G. Herbet (eds.), *Intraoperative Mapping of Cognitive Networks*,
https://doi.org/10.1007/978-3-030-75071-8_4

processes. Instead, there are large-scale networks from the posterior (parietal) region to the anterior (prefrontal) regions of the brain. Although distant at the level of the brain, these regions communicate with each other quickly and efficiently, because they are connected by "brain highways," large bundles of white matter (Fig. 4.1). These frontoparietal networks direct our attention in space, for example, towards the traffic lights before crossing the street. In general, each hemisphere of the brain directs attention towards the opposite side of space through a "dorsal" network of attention, including the superior parietal lobules, the frontal eye fields, and the dorsolateral prefrontal cortex (PFC). The pathway linking these regions is the dorsal branch of the superior longitudinal fasciculus (SLF I). However, an unforeseen and urgent event, such as the sudden arrival of the cyclist, can interrupt the current orientation and capture the subject's attention.

A second frontoparietal network deals with this important task of interrupting the ongoing attention activity, to redirect it to a new target. This second network is located lower in the brain and is thus defined as the "ventral" network of attention. It includes the inferior parietal lobule, its junction with the temporal lobe, and the ventrolateral PFC. These regions are connected by the ventral branch of the superior longitudinal fasciculus, SLF III. In most of us, the ventral network of attention is asymmetric between the cerebral hemispheres: it is mostly active in the right hemisphere (RH), the hemisphere non-dominant for language, and much less in the language-dominant left hemisphere (LH) [1]. More controversial is the possibility of a similar asymmetry for the dorsal attention network [6, 7]. An intermediate branch of the superior longitudinal fasciculus, SLF II, connects the temporoparietal part of the ventral attention network with the dorsolateral PFC, a node of the dorsal

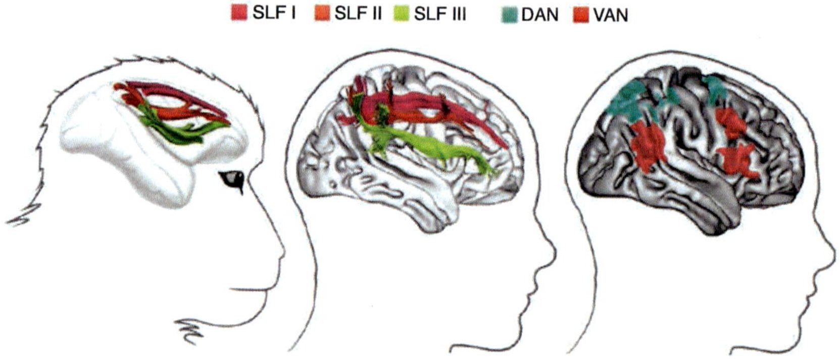

Fig. 4.1 Frontoparietal networks in the monkey (left, from [3]) and in the human right hemisphere (middle, from [4, 5]), with the three branches of the superior longitudinal fasciculus (SLF I-III). Right: dorsal (DAN) and ventral (VAN) attentional networks in the right hemisphere according to Corbetta and Shulman [1]. Figure as originally published in Frontiers in Human Neuroscience 6:110, 2012 "Brain networks of visuospatial attention and their disruption in visual neglect," by Paolo Bartolomeo, Michel Thiebaut de Schotten, Ana B. Chica. This is an open-access article distributed under the terms of the Creative Commons Attribution Non Commercial License https://www.frontiersin.org/articles/10.3389/fnhum.2012.00110/full

attention network [4]. SLF II thus allows direct communication between the ventral (SLF III) and the dorsal (SLF I) attention networks.

A further, even more ventral network is connected by the inferior fronto-occipital fasciculus (IFOF), which links the ventrolateral PFC and medial orbitofrontal cortex to the occipital cortex, and thus allows top-down influence of PFC on visual areas. The IFOF network also shows anatomical signs of asymmetry favoring the right hemisphere [5]. The right ventrolateral PFC may thus constitute a convergence zone between the visual occipitotemporal stream [8] through the IFOF, and the ventral attentional network through the SLF III. In addition to these cortical networks, subcortical structures such as the superior colliculus and the pulvinar nucleus of the thalamus also play important roles in attention processes [9]. Other subcortical nuclei, the basal ganglia, contribute to attentional processing by modulating PFC influence on visual cortex. Specifically, basal ganglia activity has been found to enhance fronto-posterior connectivity with parts of the visual cortex that process attended visual information, and to decrease fronto-posterior connectivity with portions of the visual cortex that process unattended visual information [10].

4.3 Visual Neglect, a Dramatic Clinical Consequence of Attention Network Dysfunction

Given the paramount importance of attention in our daily lives, and the asymmetries of attentional networks favoring the RH, it is not surprising that the dysfunction of these networks in the RH can have serious consequences. For example, patients with brain damage may become unable to process several stimuli when simultaneously presented (as in extinction and simultagnosia), or stimuli arising in a region of space contralateral to the brain lesion (visuospatial neglect) [11]. In these cases, the "wrong" object (i.e., an object inappropriate to the current behavioral task) may win the competition and capture the patient's attention [12]. Thus, when patients with left unilateral neglect are presented with bilateral objects, they compulsorily orient their gaze towards right-sided stimuli, as if their gaze were "magnetically" captured by these stimuli [13, 14]; afterwards, patients find it difficult to disengage their attention from these stimuli in order to explore the left part of space [15–19], so that their space exploration may remain confined to a few right-sided objects [20, 21].

4.3.1 Clinical Description

Visual, or spatial, neglect refers to patients' inability to orient their attention towards objects contralateral to their lesion (typically left-sided objects after right hemisphere damage). As a consequence, patients may behave as if the left part of the world did not exist anymore. This condition can occur in the absence of elementary sensorimotor deficits, and is severely disabling in patients' everyday life. In the acute phase of a stroke, neglect can easily be detected by examining the posture and spontaneous behavior of the patients. They stay in bed with their heads turned to the side opposite to their hemiplegia (thus, most often towards the right side), and do not respond to stimuli from the opposite, neglected space (most often the left side). For example, if someone questions them on the left side, they may not answer, or they will respond to someone else on the right side. Any task involving vision leads to an even more exaggerated deviation of the gaze, towards the right-sided objects of the visual field. The deviation of gaze gradually disappears in the days following the stroke, but the tendency to be captured by right-sided items may persist in time. At this stage, other behavioral signs may become apparent. Patients do not wash the left side of their body; they may shave or make up only the right half of the face. They forget to put their left sleeve or their left shoe, let hanging the left branch of their glasses. Neglect is often manifest in the near extra-personal space. Patients can eat only the right side of their plate, read only the right half of the newspaper titles, without bothering about their lack of meaning.

Once patients are able to perform neuropsychological tests, their behavior often remains confined to the right side of their visual space. Those of them able to stand up show disorders of the control of the posture, they may veer towards the left, probably because of impaired integration of visual, vestibular, somesthetic, or graviceptive information.

Several weeks or even months after the onset of the lesion, a substantial proportion of patients manage to compensate for neglect both in their daily lives and during neuropsychological examinations. However, even in these patients, it is possible to detect more subtle signs of attention impairment. For example, they continue to begin their exploration of space from the right side [14, 22], while most healthy controls tend to start from the left side [23]—a phenomenon perhaps related to the combined influence of brain asymmetries of the attention networks and of Western left-to-right reading habits. When patients with compensated neglect produce manual or vocal responses to lateralized objects on the right or left, they respond more slowly to left-sided targets than to right-sided ones, particularly at the beginning of the tests, as if attention were initially captured by right-sided items [24].

4.3.2 Tests of Neglect

Several paper-and-pencil tests can uncover these attention-related deficits [25]. It is very important to evaluate these capabilities in the clinic, because neglect signs can be clinically elusive; and yet diagnosis is essential because neglect patients should not be allowed to undertake activities requiring rapid reactions, such as driving for example. In addition, many of them do not fully recover from behavioral signs of neglect, which in turn can affect the recovery of their motor abilities [26].

Given the strong influence of stimulus position on neglect signs, it is important to carefully center the test sheets on the patient's midsagittal plane. Not all patients consistently show neglect on all these tests, consistent with the multi-component nature of this syndrome [27, 28], with different patterns of deficits occurring in different patients [29, 30]. To achieve good diagnostic sensitivity, it is thus important to have patients perform several visuospatial tests. Neglect tests can schematically be classified in visuo-perceptual tests, visuo-graphic tests, and representational (or imaginal) tests.

Visuo-perceptual tests are characterized by the fact that they do not require substantial motor activity towards a certain sector of space. For example, one may present patients with a lateralized version of the Wundt-Jastrow illusion [31], or ask them to identify overlapping figures [14], or to read a short text [25]. Typically, patients do not take into account information coming from the left half of the display: they do not suffer from a left-lateralized visual illusion, or omit to mention left-sided overlapping images, words, or letters.

Visuo-graphic tests can be based on activities of copy, visual search, or line bisection (Fig. 4.2).

Patients can be asked to copy geometrical or figurative drawings [33]. When copying, patients typically omit objects or details contained in the left half of the model (scene-based neglect). Sometimes, however, the patient can reproduce all the elements of the model independently of their spatial location, but neglect the left half of one or more items (object-based neglect). In visual search tests, patients are asked to find targets, such as lines [34], letters [35], stars [36], or bells [37]. Patients are asked to cancel out the target items, and typically omit to cancel left-sided targets. The difficulty of the task (e.g., when a target/distractor discrimination is

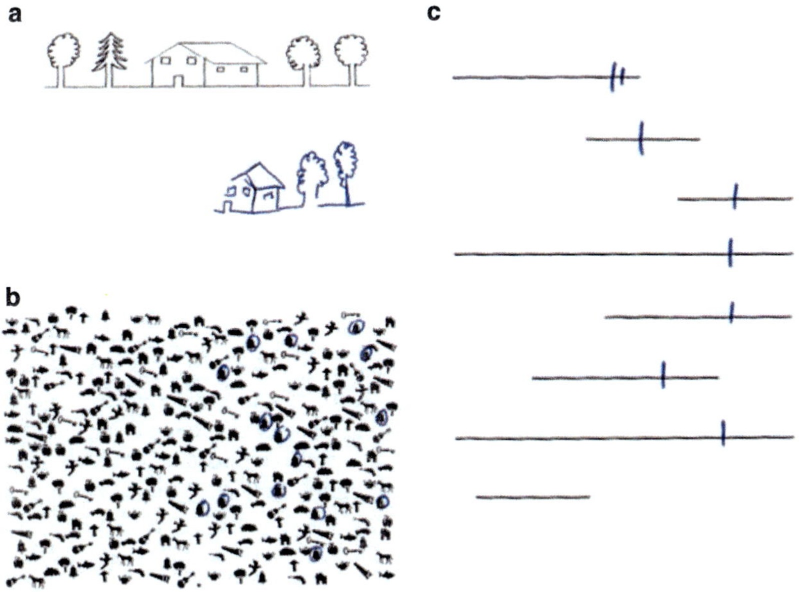

Fig. 4.2 Performance of a patient with left neglect on tests of copy (**a**), visual search (**b**), and line bisection (**c**). Figure originally published in [32]. This is an open-access article distributed under the terms of the Creative Commons Attribution Non Commercial License https://www.frontiersin.org/articles/10.3389/fnhum.2012.00110/full

required) may influence the severity of neglect, as estimated by the number of left-sided omissions: the same patients tend to omit more targets with more difficult tasks [38]. In line bisection, patients are asked to mark the midpoint of horizontal lines. They typically misplace the bisection point rightward, especially when their attention is directed on the right extremity of the line [39].

Response time tests, analogous to those used to study spatial attention in normal participants, can provide more sensitive methods to detect subclinical biases in spatial attention [40]. For example, neglect patients often compensate for neglect on paper-and-pencil tests, but can remain slower in responding to left-sided targets than to right-sided targets [24], especially when engaged in a concomitant cognitive task, such as the inhibition of inappropriate responses [41].

Visual field defects, such as left homonymous hemianopia, can sometimes co-occur with neglect, for example, when lesions damage the optic radiations or the primary visual cortex. However, they can also occur independently of neglect. Importantly, hemianopic patients without neglect try to compensate for their deficit, often to the point of paradoxically deviating towards the left on line bisection [42], whereas patients with hemianopia and neglect deviate massively towards the right [43]. Goldmann perimetry can usually distinguish between hemianopia and neglect, because neglect patients without hemianopia are typically able to detect the single targets presented in their left visual field, despite their neglect. In rare cases, however, neglect can be so severe that patients can fail to report perimetry targets (pseudohemianopia). Presumably, the mere presence of the central fixation point can induce a stimulus competition with left-sided targets, which are then neglected. In one of these patients, removal of the fixation point just before target presentation was able to restore perception of left-sided targets [44]. The possibility of neglect-related pseudohemianopia should be kept in mind especially with the now commonly used automated perimetry, where a trained perimetrist has less opportunity to interact with the patients and observe their performance. In case of doubt, lateralized ERPs can demonstrate the absence of hemianopia by showing normal response of primary visual cortex to left-sided checkerboards.

4.3.3 Models of Neglect

It has long been recognized that left neglect is a typical syndrome resulting from RH lesions [45, 46]. Early models [47, 48] held that attentional neurons of the parietal lobe, charged with spatial surveillance function, could have bilateral receptive fields in the RH, whereas they would be limited to the contralateral half of the space in the LH. According to these models, there would be little or no neglect after LH lesions because the attentional neurons of the right parietal lobe (spared by the lesion) can detect the stimuli occurring in the ipsilateral space. There would, however, be neglect for the left half of the space after RH lesions because the attentional neurons of the left parietal lobe cannot monitor the left (ipsilateral) half of the space. On the contrary, Marcel Kinsbourne [49, 50] proposed that the basic asymmetry of neglect stems from LH preferential activation in verbally mediated tests. This left activation, accompanied by a trans-callosal inhibition of the right, contralateral hemisphere, automatically gives rise to an orientation of the gaze towards the right half of the space. These phenomena would be transient in normal subjects, but could become more stable (and thus result in left neglect signs) after right brain injury. Language activities (common in clinical tests) could further interfere with this general phenomenon, by activating the LH and causing a deviation of the gaze to the right.

Neuroimaging evidence supported the Kinsbourne model, by showing a relative hyperactivation of the left superior parietal lobule as compared with its right hemisphere homolog in patients with left neglect [51]. The two structures reverted to a more balanced activity in the chronic phase, when signs of neglect had recovered. However, in the Corbetta et al.'s [51] study, other left attentional hemisphere structures, for example, in the PFC, had increased activity in the recovered phase as compared with the acute phase, thus suggesting a possible compensatory role of the undamaged LH [52]. Consistent with this mixed evidence, behavioral results did not offer definitive support for either of the rival models. For example, according to the Kinsbourne model when a group of patients with various degrees of left neglect produce speeded manual responses to left- or right-sided targets, their responses times to right-sided targets should decrease with increasing severity of neglect (as a result of increasingly stronger bias towards the right side); however, according to the Heilman/Mesulam models, these responses times should instead increase with increasing severity of neglect (as a result of less attentional resources deployed in both hemispaces). The results of such a study [20] showed that not only the responses to left targets, but also those to right targets became progressively slower as neglect increased, consistent with the hypoattention account. However, the two regression lines were not parallel. With increasing neglect, responses times to left targets increased more steeply than those to right targets did. Thus, a rightward attentional bias is present in patients with left neglect, together with left hypoattention. However, this rightward bias is one of defective, and not enhanced, attention. Also, neglect patients' performance on perceptual estimation of line lengths [53] suggests that two independent deficits contribute to neglect signs: a deficit in attentional orienting to the left, perhaps depending on impaired functioning of RH attentional networks, and a tendency for attention to be captured by right-sided stimuli, possibly resulting from the activity of an isolated LH [54] .

4.3.4 Anatomy of Neglect

Within the RH, the lesions responsible for neglect signs tend to localize in the posteroinferior portions of the parietal lobe [46, 55]. However, signs of neglect have also been reported in patients with lesions centered on the frontal lobe [56, 57], cingulate gyrus [48, 58], thalamus [59], and basal ganglia [56]. It is possible that these various focal locations have no special role per se [60], but instead result in network-based dysfunction of the attentional circuits, especially those linked by SLF II and III (recent reviews in [11, 61, 62]). Also, more ventral damage to the right-lateralized IFOF has been associated with neglect [39, 63, 64]. However, as mentioned before, damage to the LH homolog regions only rarely results in right-sided neglect [25]. Signs of right-sided neglect have been observed after bilateral hemispheric damage, whether due to vascular strokes [65, 66] or to neurodegenerative conditions [67, 68]. This finding might indicate the necessity for some degree of RH dysfunction even for signs of *right-sided* neglect to occur. The right-lateralized SLF III network is a possible candidate site of RH dysfunction in patients with right-sided neglect [7].

As detailed in the previous section, an important aspect of left neglect behavior is a bias to explore the right portions of extra-personal space. In experimental settings, this bias often translates to the production of "inappropriate" rightward saccades, i.e., saccades towards nontarget right-sided stimuli. Eye movement recordings showed that this tendency could not be completely overcome by endogenous orienting of attention, and was related to damage to SLF fibers leading to the RH FEF [13].

Recent lesion-symptom mapping studies of neglect have confirmed the presence of damage to SLF II-III and IFOF networks in the RH [64, 69–73]. Recent electrophysiological studies suggested a relative sparing of PFC activity in neglect patients. Activity in LH PFC might actually be causally related to neglect omissions: a MEG study demonstrated a specific increase of low beta synchronization activity in left frontal cortex before omissions of response to left-sided targets [74]. In an ERP study, attention-related PFC activity was preserved, but unable to counterbalance deficits in parietal-occipital activity [75]; however, in other patients PFC activity correlated with intentional, compensatory gaze shifts towards the left, neglected side [76]. Recovery from neglect has been related to the state of inter-hemispheric connectivity with the left, undamaged hemisphere [77, 78]. Evidence from diffusion-based MRI suggested an important role of the caudal portions of the corpus callosum, which connect the posterior nodes of the attentional networks, perhaps because the undamaged LH needs some access to information processed in the damaged RH to compensate for neglect signs [77, 79]. The status of more rostral portions of the corpus callosum can predict response to rehabilitation therapies such as prism adaptation: patients with chronic neglect and caudal callosal disconnection, but intact body and genu, were more likely to respond to prism adaptation therapy [80]. Prism adaptation could thus promote inter-hemispheric integration through these callosal connections (Fig. 4.3).

4.3.5 Postsurgical Neglect

Studies reporting postoperative unilateral spatial neglect after a surgical resection are scarce. We summarized in Table 4.1 a comprehensive review of the literature. We found no more than 22 cases (in eight studies: [81–88]) with signs of left spatial neglect in the immediate period (<1 week) following resection of lesions located to the right frontal, parietal, or temporal lobes. Among these cases, the deficit persisted after 3 months in 17 of them. Nakajima et al. emphasized that visuospatial cognition (assessed by the line bisection task) was the domain with the poorest chances of recovery in case of immediate postoperative deficit [88]. However, in one patient,

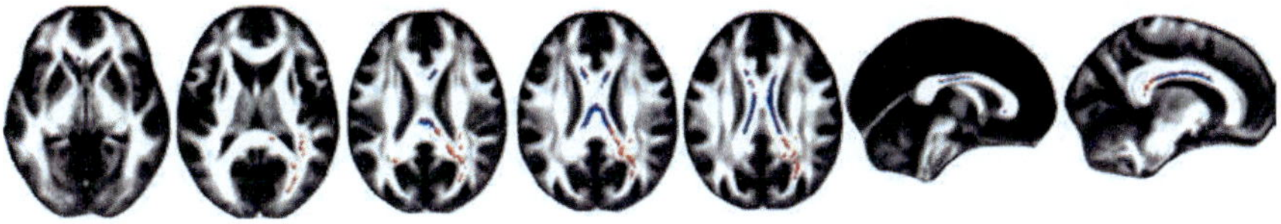

Fig. 4.3 White matter damage preventing neglect patients' recovery, as assessed by tract-based spatial statistics. Red: splenial connections whose damage prevented recovery of neglect in a longitudinal study [77]. Blue: more rostral callosal connections whose damage predicted low response to prism adaptation therapy in neglect [80]. Figure modified from [79], with permission of Oxford University Press

Table 4.1 Review of the literature about left-sided neglect following surgical resection of an hemispheric tumor

	Location	Rates of immediate deficits (<1 week)	Timing of late postop assessment	Hemianopia	Remarks
Hommet et al. [81]	R inferior parietal	1 out of 1	3 months and 2 years	No	Deficit persisted at 3 months and resolved at 2 years
Kleinman et al. [82]	R parietal	1 out of 2	NA	No	
Stone et al. [83]	R inferior frontal	1 out of 1	1 week	No	Deficit resolved after 1 week
Roux et al. [84]	R hemisphere	NA	Between 2 and 8 weeks	NA	6 adults out of 41 had a deficit at evaluation between 2 and 8 weeks postop
Emanuele et al. [85]	R hemisphere	4 out of 12	6 months	NA	Two patients with persistent deficit at 6 months postop
Talacchi et al. [86]	R parietal	1 out of 2	NA	No	Deficit resolved after 3 days
Nakajima et al. [87]	R frontal	6 out of 18	3 months	No	Deficits persisted at 3 months in the 6 cases
Nakajima et al. [88]	R hemisphere	8 out of 30	3 months	NA	Long-term deficits observed only for right-sided gliomas, located to frontal and parietal lobes

testing normalized at the 2 years assessment [81], raising the possibility of very long-term recovery. Another study also reported permanent deficits in 1 child out of 12 and 11 adults out of 27 after resection of right thalamic tumors [89]. Last but not least, one paper reported a case of permanent right spatial neglect after resection of a left parietal glioma in a patient with a reversed lateralization of language functions on functional MRI [90].

4.3.6 Intraoperative Monitoring of Spatial Cognition

Following the seminal publication introducing the line bisection task [91, 92], several authors confirmed the feasibility and efficacy of this task for intraoperative detection of sites belonging to the network of spatial awareness [84, 87, 88, 93–95].

A tablet version of target cancellation has been proposed as an alternative, especially for patients with a deficit of fine motor functions, that would interfere with the performance of the line bisection task [96]. The authors argue that target cancellation is expected to be slightly more sensitive than the line bisection to detect spatial neglect [97] and that it is independent of observer's judgment. This latter argument is no more relevant when the line bisection task is implemented in digital tablet [95, 98], a solution that should be clearly preferred to the paper-pencil version. Moreover, the target cancellation task comes with a major disadvantage: the time required to complete the task is about 20–30 s, which is rather unsuited to the intraoperative settings (stimulation should typically last less than 5 s).

In summary, a tablet version of the line bisection task, providing online automated feedback to the neuropsychologist, is currently the gold standard for intraoperative monitoring of spatial awareness.

4.3.7 Benefit of Intraoperative Line Bisection Monitoring

To the best of our knowledge, there are no studies comparing two groups of patients operated on with versus without line bisection monitoring. However, most studies reporting intraoperative line bisection monitoring with electrical stimulation at both cortical and white matter level [63, 92, 95, 96] found no cases of spatial neglect at long-term evaluations. These data fully support the recommendation to monitor the line bisection task when operating the right parietal lobe (or the left parietal lobe in case of reversed lateralization of cognitive functions, see [90]). However, one group reported that 14.3% of patients with right-sided tumors operated on in awake conditions and under line bisection monitoring still had impairments on line-bisection task at 3 months assessment [88]. These authors showed that these deficits impacted work and driving but not self-care and household activities. One explanation could be that the criteria used for defining left spatial neglect were more stringent in this study [88].

Moreover, the sensitivity and specificity of line bisection monitoring for preventing spatial neglect has been estimated by two studies. First, the importance of preserving cortical sites of line bisection deviation was questioned in a report of two cases [86]. In one of the two cases, a line bisection cortical site was removed, without inducing postoperative neglect. However, it is worth mentioning that monitoring was continued, and the resection was stopped when the patient started to show signs of neglect. Roux & al. reported the occurrence of postoperative spatial neglect (evaluated between 2 and 8 weeks postoperatively) after mapping in 41 cases. Line bisections sites were found in 27 cases, and spared in 20 cases, none of whom had a postoperative neglect. Among the 7 cases with resection of line bisection sites, 5 cases had a postoperative neglect and 2 were performing normally. It was not specified whether in these two cases the resected sites were cortical or axonal. In the 14 cases without identification of deviation sites, only 1 presented signs of neglect postoperatively. Overall, the sensitivity and specificity were 83% and 93%, respectively, further confirming the value of this monitoring.

4.3.8 Knowledge Gained from Intraoperative Mapping Studies of Line Bisection

The two largest series reporting the "line bisection" cortical sites yielded contradictory results. While Roux et al. reported sites mainly located to the inferior parietal lobe and superior temporal gyrus [84], Vallar et al. observed the highest rate of responses in the superior parietal lobule [95]. Some methodological subtleties might explain this discrepancy, such as different intensities of stimulation eliciting a response (for which there was no information in either of the two studies), or different tumor locations, resulting in distinct sampling of the parietal lobe for mapping and in distinct functional reorganization induced by plasticity. In any case, the topography of cortical hubs that would be crucial for line bisection seems to be highly variable from one patient to another and, when pooling all data from the literature, there is currently no more specific localization than the whole right parietal lobe. One possible hypothesis is that the areas supporting spatial awareness have a larger size than standard language areas, and thus require higher intensities or multifocal stimulation [99]. Of note, the frequency and amount of leftward deviations under stimulation in the right hemisphere remain unknown, and in particular it is not clear whether such sites could be safely resected or not.

At the white matter level, electrostimulation studies provided converging evidence that the frontoparietal connections, supported by the SLF II/arcuate fasciculus pathways, are essential to spatial awareness [84, 92, 95]. Several reports noted also a contribution of the IFOF (also called inferior longitudinal *system* in a new terminology, see [100]), although it is not fully demonstrated that resection within this ventral stream would systematically generate long-lasting postoperative spatial neglect [63, 84]. It is tempting to put forward the hypothesis that this ventral stream is in fact an input gate into the putamen, as it has been shown that putaminal lesions are associated with spatial neglect [101]. But striatal inputs are in general redundant: distant ipsilateral areas interconnected by associative fibers project to the same striatal territory [102], and contralateral homologous areas also project to the same striatal territory through crossing cortico-striatal fibers [103]. Such redundancy, supporting a high degree of plasticity, would explain why a unilateral putaminal disconnection would not cause by itself a long-lasting deficit. Of note, this hypothesis underlies the importance of preserving callosal fibers, a notion that is now well accepted [53]. Last but not least, the exact trajectory of thalamo-cortical fibers that would be part of the cortico-striato-thalamo-cortical loop involved in line bisection is not yet well determined. Figures 4.4 and 4.5 provide a good illustration of spatial cognition mapping in a surgical case with a right parietal tumor. In particular,

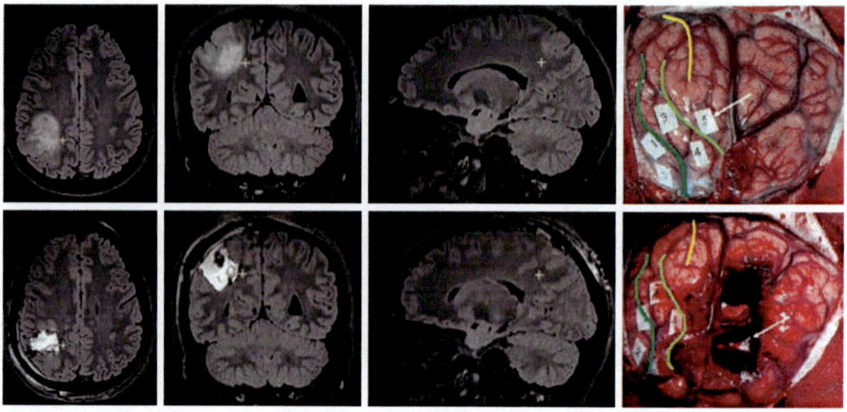

Fig. 4.4 Mapping of spatial cognition in a surgical case. Cortically, stimulation of the site tag 5 induced a mild rightward deviation but only in about half of trials. Stimulation of the white matter site tag 9 elicited systematically a strong rightward deviation. Stimulus intensity was set at 2 mA. The yellow line delineates the ascending ramus of the lateral fissure, the light green line the postcentral sulcus, and the dark green line the central sulcus. The yellow cross on the MRI matches the site tag 9

Fig. 4.5 demonstrates that fibers passing through the white matter functional site comprise SLF I-II, callosal fibers, intraparietal and temporoparietal fibers (corresponding to the posterior transverse system as defined in [100]), putaminal fibers, and thalamo-cortical fibers.

A longitudinal study of 20 patients undergoing awake brain surgery with line bisection testing before and after the removal of a low-grade glioma in the right hemisphere [104] found that the surgical resection of the right angular gyrus was associated with transient neglect signs on all tasks, whereas resection of more anterior regions correlated with transient deficits only in visual exploration or detection, but not on line bisection. However, all patients had fully recovered at follow-up 3 months after surgery, suggesting that the attentional networks showed substantial functional plasticity and reorganization. The authors attributed this pattern of recovery in terms of involvement of the contralateral left hemisphere, and of preservation of long-range white matter pathways within the right hemisphere.

In summary, electrostimulation studies have the potential to shed light on the neural basis of spatial awareness within the general framework of a cortical network-striato-thalamo-cortical network loop. To this end, electrophysiological studies offer a unique opportunity to unveil this global circuitry, by means of methods such as evoked-potentials while stimulating at 1 Hz [105] or high-frequency and afterdischarge analysis while stimulating at 60 Hz. In addition, new network-based lesion-symptom mapping could also shed light to our understanding of the link between a topographical lesion and spatial neglect [106].

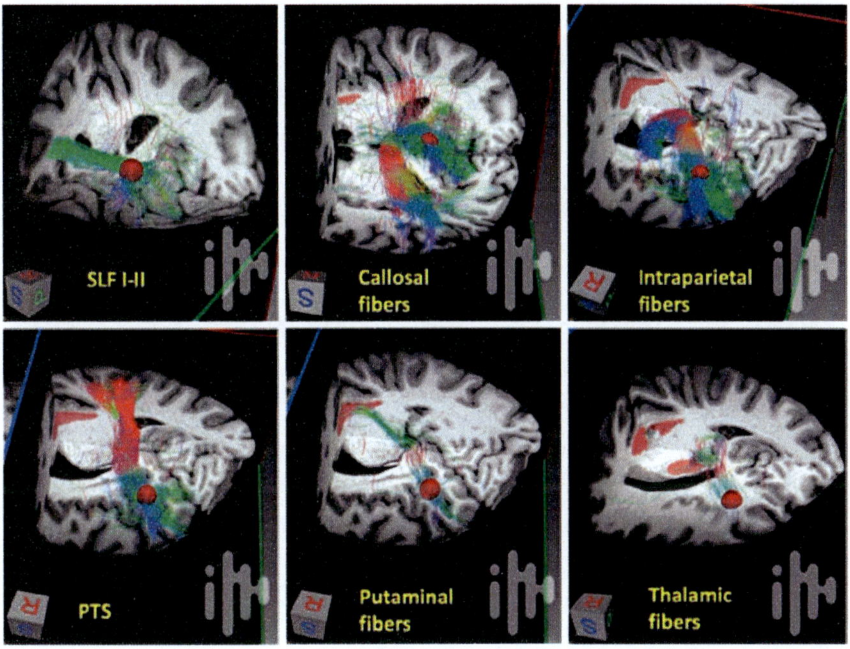

Fig. 4.5 Dissected tractogram of the white matter functional site. The red sphere corresponds to the site tag 9 and has been used as a seed. Further dissection allowed to separate fibers of the SLF I and II (linking the frontal eye field to the precuneus), callosal fibers, intraparietal and temporoparietal fibers (belonging to the posterior transverse system), and to a less extent putaminal fibers as well as thalamic fibers

Acknowledgment The work of PB is supported by the Agence Nationale de la Rercherche through ANR-16-CE37-0005 and ANR-10-IAIHU-06. EM is supported by INSERM, through the Contrat Interface.

References

1. Corbetta M, Shulman GL. Control of goal-directed and stimulus-driven attention in the brain. Nat Rev Neurosci. 2002;3:201–15.
2. Nobre AC. The attentive homunculus: now you see it, now you don't. Neurosci Biobehav Rev. 2001;25:477–96.
3. Schmahmann JD, Pandya DN. Fiber pathways of the brain, New York. Oxford university press. 2006.
4. Thiebaut de Schotten M, Dell'Acqua F, Forkel SJ, Simmons A, Vergani F, Murphy DGM, et al. A lateralized brain network for visuospatial attention. Nat Neurosci. 2011a;14:1245–6.
5. Thiebaut de Schotten M, ffytche DH, Bizzi A, Dell'Acqua F, Allin M, Walshe M, et al. Atlasing location, asymmetry and inter-subject variability of white matter tracts in the human brain with MR diffusion tractography. Neuroimage. 2011b;54:49–59.
6. Bartolomeo P. Anatomy and disorders of the spatial attention system. In: Thiebaut De Schotten M, Della Sala S, editors. Encyclopedia of behavioral neuroscience. 2nd ed. Elsevier; 2020.

7. Bartolomeo P, Seidel Malkinson T. Hemispheric lateralization of attention processes in the human brain. Curr Opin Psychol. 2019;29C:90–6.
8. Kravitz DJ, Saleem KS, Baker CI, Ungerleider LG, Mishkin M. The ventral visual pathway: an expanded neural framework for the processing of object quality. Trends Cogn Sci. 2013;17:26–49.
9. Fiebelkorn IC, Kastner S. Functional specialization in the attention network. Annu Rev Psychol. 2019;71:221–49.
10. van Schouwenburg MR, den Ouden HEM, Cools R. Selective attentional enhancement and inhibition of fronto-posterior connectivity by the basal ganglia during attention switching. Cereb Cortex. 2015;25:1527–34.
11. Bartolomeo P. Attention disorders after right brain damage: living in halved worlds. London: Springer; 2014.
12. Bartolomeo P, Urbanski M, Chokron S, Chainay, H, Moroni C, Siéroff E, Belin C. Halligan, P. Neglected attention in apparent spatial compression. Neuropsychologia. 2004;42:49–61.
13. Bourgeois A, Chica AB, Migliaccio R, Bayle DJ, Duret C, Pradat-Diehl P, et al. Inappropriate rightward saccades after right hemisphere damage: oculomotor analysis and anatomical correlates. Neuropsychologia. 2015;73:1–11.
14. Gainotti G, D'Erme P, Bartolomeo P. Early orientation of attention toward the half space ipsilateral to the lesion in patients with unilateral brain damage. J Neurol Neurosurg Psychiatry. 1991;54:1082–9.
15. Bartolomeo P, Chokron S. Orienting of attention in left unilateral neglect. Neurosci Biobehav Rev. 2002;26:217–34.
16. D'Erme P, Robertson I, Bartolomeo P, Daniele A, Gainotti G. Early rightwards orienting of attention on simple reaction time performance in patients with left-sided neglect. Neuropsychologia. 1992;30:989–1000.
17. Losier BJ, Klein RM. A review of the evidence for a disengage deficit following parietal lobe damage. Neurosci Biobehav Rev. 2001;25:1–13.
18. Posner MI, Walker JA, Friedrich FJ, Rafal RD. Effects of parietal injury on covert orienting of attention. J Neurosci. 1984;4:1863–74.
19. Rastelli F, Funes MJ, Lupiáñez J, Duret C, Bartolomeo P. Left neglect: is the disengage deficit space- or object-based? Exp Brain Res. 2008;187:439–46.
20. Bartolomeo P, Chokron S, Siéroff E. Facilitation instead of inhibition for repeated right-sided events in left neglect. Neuroreport. 1999;10:3353–7.
21. Bourgeois A, Chica AB, Migliaccio R, Thiebaut de Schotten M, Bartolomeo P. Cortical control of inhibition of return: evidence from patients with inferior parietal damage and visual neglect. Neuropsychologia. 2012;50:800–9.
22. Bartolomeo P, D'Erme P, Gainotti G. The relationship between visuospatial and representational neglect. Neurology. 1994;44:1710–4.
23. Gigliotta O, Seidel Malkinson T, Miglino O, Bartolomeo P. Pseudoneglect in visual search: behavioral evidence and connectional constraints in simulated neural circuitry. eNeuro. 2017;4:ENEURO.0154-17.2017.
24. Bartolomeo P. The novelty effect in recovered hemineglect. Cortex. 1997;33:323–32.
25. Azouvi P, Bartolomeo P, Beis JM, Perennou D, Pradat-Diehl P, Rousseaux M. A battery of tests for the quantitative assessment of unilateral neglect. Restor Neurol Neurosci. 2006;24:273–85.
26. Denes G, Semenza C, Stoppa E, Lis A. Unilateral spatial neglect and recovery from hemiplegia: a follow-up study. Brain. 1982;105:543–52.
27. Chica AB, Thiebaut de Schotten M, Toba MN, Malhotra P, Lupiáñez J, Bartolomeo P. Attention networks and their interactions after right-hemisphere damage. Cortex. 2012;48:654–63.
28. Siéroff E, Decaix C, Chokron S, Bartolomeo P. Impaired orienting of attention in left unilateral neglect: a componential analysis. Neuropsychology. 2007;21:94–113.
29. Bartolomeo P. Visual neglect. Curr Opin Neurol. 2007;20:381–6.

30. Coulthard E, Parton A, Husain M. The modular architecture of the neglect syndrome: implications for action control in visual neglect. Neuropsychologia. 2007;45:1982–4.
31. Massironi M, Antonucci G, Pizzamiglio L, Vitale MV, Zoccolotti P. The Wundt-Jastrow illusion in the study of spatial hemi-inattention. Neuropsychologia. 1988;26:161–6.
32. Bartolomeo P, Thiebaut De Schotten M, Chica AB. Brain networks of visuospatial attention and their disruption in visual neglect. Frontiers in human neuroscience. 2012;6:110.
33. Gainotti G, Messerli P, Tissot R. Qualitative analysis of unilateral spatial neglect in relation to the laterality of cerebral lesions. J Neurol Neurosurg Psychiatry. 1972;35:545–50.
34. Albert ML. A simple test of visual neglect. Neurology. 1973;23:658–64.
35. Mesulam MM. Attention, confusional states and neglect. In: Mesulam MM, editor. Principles of behavioral neurology. Philadelphia: F.A. Davis; 1985. p. 125–68.
36. Weintraub S, Mesulam MM. Right cerebral dominance in spatial attention. Further evidence based on ipsilateral neglect. Arch Neurol. 1987;44:621–5.
37. Gauthier L, Dehaut F, Joanette Y. The bells test: a quantitative and qualitative test for visual neglect. Int J Clin Neuropsychol. 1989;11:49–53.
38. Rapcsak SZ, Verfaellie M, Fleet WS, Heilman KM. Selective attention in hemispatial neglect. Arch Neurol. 1989;46:178–82.
39. Urbanski M, Bartolomeo P. Line bisection in left neglect: the importance of starting right. Cortex. 2008;44:782–93.
40. Bonato M. Neglect and extinction depend greatly on task demands: a review. Front Hum Neurosci. 2012;6:195.
41. Bartolomeo P. Inhibitory processes and compensation for spatial bias after right hemisphere damage. Neuropsychol Rehabil. 2000;10:511–26.
42. Barton JJ, Black SE. Line bisection in hemianopia. J Neurol Neurosurg Psychiatry. 1998;64:660–2.
43. Doricchi F, Angelelli P. Misrepresentation of horizontal space in left unilateral neglect: role of hemianopia. Neurology. 1999;52:1845–52.
44. Walker R, Findlay JM, Young AW, Welch J. Disentangling neglect and hemianopia. Neuropsychologia. 1991;29:1019–27.
45. Brain RW. Visual disorientation with special reference to lesion of the right brain hemisphere. Brain. 1941;64:244–72.
46. De Renzi E. Disorders of space elaboration and cognition. New York: Wiley; 1982.
47. Heilman KM, Van Den Abell T. Right hemisphere dominance for attention: the mechanism underlying hemispheric asymmetries of inattention (neglect). Neurology. 1980;30: 327–30.
48. Mesulam M-M. A cortical network for directed attention and unilateral neglect. Ann Neurol. 1981;10:309–25.
49. Kinsbourne M. A model for the mechanism of unilateral neglect of space. Trans Am Neurol Assoc. 1970;95:143–6.
50. Kinsbourne M. Orientational bias model of unilateral neglect: evidence from attentional gradients within hemispace. In: Robertson IH, Marshall JC, editors. Unilateral neglect: clinical and experimental studies. Hove: Lawrence Erlbaum Associates; 1993. p. 63–86.
51. Lecce F, Rotondaro F, Bonni S, Carlesimo A, De Schotten MT, Tomaiuolo F, Doricchi F. Cingulate neglect in humans: disruption of contralesional reward learning in right brain damage. Cortex. 2015;62:73–88.
52. Corbetta M, Kincade MJ, Lewis C, Snyder AZ, Sapir A. Neural basis and recovery of spatial attention deficits in spatial neglect. Nat Neurosci. 2005;8:1603–10.
53. Bartolomeo P, Thiebaut de Schotten M. Let thy left brain know what thy right brain doeth: inter-hemispheric compensation of functional deficits after brain damage. Neuropsychologia. 2016;93:407–12.
54. Charras P, Lupiáñez J, Migliaccio R, Toba MN, Pradat-Diehl P, Duret C, et al. Dissecting the component deficits of perceptual imbalance in visual neglect: evidence from horizontal-vertical length comparisons. Cortex. 2012;48:540–52.

55. Bartolomeo P. Spatially biased decisions: toward a dynamic interactive model of visual neglect. In: Tracy JI, Hampstead B, Sathian K, editors. Plasticity of cognition in neurologic disorders. Oxford: Oxford University Press; 2015. p. 299–322.
56. Bisiach E. Extinction and neglect: same or different? In: Paillard J, editor. Brain and space. Oxford: Oxford University Press; 1991. p. 251–7.
57. Damasio A, Damasio H, Chui H. Neglect following damage to frontal lobe or basal ganglia. Neuropsychologia. 1980;18:123–32.
58. Heilman KM, Valenstein E. Frontal lobe neglect in man. Neurology. 1972;22:660–4.
59. Watson RT, Heilman KM. Thalamic neglect. Neurology. 1979;29:690–4.
60. Bartolomeo P. The quest for the 'critical lesion site' in cognitive deficits: problems and perspectives. Cortex. 2011;47:1010–2.
61. Lunven M, Bartolomeo P. Attention and spatial cognition: neural and anatomical substrates of visual neglect. Ann Phys Rehabil Med. 2017;60:124–9.
62. Rode G, Pagliari C, Huchon L, Rossetti Y, Pisella L. Semiology of neglect: an update. Ann Phys Rehabil Med. 2017;60:177–85.
63. Herbet G, Yordanova YN, Duffau H. Left spatial neglect evoked by electrostimulation of the right inferior fronto-occipital fasciculus. Brain Topogr. 2017;30:747–56.
64. Toba MN, Migliaccio R, Batrancourt B, Bourlon C, Duret C, Pradat-Diehl P, et al. Common brain networks for distinct deficits in visual neglect. A combined structural and tractography MRI approach. Neuropsychologia. 2018a;115:167–78.
65. Ten Brink AF, Verwer JH, Biesbroek JM, Visser-Meily JMA, Nijboer TCW. Differences between left- and right-sided neglect revisited: a large cohort study across multiple domains. J Clin Exp Neuropsychol. 2017;39:707–23.
66. Weintraub S, Daffner KR, Ahern GL, Price BH, Mesulam MM. Right sided hemispatial neglect and bilateral cerebral lesions. J Neurol Neurosurg Psychiatry. 1996;60:342–4.
67. Andrade K, Samri D, Sarazin M, Cruz De Souza L, Cohen L, Thiebaut de Schotten M, et al. Visual neglect in posterior cortical atrophy. BMC Neurol. 2010;10:68.
68. Bartolomeo P, Dalla Barba G, Boissé MT, Bachoud-Lévi AC, Degos JD, Boller F. Right-side neglect in Alzheimer's disease. Neurology. 1998;51:1207–9.
69. Carter AR, McAvoy MP, Siegel JS, Hong X, Astafiev SV, Rengachary J, et al. Differential white matter involvement associated with distinct visuospatial deficits after right hemisphere stroke. Cortex. 2017;88:81–97.
70. Chechlacz M, Rotshtein P, Humphreys GW. Neuroanatomical dissections of unilateral visual neglect symptoms: ALE meta-analysis of lesion-symptom mapping. Front Hum Neurosci. 2012;6:230.
71. Molenberghs P, Sale MV, Mattingley JB. Is there a critical lesion site for unilateral spatial neglect? A meta-analysis using activation likelihood estimation. Front Hum Neurosci. 2012;6:78.
72. Toba MN, Rabuffetti M, Duret C, Pradat-Diehl P, Gainotti G, Bartolomeo P. Component deficits of visual neglect: "magnetic" attraction of attention vs. impaired spatial working memory. Neuropsychologia. 2018b;109:52–62.
73. Umarova RM, Beume L, Reisert M, Kaller CP, Kloppel S, Mader I, et al. Distinct white matter alterations following severe stroke: longitudinal DTI study in neglect. Neurology. 2017;88:1546–55.
74. Rastelli F, Tallon-Baudry C, Migliaccio R, Toba MN, Ducorps A, Pradat-Diehl P, et al. Neural dynamics of neglected targets in patients with right hemisphere damage. Cortex. 2013;49:1989–96.
75. Lasaponara S, D'Onofrio M, Pinto M, Dragone A, Menicagli D, Bueti D, et al. EEG correlates of preparatory orienting, contextual updating and inhibition of sensory processing in left spatial neglect. J Neurosci. 2018;38:2817–7.
76. Takamura Y, Imanishi M, Osaka M, Ohmatsu S, Tominaga T, Yamanaka K, et al. Intentional gaze shift to neglected space: a compensatory strategy during recovery after unilateral spatial neglect. Brain. 2016;139:2970–82.

77. Lunven M, Thiebaut De Schotten M, Bourlon C, Duret C, Migliaccio R, Rode G, et al. White matter lesional predictors of chronic visual neglect: a longitudinal study. Brain. 2015;138:746–60.
78. Umarova RM, Nitschke K, Kaller CP, Klöppel S, Beume L, Mader I, et al. Predictors and signatures of recovery from neglect in acute stroke. Ann Neurol. 2016;79:673–86.
79. Bartolomeo P. Visual neglect: getting the hemispheres to talk to each other. Brain. 2019;142:840–2.
80. Lunven M, Rode G, Bourlon C, Duret C, Migliaccio R, Chevrillon E, et al. Anatomical predictors of successful prism adaptation in chronic visual neglect. Cortex. 2019;120:629–41.
81. Hommet C, Bardet F, de Toffol B, Perrier D, Biraben A, Vignal JP, et al. Unilateral spatial neglect following right inferior parietal cortectomy. Epilepsy Behav. 2004;5:416–9.
82. Kleinman JT, Sepkuty JP, Hillis AE, Lenz FA, Heidler-Gary J, Gingis L, et al. Spatial neglect during electrocortical stimulation mapping in the right hemisphere. Epilepsia. 2007;48:2365–8.
83. Stone JJ, Reynolds MR, Leuthardt EC. Transient hemispatial neglect after surgical resection of a right frontal lobe mass. World Neurosurg. 2011;76:361.e7–10.
84. Roux F-E, Dufor O, Lauwers-Cances V, Boukhatem L, Brauge D, Draper L, et al. Electrostimulation mapping of spatial neglect. Neurosurgery. 2011;69:1218–31.
85. Emanuele B, Santini B, Talacchi A, Gerosa M, Savazzi S. Pre- and post-operative assessment of visuo-spatial functions in right hemisphere tumour patients: a pilot study. J Neurooncol. 2012;108:261–7.
86. Talacchi A, Squintani GM, Emanuele B, Tramontano V, Santini B, Savazzi S. Intraoperative cortical mapping of visuospatial functions in parietal low-grade tumors: changing perspectives of neurophysiological mapping. Neurosurg Focus. 2013;34:E4.
87. Nakajima R, Kinoshita M, Miyashita K, Okita H, Genda R, Yahata T, et al. Damage of the right dorsal superior longitudinal fascicle by awake surgery for glioma causes persistent visuospatial dysfunction. Sci Rep. 2017;7:17158.
88. Nakajima R, Kinoshita M, Okita H, Yahata T, Nakada M. Glioma surgery under awake condition can lead to good independence and functional outcome excluding deep sensation and visuospatial cognition. Neurooncol Pract. 2019;6:354–63.
89. Billingsley RL, Lang FF, Slopis JM, Schrimsher GW, Ater JL, Moore BD. Visual-spatial neglect in a child following sub-cortical tumor resection. Dev Med Child Neurol. 2002;44:191–200.
90. Mandonnet E, Mellerio C, Barberis M, Poisson I, Jansma JM, Rutten G-J. When right is on the left (and vice versa): a case series of glioma patients with reversed lateralization of cognitive functions. J Neurol Surg A Cent Eur Neurosurg. 2020a;81:138–46.
91. Bartolomeo P, Thiebaut de Schotten M, Duffau H. Mapping of visuospatial functions during brain surgery: a new tool to prevent unilateral spatial neglect. Neurosurgery. 2007;61:E1340.
92. Thiebaut de Schotten M, Urbanski M, Duffau H, Volle E, Lévy R, Dubois B, et al. Direct evidence for a parietal-frontal pathway subserving spatial awareness in humans. Science. 2005;309:2226–8.
93. Kitabayashi T, Nakada M, Kinoshita M, Sakurai H, Kobayashi S, Okita H, et al. [Awake surgery with line bisection task for two cases of parietal glioma in the non-dominant hemisphere]. No Shinkei Geka. 2012;40:1087–93.
94. Mandonnet E, De Witt Hamer P, Poisson I, Whittle I, Bernat A-L, Bresson D, et al. Initial experience using awake surgery for glioma: oncological, functional, and employment outcomes in a consecutive series of 25 cases. Neurosurgery. 2015;76:382–9; discussion 389.
95. Vallar G, Bello L, Bricolo E, Castellano A, Casarotti A, Falini A, et al. Cerebral correlates of visuospatial neglect: a direct cerebral stimulation study. Hum Brain Mapp. 2014;35:1334–50.
96. Conner AK, Glenn C, Burks JD, McCoy T, Bonney PA, Chema AA, et al. The use of the target cancellation task to identify eloquent visuospatial regions in awake craniotomies: technical note. Cureus. 2016;8:e883.
97. Molenberghs P, Sale MV. Testing for spatial neglect with line bisection and target cancellation: are both tasks really unrelated? PLoS One. 2011;6:e23017.

98. Mandonnet E, Cerliani L, Siuda-Krzywicka K, Poisson I, Zhi N, Volle E, et al. A network-level approach of cognitive flexibility impairment after surgery of a right temporo-parietal glioma. Neurochirurgie. 2017;63:308–13.
99. Gonen T, Gazit T, Korn A, Kirschner A, Perry D, Hendler T, et al. Intra-operative multi-site stimulation: expanding methodology for cortical brain mapping of language functions [Internet]. PLoS One. 2017;12:e0180740. [Cited 2019 Apr 11]. https://www.ncbi.nlm.nih.gov/pmc/articles/PMC5507257/.
100. Mandonnet E, Sarubbo S, Petit L. The nomenclature of human white matter association pathways: proposal for a systematic taxonomic anatomical classification. Front Neuroanat. 2018;12:94.
101. Karnath HO, Himmelbach M, Rorden C. The subcortical anatomy of human spatial neglect: putamen, caudate nucleus and pulvinar. Brain. 2002;125:350–60.
102. Yeterian EH, Van Hoesen GW. Cortico-striate projections in the rhesus monkey: the organization of certain cortico-caudate connections. Brain Res. 1978;139:43–63.
103. De Benedictis A, Petit L, Descoteaux M, Marras CE, Barbareschi M, Corsini F, et al. New insights in the homotopic and heterotopic connectivity of the frontal portion of the human corpus callosum revealed by microdissection and diffusion tractography. Hum Brain Mapp. 2016;37:4718–35.
104. Charras P, Herbet G, Deverdun J, de Champfleur NM, Duffau H, Bartolomeo P, et al. Functional reorganization of the attentional networks in low-grade glioma patients: a longitudinal study. Cortex. 2015;63:27–41.
105. Matsumoto R, Nair DR, LaPresto E, Bingaman W, Shibasaki H, Lüders HO. Functional connectivity in human cortical motor system: a cortico-cortical evoked potential study. Brain. 2007;130:181–97.
106. Mandonnet E, Thirion B. Tackling the complexity of lesion-symptoms mapping: how to bridge the gap between data-scientists and clinicians? In: machine learning in clinical neuroscience: foundations and applications. Springer nature publishing. 2021.

Part II

Language Functions

5 Lexical Retrieval

Sylvie Moritz-Gasser and Guillaume Herbet

5.1 Introduction

Accessing words efficiently and adequately in our mental lexicon is core to produce and understand language. This complex process of lexical retrieval entails multiple activation and selection mechanisms of conceptual semantic and phonological representations. Thus, when a person wants to produce or understand a word, associated semantic features and phonological units have to be activated in order to select the target word, which will be produced aloud where appropriate thanks to planning and execution of articulatory programs [1, 2]. Word form retrieval deficit, expressed by anomia or word-finding difficulties, apart from semantic or phonological impairments, is a universal feature of acquired language disorders, irrespective of their etiologies [3, 4]. Exploring the neurobiological underpinnings of this core stage of language processing is then of paramount importance to understand clinical presentations of brain-lesioned patients and adapt rehabilitation strategies, and, in the particular context of patients harboring a diffuse low-grade glioma (DLGG) and undergoing an awake surgery, to prevent residual long-lasting word retrieval impairments thanks to a sound-designed intraoperative language monitoring. In this chapter, we propose to underline, after a brief review of current knowledge about the neural bases of word retrieval, the unsurpassed clinical value of intraoperative word retrieval mapping, the means to achieve it and its contribution to improve anatomo-functional knowledge.

S. Moritz-Gasser (✉) · G. Herbet
Institute of Functional Genomics, University of Montpellier, INSERM U1191, Team "Plasticity, Stem Cells and Glial Tumors", Montpellier, France

Gui de Chauliac Hospital, Montpellier, France
e-mail: sylvie.gasser@umontpellier.fr; guillaume.herbet@umontpellier.fr, guillaume.herbet@igf.cnrs.fr

E. Mandonnet, G. Herbet (eds.), *Intraoperative Mapping of Cognitive Networks*,
https://doi.org/10.1007/978-3-030-75071-8_5

5.2 Neural Bases of Lexical Retrieval: A Brief Review

Recent neuroscientific literature highlights the implication of many left-sided brain areas in word retrieval, including the posterior part of the middle and inferior temporal gyri (MTG and ITG), the superior temporal gyrus (STG), the inferior parietal lobule (IPL), the inferior temporo-occipital junction, the fusiform gyrus, the middle and inferior frontal gyri (MFG and IFG), and medial frontal regions [5–13]. It is worth noting here that middle temporal and inferior frontal regions seem to be differentially involved in, respectively, activation and selection subprocesses of word retrieval [14, 15].

Studies aiming to highlight the white matter connectivity underpinning this distributed cortical network suggest the involvement of tracts belonging to both the dorsal and the ventral stream of language processing [16], including the superior longitudinal fasciculus/arcuate fasciculus (SLF/AF), the ILF, the uncinate fasciculus (UF), and the inferior fronto-occipital fasciculus (IFOF) [17–21]. Different types of naming errors in post-stroke aphasic persons may thus be related to axonal loss either in the dorsal stream (phonemic errors) or in the ventral stream (semantic errors) [22].

This complex distributed cortico-subcortical network involved in word retrieval is not surprising given the number of particularly nested processes required in this ability, as mentioned above. Among them, it is challenging to distinguish the particular stage of retrieval of the word form but studies based on intraoperative mapping, as shown in the last section of this chapter, contributed greatly to shed light on the network involved specifically in this stage, showing notably that the left ITG and the underlying ILF are of vital importance for the particular step of word finding.

Note that if the predominance of left-lateralized brain regions in lexical processing in general has no longer to be proven, a number of neuroimaging studies suggested the co-involvement of right-lateralized regions [23–25], possibly associated with domain-general attentional and control processes, involved but not specifically associated with linguistic processes [26, 27].

A complex and distributed network is then involved in lexical retrieval, requiring a systematic intraoperative monitoring of this function in DLGG patients, whatever the tumor location, in order to avoid long-lasting debilitating impairments. As shown below, to use or not to use intraoperative lexical retrieval mapping makes the difference for long-term recovery.

5.3 Evidence of Long-Lasting Lexical Retrieval Difficulties in Intraoperatively Unmapped Brains

A few studies compared functional outcomes in DLGG patients operated on without and with intraoperative mapping. Duffau et al. [28] aimed to quantify the contribution of intraoperative functional mapping by comparing two consecutive series of DLGG patients operated on in the same institution without or with use of direct electrical stimulation (DES): they showed that 3 months after the surgery, beyond the fact that resection was significantly greater in the group with use of DES, especially in eloquent areas, severe permanent deficits, including naming impairments, were almost three times fewer in this group than in that without use of DES. A recent meta-analysis of 90 observational studies showed in the same vein that using intraoperative stimulation mapping during glioma resection was associated with a significant reduction of late severe deficits in naming and motor functions, added to a more extensive resection involving more frequently eloquent locations [29].

More specifically, reports of lexical retrieval outcomes after surgery without intraoperative mapping come essentially from the field of epilepsy surgery, which concerns mostly resections in the temporal lobe. A recent systematic review highlights that long-term postsurgical naming performances are impaired compared to preoperatively in about a third of patients with left-sided temporal resections, this decline appearing to be higher for patients with the largest resections [30]. Some studies show furthermore that preoperative fMRI seems to be able to predict these postoperative naming deficits [31] and suggest that persistent postoperative decline in naming performances is associated with resection in the ventral left temporal lobe, mainly in the fusiform gyrus [32]. Moreover, a recent fMRI study reveals that preoperative activation of the left posterior ITG/fusiform gyrus during naming seems to be related to greater postoperative naming decline, in case of standard anterior temporal lobe resection (ATLR) for epilepsy, sparing these more posterior regions. The authors postulate that naming decline despite preservation of posterior ITG/fusiform gyrus may be the result of a diaschisis/disconnection effect following the ATLR [33], as the posterior ITG/fusiform gyrus is interconnected with the anterior temporal structures in normal physiological circumstances via the inferior longitudinal fasciculus.

It thus proves undeniably that intraoperative lexical retrieval monitoring is indispensable and should be part of the gold standard of care for DLGG surgery [34–36]. However, given the complexity of the brain lexical network, as briefly reviewed above, and the interindividual variability increased by tumor-induced brain plasticity, this intraoperative mapping must be performed whatever the location of the lesion, especially but not exclusively in the left hemisphere, and must concern cortical areas of this network as well as underlying white matter connectivity [37–39].

5.4 Locations at Risk: Knowledge Gained from Lesion Mapping Studies Conducted with Glioma Patients

While lesion studies assessing the functional consequences of tumors (both the lesion and its resection) on language processing in general are rather common (e.g., [40–45]), those focusing on lexical retrieval in particular are to the very least scarce. To the best of knowledge, only one large-scale neuropsychological study has provided an attempt to identify which structures, both cortical and subcortical, may be especially vulnerable to the surgical procedure in terms of lasting lexical retrieval deficits [46]. In this study, 110 patients with a histopathologically proven, left-sided diffuse low-grade glioma were assessed with a simple object naming task in the postoperative period (superior or equal to 3 months after surgery). To specifically tap into the process of lexical retrieval, the effect of semantic and phonological paraphasia as well as the variance associated with sociodemographic factors were partialed out from the number of anomia observed and from the average response time to name the object seen. These two regressed behavioral measures were used as inputs for both voxelwise and tract-oriented brain–behavioral analyses. As expected, patients performed poorly compared to neurologically healthy participants, especially concerning anomia, semantic paraphasia, and response time. Crucially, resections located in the posterior part of the ITG were strongly associated with the two measures of lexical access (Fig. 5.1). Furthermore, the amount of lesion infiltration into the ILF was strongly correlated with the same behavioral measures, even after controlling for the infiltration of other association white matter tracts. Importantly, statistical models combining both the effect of surgical resections and lesion infiltrations had a better predictive value, suggesting that both the resection of the posterior inferotemporal gyrus and the degree with which the ILF was damaged significantly contributed to long-lasting lexical retrieval difficulties after surgery. All-in-all, this study demonstrates that the posteriormost part of the ITG and its underlying white matter connections, in particular the ILF, are crucial in the network allowing individuals to retrieve the phonological form of a word. From a theoretical standpoint, this finding is unsurprising as the posterior ITG probably acts as an interfacing area between the ventral and the dorsal language network because of receiving connective inputs from three well-known language-related association tracts, including the ILF, the inferior fronto-occipital fasciculus, and arcuate fasciculus [47–49].

A longitudinal study by Wilson et al. [45] has given support to the central role of the inferior/basal temporal cortex in lexical retrieval but indirectly—since a "pure" measure of lexical retrieval was not used. More specifically, the authors provided a voxelwise lesion-symptom analysis with the aim to identify potential relationships between the location of resection sites in the left hemisphere and various language measures, including naming, fluency, comprehension, and repetition. All patients recruited in this study were operated on under local anesthesia but different lesional etiologies were included, including low-grade and high-grade glioma, epilepsy focus, and vascular malformation among the most frequent. Brain–behavioral analyses were performed with the performances obtained 2–3 days after surgery, and those gained at 1 month postsurgery. Interestingly, naming performances were associated with a large portion of the ventral temporal cortex, including the inferior and middle temporal gyri but also the fusiform and para-hippocampal gyri. Along with the results from Herbet et al. [46], further ROI-based linear analyses revealed that the amount of damage of both the middle and posterior part (not the anterior one) of the ITG predicted naming deficits. Interestingly, at 1 month postsurgery the same brain–behavior relationships remained, and picture naming was the only language measure that did not fully recover compared to the baseline preoperative assessment.

As regard to white matter connectivity, other works have corroborated the crucial role of the left ILF in lexical retrieval. As mentioned elsewhere in more detail,

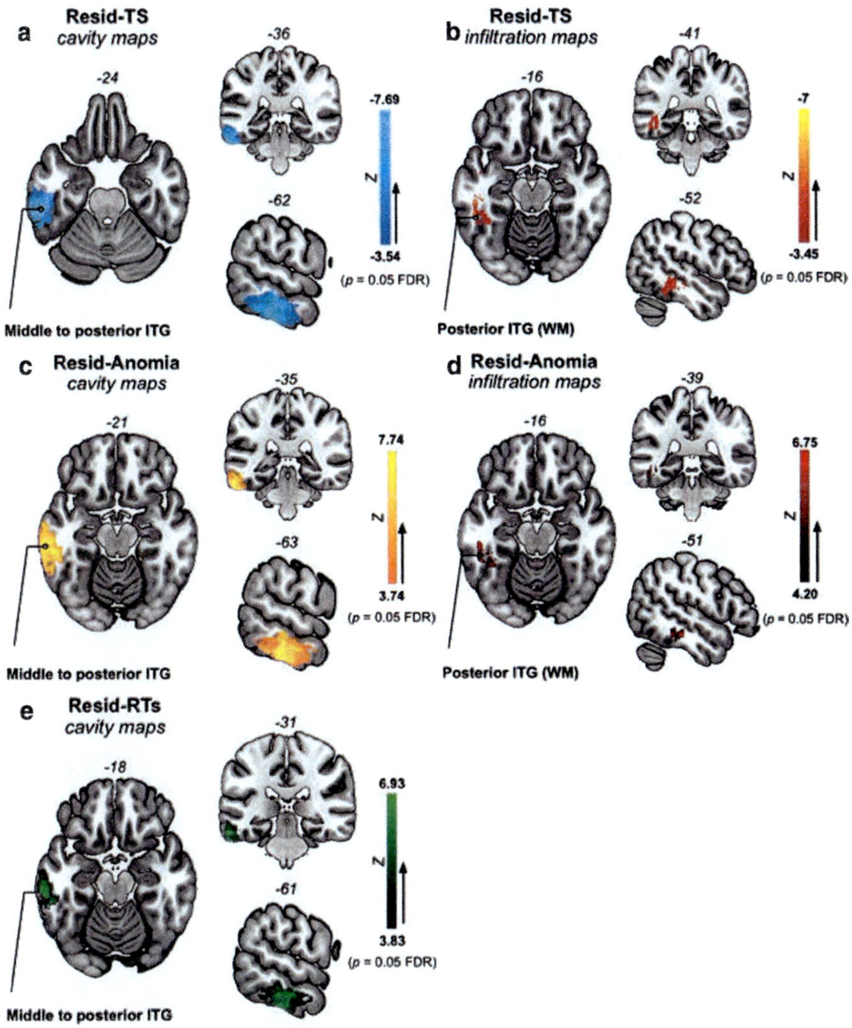

Fig. 5.1 Voxels associated with impaired picture naming performance following surgery for diffuse low-grade glioma. Significant voxels between the naming total scores and the resection cavity maps (**a**) and the residual infiltration maps (**b**). Significant voxels between the regressed measure of anomias and the resection cavity maps (**c**) and the residual infiltration maps (**d**). Significant voxels between the regressed measure of naming response times and the resection cavity maps (**e**). From Herbet et al. [46] with permission

electrostimulation of this tract systematically elicits pure anomia when the temporal pole is not overwhelmed by the tumor [50] (Fig. 5.2). As a matter of fact, transection of this ventral tract can lead to anomic aphasia, once again, when the temporal pole is not lesioned [50] (Fig. 5.3). More indirectly, a recent study mainly conducted with patients presenting with either a glioblastoma or an anaplastic glioma showed

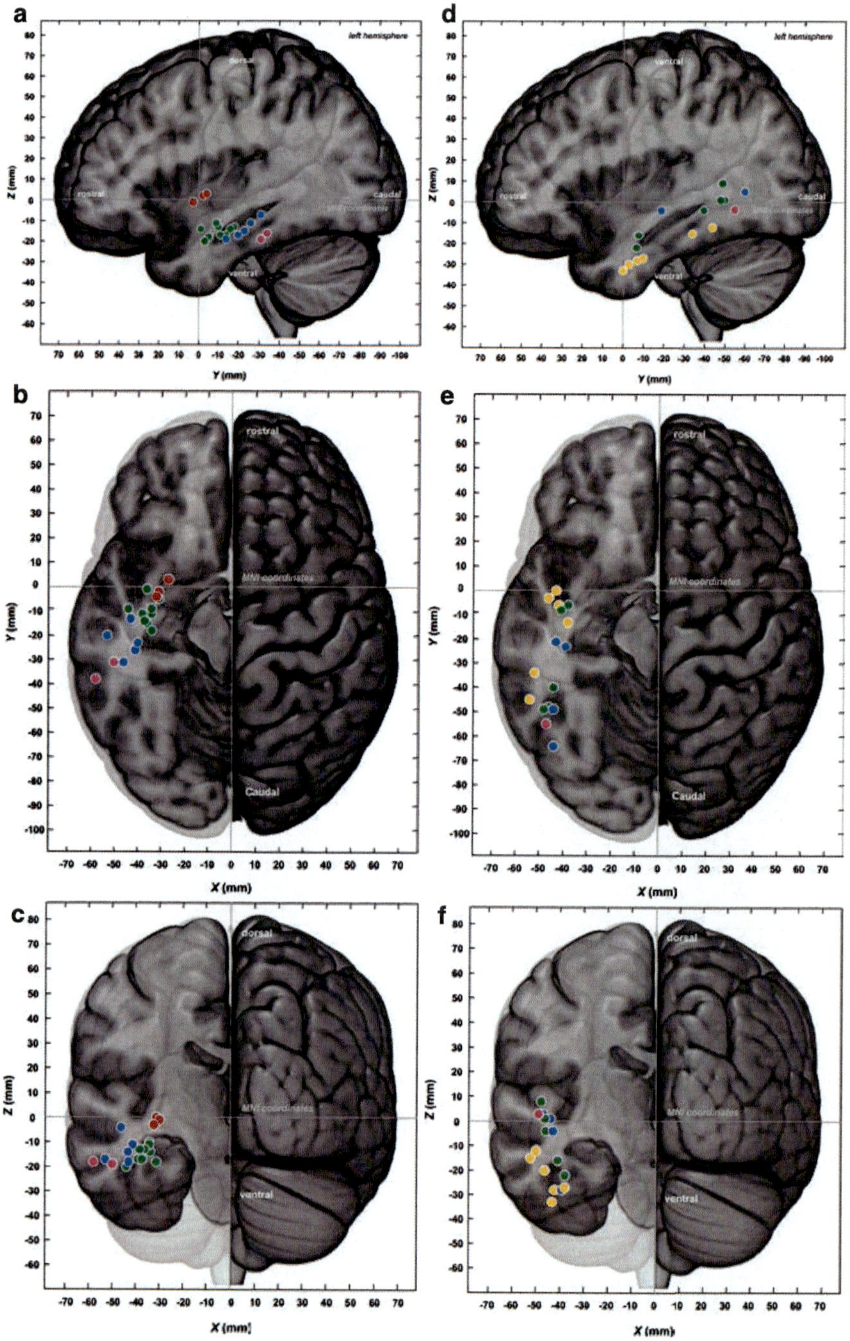

Fig. 5.2 Subcortical mapping from patients with (**a–c**) versus without (**d–f**) an infiltration of the left anterior temporal structures. Yellow: pure anomia; green: semantic paraphasia; blue: phonological paraphasia; purple: word-reading difficulties. From Herbet et al. [50] with permission

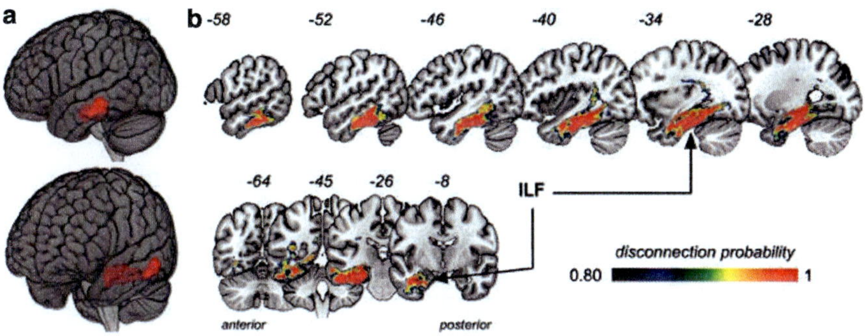

Fig. 5.3 Patient who developed an anomic aphasia due to the transection of the left ILF for surgically accessing the medial temporal structures infiltrated by the tumor. (**a**) 3D-rendering of the location of the surgical resection. (**b**) Disconnection probabilities of white matter fibers impaired by the surgical resection. From Herbet et al. [50] with permission

that general naming abilities (as measured by the Boston naming test) were associated with voxels mainly situated in the inferior and middle temporal gyri, both cortically and subcortically [43]. Moreover, the naming scores were strongly correlated with damage of the left ILF, in terms of both damaged proportion and disconnection probability, although other ventral tracts were also correlated with a lesser extent. Further, a study performed on mainly stroke patients found that a breakdown of the left ILF was predictive of a naming impairment for non-unique entities [20].

To resume this part of the chapter, powered lesion-mapping studies assessing word-finding difficulties in the context of glioma surgery are scarce. However, they strongly suggest that the most posterior part of the ITG along with the ILF is a network that should be the target of special attention during intraoperative mapping of language abilities.

5.5 Monitoring of Word Retrieval: Intraoperative Tasks

Word retrieval ability is traditionally assessed by means of picture naming tasks, consisting in naming pictures belonging to various semantic/syntactic categories. In this context, pure anomia is defined as the inability to name a picture, whereas the patient is able to speak, to repeat, and to access associated semantic features. Picture naming (e.g., DO80, [51]) remains the reference for assessing lexical abilities intraoperatively because, beyond the fact that it is perfectly suited to intraoperative time constraints, it enables to detect transient impairments in each subcomponent of lexical processing induced by DES including anomia, semantic, and phonemic paraphasia. However, given the number of processes involved in picture naming (i.e., visual recognition of the picture, identification and retrieval of associated semantic features, retrieval of the corresponding lexical unit and phonological word form, planning and execution of articulatory programs), the inability for the patient to name a picture intraoperatively following direct electrical stimulation (DES) may arise from the disruption of any of these processes. Thus, in order to identify the most accurately as possible which process is impaired when the patient is unable to name a picture intraoperatively, and then to draw relevant interpretations, it is essential to adopt a rigorous methodology and implement the following recommendations:

- Naming abilities are assessed before, during, and a few days after the surgery by the *same* trained speech-language therapist/neuropsychologist.
- Pre- and postoperative testing is timed in order to highlight a possible slowdown in lexical access.
- Only pictures that are correctly named during preoperative testing are used intraoperatively.
- Each picture is presented intraoperatively on a computer screen during 4–5 s (duration of the effect of a DES) and preceded by a sound cue, in order for the neurosurgeon to apply timely DES.
- Naming testing is performed while moving continuously the contralateral upper limb, in order to assess lexical retrieval in the context of dual task.
- The patient is asked to introduce the name of each picture by the short sentence: "this is a," in order to be able to distinguish a speech arrest (no production at all: impairment in planning motor articulatory programs) from an anomia ("this is a …?": lexical retrieval impairment) (see [52]).
- Tasks of semantic processing (e.g., non-verbal semantic association PPTT, [53]) or phonological processing (e.g., asking the patient to repeat the target name, or giving him/her a phonological cue) are added in order to characterize the deficit underlying the inability to name a picture during the DES of a given brain structure belonging either to the semantic ventral network or to the phono-articulatory dorsal network: if the DES of the same brain structure entails reproducibly an anomia but no semantic or phonological impairments, one may reasonably assume that this structure is involved in lexical retrieval per se.
- Intraoperative mapping must concern cortical areas of the lexical network as well as underlying white matter connectivity.

Some teams suggest to add other types of naming tasks, shown to—or supposed to—be more sensitive in certain cases than a "simple" object naming task. For instance, it is proposed to use an action naming task in patients with frontal DLGG—(see Chap. 11 and [54, 55]), a naming to definition task (i.e., with an auditory rather than visual input) in patients with temporal DLGG [56, 57], or a famous faces naming task in patients with DLGG involving the temporal pole/uncinate fasciculus (see Chap. 13 and [58, 59]). Others underline the importance to use naming tasks in which pictures and expected words are controlled for a number of variables, including visual complexity, imageability, word length, semantic category (biological/artifactual), and grammatical category (verbs/nouns), in order to interpret more accurately the results of perioperative assessments [60].

In sum, even if intraoperative picture naming enables to assess each subcomponent of lexical processing, it is essential to add other tasks in order to achieve accurate interpretations of DES-induced disorders. Concerning the design of naming tasks, and the question of choosing to use one or the other of these tasks according to lesion location, further dedicated longitudinal studies are absolutely needed in order to assess long-term outcomes in general/specific domains of lexical retrieval (e.g., verbs vs. nouns; proper vs. common nouns; biological vs. artefactual entities; auditory vs. visual input) (e.g., [61]) and to estimate the impact of possible long-lasting specific deficits on patients' quality of life [62]. It is indeed undeniable that anatomo-functional correlations drawn from intraoperative observations constitute a powerful and irreplaceable tool of brain functioning study, from both a clinical and neuroscientific point of view, but knowledge gained from intraoperative mapping studies has to be primarily reinvested in the improvement of DLGG patients surgical management, aiming to maximize the resection while preserving quality of life. Thus, implementation of new designed intraoperative naming tasks, based on advances in cognitive neuroscience gained from intraoperative mapping studies [63], should be guided by the onco-functional balance [64], in order to move towards an "optimized strategy" for lexical retrieval intraoperative mapping [52].

5.6 Additional Anatomo-Functional Knowledge Gained from Intraoperative Mapping Studies in Diffuse Glioma Patients

Lexical retrieval is a process in word production which is hardly distinguishable from others by using a simple naming task in the operating theater. Object naming indeed requires a number of processes (see above); the disruption of each of them can potentially lead to anomia—one of the most frequent language impairments observed during the monitoring of language abilities in "awake" surgery. Pure anomia, which is by definition not related to a disruption of semantic or phonological processing, is generally viewed as a prototypical manifestation of a defect in retrieving a word. However, for the reason mentioned above, it is not straightforward to identify which process is impaired when an anomia arises following stimulation. Theoretically, a brain structure which is repeatedly stimulated and uniquely associated with anomia may be assumed to belong to the lexical retrieval network, while structures associated with both anomia and semantic paraphasia may be rather considered as belonging to the verbal semantic network. For example, it is well known that stimulation of the left arcuate fasciculus in right-handers can lead to either phonological paraphasia or anomia (the dorsal pathway) [39], while stimulation of the left inferior fronto-occipital fasciculus can lead to either semantic paraphasia or anomia (the ventral pathway) [65, 66].

To the best of our knowledge, only one study has addressed the issue of lexical retrieval in "awake" surgery [50]. In this work, it was hypothesized that the ventral network underlain by the left ILF may be involved in retrieving the phonological form of a word, but uniquely in normal physiological circumstances. In particular, the authors made the assumption that the left ILF may be associated with lexical retrieval difficulties (i.e., pure anomia) if and only if the anterior temporal structures (ATL) are freed from tumoral infiltrations. Indeed, as diffuse low-grade glioma frequently affects structures in the ATL and thus the underlying connectivity [46, 67], the anterior part of the ILF is often targeted for resection during "awake surgery" with stimulation mapping. However, axonal stimulation studies have failed to identify a role of this tract in verbal language and semantics—two cognitive domains that are usually mapped and monitored in the operating theater [68]. However these negative results should not be viewed as evidence that the ILF is not involved in these functions; they do suggest that ILF functions may be dynamically compensated for by other structures—especially since DLGG is known to favor neuroplastic remodeling [38, 68, 69]. This kind of interpretation may explain why patients displaying unilateral damage to the ATL (e.g., following a vascular infarct or surgical resection for a tumor or epilepsy) show only mild to moderate impairments in semantic cognition [70], even if the ATL is thought to be critical for this function. It is most likely that both the left and right ATLs have critical roles in semantic memory and other language-related processes, and that this massive bilateral organization makes the semantic system more resistant to damage, as previously discussed [70, 71]. Indeed, the contralateral (undamaged) ATL may functionally compensate for the damaged ATL, a homotopic strategy that begins to be unveiled from functional or structural imaging works (e.g., [72]). In the event of bilateral damage to the ATL (as seen in neurodegenerative conditions), marked semantic disorders may arise. The same reasoning might apply to the ILF, which has dense cortical projections in the ATL.

In this context, Herbet et al. [50] reasoned that axonal stimulation of the anterior-to-middle part of the left ILF should induce language or semantic difficulties only when the temporal pole is not damaged by the tumor. Otherwise, no impairment should be observed for the reasons evoked above. The results obtained have substantiated this hypothesis, by showing that stimulation of the left ILF was systematically associated with pure anomia in the first scenario (semantic or phonological paraphasia was never induced), whereas no particular responses were observed in the second one. Semantic paraphasia was uniquely observed by stimulation of the IFOF, and phonological paraphasia by stimulation of the AF. As well as confirming that the left ILF is involved in lexical retrieval (see [46]), this finding suggests that the information broadcasted by this tract can be rerouted along alternative pathways when progressive tumor infiltration of the temporal pole prompts the latter to abandon its function via progressive functional compensation.

To resume, electrostimulation mapping has allowed to identify the left ILF as a keystone of the lexical retrieval network. Interestingly, stimulation of the ILF in the right hemisphere in left-handers is able to reproduce the same impairment that stimulation of left ILF does (Fig. 5.4).

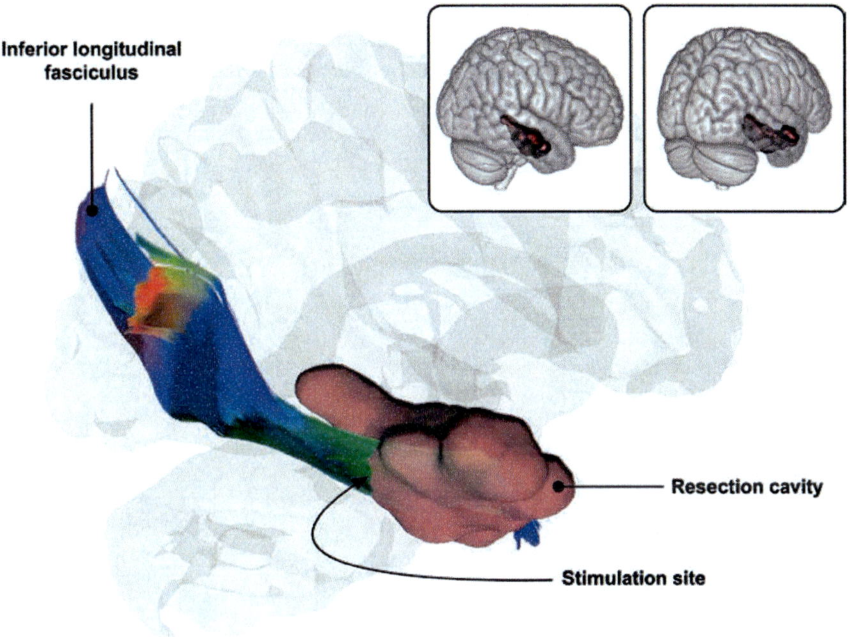

Fig. 5.4 A left-hander patient in whom pure anomia was induced by stimulating the right inferior longitudinal fasciculus. The patient's 3-month postoperative MRI was co-registered with the MNI151 template using SPM12 (https://www.fil.ion.ucl.ac.uk/spm). Then the resection cavity was mapped semi-automatically with MRIcron software. For illustrative purpose, the right inferior longitudinal fasciculus was tracked from the HCP1021 dataset (https://www.humanconnectome.org) and further overlaid with the reconstructed resection cavity onto a 3D iso-surface rendering using DSI studio (http://dsi-studio.labsolver.org/)

5.7 Conclusion

Word retrieval is core in language processing and engages a number of subprocesses involving a complex cortico-subcortical network. It should then be mapped thoroughly whatever the location of the DLGG, with a special attention paid to the most posterior part of the inferior temporal gyrus along with the inferior longitudinal fasciculus. Word retrieval ability is traditionally assessed by means of a picture naming task which is perfectly suited to intraoperative time constraints, while enabling to detect transient impairments in each subcomponent of lexical processing induced by direct electrical stimulation. However, in order to draw relevant analyses of intraoperative impairments, this task should be administered according to a rigorous methodology and be coupled with other tasks, especially semantic and phonological ones. Further dedicated longitudinal studies are undoubtedly needed to improve intraoperative monitoring of word retrieval, especially in terms of task specificity, in order to move towards an optimized and sound-designed strategy for intraoperative mapping of this ability guided by the onco-functional balance, that is, allowing to maximize the extent of DLGG resection while preserving patients quality of life by avoiding long-lasting debilitating word retrieval impairments.

References

1. Caramazza A. How many levels of processing are there in lexical access? Cogn Neuropsychol. 1997;14(1):177–208.
2. Levelt WJ. Models of word production. Trends Cogn Sci. 1999;3(6):223–32.
3. Benson DF, Davis RJ, Snyder BD. Posterior cortical atrophy. Arch Neurol. 1988;45(7):789–93.
4. Goodglass H, Wingfield A. Anomia: neuroanatomical and cognitive correlates. San Diego: Academic; 1997.
5. Price CJ. A review and synthesis of the first 20 years of PET and fMRI studies of heard speech, spoken language and reading. Neuroimage. 2012;62:816–47.
6. Damasio H, Grabowski T, Tranel D, Hichwa RD, Damasio AR. A neural basis for lexical retrieval. Nature. 1996;380:499–505.
7. Alario F-X, Chainay H, Lehericy S, Cohen L. The role of the supplementary motor area (SMA) in word production. Brain Res. 2006;1076(1):129–43.
8. Baldo JV, Arévalo A, Patterson JP, Dronkers NF. Grey and white matter correlates of picture naming: evidence from a voxel-based lesion analysis of the Boston Naming Test. Cortex. 2013;49(3):658–67.
9. DeLeon J, Gottesman RF, Kleinman JT, Newhart M, Davis C, Heidler-Gary J, et al. Neural regions essential for distinct cognitive processes underlying picture naming. Brain. 2007;130(5):1408–22.
10. Foundas AL, Daniels SK, Vasterling JJ. Anomia: case studies with lesion localization. Neurocase. 1998;4(1):35–43.
11. Gleichgerrcht E, Fridriksson J, Bonilha L. Neuroanatomical foundations of naming impairments across different neurologic conditions. Neurology. 2015;85(3):284–92.
12. Moore CJ, Price CJ. Three distinct ventral occipitotemporal regions for reading and object naming. Neuroimage. 1999;10(2):181–92.
13. Murtha S, Chertkow H, Beauregard M, Evans A. The neural substrate of picture naming. J Cogn Neurosci. 1999;11(4):399–423.
14. Piai V, Roelofs A, Jensen O, Schoffelen J-M, Bonnefond M. Distinct patterns of brain activity characterise lexical activation and competition in spoken word production. PLoS One. 2014;9(2):e88674.
15. Schnur TT, Schwartz MF, Kimberg DY, Hirshorn E, Coslett HB, Thompson-Schill SL. Localizing interference during naming: convergent neuroimaging and neuropsychological evidence for the function of Broca's area. Proc Natl Acad Sci. 2009;106(1):322–7.
16. Hickok G, Poeppel D. Dorsal and ventral streams: a framework for understanding aspects of the functional anatomy of language. Cognition. 2004;92(1–2):67–99.
17. Duffau H, Moritz-Gasser S, Mandonnet E. A re-examination of neural basis of language processing: proposal of a dynamic hodotopical model from data provided by brain stimulation mapping during picture naming. Brain Lang. 2014;131:1–10.
18. Han Z, Ma Y, Gong G, He Y, Caramazza A, Bi Y. White matter structural connectivity underlying semantic processing: evidence from brain damaged patients. Brain. 2013;136(10):2952–65.
19. Hope TM, Seghier ML, Prejawa S, Leff AP, Price CJ. Distinguishing the effect of lesion load from tract disconnection in the arcuate and uncinate fasciculi. Neuroimage. 2016;125:1169–73.

20. Mehta S, Inoue K, Rudrauf D, Damasio H, Tranel D, Grabowski T. Segregation of anterior temporal regions critical for retrieving names of unique and non-unique entities reflects underlying long-range connectivity. Cortex. 2016;75:1–19.
21. Tremblay P, Dick AS. Broca and Wernicke are dead, or moving past the classic model of language neurobiology. Brain Lang. 2016;162:60–71.
22. McKinnon ET, Fridriksson J, Basilakos A, Hickok G, Hillis AE, Spampinato MV, et al. Types of naming errors in chronic post-stroke aphasia are dissociated by dual stream axonal loss. Sci Rep. 2018;8(1):1–12.
23. Bookheimer S. Functional MRI of language: new approaches to understanding the cortical organization of semantic processing. Annu Rev Neurosci. 2002;25(1):151–88.
24. Vigneau M, Beaucousin V, Hervé P-Y, Jobard G, Petit L, Crivello F, et al. What is right-hemisphere contribution to phonological, lexico-semantic, and sentence processing?: insights from a meta-analysis. Neuroimage. 2011;54(1):577–93.
25. Bell B, Hermann B, Woodard A, Jones J, Rutecki P, Sheth R, et al. Object naming and semantic knowledge in temporal lobe epilepsy. Neuropsychology. 2001;15(4):434–43.
26. Riès SK, Dronkers NF, Knight RT. Choosing words: left hemisphere, right hemisphere, or both? Perspective on the lateralization of word retrieval. Ann N Y Acad Sci. 2016;1369(1):111.
27. Vartanian O, Goel V. Task constraints modulate activation in right ventral lateral prefrontal cortex. Neuroimage. 2005;27(4):927–33.
28. Duffau H, Gatignol P, Mandonnet E, Peruzzi P, Tzourio-Mazoyer N, Capelle L. New insights into the anatomo-functional connectivity of the semantic system: a study using cortico-subcortical electrostimulations. Brain. 2005;128(4):797–810.
29. De Witt Hamer PC, Moritz-Gasser S, Gatignol P, Duffau H. Is the human left middle longitudinal fascicle essential for language? A brain electrostimulation study. Hum Brain Mapp. 2011;32(6):962–73.
30. Sherman EM, Wiebe S, Fay-McClymont TB, Tellez-Zenteno J, Metcalfe A, Hernandez-Ronquillo L, et al. Neuropsychological outcomes after epilepsy surgery: systematic review and pooled estimates. Epilepsia. 2011;52(5):857–69.
31. Sabsevitz DS, Swanson SJ, Hammeke TA, Spanaki MV, Possing ET, Morris GL, et al. Use of preoperative functional neuroimaging to predict language deficits from epilepsy surgery. Neurology. 2003;60(11):1788–92.
32. Binder JR, Tong J-Q, Pillay SB, Conant LL, Humphries CJ, Raghavan M, et al. Temporal lobe regions essential for preserved picture naming after left temporal epilepsy surgery. Epilepsia. 2020;61(9):1939–48.
33. Trimmel K, van Graan LA, Gonzálvez GG, Haag A, Caciagli L, Vos SB, et al. Naming fMRI predicts the effect of temporal lobe resection on language decline. Ann Clin Transl Neurol. 2019;6(11):2186–96.
34. Duffau H. Surgery of low-grade gliomas: towards a 'functional neurooncology'. Curr Opin Oncol. 2009;21(6):543–9.
35. Sanai N, Berger MS. Glioma extent of resection and its impact on patient outcome. Neurosurgery. 2008;62(4):753–66.
36. Soffietti R, Baumert BG, Bello L, Von Deimling A, Duffau H, Frénay M, et al. Guidelines on management of low-grade gliomas: report of an EFNS–EANO* Task Force. Eur J Neurol. 2010;17(9):1124–33.
37. Duffau H. Contribution of cortical and subcortical electrostimulation in brain glioma surgery: methodological and functional considerations. Neurophysiol Clin. 2007;37(6):373–82.
38. Duffau H. Intraoperative cortico–subcortical stimulations in surgery of low-grade gliomas. Expert Rev Neurother. 2005;5(4):473–85.
39. Duffau H, Capelle L, Sichez N, Denvil D, Lopes M, Sichez J-P, et al. Intraoperative mapping of the subcortical language pathways using direct stimulations: an anatomo-functional study. Brain. 2002;125(1):199–214.

40. Almairac F, Herbet G, Moritz-Gasser S, de Champfleur NM, Duffau H. The left inferior fronto-occipital fasciculus subserves language semantics: a multilevel lesion study. Brain Struct Funct. 2015;220(4):1983–95.
41. Antonsson M, Longoni F, Jakola A, Tisell M, Thordstein M, Hartelius L. Pre-operative language ability in patients with presumed low-grade glioma. J Neurooncol. 2018;137(1): 93–102.
42. Banerjee P, Leu K, Harris RJ, Cloughesy TF, Lai A, Nghiemphu PL, et al. Association between lesion location and language function in adult glioma using voxel-based lesion-symptom mapping. NeuroImage Clin. 2015;9:617–24.
43. Sierpowska J, Gabarrós A, Fernández-Coello A, Camins À, Castañer S, Juncadella M, et al. White-matter pathways and semantic processing: intrasurgical and lesion-symptom mapping evidence. NeuroImage Clin. 2019;22:101704.
44. Teixidor P, Gatignol P, Leroy M, Masuet-Aumatell C, Capelle L, Duffau H. Assessment of verbal working memory before and after surgery for low-grade glioma. J Neurooncol. 2007;81(3):305–13.
45. Wilson SM, Lam D, Babiak MC, Perry DW, Shih T, Hess CP, et al. Transient aphasias after left hemisphere resective surgery. J Neurosurg. 2015;123(3):581–93.
46. Herbet G, Moritz-Gasser S, Boiseau M, Duvaux S, Cochereau J, Duffau H. Converging evidence for a cortico-subcortical network mediating lexical retrieval. Brain. 2016b;139(11):3007–21.
47. Mandonnet E, Gatignol P, Duffau H. Evidence for an occipito-temporal tract underlying visual recognition in picture naming. Clin Neurol Neurosurg. 2009;111(7):601–5.
48. Palejwala AH, O'Connor KP, Milton CK, Anderson C, Pelargos P, Briggs RG, et al. Anatomy and white matter connections of the fusiform gyrus. Sci Rep. 2020;10(1):1–12.
49. Lin Y-H, Young IM, Conner AK, Glenn CA, Chakraborty AR, Nix CE, et al. Anatomy and white matter connections of the inferior temporal gyrus. World Neurosurg. 2020;143:e656–66.
50. Herbet G, Moritz-Gasser S, Lemaitre A-L, Almairac F, Duffau H. Functional compensation of the left inferior longitudinal fasciculus for picture naming. Cogn Neuropsychol. 2019;36(3–4):140–57.
51. Metz-Lutz MN. Standardisation d'un test de denomination orale: controle des effects de l'age, du sexe et du niveau de scolarite chez des sujets adultes normaux. Rev Neuropsychol. 1991;1:73–95.
52. Mandonnet E, Sarubbo S, Duffau H. Proposal of an optimized strategy for intraoperative testing of speech and language during awake mapping. Neurosurg Rev. 2017;40(1):29–35.
53. Howard D, Patterson K. The Pyramids and Palm Trees Test: a test of semantic access from words and pictures. Pearson Assessment; 1992.
54. Lubrano V, Filleron T, Démonet J-F, Roux F-E. Anatomical correlates for category-specific naming of objects and actions: a brain stimulation mapping study. Hum Brain Mapp. 2014;35(2):429–43.
55. Rofes A, Miceli G. Language mapping with verbs and sentences in awake surgery: a review. Neuropsychol Rev. 2014;24(2):185–99.
56. Hamberger MJ, Goodman RR, Perrine K, Tamny T. Anatomic dissociation of auditory and visual naming in the lateral temporal cortex. Neurology. 2001;56(1):56–61.
57. Malow BA, Blaxton TA, Sato S, Bookheimer SY, Kufta CV, Figlozzi CM, et al. Cortical stimulation elicits regional distinctions in auditory and visual naming. Epilepsia. 1996;37(3):245–52.
58. Giussani C, Roux F-E, Bello L, Lauwers-Cances V, Papagno C, Gaini SM, et al. Who is who: areas of the brain associated with recognizing and naming famous faces. J Neurosurg. 2009;110(2):289–99.
59. Papagno C, Miracapillo C, Casarotti A, Romero Lauro LJ, Castellano A, Falini A, et al. What is the role of the uncinate fasciculus? Surgical removal and proper name retrieval. Brain. 2011;134(2):405–14.
60. Rofes A, de Aguiar V, Miceli G. A minimal standardization setting for language mapping tests: an Italian example. Neurol Sci. 2015;36(7):1113–9.
61. Papagno C, Casarotti A, Comi A, Pisoni A, Lucchelli F, Bizzi A, et al. Long-term proper name anomia after removal of the uncinate fasciculus. Brain Struct Funct. 2016;221(1):687–94.

62. Mandonnet E, Herbet G, Duffau H. Letter: Introducing New Tasks for Intraoperative Mapping in Awake Glioma Surgery: Clearing the Line Between Patient Care and Scientific Research. Neurosurgery. 2020;86(2):E256–57.
63. Rofes A, Mandonnet E, de Aguiar V, Rapp B, Tsapkini K, Miceli G. Language processing from the perspective of electrical stimulation mapping. Cogn Neuropsychol. 2019;36(3–4):117–39.
64. Duffau H, Mandonnet E. The "onco-functional balance" in surgery for diffuse low-grade glioma: integrating the extent of resection with quality of life. Acta Neurochir. 2013;155(6):951–7.
65. Herbet G, Moritz-Gasser S, Duffau H. Direct evidence for the contributive role of the right inferior fronto-occipital fasciculus in non-verbal semantic cognition. Brain Struct Funct. 2017;222(4):1597–610.
66. Moritz-Gasser S, Duffau H. The anatomo-functional connectivity of word repetition: insights provided by awake brain tumor surgery. Front Hum Neurosci. 2013;7:405.
67. Duffau H, Capelle L. Preferential brain locations of low-grade gliomas: comparison with glioblastomas and review of hypothesis. Cancer. 2004;100(12):2622–6.
68. Mandonnet E, Nouet A, Gatignol P, Capelle L, Duffau H. Does the left inferior longitudinal fasciculus play a role in language? A brain stimulation study. Brain. 2007;130(3):623–9.
69. Herbet G, Maheu M, Costi E, Lafargue G, Duffau H. Mapping neuroplastic potential in brain-damaged patients. Brain. 2016a;139(3):829–44.
70. Lambon Ralph MA, Cipolotti L, Manes F, Patterson K. Taking both sides: do unilateral anterior temporal lobe lesions disrupt semantic memory? Brain. 2010;133(11):3243–55.
71. Rice GE, Hoffman P, Ralph MAL. Graded specialization within and between the anterior temporal lobes. Ann N Y Acad Sci. 2015;1359(1):84.
72. Almairac F, Duffau H, Herbet G. Contralesional macrostructural plasticity of the insular cortex in patients with glioma: A VBM study. Neurology. 2018;91(20):e1902–08.

Spontaneous Speech

6

Djaina Satoer, Elke De Witte, and Olga Dragoy

6.1 Review: Neural Basis of Spontaneous Speech

Spontaneous speech (also called propositional speech or conversational speech) production is a complex process by which thoughts must be translated into formulated messages, syntactic frames are to be constructed with access to lexical items (harboring grammatical properties), phonological encoding and finally articulation has to be executed [1, 2]. Fillmore [3] described such a multifaceted process as "the ability to fill time with talk" (p. 93), which incorporates all stages of the expression of a speaker's idea in a fluent and coherent way by the appropriate use of lexical and grammatical devices. Spontaneous speech is a prominent faculty for a person's daily life. Thus, the importance to evaluate this component of language—the closest one to ecological conditions—peri-operatively cannot be overemphasized.

In aphasiology literature, aphasia with a specific impairment of spontaneous speech (with mostly spared naming, comprehension and repetition) is commonly referred to as "transcortical motor aphasia." This term has been introduced by Lichtheim [4], in order to describe the effects of a disconnection between the "concepts center" and the "motor center." Transcortical motor aphasia is typically observed in lesions located to the supplementary motor area (SMA) [5, 6]. Later on, Luria [7, 8] coined the term "dynamic aphasia," which pattern resembles transcortical motor aphasia, but has distinctive features, like the fact that the patient does not

D. Satoer (✉) · E. De Witte
Department of Neurosurgery, Erasmus MC—University Medical Center Rotterdam, Rotterdam, The Netherlands
e-mail: d.satoer@erasmusmc.nl

O. Dragoy
Center for Language and Brain, National Research University Higher School of Economics, Moscow, Russia
e-mail: odragoy@hse.ru

E. Mandonnet, G. Herbet (eds.), *Intraoperative Mapping of Cognitive Networks*,
https://doi.org/10.1007/978-3-030-75071-8_6

initiate to communicate (see Ardila and Lopez [9] for full list of differences between the two patterns). Luria interpreted this pattern as a failure of the transitional stage (i.e., an early stage of verbal planning), translating the "internal speech" into the linear scheme of the sentence (see also Costello and Warrington [10]). An alternative explanation viewed this syndrome as an inability to select a unique response in "open" situations, in which one out of many possible verbal responses has to be selected [11]. This type of aphasia is associated with left prefrontal dorso-lateral damage and was mostly described in the context of neurodegenerative diseases or stroke injury. The underlying mechanism of dynamic aphasia has been associated with a language specific impairment or with a more general impairment of the executive functions [12, 13]. Apart from the "classical" left hemispheric involvement in language production, there are also studies in which spontaneous speech was affected after right hemispheric damage [14, 15].

Specific microstructural linguistic aspects involved in expressive language (e.g., lexical retrieval, morphological marking, phonological encoding) are vastly distributed across various brain regions beyond the classic "Broca" and "Wernicke's areas" [16]. In addition, spontaneous speech features with fluent propositional output are also associated with the critical involvement of the left frontal/insular cortex and its white matter connections. Available lesion studies showed that cortical atrophy in the posterior inferior and middle frontal gyri correlated with reduced speech fluency, and stroke lesions in the anterior insula predicted low scores on a conversational speech metric such as the mean length of utterance—a reliable proxy for overall speech fluency [17, 18]. Wilson et al. [19] related reduced speech rate to the atrophy of both anterior (the inferior frontal and ventral precentral gyri and the SMA) and posterior cortices (the posterior superior temporal gyrus and the supramarginal gyrus), but exclusively associated articulatory agility and syntactic structure and complexity with damage to the frontal regions. Brain tumor resection in the frontal medial lobe in proximity of the SMA was also characterized by problems in propositional speech with (relatively) intact naming, repetition, and comprehension, especially in the acute postoperative stage [5, 20–22]. A central white matter structure, whose damage is consistently related to verbal fluency reduction, is the left frontal aslant tract (FAT; [23]). In individuals with post-stroke aphasia [24, 25] and primary progressive aphasia [26, 27], metrics of the FAT's integrity correlated with spontaneous speech scores, based on various verbal fluency ratings. In individuals with brain tumors, postoperative spontaneous speech fluency scores correlated with the distance between the left FAT and the resection cavity [28] and were found impaired in a case of disconnection between the posterior inferior frontal gyrus and the pre-SMA through the FAT [29]. Similarly, Dragoy et al. [30] suggested that the most consistent and prominent language deficit caused by fast-growing high-grade tumors and/or a resection in proximity of the FAT occurs at the level of discourse—that is, affecting genuine spontaneous speech.

There are mixed results about the added value of applying direct electrical stimulation (DES) near the SMA/FAT, as a large number of studies demonstrate no positively identified sites (during naming/counting) [21, 31–33]. This can be explained by the fact that the SMA can be divided into two parts, the pre-SMA and the

SMA-proper related to the common motor (speech) output system and the planning of the encoding of a linear utterance, respectively—that is, a parallel organization in the lateral frontal cortex [34]. As a result, a dissociation can be found between a purely motoric speech dysfunction where the patient is completely mute and an isolated dysfunction of spontaneous speech with intact naming, which might occur at a more “sentence planning” level. In line with this reasoning, Corrivetti et al. [35] found a difference between lexico-semantic errors and motor–speech disturbances, both at the cortical and axonal levels. They interpreted these findings as two separate language subsystems in the frontal lobe with an anterior part involved in lexico-semantic processing, and a posterior part involved in motor–speech aspects of language. Hence the used tasks may have chosen inadequately for the location in question and therefore could have been not sensitive enough for the brain location explaining negative mapping results. With application of a more specific language task, such as sentence generation, Chernoff et al. [36] found that the FAT was a key component of an interface positing a process where grammatical specifications realized as a “surface form” (see more detailed discussion in Sect. 6.2).

6.2 Intraoperative Tasks to Monitor Spontaneous Speech

Awake surgery with DES is considered the gold standard method for treatment of gliomas in language eloquent brain areas [37]. The goal is to maximize tumor resection while preserving sensori-motor, language, and other cognitive functions, and hence quality of life. The most commonly used task during cortico-subcortical stimulation to detect language functions is object naming [38]. Via electrical stimulation, speech arrests and other language errors, such as anomias, paraphasias (phonological, semantic), neologisms, and perseverations, can be elicited to draw an individual functional cartography. This serves as a guideline for the neurosurgeon to tailor the surgical route for tumor resection and to detect the functional boundaries defining the end of resection. Since cortical stimulation cannot last more than 4 s, all language tasks should ideally be performed within this time frame. Object naming and word repetition are perfectly suitable within 4 s. However, certain tasks measuring other important language aspects such as sentence judgment tasks (language perception) are not feasible within this time frame. Since these tasks provide valuable information, they are often used during resection in between stimulations [39].

Although spontaneous speech is the most salient and ecologically valid way to measure language abilities, it is not often reported to be structurally monitored during awake surgeries. In Satoer et al. [40] they mentioned that during the tumor resection, besides repetition and naming, also the spontaneous speech of patients was monitored by a linguist. Topics of discussion were mainly autobiographic (as agreed on with the patient preoperatively). The linguist checked whether the patient was still able to speak fluently and whether he/she was able to start a conversation. In case of change of the quality of the spontaneous speech (e.g., word finding problems or paraphasias), more specific language production or comprehension tasks focusing on specific linguistic levels (e.g., phonology, semantics, syntax) were selected to control more adequately for language disturbances. Hence, spontaneous speech was used as a guideline throughout the resection (e.g., with the occurrence of phonological paraphasias during resection, a word repetition task is selected to evaluate more specifically the level of phonological deterioration). Unfortunately, correlations between intraoperative findings (language deterioration and the occurrence of paraphasias) and postoperative language outcome were not investigated.

De Witte et al. [41] also underlined spontaneous speech monitoring in addition to standardized tasks during the awake procedure. In one case with a temporo-parietal tumor, no positive sites were found at the subcortical level during object naming and reading. However, auditory comprehension deficits occurred (auditory instructions could not be followed), as identified during spontaneous speech monitoring, which served as a resection boundary. A dissociation between spontaneous speech and object naming during the course of the resection was also found in a 71-year-old right-handed lady operated at the Lariboisière Hospital (E. Mandonnet, personal communication, September 1, 2020) for a glioblastoma in the caudal part of the left superior frontal gyrus, see Figs. 6.1 and 6.2.

In the course of the resection, this patient stopped producing spontaneous speech, despite intact object naming. In the immediate postoperative period, spontaneous speech was severely impaired, but at the 4-months follow-up evaluation, no language deficits were detected. However, no detailed spontaneous speech analyses or other specific semi-spontaneous speech tasks were conducted (see also Sect. 6.4 with a description of patient K.O. by Satoer et al. [42] for a dissociation between isolated language functions and spontaneous speech).

Apart from monitoring "pure" spontaneous speech, it is also possible to use language tasks at the sentence level in order to elicit a so-called "spontaneous speech in context." In 1979, Ojemann and Mateer [43] already described application of a sentence completion task in addition to object naming. They found a dissociation

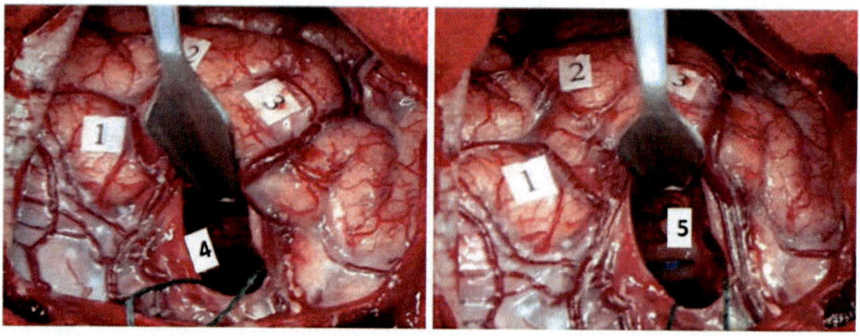

Fig. 6.1 Cortical mapping evidenced three positive sites: (1) wrist motor area, (2) face motor area, (3) anomia. Two sites were identified in the white matter (respectively on the left and right part of the figure): (4) complete motor arrest in the posterior wall (i.e., stopping both superior limb movement and counting) and (5) anomia in the lateral wall

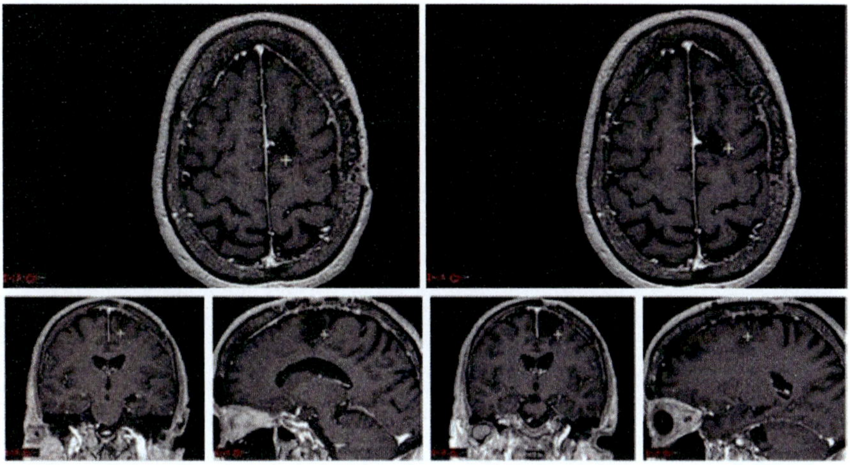

Fig. 6.2 Postoperative MRI. The yellow cross locates tag 4 on the left and tag 5 on the right

between grammatical sentence production in the sentence completion task and word retrieval during naming. A systematic review by Zanin et al. [44] investigated the application of tasks at the sentence level. They divided their results into three different groups: (1) studies that overtly assessed morpho-syntactic processes, (2) studies that did not focus overtly on syntactic processes, but their stimuli required clear morpho-syntactic processing, and (3) studies that did not overtly focused on syntactic processes, and their stimuli did not structurally elicited morpho-syntactic processing. They found that the administration of "real" syntactic tasks during the awake procedure is scarce (see Chap. 10), as most studies applied morpho-syntactic tasks (e.g., action naming at the word level). The clearest task that tapped into propositional syntactic processes not restricted to the word level appeared to be sentence completion and generation [30, 36, 41, 45].

Sentence completion (closed and broad context) was first added as a task to the Dutch Linguistic Intraoperative Protocol (DuLIP) [39] to assess language functions pre-, intra-, and postoperatively to measure language dynamics/spontaneous speech in context. In both the "closed context" sentence completion task and "broad context" sentence completion task patients were asked to read sentences out loud and complete them in a meaningful way. In the "closed context version" the patient only needed to complete the sentence with one or two words, e.g., "De bakker verkoopt … - brood" (The baker sells … - bread). This closed version can be used during cortical stimulation where the time for reading and completing the sentence is limited to 4 s. In the "broad context" version a phrase/constituent instead of a single word has to be added and the sentence has to be grammatically correct (with conjugated verbs and correct word order). For example, "Om 5 uur …. -rijdt de buurman naar zijn werk" (At 5 O'clock …. - the neighbor drives to his work) is a correct answer. In this task, the sentences do not strongly trigger a particular semantic response but allow a diversity of answers. The broad context sentence completion can also be performed during subcortical stimulation and resection. In a selection of left glioma patients ($N = 4$) from the cohort of De Witte et al. [46], the sentence completion task was used intraoperatively. Positive sites were found in all cases during intraoperative stimulation which served as a resection boundary. In two cases with a tumor located in the left SMA area, a sentence completion and an object naming task were used intraoperatively. A task dissociation was found, meaning that these patients were able to name the object during DES in the SMA area whereas they were not able to complete the sentence.

Other tasks at the sentence level have also been developed and applied during surgery. Chernoff et al. [36] described a case in which elicitation of sentences by means of various presentations of geometrical forms in colors ("the red square is above the green circle," "the two black triangles are below the blue square") was used in addition to object naming during DES of the FAT. In the sentence generation paradigm during DES versus no DES they found an effect of accuracy (patient produced an incorrect preposition—e.g., "above" instead of "below," or incorrect geometric shape—e.g., "circle" instead of "square," or speech arrests) and an effect of latency on sentence position (but not articulation time of individual words), e.g., Noun Phrase, Verb Phrase, Noun Phrase, and word within that position only at the beginning (e.g., "the" or "a"). Unfortunately, a comparison with object naming was not further discussed. Ries et al. [45] applied a sentence generation task in comparison to a word picture inference paradigm during DES. More errors were elicited during the sentence generation task in the dorsal steam, whereas the word picture interference task was more sensitive in the ventral stream. However, a discussion of the sentence generation task in comparison to object naming was not provided.

Recently, Dragoy et al. [30] suggested that sentence completion in closed context and picture-based sentence generation or that with pre-learnt lexical items [36] are suboptimal for intraoperative mapping of spontaneous speech fluency. They used a sentence completion task in a semi-broad context (e.g., "A piggy is chewing… - grass") in comparison to action naming with a sentence ("Here, s/he is … - singing") and found a task dissociation in the majority of patients. Patients were able to name the action during DES of the cortical terminations of left FAT in the inferior frontal gyrus and (pre-)SMA, whereas they were not able to come up with an appropriate sentence completion (but could read aloud the given context), see Fig. 6.3 for an illustration of this dissociation (patients 1 and 5 from Dragoy et al. [30]).

The authors explained the effect by the active context-relevant conceptual planning, lexical access, and syntactic sequencing involved in broad-context sentence completion, but not in the control action naming task. As shown, the latter was significantly less sensitive to FAT mapping and resulted in numerous obvious false negatives. Thus, it was proposed that contexts with less constrained completion are more optimal to map the brain substrate of genuine propositional spontaneous speech.

In summary, there is no gold standard about which task to use at the sentence level during the awake procedure as a proxy to spontaneous speech production. Most studies still apply morpho-syntactic tasks, which assess syntactic abilities

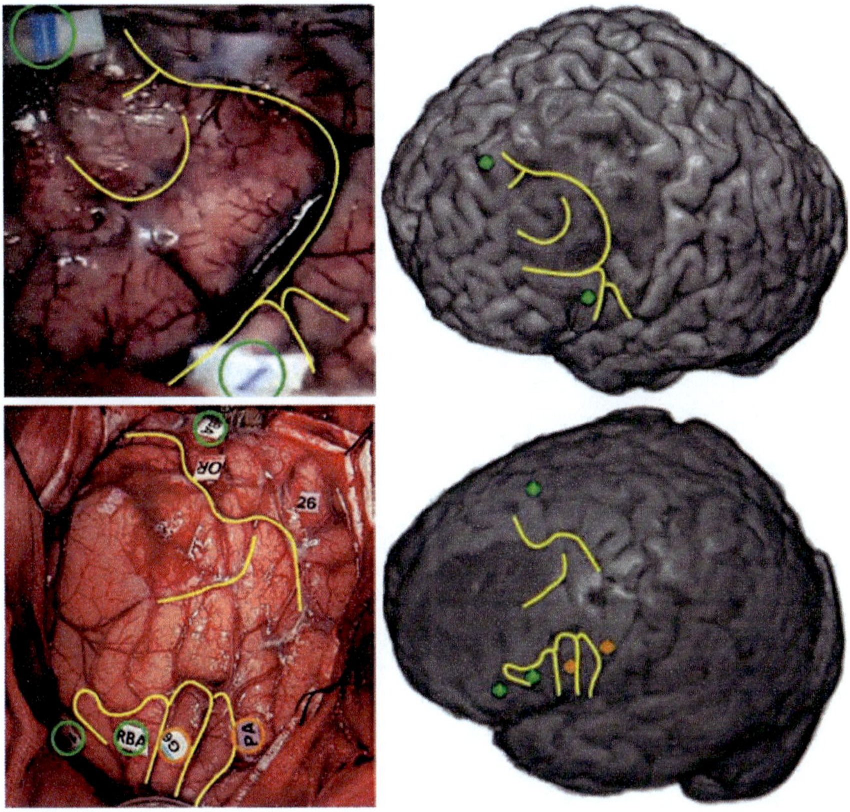

Fig. 6.3 Dissociation sentence completion and action naming. Patient 1 (left) and patient 5 (right). Green circles represent positive sites responsive to sentence completion only with spared action naming, orange dots represent positive sites responsive to sentence completion and action naming. (From Dragoy et al. [30], with permission)

only at the word level. However, there is growing evidence that sentence completion in a broad context seems to be a good alternative to monitor spontaneous speech abilities; long-term follow-up studies are needed to prove its value for language outcome.

6.3 Postoperative Deficits of Spontaneous Speech in Glioma Patients

Surprisingly, relatively few studies thoroughly investigated long-lasting spontaneous speech deficits in glioma patients (see Table 6.1 for an extensive peri-operative literature overview). Satoer et al. [52] first reported complaints of spontaneous speech at the evaluation performed 3 months after surgery. The quality of verbal

Table 6.1 Overview of studies with peri-operative spontaneous speech monitoring/tests

Study	N	Intraoperative spontaneous speech/test	Cortical positive sites	Subcortical positive sites/ resection	Short-term language outcome	Long-term language outcome	Conclusion
Dragoy et al. [30]	12	Action naming	SFG, MFG	AF	6/12 pts stable 4/12 pts declined 2/12 pts severely declined	3/12 fully recovered 3/12 pts selectively recovered 6/6 pts stable	Task dissociation in 10/12 pts with action naming vs sentence completion in left FAT
		Sentence completion	SFG, MFG	AF, FAT			
Chivukula et al. [47]	2	Spontaneous speech	No details	SMA	Pt 1: mute Pt 2: reduced spontaneous speech	Both pts recovered	SMA syndrome with loss of fluency with full recovery at long-term
Satoer et al. [48]	18	Object naming	No details	Eloquent areas	Stable in spontaneous speech and at test-level	Group level: 4/5 spontaneous speech variables deteriorate. Group level: stable at test-level	Surgery with spontaneous speech monitoring appeared to have deteriorated quality of daily speech only at long-term. Spontaneous speech has added value to standardized language tests
		Repetition	No details	No details			
		Spontaneous speech	No details	No details			

Study	N	Intraoperative spontaneous speech/test	Cortical positive sites	Subcortical positive sites/ resection	Short-term language outcome	Long-term language outcome	Conclusion
Satoer et al. [49]	4	Object naming			Pt 3: stable Pt 4: decline in repetition	Pt 3: stable Pt 4: improved to normal	After detection of perseverations during subcortical resection both decline and stability of language functions at short-term postoperatively is possible. Long-term recovery was observed
		Repetition					
		DuLIP tasks					
		Spontaneous speech		P3 and P4 near AF			
De Witte et al. [41]	3	Counting			3/3 pts deteriorated	2/3 pts recovered	Use of multimodal tests and spontaneous speech is necessary to identify specific language eloquent areas to avoid permanent aphasia
		Object naming	L temporo-parietal, L fronto-temporal, L parieto-occipital	L IFOF			
		DuLIP sentence completion[a]		L AF, SLF			
		Spontaneous speech		Subcortical area L temporo-parietal			

(continued)

Table 6.1 (continued)

Study	*N*	Intraoperative spontaneous speech/test	Cortical positive sites	Subcortical positive sites/ resection	Short-term language outcome	Long-term language outcome	Conclusion
De Witte et al. [39]	5	DuLIP tasks			Pt 1: stable Pt 2: decline Pt 3: dynamic aphasia Pt 4: severely declined Pt 5: declined	Pt 1: stable Pt 2: recovered Pt 3: recovered Pt 4: mild decline Pt 5: recovered	Intraoperative language task selection must be patient-tailored according to language level and tumor location. Surgery induced short-term decline with almost full recovery at long-term
		– Repetition	IFG	AF, CST			
		– Object naming	ant. MTG, ITG				
		– Action naming	IFG				
		– Semantic odd picture out	AG, SMG	IFOF			
		– Sentence completion	SMA	IFOF, SLF			
Satoer et al. [40]	1	Object naming	No	No	Decline in spontaneous speech	Slight decline in spontaneous speech	Intraoperative spontaneous speech monitoring was more sensitive than standard language tasks near SMA
		Repetition	No	No			
		Spontaneous speech	No	SMA			
Satoer et al. [40]	27	Object naming	No details	Eloquent areas	Group level: stable in spontaneous speech and at test-level	n/a	Spontaneous speech analyses are an addition to formal language tests to detect deviancies in speech
		Repetition	No details	No details			
		Spontaneous speech	No details	No details			
Ries et al. [45]	17	Sentence generation	Dorsal region	Dorsal region	n/a	n/a	Dorsal regions are critical for organizing words in a sequence and ventral regions are critical for processing semantic dependencies
		Word picture interface	Ventral region	Ventral region			

Study	*N*	Intraoperative spontaneous speech/test	Cortical positive sites	Subcortical positive sites/ resection	Short-term language outcome	Long-term language outcome	Conclusion
Chernoff et al. [36]	1	Object naming	No details	No details	n/a	n/a	Latency effect at the onset of a grammatical boundary was found in FAT
		Sentence generation	No details	FAT			
Chang et al. [69]	14	Counting	(other?)	n/a	n/a	n/a	Dissociation of **syntactic errors** during sentence production task in IFG in comparison to counting, naming, and repetition. Specification of intraoperative errors appears to be necessary
		Object naming	IFG, STG, MTG	n/a			
		Repetition	IFG, STG, MTG	n/a			
		Sentence production	IFG, STG	n/a			
Ojemann and Mateer [43]	4	Object naming	Perisylvian cortex	n/a	n/a	n/a	Dissociation between grammatical sentence production and word retrieval
		Sentence completion	IFG, post. STG	n/a			

(continued)

Table 6.1 (continued)

Study	*N*	Intraoperative spontaneous speech/test	Cortical positive sites	Subcortical positive sites/ resection	Short-term language outcome	Long-term language outcome	Conclusion
Rofes et al. [50]	5	n/a	n/a	n/a	All cases decline: – BADA – Spontaneous speech variables	Pt 1: decline both measures Pt 2: decline SS Pt 3: selected improvement test-level Pt 4: decline both measures Pt 5: selected recovery SS, selected decline test-level	Both measures are (selectively) sensitive to detect impairments/ decline in patients with left perisylvian tumors Full recovery/improvement at long-term was only observed in 1/5 pts
McCarron et al. [51]	43	n/a	n/a	n/a	Group level: decline – Boston Naming Test (short version) – 10/10 semi-spontaneous speech variables (Picnic scene Western Aphasia Battery)	Group level: improvement – 8/10 SS variables – Slight decline BNT	Both measures were sensitive to detect impairments in LH tumors short-term postoperatively with almost full recovery at long-term

n/a not administered, *IFG* Inferior Frontal Gyrus, *MTG* Middle Temporal Gyrus, *STG* Superior Temporal Gyrus, *SMA* Supplementary Motor Area, *AF* Arcuate Fasciculus, *IFOF* Inferior Fronto-Occipital Fasciculus, *SLF* Superior Longitudinal Fasciculus, *CST* Cortical Spinal Tract, *FAT* Frontal Aslan Tract, *LH* left hemisphere, *BADA* Batteria per l'Analisi dei Deficit Afasici

[a]As part of Quick Mixed Task

communication (based on a spontaneous speech sample of 10 min) was judged with the Aphasia Severity Rating Scale (ASRS) [53], a six-point scale varying from "0—no usable speech or auditory comprehension" to "5—minimal discernable speech handicap." Also, self-reports of language complaints during anamneses were collected. See Fragment 1 for illustration.

Fragment 1
Patient 79: "yes well, I guess everyone is looking for a word now and then, right? What, what, what was it again, but really a speech arrest I experienced that struck me, that was eh what I said, twice on the telephone and in particular that time when I was sitting at the pulmonologist, I really couldn't find the right words." (Satoer [54], page 15).

Both before and after surgery patients were rated with defective communication according to the ASRS scale 3 and 4, 9/23 and 11/21 patients, respectively. However, during anamnesis more patients complained about problems in daily conversational speech, 13/23 before operation and 13/21 after operation. Hence, more than half of the patients had word finding complaints in everyday communication pre- and postoperatively. A remarkable finding was that most of the patients with words finding complaints were scaled as having normal speech (scale 5) to a minimal discernible speech handicap (scale 4). However, it was not clear whereas there was a clear dissociation between the object naming score and the rating scale for spontaneous speech. Moreover, the level of recovery might have been hampered in patients with high-grade glioma (adjuvant treatment related morbidity or tumor continuous evolution) or in patients who did not benefit from intensive language rehabilitation. This finding suggested that word finding problems cannot always be objectified by existing standard language evaluations and needed more attention in the future, especially when surgery near speech areas has to be performed.

Therefore, a more detailed spontaneous speech analysis via transcriptions was conducted by Satoer et al. [40] and they found that glioma patients suffered from more incomplete sentences in their speech samples in comparison to healthy controls both pre- and postoperatively. After surgery, patients' mean utterance length was also shorter. It was argued that the underlying deficit could have been lexical (incomplete sentence with missing word) or syntactic (simplified/shorter phrase/utterance length or missing constituents in sentences). The majority of the spontaneous speech variables did not correlate with object naming and verbal fluency, standard language tests at the word level. An update study from the same group [48] found similar impairments in spontaneous speech variables, but no significant deterioration in spontaneous speech was found between the preoperative and the 3 months or 1 year postoperative evaluations, while a decline was demonstrated between 3 months and 1 year after surgery, suggesting once more that additional impact of the adjuvant treatments could have blurred the analysis. However, it is again remarkable that most spontaneous speech variables did not correlate with standardized tests, naming and verbal fluency, usually administered in glioma patients. These studies demonstrate that a spontaneous speech analysis seems to be more sensitive than "traditional" standardized language tests for the detection of more subtle long-term language deficits. However, transcription and analysis of spontaneous speech samples is a very time-consuming activity. Correlation analyses between incomplete sentence parameters in spontaneous speech and results from incomplete sentence tasks (closed and broad) may add to our understanding about the underlying mechanism (lexical or more syntactic problem) of their deviating daily speech.

On the other hand, Rofes et al. [50] reported a case series of glioma patients in which spontaneous speech and standardized language tasks were assessed preoperatively, and 1 week and 7 months postoperatively. Spontaneous speech analyses and standardized language tests appeared to be equally sensitive. However, the outcome of language functions was variable. The authors recommend spontaneous speech analyses for patients in which there is a restricted testing time or when the patients is too tired to undergo an entire test-battery, especially if automated speech analyses becomes more readily available (see also Nevler et al. [55]). A study by McCarron et al. [51] also found that both spontaneous speech analysis and a shortened naming test were equally sensitive to detect impairments. At short-term postoperatively a deterioration was found for both tasks followed by almost full recovery at long-term postoperatively. It has to be noted that the authors used a semi-spontaneous speech task (picture description) which could have been too "easy" to measure deviancies in comparison to patients' actual daily spontaneous speech.

In a cohort study of De Witte et al. [46] a selection of patients ($N = 24$) were assessed with sentence completion tasks which aims to assess spontaneous speech in context (closed and broad context, see also Sect. 6.3) preoperatively and at 6 weeks and 6 months postoperatively. At 6 weeks postoperatively performance on a sentence completion task (broad context) deteriorated while at 6 months postoperatively recovery to preoperative level was found. Although no long-term deficits were found, language dynamics were clearly impaired short-term after surgery. The authors state that similar to the recovery of other language tests at 6 months postoperatively, the language improvement during follow-up could be explained by brain reorganization mechanisms including functional compensation. On the other hand, a patient-reported questionnaire administered in 10 out of these 24 patients at 6 months postoperatively revealed that 3 out of 10 still complained of difficulties with finding the right words and initiating language although none of them showed language deficits in the test-scores. As in the studies by Satoer et al. [40, 48, 52] these findings underline the importance of sensitive language assessments, detailed spontaneous speech analyses, and self-reported language complaints.

6.4 Intraoperative Spontaneous Speech Monitoring: Long-Term Deficits or Benefits?

Studies in which both (detailed) intraoperative spontaneous speech monitoring and long-term language outcome are reported are scarce. The occurrence of a spontaneous speech disorder (dynamic aphasia) is often mentioned with spontaneous recovery within a few days or weeks [5]. However, the evaluation of the quality of spontaneous speech is almost always based on clinical observations without detailed linguistic analyses.

In the observational spontaneous speech studies by Satoer et al. [40, 48] no significant deterioration of the selected spontaneous speech variables compared to the preoperative level were found, suggesting that patients may have benefitted from the intraoperative procedure with spontaneous speech monitoring. Similarly, in a small selection of patients of the cohort of De Witte et al. [46] no long-term deficits were found in patients ($N = 4$) who were monitored with sentence completion during DES and spontaneous speech monitoring intraoperatively.

In a case report of Satoer et al. [42], K.O. was treated for a glioma near the SMA. During awake craniotomy, typically no positive stimulation sites were found in the region of resection. At the end of the resection, K.O. developed a strong reduction of the spontaneous speech (dynamic aphasia) in the context of intact naming, repetition, and comprehension. The authors compared results of an extensive neuropsychological and linguistic protocol of K.O. to other glioma patients and to healthy participants (as described in Satoer et al. [40, 52]) and found that K.O. represented a different cognitive profile mainly characterized by a deviant quality of the spontaneous speech, slower reaction time on the "Dynamic Aphasia Test,"[1] and impaired verbal fluency with intact naming, repetition, and comprehension. Most recovery in K.O.'s spontaneous speech took place between 7 weeks and 3 months postoperatively, but failed to reach baseline level within 1 year (incomplete sentences remained impaired and more repetitions—compared to other glioma patients and healthy participants—occurred in spontaneous speech). The same recovery course was found for the reaction times in the Dynamic Aphasia Test, with a surprising deterioration at 1 year. At all test-moments, K.O.'s performance at cognitive tests was better than that of other glioma patients. In this patient, the authors argued that difficulties in selecting speech act intentions/plan were the underlying cause of his impairments. The inability to search the lexicon with a semantic strategy (word finding) may also have interfered [58] accompanied by a selective attention deficit. In contrast, some (case) reports with extensive test-batteries document a recovery

[1] The Dynamic Aphasia Test consists of sentence completion with word and constituents, sentence generation with a given word or sentence cue, picture description and spontaneous speech in daily situations based on Bloom and Fischler [55], Blomert et al. [56] and Robinson et al. [13].

to baseline level [30, 39, 47]. There are two case reports where only motor mapping was conducted for tumor resection in the superior frontal gyrus which resulted in loss of speech initiation with intact comprehension directly after surgery followed by a spontaneous recovery as assessed about 3 months postoperatively. However, no detailed spontaneous speech analyses were conducted [59, 60]. Ultimately, as was raised earlier, in addition to formal testing and/or spontaneous speech analyses, self-reported language complaints in the (preoperative and) long-term follow-up period need to be taken into account as well.

A small study ($N = 15$) investigating the occurrence of language disorders with a test-battery for mild aphasia (Diagnostic Instrument for Mild Aphasia) including sentence completion [61] and self-reported language complaints were registered in low-grade glioma patients before awake surgery until 1 year after awake surgery [62]. In the intraoperative procedure, spontaneous speech was monitored as described by Satoer et al. [40, 48]. They found that before surgery 53% of patients (8/15) reported language complaints, of whom 5 had difficulties at the sentence level. Two months after surgery 67% (10/15) reported complaints, of whom 9 had difficulties at the sentence level. One year after surgery 62% (8/15) reported complaints, of whom 6 had difficulties at the sentence level. However, only before surgery the incidence of the self-reported language complaints significantly correlated with the presence of a language impairments at test-level (including a sentence completion task). Wolthuis et al. explained this phenomenon due to high variability in the patient group underlining an extensive patient-tailored language assessment including a detailed anamnesis about language use in daily life. A weak relation between subjective complaints and objective test-results after brain tumor surgery has previously been reported for executive functioning [63]. For language functioning, this has only been observed before brain tumor surgery [64, 65]. Remarkably, the difference between self-reported information and test performance did not concern one particular language level or domain (word retrieval, speech production at sentence level, comprehension, reading, and writing). This may be due to under- or overestimation of patients' own skills [66], the gap between daily language and artificial tests [48], or particular patient characteristics [67]. Currently, Satoer and colleagues are working on a standardized questionnaire for mild language complaints. This can be used as an additional tool to select specific language tasks, to conduct more extensive spontaneous speech analyses, and, if necessary, to refer to a speech language therapist.

In summary, there is currently insufficient evidence that monitoring of spontaneous speech during awake glioma surgery confers a significant advantage in late outcomes. However, more than a decade of clinical experience supports the importance and sensitivity of spontaneous speech monitoring peri-operatively to be warranted for (further) deterioration. Of note, it should be kept in mind that the reverse is not true: purely anomic aphasia has been reported when operating the posterior basal/inferior temporal cortex, despite effective spontaneous speech [68]. Long-term follow-up studies with extensive intraoperative recordings and analyses of spontaneous speech and/or sentence completion tasks are still necessary to elucidate its added value for outcome.

6.5 Conclusions

Spontaneous speech is the most important aspect of language, as everyone needs to convey a message in daily conversation. Until now there is convincing evidence from neuroimaging and intraoperative mapping that spontaneous speech can be dissociated from isolated language abilities, such as word retrieval. However, adequate and sensitive assessment of spontaneous speech in clinical settings still remains a challenge as it is still not yet fully understood in what exact way glioma patients show impairments and suffer from it in the perioperative phase (due to large variability). Also there are often time constraints in clinical test-settings, as transcription of speech is effortful. Notwithstanding, the findings underline the relevance of adding evaluation of daily speech to the peri-operative language test-protocol, ideally in combination with tests at the sentence level, such as sentence completion in (semi-)broad context. By only monitoring language functions in isolation, "subtle" yet devastating linguistic impairments could be missed, increasing the risk for long-term postoperative impairments with negative effects on daily life.

References

1. Caramazza A. How many levels of processing are there in lexical access? Cogn Neuropsychol. 1997;14:177–208.
2. Dell GS, Schwartz MF, Martin N, Saffran EM, Gagnon DA. Lexical access in aphasic and nonaphasic speakers. Psychol Rev. 1997;104(4):801–38.
3. Fillmore CJ. On fluency. In: Fillmore DKCJ, Wang WSJ, editors. Individual differences in language ability and language behavior. New York: Academic; 1979. p. 85–101.
4. Lichtheim L. On aphasia. Brain. 1885;7:433–84.
5. Krainik A, Lehéricy S, Duffau H, Capelle L, Chainay H, Cornu P, Cohen L, Boch AL, Mangin JF, Le Bihan D, Marsault C. Postoperative speech disorder after medial frontal surgery: role of the supplementary motor area. Neurology. 2003;60(4):587–94.
6. Naeser MA, Hayward RW. Lesion localization in aphasia with cranial computed tomography and the Boston Diagnostic Aphasia Exam. Neurology. 1978;28(6):545–51.
7. Luria AR. raumaticheskaya Aphasia. Klinika, semantika i vosstanovitelnaya terapiya [Traumatic aphasia]. Academia Meditsintskikh Nauk SSSR. 1947.
8. Luria AR, Tsvetkova LS. The mechanism of 'dynamic aphasia'. Found Lang. 1968;4(3): 296–307.
9. Ardila A, Lopez MV. Transcortical motor aphasia: one or two aphasias? Brain Lang. 1984;22(2):350–3.
10. Costello AL, Warrington EK. Dynamic aphasia: the selective impairment of verbal planning. Cortex. 1989;25(1):103–14.
11. Robinson G, Blair J, Cipolotti L. Dynamic aphasia: an inability to select between competing verbal responses? Brain. 1998;121(Pt 1):77–89.
12. Esmonde T, Giles E, Xuereb J, Hodges J. Progressive supranuclear palsy presenting with dynamic aphasia. J Neurol Neurosurg Psychiatry. 1996;60(4):403–10.
13. Robinson G, Shallice T, Cipolotti L. Dynamic aphasia in progressive supranuclear palsy: a deficit in generating a fluent sequence of novel thought. Neuropsychologia. 2006;44(8):1344–60.
14. Jehna M, Becker J, Zaar K, von Campe G, Mahdy Ali K, Reishofer G, Payer F, Synowitz M, Fazekas F, Enzinger C, Deutschmann H. Symmetry of the arcuate fasciculus and its impact on

language performance of patients with brain tumors in the language-dominant hemisphere. J Neurosurg. 2017;127(6):1407–16.
15. Thomson AM, Taylor R, Whittle IR. Assessment of communication impairment and the effects of resective surgery in solitary, right-sided supratentorial intracranial tumours: a prospective study. Br J Neurosurg. 1998;12(5):423–9.
16. Tremblay P, Dick AS. Broca and Wernicke are dead, or moving past the classic model of language neurobiology. Brain Lang. 2016;162:60–71.
17. Borovsky A, Saygin AP, Bates E, Dronkers N. Lesion correlates of conversational speech production deficits. Neuropsychologia. 2007;45(11):2525–33.
18. Rogalski E, Cobia D, Harrison TM, Wieneke C, Thompson CK, Weintraub S, Mesulam MM. Anatomy of language impairments in primary progressive aphasia. J Neurosci. 2011;31(9):3344–50.
19. Wilson SM, Henry ML, Besbris M, Ogar JM, Dronkers NF, Jarrold W, Miller BL, Gorno-Tempini ML. Connected speech production in three variants of primary progressive aphasia. Brain. 2010;133(Pt 7):2069–88.
20. Bohland JW, Guenther FH. An fMRI investigation of syllable sequence production. Neuroimage. 2006;32(2):821–41.
21. Duffau H, Lopes M, Denvil D, Capelle L. Delayed onset of the supplementary motor area syndrome after surgical resection of the mesial frontal lobe: a time course study using intraoperative mapping in an awake patient. Stereotact Funct Neurosurg. 2001;76(2):74–82.
22. Laplane D, Talairach J, Meininger V, Bancaud J, Orgogozo JM. Clinical consequences of corticectomies involving the supplementary motor area in man. J Neurol Sci. 1977;34(3):301–14.
23. Catani M, Dell'acqua F, Vergani F, Malik F, Hodge H, Roy P, Valabregue R, Thiebaut de Schotten M. Short frontal lobe connections of the human brain. Cortex. 2012;48(2):273–91.
24. Basilakos A, Fillmore PT, Rorden C, Guo D, Bonilha L, Fridriksson J. Regional white matter damage predicts speech fluency in chronic post-stroke aphasia. Front Hum Neurosci. 2014;8:845.
25. Li M, Zhang Y, Song L, Huang R, Ding J, Fang Y, Xu Y, Han Z. Structural connectivity subserving verbal fluency revealed by lesion-behavior mapping in stroke patients. Neuropsychologia. 2017;101:85–96.
26. Catani M, Mesulam MM, Jakobsen E, Malik F, Martersteck A, Wieneke C, Thompson CK, Thiebaut de Schotten M, Dell'Acqua F, Weintraub S, Rogalski E. A novel frontal pathway underlies verbal fluency in primary progressive aphasia. Brain. 2013;136(Pt 8):2619–28.
27. Mandelli ML, Caverzasi E, Binney RJ, Henry ML, Lobach I, Block N, Amirbekian B, Dronkers N, Miller BL, Henry RG, Gorno-Tempini ML. Frontal white matter tracts sustaining speech production in primary progressive aphasia. J Neurosci. 2014;34(29):9754–67.
28. Kinoshita M, de Champfleur NM, Deverdun J, Moritz-Gasser S, Herbet G, Duffau H. Role of fronto-striatal tract and frontal aslant tract in movement and speech: an axonal mapping study. Brain Struct Funct. 2015;220(6):3399–412.
29. Chernoff BL, Teghipco A, Garcea FE, Sims MH, Paul DA, Tivarus ME, Smith SO, Pilcher WH, Mahon BZ. A role for the frontal aslant tract in speech planning: a neurosurgical case study. J Cogn Neurosci. 2018;30(5):752–69. https://doi.org/10.1162/jocn_a_01244. PMID: 29569513.
30. Dragoy O, Zyryanov A, Bronov O, Gordeyeva E, Gronskaya N, Kryuchkova O, Klyuev E, Kopachev D, Medyanik I, Mishnyakova L, Pedyash N, Pronin I, Reutov A, Sitnikov A, Stupina E, Yashin K, Zhirnova V, Zuev A. Functional linguistic specificity of the left frontal aslant tract for spontaneous speech fluency: evidence from intraoperative language mapping. Brain Lang. 2020;208:104836.
31. Lüders HO, Dinner DS, Morris HH, Wyllie E, Comair YG. Cortical electrical stimulation in humans. The negative motor areas. Adv Neurol. 1995;67:115–29.
32. Rostomily RC, Berger MS, Ojemann GA, Lettich E. Postoperative deficits and functional recovery following removal of tumors involving the dominant hemisphere supplementary motor area. J Neurosurg. 1991;75(1):62–8.

33. Schucht P, Moritz-Gasser S, Herbet G, Raabe A, Duffau H. Subcortical electrostimulation to identify network subserving motor control. Hum Brain Mapp. 2013;34(11):3023–30.
34. Alario FX, Chainay H, Lehericy S, Cohen L. The role of the supplementary motor area (SMA) in word production. Brain Res. 2006;1076(1):129–43.
35. Corrivetti F, de Schotten MT, Poisson I, Froelich S, Descoteaux M, Rheault F, Mandonnet E. Dissociating motor-speech from lexico-semantic systems in the left frontal lobe: insight from a series of 17 awake intraoperative mappings in glioma patients. Brain Struct Funct. 2019;224(3):1151–65.
36. Chernoff BL, Sims MH, Smith SO, Pilcher WH, Mahon BZ. Direct electrical stimulation of the left frontal aslant tract disrupts sentence planning without affecting articulation. Cogn Neuropsychol. 2019;36(3–4):178–92. https://doi.org/10.1080/02643294.2019.1619544.
37. De Witt Hamer PC, Robles SG, Zwinderman AH, Duffau H, Berger MS. Impact of intraoperative stimulation brain mapping on glioma surgery outcome: a meta-analysis. J Clin Oncol. 2012;30(20):2559–65.
38. De Witte E, Mariën P. The neurolinguistic approach to awake surgery reviewed. Clin Neurol Neurosurg. 2013;115(2):127–45.
39. De Witte E, Satoer D, Robert E, Colle H, Verheyen S, Visch-Brink E, Mariën P. The Dutch Linguistic Intraoperative Protocol: a valid linguistic approach to awake brain surgery. Brain Lang. 2015a;140:35–48.
40. Satoer D, Vincent A, Smits M, Dirven C, Visch-Brink E. Spontaneous speech of patients with gliomas in eloquent areas before and early after surgery. Acta Neurochir (Wien). 2013;155(4):685–92.
41. De Witte E, Satoer D, Colle H, Robert E, Visch-Brink E, Mariën P. Subcortical language and non-language mapping in awake brain surgery: the use of multimodal tests. Acta Neurochir (Wien). 2015b;157(4):577–88.
42. Satoer D, Kloet A, Vincent A, Dirven C, Visch-Brink E. Dynamic aphasia following low-grade glioma surgery near the supplementary motor area: a selective spontaneous speech deficit. Neurocase. 2014;20(6):704–16.
43. Ojemann G, Mateer C. Human language cortex: localization of memory, syntax, and sequential motor-phoneme identification systems. Science. 1979;205(4413):1401–3.
44. Zanin E, Riva M, Bambini V, Cappa SF, Magrassi L, Moro A. The contribution of surgical brain mapping to the understanding of the anatomo-functional basis of syntax: a critical review. Neurol Sci. 2017;38(9):1579–89.
45. Ries SK, Piai V, Perry D, Griffin S, Jordan K, Henry R, Knight RT, Berger MS. Roles of ventral versus dorsal pathways in language production: an awake language mapping study. Brain Lang. 2019;191:17–27.
46. De Witte E, Satoer D, Visch-Brink E, Mariën P. Cognitive outcome after awake surgery for left and right hemisphere tumours. In: Academy of Aphasia 53rd Annual Meeting. 2015c.
47. Chivukula S, Pikul BK, Black KL, Pouratian N, Bookheimer SY. Contralateral functional reorganization of the speech supplementary motor area following neurosurgical tumor resection. Brain Lang. 2018;183:41–6.
48. Satoer D, Vincent A, Ruhaak L, Smits M, Dirven C, Visch-Brink E. Spontaneous speech in patients with gliomas in eloquent areas: evaluation until 1 year after surgery. Clin Neurol Neurosurg. 2018;167:112–6.
49. Satoer D, De Witte E, Smits M, Bastiaanse R, Vincent A, Mariën P, Visch-Brink E. Differential effects of awake glioma surgery in "critical" language areas on cognition: 4 case studies. Case Rep Neurol Med. 2017;2017:6038641.
50. Rofes A, Talacchi A, Santini B, Pinna G, Nickels L, Bastiaanse R, Miceli G. Language in individuals with left hemisphere tumors: is spontaneous speech analysis comparable to formal testing? J Clin Exp Neuropsychol. 2018;40(7):722–32. https://doi.org/10.1080/13803395.2018.1426734.
51. McCarron A, Chavez A, Babiak M, Berger MS, Chang EF, Wilson SM. Connected speech in transient aphasias after left hemisphere resective surgery. Aphasiology. 2017;31(11):1266–81.

52. Satoer D, Vork J, Visch-Brink E, Smits M, Dirven C, Vincent A. Cognitive functioning early after surgery of gliomas in eloquent areas. J Neurosurg. 2012;117(5):831–8.
53. Goodglass H, Kaplan E. The assessment of aphasia and related disorders. Philadelphia: Lea & Febiger; 1983.
54. Satoer D. Speaking on the edge: the protection of cognition after glioma surgery in eloquent areas. Unpublished doctoral dissertation. Erasmus University, Rotterdam. 2014.
55. Nevler N, Ash S, Irwin DJ, Liberman M, Grossman M. Validated automatic speech biomarkers in primary progressive aphasia. Ann Clin Transl Neurol. 2019;6(1):4–14.
56. Bloom PA, Fischler I. Completion norms for 329 sentence contexts. Mem Cogn. 1980;8(6):631–42.
57. Blomert L, Kloster C, Kean ML. Amsterdam-Nijmegen test voor Alledaagse Taalvaardigheden. (ANTAT). Swets & Zeitlinger; 1995.
58. Gold M, Nadeau SE, Jacobs DH, Adair JC, Rothi LJ, Heilman KM. Adynamic aphasia: a transcortical motor aphasia with defective semantic strategy formation. Brain Lang. 1997;57(3):374–93.
59. Quirarte JA, Kumar VA, Liu HL, Noll KR, Wefel JS, Lang FF. Language supplementary motor area syndrome correlated with dynamic changes in perioperative task-based functional MRI activations: case report. J Neurosurg. 2020:1–5.
60. Young JS, Morshed RA, Mansoori Z, Cha S, Berger MS. Disruption of frontal aslant tract is not associated with long-term postoperative language deficits. World Neurosurg. 2020;133:192–5.
61. Satoer D, de Witte E, Bastiaanse R, Vincent A, Mariën P, Visch-Brink E. Diagnostic Instrument for Mild Aphasia (DIMA): standardization and clinical application. In: Academy of Aphasia 55th Annual Meeting. 2019.
62. Wolthuis N. Language impairments and resting-state EEG in brain tumour patients: Revealing connections. University of Groningen. 2021. https://doi.org/10.33612/diss.159333388.
63. van der Linden SD, Gehring K, De Baene W, Emons WHM, Rutten GM, Sitskoorn MM. Assessment of executive functioning in patients with meningioma and low-grade glioma: a comparison of self-report, proxy-report, and test performance. J Int Neuropsychol Soc. 2020;26(2):187–96.
64. Antonsson M, Longoni F, Jakola A, Tisell M, Thordstein M, Hartelius L. Pre-operative language ability in patients with presumed low-grade glioma. J Neurooncol. 2018;137(1):93–102.
65. Pranckeviciene A, Deltuva VP, Tamasauskas A, Zegliene J, Bunevicius A. Clinical and biological correlates of preoperative cognitive functioning of glioma and meningioma patients. Biomed Res Int. 2020;2020:2054859.
66. Kruger J, Dunning D. Unskilled and unaware of it: how difficulties in recognizing one's own incompetence lead to inflated self-assessments. J Pers Soc Psychol. 1999;77(6):1121–34.
67. Gehring K, Taphoorn MJ, Sitskoorn MM, Aaronson NK. Predictors of subjective versus objective cognitive functioning in patients with stable grades II and III glioma. Neurooncol Pract. 2015;2(1):20–31.
68. Herbet G, Moritz-Gasser S, Duffau H. Electrical stimulation of the dorsolateral prefrontal cortex impairs semantic cognition. Neurology. 2018;90(12):e1077–84.
69. Chang EF, Kurteff G, Wilson SM. Selective interference with syntactic encoding during sentence production by direct electrocortical stimulation of the inferior frontal gyrus. J Cogn Neurosci. 2018;30(3):411–20.

Reading

7

Ilyess Zemmoura, Emmanuel Mandonnet,
and Laurent Cohen

7.1 Neural Basis of Reading

Reading a word requires several steps of processing that begin by the recognition of letters by the visual system, and that ends with the pronunciation of a meaningful word.

Although the anatomy of cortical areas, and even more of their connectivity, that sustains reading processes still lacks robust evidence, a dual-route computational model of reading is currently widely accepted. The first descriptions of a dual-route model were based on findings from brain-damaged patients with acquired dyslexia [1–4]. These dual-route models dissociate a ventral lexical-semantic pathway devoted to the reading of meaningful words (this route subserves the so-called "addressed phonology") and the dorsal phonological pathway devoted to the reading of nonwords and pseudo-words (this one is devoted to the so-called "assembled phonology") [5–10].

The first steps of reading are supported by a visual word form system that connects the extrastriate occipital cortex to the cortex of the left lateral

I. Zemmoura (✉)
UMR 1253, iBrain, Université de Tours, Inserm, Tours, France

Department of Neurosurgery, CHRU de Tours, Tours, France
e-mail: ilyess.zemmoura@univ-tours.fr

E. Mandonnet
Department of Neurosurgery, Lariboisière Hospital, Paris Brain Institute (ICM) and Université de Paris, Paris, France

Institut du Cerveau, CNRS UMR 7225, INSERM U1127, Paris, France
e-mail: emmanuel.mandonnet@aphp.fr

L. Cohen
Institut du Cerveau, CNRS UMR 7225, INSERM U1127, Paris, France

Department of Neurology, Pitié-Salpêtrière Hospital, Paris, France

Sorbonne Université, Paris, France

E. Mandonnet, G. Herbet (eds.), *Intraoperative Mapping of Cognitive Networks*,
https://doi.org/10.1007/978-3-030-75071-8_7

occipitotemporal sulcus, at the anterolateral aspects of the left fusiform gyrus. This latter region is known as the visual word form area (VWFA) [11–14]. It receives visual input from the foveal region of both hemifields, via the inferior longitudinal fasciculus (ILF) and the splenium of the corpus callosum, with right-hemifield predominance.

The VWFA supports orthographic analysis, that is, the identification of letters and groups of letters, and the encoding of their order, possibly through a neural hierarchy [15, 16], similar to the one supporting face [17] or object [18] processing.

Then, for both familiar words and pseudo-words, orthographic representations may be translated into phonological representations based on the statistics of letters-to-sounds correspondences, corresponding to the "assembled phonology" pathway. For real words, reading may also proceed through access to the pronunciation stored in memory among other word-related knowledge ("addressed phonology" pathway) [15, 19, 20].

The anatomical connections of the VWFA are still a matter of debate. This is mostly due to the numerous fiber crossings encountered in the occipitotemporal area which cannot be entirely resolved either by diffusion tractography or by fiber dissections (the two main exploration tools of human brain anatomical connectivity available at the time), even less by extrapolation techniques based on primates anatomy, such as autoradiography, given the huge difference between the anatomy of humans and nonspeaking primates. In addition to the fibers of the tapetum that form the posterior corpus callosum, at least five association fiber tracts cross or terminate in the region of the VWFA, namely, according the recent nomenclature [21], the basal longitudinal system (BLS), the inferior longitudinal system (ILS), the arcuate fascicle (AF), the posterior transverse system comprising the vertical temporoparietal fasciculus (VTPF), and the vertical occipital fascicle (VOF) (respectively inferior longitudinal fasciculus (ILF), inferior fronto-occipital fasciculus (IFOF), arcuate fasciculus, posterior arcuate fasciculus, and vertical occipital fasciculus in the historical nomenclature) (Fig. 7.1).

Bouhali et al. used tractography to assess the anatomical connections of the VWFA [22]. Based on the hypothesis of a hierarchically organized VWFA, they segmented the VWF system into multiple regions along the antero-posterior axis. They found that the anterior sector of the VWFA was mostly connected with perisylvian language cortical areas, orbitofrontal and anterior temporal regions while the posterior sector was mostly connected to the homolateral calcarine fissure via the BLS/ILF, and to the contralateral occipital cortex via the splenium of the corpus callosum.

These tracts allow bottom-up and top-down processing of words by the orthographic, phonological, and semantic systems. Their interplay is not entirely understood nor explained by the proposed neurocognitive models of reading [1, 5, 6, 9, 23–25]. Indeed, most of the anatomical data concerning the neural bases of reading have been provided by functional MRI (fMRI) [7, 11, 13, 19, 26–32], event-related potentials (ERP) [8], or magnetoencephalography (MEG) [33]. As a consequence, the dorsal phonological and ventral lexico-semantic routes of reading are concepts mainly supported by cortical activations in regions that have been related to

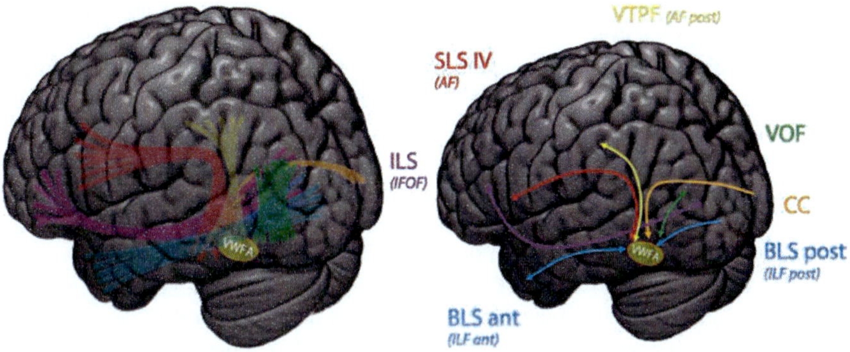

Fig. 7.1 Left lateral oblique posterior view of the brain, showing the main fiber tracts connected with the visual word form area (VWFA). The VWFA is located inside the left lateral occipitotemporal sulcus (at the lateral aspect of the fusiform gyrus). It receives visual inputs from the homolateral and contralateral visual cortex via, respectively, the posterior portion of the basal longitudinal system (BLS post, in blue, the BLS being also known as the inferior longitudinal fasciculus or ILF) and the corpus callosum (CC, in orange). Letters and their order are identified inside the VWFA. Afterwards, the meaning and pronunciation of the decoded words are accessed through the dorsal phonological stream—mainly the arcuate branch of the superior longitudinal system (SLS IV, in red, also known as the arcuate fasciculus or AF), the vertical temporoparietal fasciculus (VTPF, in yellow, also known as the posterior vertical segment of the arcuate fasciculus or AF post), and the vertical occipital fasciculus (VOF, in green)—and the ventral semantic system via the anterior portion of the BLS and the inferior longitudinal system (ILS, in purple, also known as the inferior fronto-occipital fasciculus or IFOF)

different reading tasks involving either phonological or semantic processing. For example, Jobard et al. [26] found that cortical activations of the middle temporal gyrus (MTG), basal temporal region, and pars triangularis of the inferior frontal gyrus (PTr) are related to lexical processing, while cortical activations of the superior temporal gyrus (STG), MTG, supramarginalis gyrus (SMG), and pars opercularis of the inferior frontal gyrus (POp) have been related to phonological processing of reading words. These two patterns of cortical activations correspond to the cortical connection of, respectively, the ILS/IFOF and AF.

All these data provide strong but indirect evidence that the ventral lexico-semantic pathway of reading might be subserved by the ILS/IFOF and the dorsal phonological pathway by the AF [34–38].

A few recent studies directly focused on fiber connections of the VWFA using diffusion tractography [39–41] and direct electrical stimulation during awake surgery [20]. The only tract that has been demonstrated to be a posterior connection to the VWFA is the BLS/ILF [20, 39], whose interruption causes pure alexia (namely, alexia without agraphia nor anomia). Also considered downstream are the inputs from the contralateral temporo-occipital cortex, through the fibers of the splenium of the corpus callosum, whose disconnection is known to cause left hemialexia (see [11] and references therein). Other supposed connections to the VWFA are the VTPF/AFpost and the VOF. The VTPF/AFpost has been found to be connected to the VWFA in diffusion tractography studies [39, 40] and its involvement in reading is supported by the correlation between its fractional anisotropy and reading skills [42]. Moreover disconnection of the VTPF/AFpost from the VWFA results in a deficit of assembled phonology (alexia of pseudo-words) [20]. Finally it has been proposed that a lesion of the VOF might result in the so-called "subangular alexia" [40], a rare impairment similar to pure alexia but associated with parietal lesions [2, 43].

Disruption of the anterior connectivity of the VWFA through the anterior portion of the BLS/ILF (BLSa/ILFa), the ILS/IFOF, or the AF has not been reported to cause reading disturbances, probably due to the divergence and redundancy of the output connections from the VWFA. However, normal word reading does not rule out impaired reading comprehension, and some of these tracts could be implicated in narrative-level reading (for example, it has been shown that diffusion-weighted imaging of the BLS/ILF and the AF correlated with comprehension scores [44]).

7.2 Evidence of Long-Term Dyslexia in Patients Without Intraoperative Reading Testing

The first series of patients suffering from alexia following left occipital lobectomies dates back to 1952 [45]. In this seminal paper, authors nicely described in a series of seven patients the time pattern of the deficit evolution. In the very acute period, complete alexia was observed, before the patient started to read single letters or syllables, around 10 days after surgery. The next step was noted around 8 weeks after surgery: the patients were then able to read slowly, through a letter-by-letter strategy. Four to five months after surgery, this letter-by-letter reading was faster, but reading remained effortful and ineffective. Later on, Greenblatt [46] reported two cases with alexia following occipital lobectomies, the extent of which was demonstrated with postoperative computed tomography. The author also retrospectively discussed the cases of Hécaen et al. [45] and refined the connectionist anatomical model of Déjerine [47], introducing the idea that a resection that would preserve the lateral aspect of the occipital lobe would promote better recovery. However, this hypothesis was subsequently invalidated by several case reports. First, Kamada et al. reported a case of permanent dyslexia following resection of a glioma located to the fusiform gyrus, parahippocampal gyrus, and hippocampus [48]. Interestingly, pre- and postoperative MEG during a reading task demonstrated that dipole activity in the fusiform gyrus completely disappeared after surgery. Then, Gaillard et al. documented a case of alexia following a small surgical resection in the vicinity of the VWFA [49], as delineated preoperatively with functional MRI and stereoencephalography (SEEG). Ultimately, it was demonstrated that the VWFA was preserved, but disconnected from the occipital pole, due to a damage at the level of the posterior BLS/ILF and callosal fibers [39]. More recently, two cases were reported in which surgery disconnected the BLS/ILF afferences of the VWFA [50]. Surprisingly, the two patients had no long-lasting alexia, contrasting with the outcome reported in Gaillard et al. [39], thus emphasizing the importance of keeping callosal fibers intact during surgery.

In summary, there is ample evidence that resections around the VWFA in the left basal temporo-occipital region yields substantial risk of long-lasting deficits in reading.

7.3 Review of the Different Tasks Newly Designed to Monitor Reading Intraoperatively

None of the currently available reading tasks has been validated for intraoperative testing. In the literature, only four studies assessed reading intraoperatively [20, 51–53]. In these four studies, the reading tasks used have been specifically designed for intraoperative testing but, to our knowledge, have never been further validated.

Roux et al. [51] used a set of 30 sentences featuring various syntactic structures and word types (verbs, grammatical words, etc.). Mani et al. [52] asked patients to read a story aloud, and they added, for one patient, a "reading material with an escalating degree of complexity and also (...) single and multidigit numbers." Motomura et al. [53] used two reading aloud tasks. The first one was administered during cortical mapping before tumor resection, and consisted in reading aloud words written either with "kanji" (Japanese morphograms) or with "kana" (Japanese syllabograms). The second task was administered after tumor resection, during direct electrical stimulation of the surgical cavity boundaries. It consisted in reading aloud full Japanese sentences. Zemmoura et al. [20] displayed a series of consecutive printed words—successively a regular word, an irregular word, and a pseudo-word—, for 4 s each.

Each method has advantages and limitations. Reading a sentence during awake surgery, as proposed by Roux et al. and by Mani et al., is more ecological than just reading a succession of words, and allows for the assessment of complex reading processes. Nonetheless, with such a task it is almost impossible to characterize the type of errors induced by the electrical stimulation, as multiple processes take place simultaneously during sentence reading. Contrariwise, reading a unique word does not require syntactic and/or grammatical processing, and offers the clinicians a robust method to rapidly identify areas critically involved in reading.

Asking patients to read aloud both sentences and letters/syllables/words should be considered, in order to achieve both sufficient sensitivity and selectivity, in as much as the time spent to collect such data remains manageable. Of course, the use of reading tasks, performed on top of classical motor and language tasks, should be discussed depending on the patient's reading skills, and on the impact which alexia could have on his/her daily life, professional and personal activities.

7.4 Evidence of Functional Improvement in Patients Operated on with Reading Monitoring

There are only few papers reporting the preservation of reading abilities by means of intraoperative identification of alexia sites. Mandonnet et al. observed a patient with intraoperative identification of a cortical site (visual object form area—VOFA) and of a white matter site (within the BLS/ILF) whose stimulation generated visual paraphasia [54]. The patient presented a reading deficit in the immediate postoperative period, suggesting that the VWFA and/or its connections were damaged. Six months after the surgery, the patient fully recovered reading abilities, suggesting a certain degree of functional overlap between the VWFA and the VOFA and the possibility to recycle the VOFA for reading, thanks to postoperative plasticity, enhanced by rehabilitation training. This case contrasts with the case reported by Gaillard et al. [49], who was operated on without any intraoperative mapping, and who had still letter-by-letter reading 6 months after surgery. This plasticity of the VOFA/VWFA was later confirmed in a study reporting three cases [55]. Sites whose stimulation generated visual recognition disorders were identified in these three cases and surgically spared. Again, despite severe reading impairment in the immediate postoperative period, all patients recovered normal reading at 6 months. Finally, Zemmoura et al. studied a series of seven patients with intraoperative mapping of sites involved in a reading task [20]—see also Fig. 7.2.

This task consisted in reading successively one regular, one irregular, and one pseudo-word, written on a laptop screen. Despite severe alexia in the immediate postoperative period, all patients recovered normal scores in regular word reading, albeit with a certain degree of slowness in two of them. However, five patients had

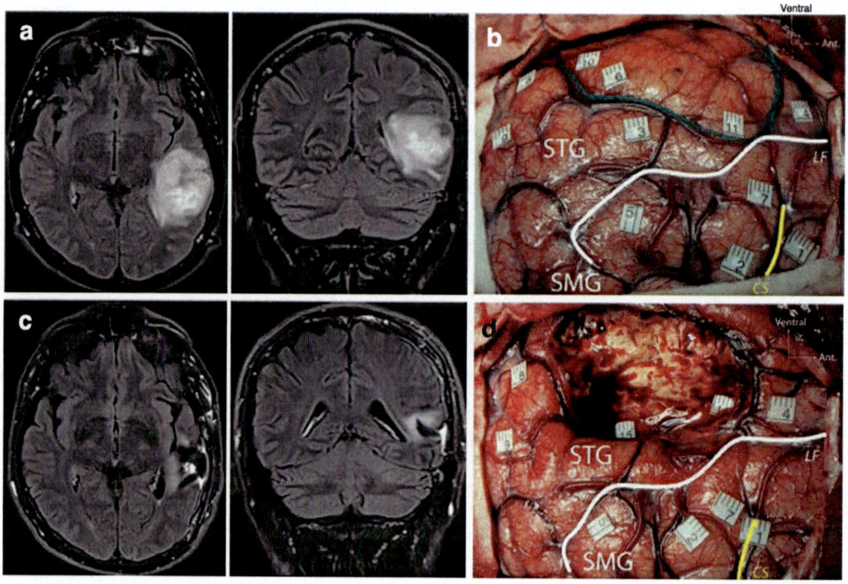

Fig. 7.2 Illustrative case of a 37-year-old man, working as a cook. (**a**) Preoperative flair MRI. (**b**) Pre-resection mapping. Stimulation of tags 8 and 9 elicited alexia of irregular words. (**c**) Postoperative flair MRI. (**d**) Post-resection mapping, demonstrating the preservation of tags 8 and 9. Patient had immediate postoperative alexia, which partially recovered at the 3-month postoperative evaluation and fully recovered at the 9-month postoperative evaluation. *CS* central sulcus, *LF* lateral fissure, *SMG* supramarginalis gyrus, *STG* superior temporal gyrus

persisting difficulties with pseudo-words. Among them, one was not tested for irregular words, two had also difficulties with irregular words (6 or 5 words out of 7 correctly read), and two showed good performance (7/7), but with some slowness.

7.5 Anatomo-Functional Knowledge Gained from Intraoperative Mapping Studies of Reading

Roux et al. demonstrated the segregation, at the cortical level, between sites involved in sub-lexical versus lexical processing in reading [56]. To this end, they used a reading task combining only irregular words and pseudo-words. Pseudo-words specific sites were detected when stimulating the anterior supramarginal gyrus, and irregular words specific sites were observed in the posterior supramarginal gyrus/superior temporal gyrus. Of note, these sites largely overlapped with sites inducing errors with both types of words. Unfortunately, it is unclear in this study if the disturbances were truly specific to reading. Indeed, although it was stated that "it must be emphasized that, when we qualified a reading site as "pseudo-word specific reading" it meant that neither picture naming nor (irregular) word reading interferences were found in this area," the same statement was not explicitly made for irregular words. As naming (or even counting) sites were not reported, it is not clear that reading sites were actually distinct from picture naming sites.

Zemmoura et al. proposed a new model of the connectivity of the VWFA. In particular, in order to explain that stimulation of the white matter superiorly to the VWFA impaired reading of both irregular and pseudo-words (but not of regular words), they proposed that the inferior parietal lobule modulates from top-down the balance between the lexical and sub-lexical routes, through the posterior transverse system [21, 57, 58]. This model has been further formalized by Mandonnet and Duffau [59] and linked to connectionist computational models of reading. It was argued that the atypical pattern observed by Zemmoura et al. (that is impairment for irregular and pseudo-words only) was indeed caused by a damage to the system weighting the balance between the sub-lexical and lexical pathways. The anatomy of this regulatory system between the two routes was not clearly established. An alternative explanation of this atypical pattern would be that the sub-lexical and lexical routes are both partially damaged. For regular words, the converging responses of the two routes would potentialize each other, while such synergy would not exist for irregular and pseudo-words. This latter hypothesis would explain why reading pseudo-words is more fragile than reading regular or irregular words: the phonological and articulatory processes required for pseudo-words are restricted to the left hemisphere, while the lexical stream might have bilateral components, from the right and left VWFA to the bilaterally represented semantic system. From the semantic system, phonological codes could be retrieved in a second step. The price to pay for this indirect semantically mediated access would be slower reading time. In accordance with this view, the participation of the right VWFA has been hypothesized to explain the capacity of the so-called implicit reading observed in some alexic patients [60, 61].

7.6 Conclusion

Reading is a fundamental cognitive function, which highly impacts patients' quality of life when impaired. Recent advances in the knowledge of the reading network allows for the systematic intraoperative testing of this function when surgery involves the posterior aspects of the left temporal lobe and/or the left occipital lobe, i.e., around the usual location of the VWFA (which is found inside the lateral occipitotemporal sulcus, separating the fusiform gyrus from the inferior temporal gyrus).

There is currently no consensus about the task to administrate intraoperatively. Nonetheless, the tasks appearing to have to best efficiency trade-off of sensitivity and duration are word reading tasks. To obtain a good sensitivity and specificity, the set of words administered during the surgical procedure should comprise irregular and pseudo-words, but not necessarily regular words, as these are not expected to be impaired if both irregular and pseudo-words are spared.

These recommendations might evolve in the next years, as they are based on only four published reports. In particular, there are no reports assessing reading comprehension in patients with normal word-level reading abilities. This lack of data is mostly due to the lack of evidence that testing reading provides better results in terms of postoperative reading deficit, but also to the relative rarity of low-grade glioma involving the left temporo-occipital junction. Testing reading systematically should help us to better understand the reading network and to better choose the type of tasks to administer intraoperatively.

References

1. Marshall JC, Newcombe F. Patterns of paralexia: a psycholinguistic approach. J Psycholinguist Res. 1973;2(3):175–99.
2. Greenblatt SH. Subangular alexia without agraphia or hemianopsia. Brain Lang. 1976;3(2):229–45.
3. Damasio A, Damasio H, Chui H. Neglect following damage to frontal lobe or basal ganglia. Neuropsychologia. 1980;18:123–32.
4. Shallice T, Warrington E. Single and multiple component central dyslexic syndromes. In: Coltheart M, Patterson K, Marshall JC, editors. Deep dyslexia. London: Routledge and Kegan Paul; 1980. p. 119–45.
5. Zorzi M, Houhgton G, Butterworth B. Two routes or one in reading aloud? A connectionist dual-process model. J Exp Psychol Hum Percept Perform. 1998;24:1131–61.
6. Coltheart M, Rastle K, Perry C, Langdon R, Ziegler J. DRC: a dual route cascaded model of visual word recognition and reading aloud. Psychol Rev. 2001;108(1):204–56.
7. Simos PG, Breier JI, Fletcher JM, Foorman BR, Castillo EM, Papanicolaou AC. Brain mechanisms for reading words and pseudowords: an integrated approach. Cereb Cortex. 2002;12(3):297–305.
8. Proverbio AM, Vecchi L, Zani A. From orthography to phonetics: ERP measures of grapheme-to-phoneme conversion mechanisms in reading. J Cogn Neurosci. 2004;16(2):301–17.
9. Perry C, Ziegler JC, Zorzi M. Nested incremental modeling in the development of computational theories: the CDP+ model of reading aloud. Psychol Rev. 2007;114(2):273–315.

10. Perry C, Ziegler JC, Zorzi M. Beyond single syllables: large-scale modeling of reading aloud with the Connectionist Dual Process (CDP++) model. Cogn Psychol. 2010;61(2):106–51.
11. Cohen L, Dehaene S, Naccache L, Lehéricy S, Dehaene-Lambertz G, Hénaff MA, et al. The visual word form area: spatial and temporal characterization of an initial stage of reading in normal subjects and posterior split-brain patients. Brain. 2000;123(Pt 2):291–307.
12. Dehaene S, Le Clec'H G, Poline J-B, Le Bihan D, Cohen L. The visual word form area: a prelexical representation of visual words in the fusiform gyrus. Neuroreport. 2002;13(3):321–5.
13. Dehaene S, Cohen L. The unique role of the visual word form area in reading. Trends Cogn Sci (Regul Ed). 2011;15(6):254–62.
14. Le R, Witthoft N, Ben-Shachar M, Wandell B. The field of view available to the ventral occipito-temporal reading circuitry. J Vis. 2017;17(4):6.
15. Dehaene S, Cohen L, Sigman M, Vinckier F. The neural code for written words: a proposal. Trends Cogn Sci (Regul Ed). 2005;9(7):335–41.
16. Vinckier F, Dehaene S, Jobert A, Dubus JP, Sigman M, Cohen L. Hierarchical coding of letter strings in the ventral stream: dissecting the inner organization of the visual word-form system. Neuron. 2007;55(1):143–56.
17. Freiwald WA, Tsao DY. Functional compartmentalization and viewpoint generalization within the macaque face-processing system. Science. 2010;330(6005):845–51.
18. Yamins DLK, Hong H, Cadieu CF, Solomon EA, Seibert D, DiCarlo JJ. Performance-optimized hierarchical models predict neural responses in higher visual cortex. Proc Natl Acad Sci U S A. 2014;111(23):8619–24.
19. Twomey T, Kawabata Duncan KJ, Price CJ, Devlin JT. Top-down modulation of ventral occipito-temporal responses during visual word recognition. Neuroimage. 2011;55(3):1242–51.
20. Zemmoura I, Herbet G, Moritz-Gasser S, Duffau H. New insights into the neural network mediating reading processes provided by cortico-subcortical electrical mapping. Hum Brain Mapp. 2015;36(6):2215–30.
21. Mandonnet E, Sarubbo S, Petit L. The nomenclature of human white matter association pathways: proposal for a systematic taxonomic anatomical classification. Front Neuroanat. 2018;12:94.
22. Bouhali F, Thiebaut de Schotten M, Pinel P, Poupon C, Mangin J-F, Dehaene S, et al. Anatomical connections of the visual word form area. J Neurosci. 2014;34(46):15402–14.
23. Seidenberg MS, McClelland JL. A distributed, developmental model of word recognition and naming. Psychol Rev. 1989;96(4):523–68.
24. Plaut DC, McClelland JL, Seidenberg MS, Patterson K. Understanding normal and impaired word reading: computational principles in quasi-regular domains. Psychol Rev. 1996;103(1):56–115.
25. Ans B, Carbonnel S, Valdois S. A connectionist multiple-trace memory model for polysyllabic word reading. Psychol Rev. 1998;105(4):678–723.
26. Jobard G, Crivello F, Tzourio-Mazoyer N. Evaluation of the dual route theory of reading: a metanalysis of 35 neuroimaging studies. Neuroimage. 2003;20(2):693–712.
27. Mechelli A, Gorno-Tempini ML, Price CJ. Neuroimaging studies of word and pseudoword reading: consistencies, inconsistencies, and limitations. J Cogn Neurosci. 2003;15(2):260–71.
28. Mechelli A, Crinion JT, Long S, Friston KJ, Lambon Ralph MA, Patterson K, et al. Dissociating reading processes on the basis of neuronal interactions. J Cogn Neurosci. 2005;17(11):1753–65.
29. Henry C, Gaillard R, Volle E, Chiras J, Ferrieux S, Dehaene S, et al. Brain activations during letter-by-letter reading: a follow-up study. Neuropsychologia. 2005;43(14):1983–9.
30. Vinckier F, Naccache L, Papeix C, Forget J, Hahn-Barma V, Dehaene S, et al. "What" and "where" in word reading: ventral coding of written words revealed by parietal atrophy. J Cogn Neurosci. 2006;18(12):1998–2012.
31. Dehaene S, Pegado F, Braga LW, Ventura P, Nunes Filho G, Jobert A, et al. How learning to read changes the cortical networks for vision and language. Science. 2010;330(6009):1359–64.
32. Tsapkini K, Vindiola M, Rapp B. Patterns of brain reorganization subsequent to left fusiform damage: fMRI evidence from visual processing of words and pseudowords, faces and objects. Neuroimage. 2011;55(3):1357–72.

33. Marinkovic K, Dhond RP, Dale AM, Glessner M, Carr V, Halgren E. Spatiotemporal dynamics of modality-specific and supramodal word processing. Neuron. 2003;38(3):487–97.
34. Catani M, Jones DK, Ffytche DH. Perisylvian language networks of the human brain. Ann Neurol. 2005;57(1):8–16.
35. Duffau H, Herbet G, Moritz-Gasser S. Toward a pluri-component, multimodal, and dynamic organization of the ventral semantic stream in humans: lessons from stimulation mapping in awake patients. Front Syst Neurosci. 2013;7:44.
36. Martino J, De Witt Hamer PC, Berger MS, Lawton MT, Arnold CM, de Lucas EM, et al. Analysis of the subcomponents and cortical terminations of the perisylvian superior longitudinal fasciculus: a fiber dissection and DTI tractography study. Brain Struct Funct. 2013;218(1):105–21.
37. Martino J, da Silva-Freitas R, Caballero H, Marco de Lucas E, García-Porrero JA, Vázquez-Barquero A. Fiber dissection and diffusion tensor imaging tractography study of the temporoparietal fiber intersection area. Neurosurgery. 2013;72(1 Suppl Operative):87–97; discussion 97–8.
38. Sarubbo S, De Benedictis A, Maldonado IL, Basso G, Duffau H. Frontal terminations for the inferior fronto-occipital fascicle: anatomical dissection, DTI study and functional considerations on a multi-component bundle. Brain Struct Funct. 2013;218(1):21–37.
39. Epelbaum S, Pinel P, Gaillard R, Delmaire C, Perrin M, Dupont S, et al. Pure alexia as a disconnection syndrome: new diffusion imaging evidence for an old concept. Cortex. 2008;44(8):962–74.
40. Yeatman JD, Rauschecker AM, Wandell BA. Anatomy of the visual word form area: adjacent cortical circuits and long-range white matter connections. Brain Lang. 2013;125(2):146–55.
41. Cummine J, Dai W, Borowsky R, Gould L, Rollans C, Boliek C. Investigating the ventral-lexical, dorsal-sublexical model of basic reading processes using diffusion tensor imaging. Brain Struct Funct. 2015;220(1):445–55.
42. Thiebaut de Schotten M, Cohen L, Amemiya E, Braga LW, Dehaene S. Learning to read improves the structure of the arcuate fasciculus. Cereb Cortex. 2014;24(4):989–95.
43. Iragui VJ, Kritchevsky M. Alexia without agraphia or hemianopia in parietal infarction. J Neurol Neurosurg Psychiatry. 1991;54(9):841–2.
44. Horowitz-Kraus T, Wang Y, Plante E, Holland SK. Involvement of the right hemisphere in reading comprehension: a DTI study. Brain Res. 2014;1582:34–44.
45. Hécaen H, De Ajuriaguerra J, David M. [Functional deficits after occipital lobectomy]. Monatsschr Psychiatr Neurol. 1952;123(4–5):239–91.
46. Greenblatt SH. Left occipital lobectomy and the preangular anatomy of reading. Brain Lang. 1990;38(4):576–95.
47. Déjerine J. Comptes rendus des séances de la Société de biologie et de ses filiales [Internet]. Gallica. 1892 [cité 27 oct 2020]. Disponible sur https://gallica.bnf.fr/ark:/12148/bpt6k6474243s.
48. Kamada K, Sawamura Y, Takeuchi F, Houkin K, Kawaguchi H, Iwasaki Y, et al. Gradual recovery from dyslexia and related serial magnetoencephalographic changes in the lexicosemantic centers after resection of a mesial temporal astrocytoma. Case report. J Neurosurg. 2004;100(6):1101–6.
49. Gaillard R, Naccache L, Pinel P, Clémenceau S, Volle E, Hasboun D, et al. Direct intracranial, FMRI, and lesion evidence for the causal role of left inferotemporal cortex in reading. Neuron. 2006;50(2):191–204.
50. Lopes R, Nunes RG, Simões MR, Secca MF, Leal A. The Visual Word Form Area remains in the dominant hemisphere for language in late-onset left occipital lobe epilepsies: a postsurgery analysis of two cases. Epilepsy Behav. 2015;46:91–8.
51. Roux F-E, Lubrano V, Lauwers-Cances V, Trémoulet M, Mascott CR, Démonet J-F. Intra-operative mapping of cortical areas involved in reading in mono- and bilingual patients. Brain. 2004;127(Pt 8):1796–810.
52. Mani J, Diehl B, Piao Z, Schuele SS, Lapresto E, Liu P, et al. Evidence for a basal temporal visual language center: cortical stimulation producing pure alexia. Neurology. 2008;71(20):1621–7.

53. Motomura K, Fujii M, Maesawa S, Kuramitsu S, Natsume A, Wakabayashi T. Association of dorsal inferior frontooccipital fasciculus fibers in the deep parietal lobe with both reading and writing processes: a brain mapping study. J Neurosurg. 2014;121(1):142–8.
54. Mandonnet E, Gatignol P, Duffau H. Evidence for an occipito-temporal tract underlying visual recognition in picture naming. Clin Neurol Neurosurg. 2009;111(7):601–5.
55. Gil-Robles S, Carvallo A, Jimenez MDM, Gomez Caicoya A, Martinez R, Ruiz-Ocaña C, et al. Double dissociation between visual recognition and picture naming: a study of the visual language connectivity using tractography and brain stimulation. Neurosurgery. 2013;72(4):678–86.
56. Roux F-E, Durand J-B, Jucla M, Réhault E, Reddy M, Démonet J-F. Segregation of lexical and sub-lexical reading processes in the left perisylvian cortex. PLoS One. 2012;7(11):e50665.
57. Burks JD, Boettcher LB, Conner AK, Glenn CA, Bonney PA, Baker CM, et al. White matter connections of the inferior parietal lobule: a study of surgical anatomy. Brain Behav [Internet]. 2017;7(4) [cité 23 déc 2017]. Disponible sur https://www.ncbi.nlm.nih.gov/pmc/articles/PMC5390831/.
58. Bullock D, Takemura H, Caiafa CF, Kitchell L, McPherson B, Caron B, et al. Associative white matter connecting the dorsal and ventral posterior human cortex. Brain Struct Funct. 2019;224(8):2631–60.
59. Mandonnet E, Duffau H. Setting the balance between the lexical and sublexical pathways of dual-route models of reading: insight from atypical dyslexia in surgical glioma patients. Front Psychol. 2016;7:1730.
60. Coslett HB, Saffran EM. Evidence for preserved reading in "pure alexia". Brain. 1989;112(Pt 2):327–59.
61. Cohen L, Dehaene S. Calculating without reading: unsuspected residual abilities in pure alexia. Cogn Neuropsychol. 2000;17(6):563–83.

Handwriting

8

Franck-Emmanuel Roux, Mahamadou Niare,
Fleur Céline van Ierschot, Jean-Baptiste Durand,
Gabriele Miceli, and Jean-François Demonet

8.1 Introduction

To the best of our knowledge, the first published mention of the use of spelling tasks during awake electrostimulation mappings was in the 1959 book by Penfield and Roberts—*Speech and Brain Mechanisms* [1]—although details of their handwriting assessments were not reported. Three decades later, Lesser et al. [2] described testing handwriting and oral language in three patients by using subdural grids in the frontal lobes. They did not identify specific neural sites for handwriting, i.e., independent from the motor or other language areas. While attention to language testing in awake surgery has grown vastly in the subsequent decades, reports on the assessment of spelling tasks (including handwriting, typing, and oral spelling) have remained scarce [3] (Table 8.1). Spelling relies on multiple cognitive components

F.-E. Roux (✉) · M. Niare
CNRS (CERCO) UMR Unité 5549, Université Paul Sabatier, Toulouse, France

Pôle Neurosciences (Neurochirurgie), Centres Hospitalo-Universitaires, Toulouse, France

F. C. van Ierschot
Department of Medical Psychology, Amsterdam University Medical Center, Amsterdam, Netherlands

J.-B. Durand
CNRS (CERCO) UMR Unité 5549, Université Paul Sabatier, Toulouse, France
e-mail: jbdurand@cnrs.fr

G. Miceli
Center for Mind/Brain Sciences (CiMeC), University of Trento, Rovereto, Italy

Centro Linceo Interdisciplinare 'Beniamino Segre', Accademia dei Lincei, Rome, Italy
e-mail: gabriele.miceli@unitn.it

J.-F. Demonet
Department of Clinical Neurosciences, Leenaards Memory Center, CHUV and University of Lausanne, Lausanne, Switzerland
e-mail: jean-francois.demonet@chuv.ch

E. Mandonnet, G. Herbet (eds.), *Intraoperative Mapping of Cognitive Networks*,
https://doi.org/10.1007/978-3-030-75071-8_8

Table 8.1 Overview of studies with intraoperative handwriting during awake surgery for glioma treatment

	Patient characteristics					Tumor characteristics			Cortical stimulation	Subcortical stimulation
Authors, year	*N*	Sex	Age (years)	Hand	Language	Tumor type (grade)	Tumor site	Tumor location		
Lesser et al., 1984 [2]	3	1 F, 2 M	30, 34, 36	RH	NR	1 LGG (NS), 2 Other	LHem	Frontal: IFG	Yes	No
Roux et al., 2003 [4]	6	4 F, 2 M	$\mu = 52$	5 RH, 1 LH	French	2 HGG (III), 4 Other	5 LHem, 1 RHem	Parietal: AG	Yes	No
Lubrano et al., 2004 [5]	14	8 F, 6 M	$\mu = 47$	12 RH, 2 LH	French	6 HGG (III, IV), 1 LGG (NS), 7 Other	11 LHem, 3 RHem	Frontal: posterior SFG, MFG, IFG	Yes	No
Roux et al., 2009 [6]	12	5 F, 7 M	$\mu = 37$	10 RH, 2 LH	French	NR	11 LHem, 1 RHem	Frontal: posterior SFG, MFG, IFG	Yes	No
Magrassi et al., 2010 [7]	2	1 F, 1 M	82, 38	RH	Italian	2 HGG (III, IV)	LHem	Parietal: anterior SPL	Yes	No
Roux et al., 2014 [8]	30	9 F, 21 M	$\mu = 48$	27 RH, 3 LH	French	15 HGG (NS), 9 LGG (NS)	23 LHem, 7 RHem	Temporoparietal	Yes	No
Motomura et al., 2014 [9]	1	M	48	RH	Japanese	HGG (IV)	LHem	Parietal: IPL	Yes	Yes
Van Ierschot et al., 2018 [3]	3	2 F, 1 M	44, 34, 74	RH	Italian	2 HGG (III, IV), 1 LGG (II)	LHem	Frontal: posterior MFG, temporal: posterior MTG	Yes	No

F female, *M* male, μ mean, *RH* right handed, *LH* left handed, *NR* not reported, *NS* not specified, *LGG* low-grade glioma, *HGG* high grade glioma, *Other* metastases, cavernoma, meningioma, arteriovenous malformation, clonic seizure, cortical dysplasia, *LHem* left hemisphere, *RHem* right hemisphere, *SFG* superior frontal gyrus, *MFG* middle frontal gyrus, *IFG* inferior frontal gyrus, *SPL* superior parietal lobe, *IPL* inferior parietal lobe, *AG* angular gyrus, *MTG* middle temporal gyrus that are partly shared with and partly different from other language functions. The informative value of mapping spelling during neurosurgical procedures depends on the entire language system's integrity and several practical issues. In this chapter, we evaluate whether spelling tasks are actually useful during neurosurgical mappings in relationship with, among other factors, the brain region under evaluation. Throughout this chapter, we use the word "spelling" when referring to all the tasks requiring access to abstract knowledge of orthography, and we use "handwriting," "oral spelling," and "typing" when referring to these specific tasks.

8.2 The Writing Brain

All forms of spelling (i.e., handwriting, typing, and oral spelling) are highly dependent on at least two main brain systems: language and motor processes. Knowledge about the neuroanatomy of spelling initially came from neuropsychological studies of patients with brain lesions [10, 11] and has been expanded by neuroimaging, lesion, and electrostimulation studies (see Planton et al. [12] and van Ierschot [3] for reviews). A detailed description of the linguistic and motoric processes and their neural correlates is beyond the scope of this chapter, yet we can delineate three cortical regions that are consistently reported to be involved in handwriting: (1) the left posterotemporal lobe, (2) the parietal lobe, and (3) the region between the left superior and middle frontal gyri. Based on lesion, neuroimaging, and electrostimulation studies, these regions could support the processes specific or at least crucial to handwriting. We will describe the roles of these areas and their specificity to handwriting.

The posterotemporal lobe is involved in both alphabetic and morphosyllabic (Chinese or Japanese) spelling systems. The posterior parts of the *left superior and middle temporal gyri* are involved in several stages of the auditory-to-motor pathway of handwriting from dictation, be it through comprehension of the dictated sentences, lexico-semantic retrieval, or phonologic processing [8]. Lesion and neuroimaging studies have tied the posterior superior temporal gyrus to the sound-to-print mapping in spelling (phoneme-grapheme conversion) [13, 14], showing that disturbance of this region causes difficulty in the spelling of pseudowords or novel words. Other studies have also pointed to the posterior middle temporal gyrus for phoneme-grapheme conversion processing [15]. Lesion studies showed that damage to the superior temporal lobe may result in difficulties to write letter in the right order, particularly in longer words [16]. Another area of the left temporal lobe, the *fusiform gyrus* near the inferior occipitotemporal junction and the posterior inferior temporal lobe, has been consistently shown to be involved in the selection of the correct orthographic string from long-term memory (orthographic output lexicon) [12, 17–24]. Focal damage to this area can result in "surface" agraphia, characterized by phonologically plausible errors [21, 22, 25]. However, converging data have shown that the left fusiform area may not be spelling specific, as it is also involved in reading [26] through the "Visual Word Form Area" [27] (see Chap. 7).

Within the parietal lobe, the *left superior parietal cortex* has been proposed as a site of temporary storage of "visuokinesthetic and sequential motor engrams for letters and words" (graphemic buffer) [28], in line with the function of sensorimotor integration generally attributed to the posterior parietal lobe [29, 30]. Other studies stressed the role of the intraparietal sulcus in graphemic buffer processing [22, 31]. The *left inferior parietal cortex* (*supramarginal and angular gyrus*) also seems crucial for spelling [32], although the involvement of the supramarginal and angular gyri in spelling-specific tasks is debated in neuroimaging and lesion studies [12, 22]. The *supramarginal gyrus* has been proposed as the neural underpinning of phoneme-to-grapheme conversion procedures [33, 34], in conjunction with the opercular part of Broca's area [35, 36]. Damage to this region is associated with an inability to write pseudowords or novel words [13, 37]. Yet, the function of the supramarginal gyrus may not be restricted to spelling, as specific pseudoword reading disturbances were also observed during cortical electrostimulation in this gyrus [38]. Lesions of the *angular gyrus* are classically associated with spelling disturbances [10]. Although lexical agraphia (i.e., inability to write irregular words after orthographic output lexical disturbance) has been reported in patients with damage to the angular gyrus [33, 39], studies with more precise localization techniques have shown that the angular gyrus may not be involved in the orthographic output lexicon [20, 24]. Moreover, spelling disturbances related to Gerstmann syndrome (dysgraphia, acalculia, finger agnosia, inability to distinguish between the right and left side of the body) have been observed during electrostimulation of this gyrus [4]. Finally, neuroimaging studies have shown that in addition to the superior parietal lobe and the supramarginal gyrus, the angular gyrus may also be involved in graphemic buffer processes in reading and writing Chinese characters [40, 41].

The junction of the *left superior and middle frontal* gyri is commonly referred to as Exner's area [42]. This area (located in BA6) is located just in front of the hand area in the primary motor cortex and is generally thought of as being specifically involved in spelling. In clinical practice, pure agraphia (spelling impairment with preserved oral language) has been observed in patients with frontal lobe lesions [20, 43, 44]. Damage to BA6 has been shown to result in difficulties in spelling words with letters in the right sequential order (graphemic buffer damage) [45, 46] and in allographic processing difficulties, i.e., in the formation of letters [11, 47]. Congruently, neuroimaging studies showed BA6 activity during specific linguistic spelling tasks (e.g., long word spelling) [31, 41, 48], as well as in sensorimotor spelling tasks related to finger or hand movements [6, 34, 49, 50]. More recent neuroimaging data underlined the importance of this area as a handwriting-specific area that is involved in handwriting only and not in, for example, oral spelling [51]. The results of awake surgery studies are in line with this finding, showing that electrostimulation of BA6 could specifically impair handwriting [6]. Since these impairments were characterized by ill-formed letters, slow handwriting, or handwriting arrest, Roux et al. proposed that Exner's area could function as an interface between abstract orthographic representations and the generation of motor commands and named it the *graphemic/motor frontal area* (GMFA). A similar viewpoint was adopted by Purcell et al. [52] to account for the activation of this area in a bimanual typing task. Scarone et al. [50] also suggested that among the patients, only those with lesions of the supplementary motor area could not recover from agraphia in the postoperative period.

Finally, little is known about the subcortical pathways involved in spelling. In a single case report, Motomura et al. [9] showed that the portion of the inferior fronto-occipital fasciculus that links the frontal lobe to the superior parietal lobule plays a role in reading and writing.

In summary, as also suggested by Scarone et al. [50], the left superior parietal lobe, the intraparietal sulcus, and the region between the left superior and middle frontal gyri seem to be crucial, handwriting-specific regions (Fig. 8.1). Other regions in the left temporal and inferior parietal lobes are also important in spelling, albeit involved also in other language tasks. Subcortical pathways need to be investigated in greater detail.

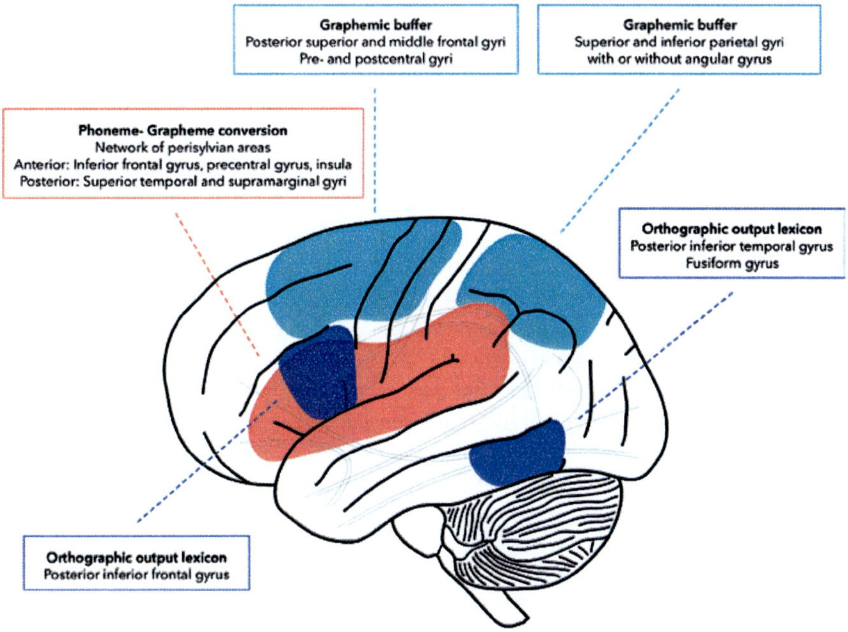

Fig. 8.1 Schematic illustration of the role of the different areas involved in handwriting. The cortical regions most consistently reported as critical for the linguistic stages of spelling in lesion and neuroanatomical studies are depicted. In frontal regions, the posterior superior and middle frontal gyri (Exner's area) have been linked with graphemic buffer processing. The posterior portion of the inferior frontal gyrus is mentioned in relation with the orthographic output lexicon and phoneme-grapheme conversion procedures. In the parietal lobe, the superior parietal gyrus, the intraparietal sulcus, and (to lesser extent) the inferior parietal gyrus are critical for graphemic buffer processing. The inferior parietal lobule (and mostly the supramarginal gyrus) is also frequently correlated with phoneme-grapheme conversion procedures. In temporal regions, the posterior superior temporal gyrus correlates with phoneme-grapheme conversion processing. The left fusiform gyrus is involved in long-term memory storage of orthographic word forms

8.3 Special Cases: Different Scripts, Bilingualism, Handedness, and Sex Differences

Most of the literature on the organization of the spelling process in the brain is based on alphabetic scripts, and brain organization could be different if different types of scripts are used. For instance, results of neuroimaging studies focused on lexical decision showed that differences between the neural substrates of alphabetic versus Chinese characters could exist in the middle frontal and the fusiform gyri [53]. Along the same lines, performance differences in kanji (morphogram) versus kana (phonogram) spelling in Japanese patients with brain lesions led Sakurai to propose that the angular gyrus, the posterior middle temporal gyrus, and the intraparietal sulcus are critical for kanji spelling, whereas the supramarginal gyrus plays a critical role in kana spelling [54]. Differences could also exist between the orthographic representations of digits (Arabic numbers) and letters (words), as suggested by Chen et al. [40] and by the finding of dissociated impairment of the two written codes in a patient with a surgical lesion of the premotor cortex reported by Anderson et al. [47]

It has also been shown that brain mapping results could be influenced by bilingualism [55–57]. The brains of bilingual individuals might host both language-shared and language-specific cortical areas [58]. More selective dissociations, such as the impairment of spelling in only one language [59, 60], have been reported. Lubrano et al. [5] mapped the areas of Exner's region that were involved in handwriting in an Arabic/French bilingual patient. In this case, the localization of areas critical for spelling was similar for French and Arabic. The small number of observations in bilingual patients leaves a lot of uncertainty as to whether spelling areas specific for each language are the rule or the exception. As it is, testing spelling skills in both languages in bilingual patients is a good option, especially when the spelling systems of the languages involved differ significantly.

Handedness is also a condition that can modify brain organization. It has been shown that the preferred hand of left- and right-handed subjects is controlled mainly by the hemisphere contralateral to that hand, whereas the non-preferred hand is controlled by both hemispheres [61]. Functional MRI also revealed that the GMFA was a common left frontal writing-specific area activated during word handwriting in left- and right-handed patients [6].

Finally, activations during handwriting tasks may differ between men and women [62]. A study on handwriting in Chinese showed that men could have a more important activation in the left posterior middle frontal gyrus than women [63]. However, the literature on potential sex-linked differences in the brain organization of spelling processes is too sparse to allow conclusions that may constrain neurosurgical mappings.

8.4 Mapping Writing Function During Awake Surgery: Practical Issues

Several issues can be debated when testing spelling during awake surgery: (1) the position of the patient during surgery and the support used, (2) her/his level of consciousness, (3) the types of tasks and/or stimuli used, (4) the analysis of the possible errors induced by electrostimulation and their significance, and (5) the reproducibility of interferences. Literature on these topics—in contrast to the well-known motor and naming tasks used during awake surgery—is scarce.

First, the usual position for writing to be upright and write by hand on a horizontal surface or to sit or stand in front of a computer and type on a keyboard. The position of the patient lying on the operating table is not ideal for writing or typing. In handwriting, the hand used by the patient must be released and adapted to the paper sheet or the tablet, which in turn must be placed in such a manner that the patient can see what (s)he is writing. Typing may be more difficult to evaluate than handwriting, as it requires the patient to freely use both hands, which is difficult to achieve in the operating room. When the patient uses only his/her dominant hand to type, typing is slower and unnatural, and interferences could be difficult to analyze and interpret.

Second, handwriting requires a high level of consciousness that cannot be taken for granted when patients are awakened from general anesthesia for awake surgery procedures. Compared to naming, pure motor, or counting tasks, writing is more complex, as it depends on multiple cognitive processes. Fatigue, stress, and persisting effects of anesthetic drugs from the initial anesthesia are all factors that can affect the patient's performance.

Third, the selection of tasks and stimuli to be administered before and during surgery—and during electrocortical mapping—is complex. Spelling can be assessed in different modalities that may have both advantages and disadvantages. As the linguistic processes of handwriting, typing, and oral spelling rely on shared processes, theoretically the linguistic aspects of spelling may be assessed by any of these tasks. Generally speaking, however, it is advisable to adapt the perioperative task(s) to the educational level of the patient and his/her daily use of spelling abilities. As writing by hand is increasingly replaced by digital spelling (associated with the use of computers, tablet devices, or mobile phones), the modality selected to assess spelling may change. As regards motoric processes, different neural regions may be involved in different tasks as shown by the fact that the left posterior parietal and anterior left premotor cortices are more active in typing than in handwriting [64]. The choice between spelling modalities is also influenced by the language of the patient. For example, native speakers of orthographically transparent languages, such as Italian, do not learn to spell orally, whereas oral spelling is a pivotal educational task in speakers of orthographically opaque languages, like English or French. Another relevant issue in task selection concerns input modality. The three most commonly used tasks are spelling in response to dictation, copying a text, and spontaneous writing. As for task selection, spelling may be assessed with words, pseudowords, or sentences. Furthermore, at each of these levels, regularity, length, frequency, and grammatical class may be varied systematically. Within an ongoing debate [3, 65], a proposal is to select the specific stimuli that, based on the functional neuroanatomy of the spelling brain, assess functions that are at greater risk of damage during surgery (see *Which Spelling Tasks for Which Location: When to Assess Spelling Intraoperatively*, later in this chapter).

Fourth, interferences may be less easy to analyze and detect in writing than in other language-related tasks. While interferences are usually identified quickly by the brain mapping team during naming or reading tasks, the numerous potential sources of spelling errors may complicate performance evaluation. For example, while writing or typing arrests are immediately seen, other spelling interferences such as phonemic or semantic interferences or motoric alterations in handwriting are more difficult to distinguish on the spot. Moreover, the patient's customary handwriting will be modified when lying on the operating table. This will make the analysis of possible interferences induced by electrostimulation difficult. It has also been observed that spelling errors can arise with some delay (sometimes more than 5 s) after electrostimulation. For this reason, from the clinical standpoint one may argue that dictating sentences (including subject/verb/other words) is more likely to elicit errors than dictating isolated words. In several studies, Roux and coworkers [5, 6, 66] mapped spelling skills by using a stimulation train of 4 or 5 s just after the beginning of a sentence and then observing possible interferences. They observed fewer interferences when stimulation was applied during the dictation of isolated words than when it was applied during the dictation of sentences (regardless of whether stimulation was delivered a few seconds before or at the beginning of word dictation). Yet, for scientific purposes, dictating words may offer a more accurate analysis of the stimulation sites and of the disruption of specific cognitive processes than sentence dictation.

Finally, regarding the validation of spelling interferences, uncertainties remain with respect to stimulation parameters and the reliability of direct electrical stimulation protocols. As with well-known tasks such as picture naming, the choice of the current intensity to be used for stimulation and the reproducibility of language trials need to be statistically reliable before one can conclude that an area is involved in spelling [67, 68]. Empirically, one could start by assuming that the intensity of stimulation (and other current parameters) needed to detect a spelling interference should be the same used for picture naming or reading tasks [68] and then test this hypothesis in a large, prospective study. However, it is important to understand that, as is the case with naming [67], electrostimulation trials in spelling assessments can produce graded patterns of positive reproducibility levels. For instance, out of three electrical stimulations in two areas, only a single spelling interference may be detected in one area, and two interferences in another. It is relatively rare for interferences to be consistently identified in response to all three of a set of stimulations delivered to a single site. The significance of the outcome of stimulation should be interpreted in the light of the baseline error rates found in the preoperative evaluation.

8.5 An Illustrative Case

A 45-year-old right-handed, bilingual (English/French) woman with a cavernoma between the left superior and middle frontal gyri was selected for awake surgery. She was born in the USA and had been living in France for 20 years. She spoke

English at home and French at work. The decision to remove the cavernoma was made after she had two partial seizures over a 3-month period. A complete preoperative evaluation of speech and non-spoken language tasks such as handwriting was performed in both French and English and revealed no abnormality. Intraoperative language mapping was performed in both languages with picture naming, word reading, and handwriting (writing sentences in response to dictation) tasks (Fig. 8.2). Three trials were performed for each task for each cortical area studied. The simulation parameters were as follows: current intensity 7 mA; biphasic square wave pulses of 1 ms duration; 60-Hz trains; and maximum train duration 6 s.

a

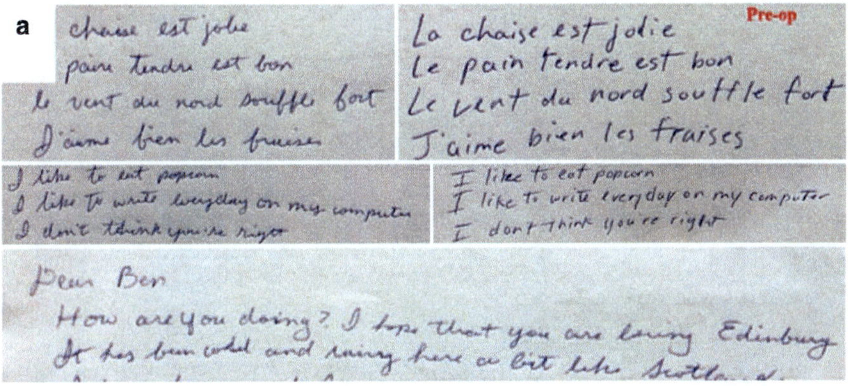

Fig. 8.2 An illustrative case: mapping spelling in a 45-year-old bilingual woman with a cavernoma close to Exner's area. (**a**) Examples of the preoperative spelling output (dictation, copying, free spelling) with different kinds of handwriting (cursive and print) in both languages. Preoperative spelling evaluation was normal. (**b**) A region involved in spelling (indicated by W) was detected in Exner's area (MNI coordinates: $x = -23.8$, $y = 3.9$, $z = 61.8$). The MNI coordinates place it close to the center of mass of the fMRI activations found in the middle frontal gyrus by the meta-analysis of Planton et al. [12] and to those of an fMRI/electrostimulation study performed in 12 patients and 12 volunteers [6]. (**c**) The W in the intraoperative photograph indicates the area of spelling error. The errors (indicated by red underscoring) were repetitive when stimulating this area (three trials in each language and interferences in each trial): letters were ill-formed, the patient stopped spelling. These spelling errors were detected in English and in French, and the type of interference was similar in both languages. When this area was stimulated, the patient showed no interference in the repetitive flexion/extension of the fingers of the right hand and no ocular movement or other motor activity. Furthermore, no reading and naming interferences were detected in this area. The spelling interference was considered as specific and localized in a patch of cortex less than 1 cm^2 (high spatial resolution of the stimulation). Stimulation of nearby cortical areas induced no response. This spelling area was spared, although the surgical approach used to remove the cavernoma was close (1 cm). There was an area of hesitation (marked H) in French naming—with three of four trials positive in this area. (**d**) Examples of spelling to dictation the same text one day after surgery show some errors. Letters are still ill-formed. (**e**) Three days after surgery no spelling errors were detected, thus reaching the preoperative baseline

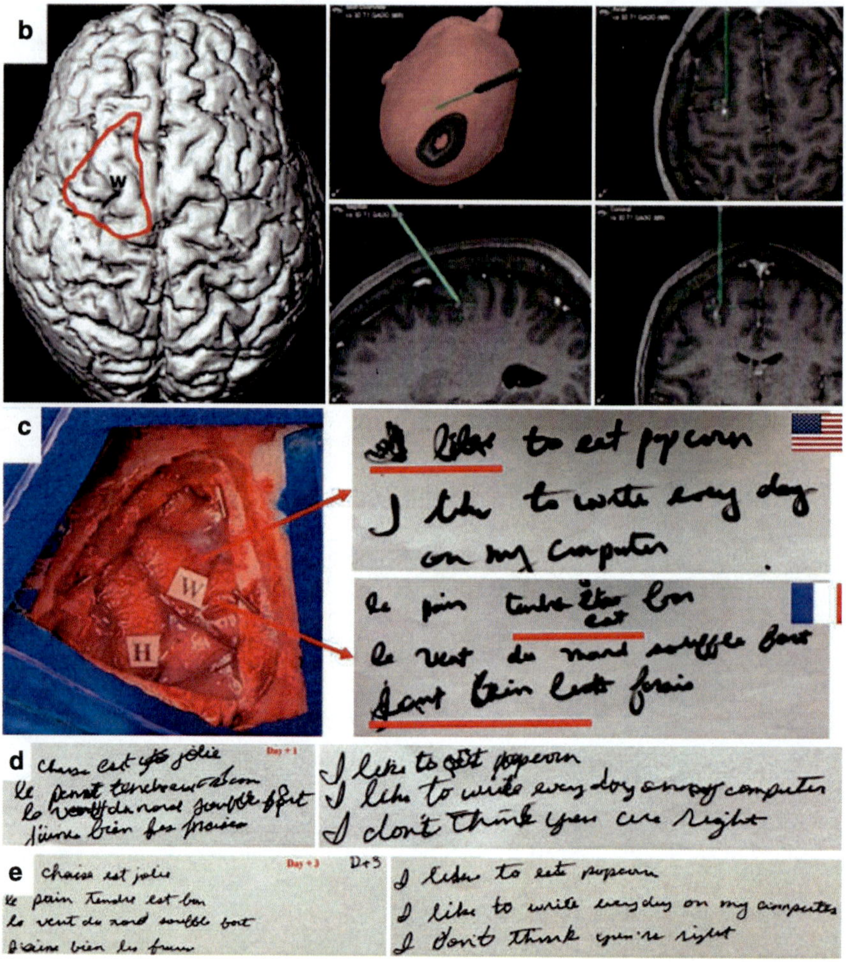

Fig. 8.2 (continued)

8.6 Which Spelling Tasks for Which Location: When to Assess Spelling Intraoperatively

The selection of tasks for brain mapping in neurosurgery is the matter of a continued debate, focused on whether testing should be carried out with the same standard tasks or tailored to the brain region to be operated upon and to the patient's preoperative skills [69, 70]. Both approaches have advantages and drawbacks. The main advantage of standard tasks such as object naming or reading is that they are simple to administer and interpret. These tasks have also been "validated" in numerous publications for many decades. On the other hand, increasing knowledge about neurofunctional correlates leads us to propose a more articulated array of tasks, according to the brain region being tested. As it is known that lesions in specific brain regions may result in the disruption of specific tasks, the functioning of that brain region may not be adequately assessed by using another task. For example, stimulation of the left superior parietal lobe may cause errors in writing but not in object naming or reading. If only naming or reading is assessed, one might inaccurately conclude that the left superior parietal lobe is not crucial for language skills and therefore may be removed. On the other hand, a main limitation of this approach is that "novel" tasks are likely to be less validated. Moreover, the more tasks one administers, the more likely it is that one will find interferences. The question is whether all these interferences are actually informative, hence useful for the patient undergoing surgery. The use of many intraoperative tasks for brain mapping in a single case may be discouraged based on surgical constraints, as it may cause the patient discomfort and/or fatigue and unduly lengthen the procedure. Spelling assessment is a typical example of a task that may induce interferences during intraoperative mapping, but whose usefulness could be questioned. Would sparing of the cortical areas for spelling detected by electrostimulation avoid deficits in the patient's ability to write? Or could permanent (or transient) deficits be induced if these areas are not spared? Because neurosurgeons would prefer in most cases to spare a detected area rather than to remove it, cases in which these areas are not spared are rare. To evaluate the possible sparing of spelling, a recent study investigated the degree of generalization across different language tasks in a small number of patients [3]. Results showed that spelling was preserved in all cases in which it was assessed intraoperatively. Nevertheless, spelling deficits could arise in the immediate postoperative period when only naming or reading (but not spelling) was assessed intraoperatively.

On the other hand, it may be argued that finding interference in a given cortical area during a task does not always make sparing of that area necessary. The area can be dispensable, its removal leading to no apparent difficulty because the brain is able to compensate (sometimes immediately) for some deficits [71]. For example, in the study of Scarone et al. [50], only patients with a SMA resection had long-lasting (>24 months) motoric dysgraphia. Also, a deficit may not be equally disabling for all patients, as the ability to write may not be equally crucial for each individual's quality of life.

Furthermore, spelling performance after surgery may not be influenced only by the preservation of spelling areas. For example, Lubrano et al. [5] found subtle spelling disturbances in postoperative evaluations after intraoperative preservation of spelling areas and suggested that these disturbances might be due to global language impairment, fatigue, or concomitant radiotherapy.

In a series of studies [5, 6, 66], areas of interference with spelling were not always found. But when detected, these areas were not deliberately removed. Whether such areas were detected or not, no pure agraphia was observed postoperatively, and spelling difficulties were associated in most cases with more global, transient language disturbances. We hope that future neurosurgical brain mapping studies will provide more data on this topic.

8.7 Conclusions

The lesion, neuroimaging, and awake surgery literature on the organization of spelling is rather sparse compared to the literature on other language functions. If the surgical team decides to assess spelling intraoperatively, the location of the tumor can be used together with preoperative neuropsychological and language evaluation to aid in the selection of tasks and stimuli. The region between the left superior and middle frontal gyri (Exner's area), the left superior parietal lobe, and the intraparietal sulcus seem more specific to spelling than other cortical areas (inferior parietal lobe and posterior temporal gyrus). We propose that intraoperative spelling tasks should be used when mapping of the spelling-specific regions is needed, while other language tasks may suffice to assess the functioning of other brain regions.

References

1. Penfield W, Roberts L. Speech and brain-mechanisms. Princeton: Princeton University Press; 1959.
2. Lesser RP, Lueders H, Dinner DS, Hahn J, Cohen L. The location of speech and writing functions in the frontal language area: results of extraoperative cortical stimulation. Brain. 1984;107:275–91. https://doi.org/10.1093/brain/107.1.275.
3. Tsapkini K, Vindiola M, Rapp B. Patterns of brain reorganization subsequent to left fusiform damage: fMRI evidence from visual processing of words and pseudowords, faces and objects. Neuroimage. 2011;55:1357–72. https://doi.org/10.1016/j.neuroimage.2010.12.024.
4. Roux FE, Boetto S, Sacko O, Chollet F, Trémoulet M. Writing, calculating, and finger recognition in the region of the angular gyrus: a cortical stimulation study of Gerstmann syndrome. J Neurosurg. 2003;99:716–27. https://doi.org/10.3171/jns.2003.99.4.0716.
5. Lubrano V, Roux FE, Démonet JF. Writing-specific sites in frontal areas: a cortical stimulation study. J Neurosurg. 2004;101:787–98. https://doi.org/10.3171/jns.2004.101.5.0787.
6. Roux FE, Dufor O, Giussani C, Wamain Y, Draper L, Longcamp M, et al. The graphemic/motor frontal area Exner's area revisited. Ann Neurol. 2009;66:537–45. https://doi.org/10.1002/ana.21804.
7. Magrassi L, Bongetta D, Bianchini S, Berardesca M, Arienta C. Central and peripheral components of writing critically depend on a defined area of the dominant superior parietal gyrus. Brain Res. 2010;1346:145–54. https://doi.org/10.1016/j.brainres.2010.05.046.
8. Roux FE, Durand JB, Réhault E, Planton S, Draper L, Démonet JF. The neural basis for writing from dictation in the temporoparietal cortex. Cortex. 2014;50:64–75. https://doi.org/10.1016/j.cortex.2013.09.012.
9. Motomura K, Fujii M, Maesawa S, Kuramitsu S, Natsume A, Wakabayashi T. Association of dorsal inferior frontooccipital fasciculus fibers in the deep parietal lobe with both reading and writing processes: a brain mapping study. Case report. J Neurosurg. 2014;121:142–8. https://doi.org/10.3171/2014.2.JNS131234.
10. Déjérine MJ. Contribution à l'étude des troubles de l'écriture chez les aphasiques. Mém Soc Biol. 1891;9:97–113.
11. Exner S. Untersuchungen über die Localisation der Functionen in der Grosshirnrinde des Menschen. Vienna: Braumüller; 1881.
12. Planton S, Jucla M, Roux FE, Démonet JF. The "handwriting brain": a meta-analysis of neuroimaging studies of motor versus orthographic processes. Cortex. 2013;49:2772–87. https://doi.org/10.1016/j.cortex.2013.05.011.

13. Henry ML, Beeson PM, Stark AJ, Rapcsak SZ. The role of left perisylvian cortical regions in spelling. Brain Lang. 2007;100:44–52. https://doi.org/10.1016/j.bandl.2006.06.011.
14. Ludersdorfer P, Kronbichler M, Wimmer H. Accessing orthographic representations from speech: the role of left ventral occipitotemporal cortex in spelling. Hum Brain Mapp. 2015;36:1393–406. https://doi.org/10.1002/hbm.22709.
15. Potgieser ARE, van der Hoorn A, de Jong BM. Cerebral activations related to writing and drawing with each hand. PLoS One. 2015;10:e0126723. https://doi.org/10.1371/journal.pone.0126723.
16. Buchwald A, Rapp B. Distinctions between orthographic long-term memory and working memory. Cogn Neuropsychol. 2009;26:724–51. https://doi.org/10.1080/02643291003707332.
17. Hillis AE, Work M, Barker PB, Jacobs MA, Breese EL, Maurer K. Re-examining the brain regions crucial for orchestrating speech articulation. Brain. 2004;127:1479–87. https://doi.org/10.1093/brain/awh172.
18. Nakamura K, Honda M, Okada T, Hanakawa T, Toma K, Fukuyama H, et al. Participation of the left posterior inferior temporal cortex in writing and mental recall of kanji orthography. A functional MRI study. Brain. 2000;123(5):954–67.
19. Purcell JJ, Turkeltaub PE, Eden GF, Rapp B. Examining the central and peripheral processes of written word production through meta-analysis. Front Psychol. 2011;2:239. https://doi.org/10.3389/fpsyg.2011.00239.
20. Rapcsak SZ, Beeson PM. The role of left posterior inferior temporal cortex in spelling. Neurology. 2004;62:2221–9. https://doi.org/10.1212/01.wnl.0000130169.60752.c5.
21. Rapcsak SZ, Arthur SA, Rubens AB. Lexical agraphia from focal lesion of the left precentral gyrus. Neurology. 1988;38:1119–23. https://doi.org/10.1212/wnl.38.7.1119.
22. Rapp B, Fischer-Baum S, Miozzo M. Modality and morphology: what we write may not be what we say. Psychol Sci. 2015;26:892–902. https://doi.org/10.1177/0956797615573520.
23. Sugihara G, Kaminaga T, Sugishita M. Interindividual uniformity and variety of the "writing center": a functional MRI study. Neuroimage. 2006;32:1837–49. https://doi.org/10.1016/j.neuroimage.2006.05.035.
24. Tomasino B, Marin D, Maieron M, D'Agostini S, Medeossi I, Fabbro F, et al. A multimodal mapping study of conduction aphasia with impaired repetition and spared reading aloud. Neuropsychologia. 2015;70:214–26. https://doi.org/10.1016/j.neuropsychologia.2015.02.023.
25. Segal E, Petrides M. The anterior superior parietal lobule and its interactions with language and motor areas during writing. Eur J Neurosci. 2012;35:309–22. https://doi.org/10.1111/j.1460-9568.2011.07937.x.
26. Beeson PM, Rapcsak S, Plante E, Chargualaf J, Chung A, Johnson S, et al. The neural substrates of writing: a functional magnetic resonance imaging study. Aphasiology. 2003;17:647–65. https://doi.org/10.1080/02687030344000067.
27. Cohen L, Dehaene S, Naccache L, Lehéricy S, Dehaene-Lambertz G, Hénaff M-A, et al. The visual word form area: spatial and temporal characterization of an initial stage of reading in normal subjects and posterior split-brain patients. Brain. 2000;123:291–307. https://doi.org/10.1093/brain/123.2.291.
28. Sakurai Y, Onuma Y, Nakazawa G, Ugawa Y, Momose T, Tsuji S, et al. Parietal dysgraphia: characterization of abnormal writing stroke sequences, character formation and character recall. Behav Neurol. 2007;18:99–114. https://doi.org/10.1155/2007/906417.
29. Andersen RA, Snyder LH, Bradley DC, Xing J. Multimodal representation of space in the posterior parietal cortex and its use in planning movements. Annu Rev Neurosci. 1997;20:303–30. https://doi.org/10.1146/annurev.neuro.20.1.303.
30. Rapp B, Lipka K. The literate brain: the relationship between spelling and reading. J Cogn Neurosci. 2011;23:1180–97. https://doi.org/10.1162/jocn.2010.21507.
31. Rapp B, Dufor O. The neurotopography of written word production: an fMRI investigation of the distribution of sensitivity to length and frequency. J Cogn Neurosci. 2011;23:4067–81. https://doi.org/10.1162/jocn_a_00109.

32. Baldo JV, Kacinik N, Ludy C, Paulraj S, Moncrief A, Piai V, et al. Voxel-based lesion analysis of brain regions underlying reading and writing. Neuropsychologia. 2018;115:51–9. https://doi.org/10.1016/j.neuropsychologia.2018.03.021.
33. Roeltgen DP, Heilman KM. Lexical agraphia: further support for the two-system hypothesis of linguistic agraphia. Brain. 1984;107:811–27. https://doi.org/10.1093/brain/107.3.811.
34. Soma Y, Sugishita M, Kitamura K, Maruyama S, Imanaga H. Lexical agraphia in the Japanese language: pure agraphia for kanji due to left posteroinferior temporal lesions. Brain. 1989;112:1549–61. https://doi.org/10.1093/brain/112.6.1549.
35. Jobard G, Crivello F, Tzourio-Mazoyer N. Evaluation of the dual route theory of reading: a metanalysis of 35 neuroimaging studies. Neuroimage. 2003;20:693–712. https://doi.org/10.1016/S1053-8119(03)00343-4.
36. Vidaković MR, Gabelica D, Vujović I, Šoda J, Batarelo N, Džimbeg A, et al. A novel approach for monitoring writing interferences during navigated transcranial magnetic stimulation mappings of writing related cortical areas. J Neurosci Methods. 2015;255:139–50. https://doi.org/10.1016/j.jneumeth.2015.08.003.
37. Alexander MP, Friedman RB, Loverso F, Fischer RS. Lesion localization of phonological agraphia. Brain Lang. 1992;43:83–95. https://doi.org/10.1016/0093-934x(92)90022-7.
38. Roux FE, Durand JB, Jucla M, Réhault E, Reddy M, Démonet JF. Segregation of lexical and sub-lexical reading processes in the left perisylvian cortex. PLoS One. 2012;7:e50665. https://doi.org/10.1371/journal.pone.0050665.
39. Roeltgen DP. Agraphia. In: Heilman KM, Valenstein E, editors. Clinical neuropsychology. 3rd ed. Oxford: Oxford University Press; 2003. p. 126–45.
40. Chen H, Pan X, Bickerton WL, Lau JK, Zhou J, Zhou B, et al. Delineating the cognitive-neural substrates of writing: a large scale behavioral and voxel based morphometry study. Sci Rep. 2019;9:1881. https://doi.org/10.1038/s41598-019-55129-3.
41. Chen HY, Chang EC, Chen SHY, Lin YC, Wu DH. Functional and anatomical dissociation between the orthographic lexicon and the orthographic buffer revealed in reading and writing Chinese characters by fMRI. Neuroimage. 2016;129:105–16. https://doi.org/10.1016/j.neuroimage.2016.01.009.
42. Roux FE, Draper L, Köpke B, Démonet JF. Who actually read Exner? Returning to the source of the frontal "writing centre" hypothesis. Cortex. 2010;46:1204–10. https://doi.org/10.1016/j.cortex.2010.03.001.
43. Gordinier HC. A case of a brain tumor at the base of the second left frontal convolution. Am J Med Sci. 1899;117:526–35.
44. Mahoudeau D, David M, Lecoeur J. Un nouveau cas d'agraphie sans aphasie révélatrice d'une tumeur métastatique du pied de la deuxieme circonvolution frontale gauche. Rev Neurol (Paris). 1951;84:159–61.
45. Hillis AE, Caramazza A. The graphemic buffer and attentional mechanisms. Brain Lang. 1989;36:208–35. https://doi.org/10.1016/0093-934x(89)90062-x.
46. Miceli G, Capasso R, Benvegnù B, Caramazza A. The categorical distinction of vowel and consonant representations: evidence from dysgraphia. Neurocase. 2004;10:109–21. https://doi.org/10.1080/13554790409609942.
47. Anderson S, Damasio A, Damasio H. Troubled letters but not numbers. Domain specific cognitive impairments following focal damage in frontal cortex. Brain. 1990;113:749–66. https://doi.org/10.1093/brain/113.3.749.
48. van Ierschot F, Bastiaanse R, Miceli G. Evaluating spelling in glioma patients undergoing awake surgery: a systematic review. Neuropsychol Rev. 2018;28:470–95. https://doi.org/10.1007/s11065-018-9391-7.
49. Katanoda K, Yoshikawa K, Sugishita M. A functional MRI study on the neural substrates for writing. Hum Brain Mapp. 2001;13:34–42. https://doi.org/10.1002/hbm.1023.
50. Scarone P, Gatignol P, Guillaume S, Denvil D, Capelle L, Duffau H. Agraphia after awake surgery for brain tumor: new insights into the anatomo-functional network of writing. Surg Neurol. 2009;72(3):223–41. https://doi.org/10.1016/j.surneu.2008.10.074.

51. Planton S, Longcamp M, Péran P, Démonet JF, Jucla M. How specialized are writing-specific brain regions? An fMRI study of writing, drawing and oral spelling. Cortex. 2017;88:66–80. https://doi.org/10.1016/j.cortex.2016.11.018.
52. Purcell JJ, Napoliello EM, Eden GF. A combined fMRI study of typed spelling and reading. Neuroimage. 2011;55:750–62. https://doi.org/10.1016/j.neuroimage.2010.11.042.
53. Vigneau M, Beaucousin V, Hervé PY, Duffau H, Crivello F, Houdé O, et al. Meta-analyzing left hemisphere language areas: phonology, semantics, and sentence processing. Neuroimage. 2006;30:1414–32. https://doi.org/10.1016/j.neuroimage.2005.11.002.
54. Sakurai Y. Kanji (morphogram) and kana (phonogram) problem in Japanese alexia and agraphia. Front Neurol Neurosci. 2019;44:53–63. https://doi.org/10.1159/000494952.
55. Ojemann GA, Whitaker HA. The bilingual brain. Arch Neurol. 1978;35:409–12. https://doi.org/10.1001/archneur.1978.00500310011002.
56. Roux FE, Lubrano V, Lauwers-Cances V, Trémoulet M, Mascott CR, Démonet JF. Intra-operative mapping of cortical areas involved in reading in mono- and bilingual patients. Brain. 2004;127:1796–810. https://doi.org/10.1093/brain/awh204.
57. Roux FE, Trétmoulet M. Organization of language areas in bilingual patients: a cortical stimulation study. J Neurosurg. 2002;97:857–64. https://doi.org/10.3171/jns.2002.97.4.0857.
58. Giussani C, Roux FE, Lubrano V, Gaini SM, Bello L. Review of language organisation in bilingual patients: what can we learn from direct brain mapping? Acta Neurochir (Wien). 2007;149:1109–16. https://doi.org/10.1007/s00701-007-1266-2.
59. Hinshelwood J. Four cases of word-blindness. Lancet. 1902;1:358–63. https://doi.org/10.1016/S0140-6736(01)81505-1.
60. Wang X, Yang J, Yang J, Mencl WE, Shu H, Zevin JD. Language differences in the brain network for reading in naturalistic story reading and lexical decision. PLoS One. 2015;10:e0124388. https://doi.org/10.1371/journal.pone.0124388.
61. Grabowska A, Gut M, Binder M, Forsberg L, Rymarczyk K, Urbanik A. Switching handedness: fMRI study of hand motor control in right-handers, left-handers and converted left-handers. Acta Neurobiol Exp (Wars). 2012;72:439–51.
62. Yang Y, Tam F, Graham SJ, Sun G, Li J, Gu C, et al. Men and women differ in the neural basis of handwriting. Hum Brain Mapp. 2020;41:2642–55. https://doi.org/10.1002/hbm.24968.
63. Yamadori A. Ideogram reading in alexia. Brain. 1975;98:231–8. https://doi.org/10.1093/brain/98.2.231.
64. Higashiyama Y, Takeda K, Someya Y, Kuroiwa Y, Tanaka F. The neural basis of typewriting: a functional MRI study. PLoS One. 2015;10:e0134131. https://doi.org/10.1371/journal.pone.0134131.
65. Kandel S, Perret C. How does the interaction between spelling and motor processes build up during writing acquisition? Cognition. 2015;136:325–36. https://doi.org/10.1016/j.cognition.2014.11.014.
66. Roux S, McKeeff TJ, Grosjacques G, Afonso O, Kandel S. The interaction between central and peripheral processes in handwriting production. Cognition. 2013;127:235–41. https://doi.org/10.1016/j.cognition.2012.12.009.
67. Roux FE, Djidjeli I, Quéhan R, Réhault E, Giussani C, Durand J. Intraoperative electrostimulation for awake brain mapping: how many positive interference responses are required for reliability? J Neurosurg. 2019. https://doi.org/10.3171/2019.6.JNS19925.
68. Roux FE, Durand JB, Djidjeli I, Moyse E, Giussani C. Variability of intraoperative electrostimulation parameters in conscious individuals: language cortex. J Neurosurg. 2017;126:1641–52. https://doi.org/10.3171/2016.4.JNS152434.
69. Coello AF, Moritz-Gasser S, Martino J, Martinoni M, Matsuda R, Duffau H. Selection of intraoperative tasks for awake mapping based on relationships between tumor location and functional networks: a review. J Neurosurg. 2013;119:1380–94. https://doi.org/10.3171/2013.6.JNS122470.

70. Rofes A, Spena G, Miozzo A, Fontanella M, Miceli G. Advantages and disadvantages of intraoperative language tasks in awake surgery: a three-task approach for prefrontal tumors. J Neurosurg Sci. 2015;59:337–49.
71. Gibb WR, Kong NW, Tate MC. Direct evidence of plasticity within human primary motor and somatosensory cortices of patients with glioblastoma. Neural Plast. 2020;2020:8893708. https://doi.org/10.1155/2020/8893708.

Repeating

9

Sylvie Moritz-Gasser

9.1 Introduction

Verbal repetition consists of the immediate or short-delayed spoken reproduction of an auditory stimulus, that is, the transcoding of an auditory input into an articulatory output, then requiring the coordinated involvement of auditory, memory, and motor processes. Therefore, this apparent simple task actually involves a complex set of subprocesses. Verbal repetition necessitates to process lexical-semantic as well as sub-lexical-phonological linguistic components, suggesting a dual-route model of processing [1] in which the two routes interact [2] albeit at various degrees depending on the nature of the verbal input to be repeated (e.g., real word/non-word/sentence) [3, 4]. Furthermore, the brief delay between input and output processes, during which the verbal input has to be temporarily maintained in memory in order to be correctly repeated, put forward the strong involvement of verbal short-term memory (STM), including two components—the phonological buffer and the articulatory loop [5]— in language repetition [6], underlining the necessary consideration of the interaction of domain-general cognitive mechanisms with language processing [7, 8] and their integration in neurocomputational models.

Verbal STM abilities, as assessed by means of non-word repetition, have further been linked to the development of vocabulary in children [9, 10], and to grammatical learning and expressive skills [11]. Repetition skills seem then to play a crucial role in language development and are considered, together with tense marking and sentence recall, as clinical markers of developmental language disorders such as specific language impairment (SLI) [12–15]. Finally, in post-stroke aphasic patients, word repetition abilities in the acute phase, as well as the initial severity of

S. Moritz-Gasser (✉)
Institute of Functional Genomics, INSERM U1191, Team "Plasticity, Stem Cells and Glial Tumors", University of Montpellier, Montpellier, France

Gui de Chauliac Hospital, Montpellier, France
e-mail: sylvie.gasser@umontpellier.fr

E. Mandonnet, G. Herbet (eds.), *Intraoperative Mapping of Cognitive Networks*,
https://doi.org/10.1007/978-3-030-75071-8_9

phonological disorders, seem to be a strong predictor of verbal long-term outcomes [16–18].

Repeating is then a critical linguistic skill and deserves a special attention during intraoperative brain mapping. After a review of brain structures involved in this ability, we describe in this chapter knowledge gained from lesion-symptom and intraoperative mapping studies, and then propose a relevant protocol that may be used for intraoperative mapping of verbal repetition.

9.2 Neural Bases of Verbal Repetition

In the context of the dual-stream model of language processing [19], it is well known that phonological-articulatory processes (linking sound to articulation) are mediated by a left dorsal stream underlain by the arcuate/superior longitudinal fasciculi (AF-SLF) while semantic processes (linking sound to meaning) are mediated by a ventral stream underlain by the inferior fronto-occipital/inferior longitudinal/uncinate fasciculi (IFOF-ILF-UF) [20–23]. It is then traditionally claimed that verbal repetition, consisting in transcoding an auditory input into an articulatory output, activates predominantly the dorsal components of this network, underlain by the left AF-SLF. The role of the dorsal stream in this skill has indeed been widely demonstrated [20, 24, 25], with the long medial AF—connecting the middle and inferior temporal gyri (MTG, ITG) with precentral gyrus and pars opercularis of the inferior frontal gyrus (IFG), crucially involved in decoding and encoding phonological representations (phonological buffer), and the anterolateral SLFIII—connecting the supramarginalis gyrus (SMG) and superior temporal gyrus (STG) with the precentral gyrus [26–28], essential in linking phonological information to articulatory-based representations (articulatory loop) [29–31]. Studies of patients with the logopenic variant of primary progressive aphasia (lvPPA), notably characterized by frequent pauses in spoken language and impairments in sentence repetition attributed to a deficit in the phonological loop component of STM, have besides identified a pattern of damage affecting primarily the left temporo-parietal junction and loss of volume in long underlying association dorsal tracts [32]. Furthermore, it has been shown that AF lesion load in chronic post-stroke aphasic patients significantly predicted rate, informativeness, and overall efficiency of speech [33].

Yet, pioneering works by Wernicke [34, 35] and Lichtheim [36] already suggested the involvement of both the dorsal and the ventral stream in repetition, on the basis of predictions drawn from the observation of two different types of repetition disorders in aphasic individuals: inability to repeat real words and pseudowords, associated with production of phonological paraphasia along with attempts to correct ("*conduites d'approche*") known as *conduction aphasia*, which could be due to a failure in the direct phonological pathway, or production of semantically related errors in real words repetition, associated with difficulties in repeating pseudowords, currently termed *deep dysphasia* [37], which in contrast could be due to a failure in the indirect lexical-semantic pathway [38]. These predictions have been further confirmed by more recent neuropsychological, neurostimulation, imaging, and lesion based studies, specifying besides the neural underpinnings of verbal repetition. Hanley et al. [4] suggested that dissociated repetition impairment patterns in aphasic patients (e.g., production of semantic paraphasia in real-word repetition tasks/production of phonological paraphasia in repetition of real word of low imageability only, both accompanied by difficulties in repeating pseudoword) support the existence of both lexical and sublexical repetition routes interacting with each other, consistent with the dual-route model of repetition [1], and the "summation" hypothesis [2]. Another evidence for the role of both routes and their interaction in repetition is *conduites d'approche* behavior, i.e., successive phonological attempts to correct, typically observed in patients with *conduction aphasia* associated with damage to the AF in whom activation from the ventral semantic pathway has been shown to increase the rate of successful *conduites d'approche* in real-word repetition tasks [39]. Therefore, this deceptively simple skill appears to be supported by a widely distributed network of mainly—but not exclusively—left-sided regions belonging predominantly to the dorsal route underlain by the AF/SLF and interacting with the ventral route, including notably the superior temporal sulcus (STS), parieto-temporal junction (PTJ, in particular area Sylvian-parietal-temporal Spt), inferior parietal lobe (IPL, especially SMG), pars orbitalis and opercularis of the IFG, ventral premotor cortex (vPMC), supplementary motor area (SMA), anterior insula, putamen, and posterior part of the MTG and ITG [24, 40–45]. It is worth noting that a few studies highlighted repetition deficits in right-sided brain lesioned patients [46, 47], as well as lack of repetition impairments or successful recovery of repetition skills in patients with damage to the left AF [48–51], suggesting a possible involvement of the right hemisphere in verbal repetition in right-handers, presumed to depend however on inter-individual variability in the hemispheric lateralization of the AF [3, 52]. Furthermore, in order to perform the maintenance of verbal information, domain-general processes are synchronously recruited along with linguistic processes (including verbal STM) in a flexible manner depending on the load of the verbal material to be repeated (single real word/pseudoword varying in imageability/complexity, word list, sentence) and on time constraints (immediate/delayed repetition) [8]. Serial order and attentional processing systems are thus implicated in verbal repetition, likely involving a bilateral fronto-parietal network, in order to maintain and coordinate linguistic representations temporarily activated in the dorsal and ventral language processing networks [6]. Finally, if repetition of single words and word lists may result from activation of both hemispheres in temporo-parietal and premotor cortices, it has been shown that *non-word* repetition likely involves the same pattern of activation but only in the left hemisphere [22, 50], and that damage to specifically the white matter connectivity underlying this left dorsal network (AF/SLF) correlates significantly with repetition deficits [24, 25, 53]. This dissociation of activation patterns may be easily explained by the fact that, unlike real words, non-words are not associated with semantic representations and their repetition, which cannot be facilitated by word recognition, is consequently entirely reliant on phonological processing, involving in turn STM mechanisms [8, 53].

9.3 Knowledge Gained from Lesion-Symptom Mapping Studies in Glioma Patients

Among the rather large amount of studies assessing language processing in glioma patients, those focusing specifically on repetition abilities are quite scarce to date. In a recent study aiming to analyze the relationships between specific white matter pathways and language deficits, in order to determine which pathways are predictive of long-term language deficits following awake surgery, 35 left-sided glioma patients with pre- and postoperative high angular resolution diffusion-weighted imaging (HARDI q-ball) fiber tracking were included. Using a rating scale to estimate the degree of pathway injury, the authors found that the AF and/or temporo-parietal part of the SLF were significantly affected in patients with immediate postoperative language deficits, and that damage to these two pathways was predictive of long-term language deficit [54]. It is worth noting however that persistent language impairments were found only in high-grade glioma patients. In the same vein, a study based on preoperative diffusion tensor imaging with deterministic tractography of the AF, IFOF, and UF in 77 presumed low-grade glioma patients (62 left-sided) aimed to determine whether preoperative cognitive functioning, including language, would be associated with changes in white matter tracts microarchitecture. Among other results, a strong significant correlation was notably found between fractional anisotropy in the AF and phoneme/word/sentence repetition performances [55]. Finally, in a recent multimodal case study, Chernoff et al. [56] investigated notably whether longitudinal changes in inter-hemispheric connectivity relates to functional language recovery in a patient with a left inferior parietal glioma infiltrating the posterior part of the long segment of the AF. They found that, in addition to a reduction in the structural integrity of the left AF after surgery compared to before, left intra-hemispheric functional connectivity was reduced while inter-hemispheric connectivity increased between left hemisphere language regions and their right hemisphere homologues, and that these changes in functional connectivity were coincident with the patient recovery from a postoperative selective sentence repetition impairment, three and a half months after the surgery. The authors mentioned that sentence repetition difficulties already emerged at the end of the surgery, suggesting that it was not the cortical resection but rather the subcortical resection along the AF that caused them. They concluded that functional recovery may be facilitated by an increased synchrony between hemispheres.

9.4 Additional Anatomo-functional Knowledge Gained from Intraoperative Mapping Studies

Even if repetition is not routinely assessed during intraoperative brain mapping, current literature reporting results of electrostimulation-based studies combined with perioperative language evaluations offers valuable anatomo-functional insights concerning this skill. Leonard et al. [57] addressed the dynamics of neural processes underlying verbal (real word and non-word) repetition during electro-cortical stimulation in 58 patients undergoing an awake surgery for either epilepsy or glioma. By analyzing the type of errors transiently induced (e.g., phonological paraphasia, phonetic distortion, no response, perseveration) and the influence of psycholinguistic variables, such as word length and lexical frequency, they suggested that verbal repetition involves a distributed set of overlapping cortical regions, including the posterior STG, the SMG, and precentral gyrus, processing specific types of information (perceptual, phonological, speech-related) strongly influenced by psycholinguistic variables. More specifically, the role of the temporoparietal junction (TPJ) in language has been investigated in studies involving patients undergoing an awake surgery for a glioma located in the left IPL. In the first one, anomia was the most frequent cortical DES-induced impairment (9 cases out of 14) at the posterior part of the STG and MTG. At the subcortical level, articulatory disorders were induced by stimulation of white matter in the anterior and lateral part of the surgical cavity (11 cases out of 14), corresponding to the horizontal portion of the lateral segment of the SLF (SLF III). Deeper and superiorly, phonological paraphasia (in both naming and repetition) was induced in 12 cases out of 14, by DES of the postero-superior portion of the AF. All these structures were then surgically preserved and no patient retained a speech or language deficit 3 months postoperatively [30]. In the second one, the authors compared the rate of long-term language deficits in patients having undergone an awake surgery for a glioma invading the left IPL with intraoperative cortical (17 patients) and subcortical (8 patients) language mapping, and found that a significant higher rate of mild to moderate long-term language deficits (word finding difficulties, impaired repetition, paraphasia, alexia) was observed in patients who exhibited positive cortical language sites, as compared with patients who did not. They then concluded that, on the one hand, the absence of positive cortical stimulation sites overlying the tumor and resection cavity would be predictive of good language outcomes, and, on the other hand, the presence of long-term new postoperative language deficits in some patients would suggest that alternative protocols for subcortical stimulation mapping should be considered specifically for IPL glioma resection [58]. It is worth noting that in this study, a positive subcortical site eliciting anomia was found in the posterior portion of the AF, as reported in the first study. Therefore, these studies both confirm, if still needed, the crucial role of the AF in phonological processes, involved in naming as well as in repetition, underlining consequently the major importance of its monitoring during awake surgery, and the need for relevant tools to achieve it. An illustrative case is provided in Fig. 9.1, depicting intraoperative cortical and subcortical mapping in a patient with a left SMG glioma.

In this state of mind, Sierpowska et al. [59] conducted a study focusing on the monitoring of the AF function in 12 patients undergoing awake brain surgery for tumor resection in the AF vicinity. They aimed to compare the respective efficiency of a non-word repetition task (NWR) vs. real-word repetition task (WR) vs. naming task in detecting intraoperative phonological disorders, and then monitoring AF function. They thus designed a WR and NWR task (40 items in each) that they administered to the patients pre- and postoperatively, in addition to a standard neuropsychological assessment, and intraoperatively, in addition to a standard naming

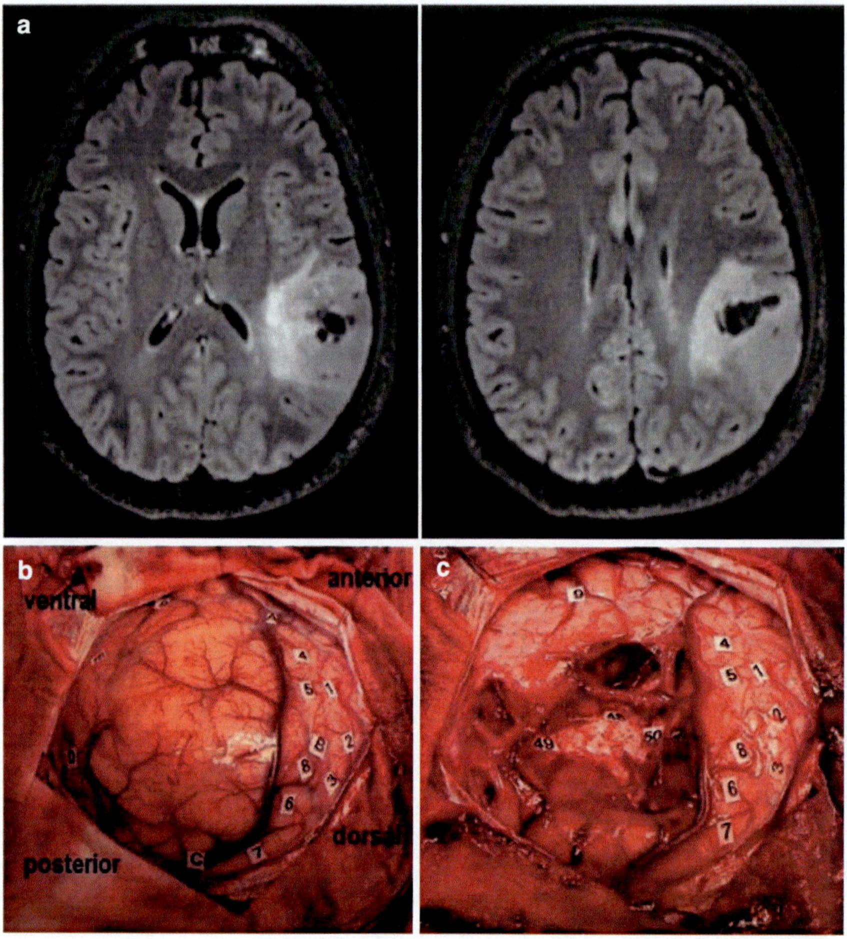

Fig. 9.1 Illustrative case involving a left SMG glioma. Preoperative axial FLAIR MRI (**a**). Cortical and subcortical intraoperative mapping before (**b**) and after (**c**) resection. At the cortical level, stimulation of the site labeled 9 elicited anomia during the naming task, no other cortical site elicited language disorders. At the subcortical level, stimulation of the site labeled 50 (posterior part of the SLF horizontal segment: SLF III) elicited articulatory disorders and syllabification during the naming task; stimulation of the sites labeled 48 and 49 (postero-superior part of the AF) elicited phonological paraphasia and spelling of the target word, during both naming and WR. *SMG* supra marginalis gyrus, *SLF* superior longitudinal fasciculus, *AF* arcuate fasciculus, *WR* word repetition

task. At the 3 times of evaluation, they detected significantly more errors using the NWR task than the WR task, and observed that intraoperative disorders in NWR could occur whereas naming was not marred by phonological paraphasias. The authors then propose to introduce a NWR task in addition to WR and naming tasks during awake brain mapping in the vicinity of the AF, in order to increase the accuracy of AF function monitoring. The need to use a NWR task in addition to WR was previously suggested in an opinion article based on the analysis of DES-induced disorders and perioperative examinations in 200 glioma patients [31]. In this article, the authors highlighted besides a strong interaction between the dorsal phonological stream and the ventral semantic stream in verbal repetition, the latter one being likely involved in control mechanisms of semantic activations during WR, consistent with the reported relation between increased rate of successful *conduites d'approche* and activation from the ventral semantic pathway during WR in patients with conduction aphasia [39].

We may summarize the above sections as follows:

By converting auditory inputs into articulatory outputs, verbal repetition involves strongly the phonological buffer and the articulatory loop of verbal STM; repetition abilities are linked to lexical/grammatical learning and expressive skills in developmental conditions, and are predictive of language recovery in acquired pathological conditions; repetition is anatomically heavily supported by the dorsal phonological network, involving a distributed set of peri-sylvian cortical regions, underlain by the AF-SLF, interacting with the ventral semantic network; damage to this dorsal network in the context of brain tumor, and seemingly to the postero-superior part of the AF especially, is particularly deleterious for phonological processing and predictive of postoperative long-term language impairment; a NWR task seems to be more sensitive than a WR or naming task in detecting phonological disorders.

9.5 Monitoring Repetition Intraoperatively: Proposal of a Relevant Protocol

As for any function, intraoperative monitoring of repetition abilities should be performed with the unique goal of achieving a maximal tumor resection while avoiding long-lasting deficits. It is therefore not relevant to assess repetition per se during brain mapping, but only with regard to the meaning of a reproducible stimulation-induced repetition deficit, that is, to cognitivo-linguistic disorders that may lead to or be caused by a deficit in repetition abilities. As described above, verbal repetition is supported by both a lexical and a sublexical route interacting with each other: since lexical processes are routinely assessed intraoperatively by means of a naming task, is there a need for adding a repetition task? In other words, does a repetition task bring a genuine contribution compared to a naming task? Given the link between repetition skills and verbal STM and the role they consequently seem to play, as specified above, in language development as well as in the prediction of verbal long-term outcomes in aphasic patients, we may answer yes to both questions. Furthermore, as described by Sierpowska et al. [59], intraoperative phonological impairments may emerge during NWR whereas no phonological paraphasia is produced in picture-naming. Likewise, if cases of preserved repetition despite impaired naming are common, converse cases of impaired repetition despite preserved naming, albeit rare, have been reported [47], emphasizing the need to add a repetition task to the standard picture-naming task, as a highly informative task for monitoring sensory, cognitive, linguistic, as well as speech-related motor functions [57]. Lastly, given the strong involvement of verbal STM in language repetition, adding a repetition task is also of great interest for assessing STM performances (see Chap. 12). It has further been shown at this regard that span tasks using non-words would provide a more sensitive measure of phonological STM capacity than tasks involving real words or digits, because of the absence of lexical-semantic information associated with non-words [8]. Therefore, taking also into account awake brain mapping time constraints, knowledge gained from glioma patients studies, and provided that speech-related motor functions, lexical retrieval, and semantic processing are monitored in a sound-designed fashion (see Chaps. 5 and 15), intraoperative repetition mapping might be performed according to the following criteria:

- Assessment of repetition abilities before, just after, and at least 3 months after the surgery by means of WR varying in frequency, length, and imageability, NWR varying in length, and sentences repetition varying in length and level of plausibility, in addition to the standard neuropsychological evaluation.
- Left-sided glioma: Intraoperative mapping of repetition in case of impaired naming resulting in anomia, consisting in repeating the target word and, in the same stimulation site, repeating non-words.
- Left- and right-sided glioma infiltrating the posterior dorsal network (IPL, post STG, postero-superior AF): systematic intraoperative mapping of repetition in addition to the standard naming task, even in case of preserved naming, with WR and NWR tasks.

9.6 Conclusion

Repeating is a critical linguistic skill that deserves a special attention during intraoperative brain mapping. The review of literature provided in this chapter underlines the link between repetition abilities, verbal short-term memory, language processing, and overall efficiency of spontaneous discourse, and the critical role of the dorsal phonological network in this skill, involving a set of cortical peri-sylvian areas and sustained by the arcuate fasciculus, especially in its postero-superior portion. Given knowledge gained from this literature but also time constraints of awake brain mapping, performed with the unique goal of achieving a maximal tumor resection while avoiding long-lasting impairments, a relevant protocol of intraoperative repetition monitoring is needed in addition to standard naming tasks, in order to avoid repetition deficits, and then to strengthen postoperative language outcomes and to promote speech-language and cognitive rehabilitation strategies.

References

1. McCarthy R, Warrington EK. A two-route model of speech production. Evidence from aphasia. Brain. 1984;107:463–85.
2. Hillis A, Caramazza A. Mechanisms for accessing lexical representations for output: evidence from a category specific semantic deficit. Brain Lang. 1991;40:106–44.
3. Berthier ML, Froudist Walsh S, Dávila G, Nabrozidis A, Juárez Y, Ruiz de Mier R, Gutiérrez A, De-Torres I, Ruiz-Cruces R, Alfaro F, García-Casares N. Dissociated repetition deficits in aphasia can reflect flexible interactions between left dorsal and ventral streams and gender-dimorphic architecture of the right dorsal stream. Front Hum Neurosci. 2013;7:873.
4. Hanley JR, Kay J, Edwards M. Imageability effects, phonological errors, and the relationship between auditory repetition and picture naming: implications for models of auditory repetition. Cogn Neuropsychol. 2002;19(3):193–206.
5. Baddeley A, Lewis V, Vallar G. Exploring the articulatory loop. Q J Exp Psychol Sect A. 1984;36(2):233–52.
6. Majerus S. Language repetition and short-term memory: an integrative framework. Front Hum Neurosci. 2013;7:357.
7. Friederici AD. The cortical language circuit: from auditory perception to sentence comprehension. Trends Cogn Sci. 2012;16:262–8.
8. Jacquemot C, Scott SK. What is the relationship between phonological short-term memory and speech processing? Trends Cogn Sci. 2006;10(11):480–6.
9. Baddeley A, Gathercole S, Papagno C. The phonological loop as a language learning device. Psychol Rev. 1998;105(1):158–73.
10. Gathercole SE, Baddeley A. Evaluation of the role of phonological STM in the development of vocabulary in children: a longitudinal study. J Mem Lang. 1989;28:200–13.
11. Adams A, Gathercole S. Phonological working memory and speech production in preschool children. J Speech Hear Res. 1995;38:403–14.
12. Conti-Ramsden G. Processing and linguistic markers in young children with specific language impairment (SLI). J Speech Lang Hear Res. 2003;46(5):1029–37.
13. Montgomery JW. Working memory and comprehension in children with specific language impairment: what we know so far. J Commun Disord. 2003;36(3):221–31.
14. Redmond SM, Thompson HL, Goldstein S. Psycholinguistic profiling differentiates specific language impairment from typical development and from attention-deficit/hyperactivity disorder. J Speech Lang Hear Res. 2011;54(1):99–117.
15. Tager-Flusberg H. Defining language impairments in a subgroup of children with autism spectrum disorder. Sci China Life Sci. 2015;58(10):1044–52.
16. El Hachioui H, Lingsma HF, van de Sandt-Koenderman MW, Dippel DW, Koudstaal PJ, Visch-Brink EG. Long-term prognosis of aphasia after stroke. J Neurol Neurosurg Psychiatry. 2013;84(3):310–5.
17. Glize B, Villain M, Richert L, Vellay M, de Gabory I, Mazaux JM, Dehail P, Sibon I, Laganaro M, Joseph PA. Language features in the acute phase of poststroke severe aphasia could predict the outcome. Eur J Phys Rehabil Med. 2017;53(2):249–55.
18. Tábuas-Pereira M, Beato-Coelho J, Ribeiro J, Nogueira AR, Cruz L, Silva F, Sargento-Freitas J, Cordeiro G, Santana I. Single word repetition predicts long-term outcome of aphasia caused by an ischemic stroke. J Stroke Cerebrovasc Dis. 2020;29(2):104566.
19. Hickok G, Poeppel D. Dorsal and ventral streams: a framework for understanding aspects of the functional anatomy of language. Cognition. 2004;92(1–2):67–99.
20. Duffau H. The anatomo-functional connectivity of language revisited: new insights provided by electrostimulation and tractography. Neuropsychologia. 2008;46:927–34.
21. Duffau H, Moritz-Gasser S, Mandonnet E. A re-examination of neural basis of language processing: proposal of a dynamic hodotopical model from data provided by brain stimulation mapping during picture naming. Brain Lang. 2014;131:1–10.

22. Saur D, Kreher BW, Schnell S, Kümmerer D, Kellmeyer P, Vry MS, et al. Ventral and dorsal pathways for language. Proc Natl Acad Sci U S A. 2008;105(46):18035–40.
23. Tremblay P, Dick AS. Broca and Wernicke are dead, or moving past the classic model of language neurobiology. Brain Lang. 2016;162:60–71.
24. Fridriksson J, Kjartansson O, Morgan PS, Hjaltason H, Magnusdottir S, Bonilha L, Rorden C. Impaired speech repetition and left parietal lobe damage. J Neurosci. 2010;30(33):11057–61.
25. Kümmerer D, Hartwigsen G, Kellmeyer P, Glauche V, Mader I, Klöppel S, Suchan J, Karnath HO, Weiller C, Saur D. Damage to ventral and dorsal language pathways in acute aphasia. Brain. 2013;136(Pt 2):619–29.
26. Bernard F, Zemmoura I, Ter Minassian A, Lemée JM, Menei P. Anatomical variability of the arcuate fasciculus: a systematical review. Surg Radiol Anat. 2019;41(8):889–900.
27. Makris N, Kennedy DN, McInerney S, Sorensen AG, Wang R, Caviness VS Jr, et al. Segmentation of subcomponents within the superior longitudinal fascicle in humans: a quantitative, in vivo, DT-MRI study. Cereb Cortex. 2005;15:854–69.
28. Martino J, De Witt Hamer PC, Berger MS, Lawton MT, Arnold CM, de Lucas EM, Duffau H. Analysis of the subcomponents and cortical terminations of the perisylvian superior longitudinal fasciculus: a fiber dissection and DTI tractography study. Brain Struct Funct. 2013;218(1):105–21.
29. Duffau H, Gatignol P, Denvil D, Lopes M, Capelle L. The articulatory loop: study of the subcortical connectivity by electrostimulation. Neuroreport. 2003;14:2005–8.
30. Maldonado IL, Moritz-Gasser S, de Champfleur NM, Bertram L, Moulinié G, Duffau H. Surgery for gliomas involving the left inferior parietal lobule: new insights into the functional anatomy provided by stimulation mapping in awake patients. J Neurosurg. 2011;115(4):770–9.
31. Moritz-Gasser S, Duffau H. The anatomo-functional connectivity of word repetition: insights provided by awake brain tumor surgery. Front Hum Neurosci. 2013;7:405.
32. Henry ML, Gorno-Tempini ML. The logopenic variant of primary progressive aphasia. Curr Opin Neurol. 2010;23(6):633–7.
33. Marchina S, Zhu LL, Norton A, Zipse L, Wan CY, Schlaug G. Impairment of speech production predicted by lesion load of the left arcuate fasciculus. Stroke. 2011;42(8):2251–6.
34. Wernicke C. Der aphasische Symptomenkomplex. Eine psychologische Studie auf Anatomischer Basis. Breslau: Cohn und Weigert; 1874.
35. Wernicke C. The symptom complex of aphasia. Monatsschr Psychiatr Neurol. 1903;4:265–324.
36. Lichtheim L. On aphasia. Brain. 1885;7:433–84.
37. Michel F, Andreewsky E. Deep dysphasia—an analog of deep dyslexia in the auditory modality. Brain Lang. 1983;18:212–23.
38. Eggert GH. Wernicke's works on aphasia: a source book and review. The Hague: Mouton; 1977.
39. Ueno T, Lambon Ralph MA. The roles of the "ventral" semantic and "dorsal" pathways in *conduite d'approche*: a neuroanatomically-constrained computational modelling investigation. Front Hum Neurosci. 2013;7:422.
40. Baldo JV, Katseff S, Dronkers NF. Brain regions underlying repetition and auditory-verbal short-term memory deficits in aphasia: evidence from voxel-based lesion symptom mapping. Aphasiology. 2012;26(3–4):338–54.
41. Forkel SJ, Rogalski E, Drossinos Sancho N, D'Anna L, Luque Laguna P, Sridhar J, Dell'Acqua F, Weintraub S, Thompson C, Mesulam MM, Catani M. Anatomical evidence of an indirect pathway for word repetition. Neurology. 2020;94(6):e594–606.
42. Fridriksson J, den Ouden DB, Hillis AE, Hickok G, Rorden C, Basilakos A, Yourganov G, Bonilha L. Anatomy of aphasia revisited. Brain. 2018;141(3):848–62.
43. Geschwind N. Disconnection syndromes in animals and man. Brain. 1965;88:237–94.
44. Hickok G, Buchsbaum B, Humphries C, Muftuler T. Auditory-motor interaction revealed by fMRI: speech, music, and working memory in area Spt. J Cogn Neurosci. 2003;15(5):673–82.
45. Hope TMH, Prejawa S, Parker Jones O, Oberhuber M, Seghier ML, Green DW, Price CJ. Dissecting the functional anatomy of auditory word repetition. Front Hum Neurosci. 2013;8:246.

46. De-Torres I, Dávila G, Berthier ML, Walsh SF, Moreno-Torres I, Ruiz-Cruces R. Repeating with the right hemisphere: reduced interactions between phonological and lexical-semantic systems in crossed aphasia? Front Hum Neurosci. 2013;7:675.
47. Pandey AK, Heilman KM. Conduction aphasia with intact visual object naming. Cogn Behav Neurol. 2014;27(2):96–101.
48. Abo M, Senoo A, Watanabe S, Miyano S, Doseki K, Sasaki N, et al. Language-related brain function during word repetition in post-stroke aphasia. Neuroreport. 2004;15(12):1891–4.
49. Bernal B, Ardila A. The role of the arcuate fasciculus in conduction aphasia. Brain. 2009;132(Pt 9):2309–16.
50. Berthier ML, Lambon Ralph MA, Pujol J, Green C. Arcuate fasciculus variability and repetition: the left sometimes can be right. Cortex. 2012;48(2):133–43.
51. Weiller C, Isensee C, Rijntjes M, Huber W, Müller S, Bier D, et al. Recovery from Wernicke's aphasia: a positron emission tomographic study. Ann Neurol. 1995;37(6):723–32.
52. Catani M, Mesulam M. The arcuate fasciculus and the disconnection theme in language and aphasia: history and current state. Cortex. 2008;44(8):953–61.
53. Parker Jones O, Prejawa S, Hope TM, Oberhuber M, Seghier ML, Leff AP, Green DW, Price CJ. Sensory-to-motor integration during auditory repetition: a combined fMRI and lesion study. Front Hum Neurosci. 2014;8:24.
54. Caverzasi E, Hervey-Jumper SL, Jordan KM, Lobach IV, Li J, Panara V, Racine CA, Sankaranarayanan V, Amirbekian B, Papinutto N, Berger MS, Henry RG. Identifying preoperative language tracts and predicting postoperative functional recovery using HARDI q-ball fiber tractography in patients with gliomas. J Neurosurg. 2016;125(1):33–45.
55. Incekara F, Satoer D, Visch-Brink E, Vincent A, Smits M. Changes in language white matter tract microarchitecture associated with cognitive deficits in patients with presumed low-grade glioma. J Neurosurg. 2019;130:1538–46.
56. Chernoff BL, Teghipco A, Garcea FE, Belkhir R, Sims MH, Paul DA, Tivarus ME, Smith SO, Hintz E, Pilcher WH, Mahon BZ. Reorganized language network connectivity after left arcuate fasciculus resection: a case study. Cortex. 2020;123:173–84.
57. Leonard MK, Cai R, Babiak MC, Ren A, Chang EF. The peri-Sylvian cortical network underlying single word repetition revealed by electrocortical stimulation and direct neural recordings. Brain Lang. 2019;193:58–72.
58. Southwell DG, Riva M, Jordan K, Caverzasi E, Li J, Perry DW, Henry RG, Berger MS. Language outcomes after resection of dominant inferior parietal lobule gliomas. J Neurosurg. 2017;127(4):781–9.
59. Sierpowska J, Gabarrós A, Fernandez-Coello A, Camins À, Castañer S, Juncadella M, Morís J, Rodríguez-Fornells A. Words are not enough: nonword repetition as an indicator of arcuate fasciculus integrity during brain tumor resection. J Neurosurg. 2017;126(2):435–45.

Syntax 10

Ryuta Kinno, Edward Chang, and Angela D. Friederici

10.1 Review of the Neural Basis of Syntax

Language is a complex cognitive system that contains different subsystems closely working together to ensure smooth language production and comprehension.

10.1.1 Syntax

Within the language system, syntax refers to the process that governs the word order structure of sentences in a given language. At the linguistic theoretical level Chomsky [1] was the first to propose a generative approach characterizing syntax in a systematic structural manner and, moreover, to define language as a biological "organ." Developments within the generative framework more recently put forward the view that syntax is based on a single computational mechanism called *Merge* which when recursively applied generates all possible phrases and sentences [2, 3]. Merge is defined as a computation bringing together two syntactic units to form a new one. For example, a determiner */the/* and the noun */man/* are combined to a new

R. Kinno (✉)
Division of Neurology, Department of Internal Medicine, Showa University Northern Yokohama Hospital, Yokohama, Japan
e-mail: kinno@med.showa-u.ac.jp

E. Chang
Department of Neurological Surgery, University of California, San Francisco, CA, USA
e-mail: Edward.Chang@ucsf.edu

A. D. Friederici
Department of Neuropsychology, Max Planck Institute for Human Cognitive and Brain Sciences, Leipzig, Germany
e-mail: friederici@cbs.mpg.de

E. Mandonnet, G. Herbet (eds.), *Intraoperative Mapping of Cognitive Networks*,
https://doi.org/10.1007/978-3-030-75071-8_10

syntactic unit, i.e., a determiner phrase /*the men*/. The determiner phrase /*the men*/ can be brought together with a verb /*sing*/ to make up a sentence /*the men sing*/. By applying this computation recursively, complex sentences can be generated.

10.1.2 Functional Imaging Studies

The description of the language-brain relationship was greatly improved and became more fine-grained with the advent of brain imaging. Initially, imaging studies focussed on semantic and phonological processes at the word level [4–8] and then also on syntactic processes [9–12]. Further imaging studies on syntactic processing reviewed in Friederici [13] systematically investigated different types of syntactically complex sentences in English, German, Hebrew, as well as Japanese and they all found activation in the left inferior frontal gyrus (IFG) to increase as a function of increased syntactic complexity. In addition to the frontal activations, increased activation was found in the left posterior temporal cortex mostly in the superior temporal gyrus (STG) and superior temporal sulcus (STS), but also in the middle temporal gyrus (MTG). Additional imaging studies in other languages support this view in general: Dutch [14]; Italian [15]; French [16]; and Chinese [17].

Guided by psycholinguistic theory, a study in German has shown that the systematic increase over complexity as implicated by the number of moved constituents lead to a parametric increase of left pars opercularis [18] and in the posterior STG/STS [19]. A study in French demonstrated that the increased size of the constituents resulted in increased activation in the left pars triangularis and the posterior temporal cortex [16]. It was demonstrated that these studies suggest that syntactic processes during comprehension recruit the left IFG and the left posterior STG/STS. These regions are functionally connected during sentence processing [20, 21].

Thus, these functional imaging studies provide a decent localization of syntactic processes for processing complex sentences. However, for a surgery-relevant test there are two issues that have to be considered: first, the reported imaging data are group data and second, the stimuli used are often too long for a presentation during surgery.

It has therefore been proposed to use verb processing tasks as stimuli for language and syntax mapping in awake surgery [22]. This is a valid proposal as the verb is a linguistic unit that carries syntactic information (verb-argument structure) in addition to its semantics. But verbs as such do not cover the core aspect of syntax, which is the rule-based combination of syntactic units, such as the computation *Merge*.

Stepping away from investigating syntactic processing by means of complex sentence structures, a recent approach focussed on the most basic computation *Merge*. It was demonstrated the basic linguistic computation can be localized in the posterior portion of Broca's area, the pars opercularis also called Brodmann Area (BA) 44 [23]. The stimulus material used in this study consisted of two-word sequences which either allowed the syntactic computation *Merge* (determiner and noun [in this case a pseudonoun] /*this flirk*/) or not (due to the missing determiner). The resulting activation was localized in a very confined subpart of BA 44, the most anterior-ventral part of BA 44, and, moreover, the variability across participants was very low. Conversely, the frontal operculum/anterior insula, a phylogenetically older and less specialized region, was found to be equally active for both phrasal structures and unstructured word-lists, not discriminating between these. Additional studies using this paradigm [17, 24] confirmed the functional localization of *Merge*. These data together with the findings from the studies on sentence processing indicate that BA 44 in the IFG supports syntactic processes at all levels of complexity, the most basic level [25] and the most complex levels [18, 26]. Thus, the two-word phrase paradigm provides a good candidate for syntax mapping during surgery.

To summarize it appears that functional imaging studies provide a more fine-grained syntax mapping than studies with stroke patients. Lesions in stroke patients are less confined and also vary in size from patient to patient. However, the studies agree in that the left IFG is important for syntactic processes in production and comprehension. It appears that within the IFG phrase structure building relies on the pars opercularis (BA 44), but that the pars triangularis (BA 45) comes into play when stimuli or tasks do not focus on purely syntactic information. Neuroimaging data suggest that the posterior portion of the superior temporal gyrus, moreover, plays a crucial role for sentence comprehension.

10.2 Review About Evidence of Long-Term Deficits in Patients Who Did Not Benefit from Intraoperative Monitoring of Syntax

Only few studies have carefully documented long-term deficits in patients who did not benefit from intraoperative monitoring of syntax. Syntax is not routinely assessed and not part of standard intraoperative language mapping. However, there have been studies carried out on patients with brain injuries that have resulted in syntactic deficits such as agrammatism.

Early localization models resulted in the classical view of Broca's area subserving language/speech production [27] and Wernicke's area subserving language/speech comprehension [28] that lasted for almost a century. Then the formulation of the linguistic theory by Chomsky [1] triggered new psycholinguistic and neurolinguistic thinking. In the 1970s, the idea emerged that syntax as a core subsystem of language may not only subserve language production, but also syntactic processes in language comprehension. This led to the prediction that a lesion causing the aphasic syndrome of agrammatic Broca's aphasia should also cause syntactic deficits in comprehension which was indeed demonstrated by Zurif and colleagues [29, 30]. Broca's aphasics were shown to comprehend complex sentences only when the interpretation was possible on the basis of semantic information /*the apple that the boy is eating is red*/, but not when it was dependent on the syntactic cues only /*the man that the woman is hugging is happy*/.

Similar results with patients were found in different languages for different sentence constructions in which assignment of the actor and the undergoer depends on syntactic cues. For English, comparable effects were found for passive constructions such as /*the boy was hugged by the woman*/ vs. /*the apple was eaten by the woman*/ in most cases of agrammatic patients [31]. For Dutch—a language with less strict word order than English—it was shown, however, that passive sentences are processes quite well by Broca's aphasics. As this holds independent of the position of the prepositional phrase (by-phrase) which indicates the actor role it appears that the lexical element "by" is used for subject-assignment in Dutch [32]. For German—a word order free, case marking language—respective effects were found for sentences in which subject and object nouns are coded by case marking in the determiner with nominative (NOM) case marking the subject noun and accusative (ACC) case marking the object noun /*der (NOM) Polizist sieht den (ACC) Räuber*/ vs. /*den (ACC) Räuber sieht der (NOM) Polizist*/, both sentences meaning /*the policeman sees the robber*/ [33]. Such sentences in particular the accusative-first construction require syntactic knowledge in order to understand who is doing what to whom as for these semantic reversible sentences semantic cues do not help.

For Japanese, lesions in the pars opercularis (BA 44) and pars triangularis (BA 45) are also reported to affect processing passive sentences [34]. In Japanese sentences—in contrast to English sentences—the verb is in sentence final position following the two argument nouns which are case marked, though the underlying syntactic structure remains ambiguous until the verb is encountered. Due to the sentence final position of the verb which is crucial for the construction of the underlying syntactic structure, the observed deficit in processing passive sentences reflects processes of syntactic reanalysis (see also [35]).

From these findings we have to conclude two things. First, in order to test syntactic abilities, one has to consider the specifics of the language under investigation. Second, one has to control the stimulus material well and prevent interaction with possible semantic cues which might allow to circumvent syntactic processes.

The likelihood of incurring temporary or permanent language dysfunction has been addressed by one study that retrospectively analyzed outcomes in 43 patients with gliomas that predominantly involved the dominant frontal operculum [36]. Transient deficits occurred in 12 patients (27.9%), while 4 patients (9.8%) had persistent deficits involving language. Individuals with preoperative language deficits and patients with seizures characterized by speech dysfunction appear to be at the highest risk to develop a deficit (relative risks 3.09 and 1.75, respectively). No patient with a tumor involving the pars orbitalis experienced a persistent deficit. Given the low rate of language morbidity reported in this group of patients, resection of gliomas within the dominant frontal operculum is well tolerated with acceptable morbidity and, in this particular location, it is not thought to be a deterrent in the overall management of these tumors.

10.3 Lesion-Symptom Mapping Studies for Syntactic Abilities of Patients with a Glioma

Although several lesion-symptom studies for patients with a glioma have been performed, there are a limited number of studies that have examined language function including syntactic processing. The first study that focused on the syntactic abilities of patients with a glioma was published in 2009 [34]. In this study, patients with a glioma in the left frontal cortex but with no apparent disability in verbal/written communication or intelligence quotient were examined by the picture–sentence verification task (Fig. 10.1) [37]. This task included three main conditions distinguished by sentence types: canonical/subject-initial active sentences, noncanonical/subject-initial passive sentences, and noncanonical/object-initial active sentences. Under these conditions, each sentence had a *transitive* verb and two arguments (phrases associated with the predicate) with different grammatical relations, i.e., which is the subject (S) of the verb (V), and which is its indirect object (IO) or direct object (DO). Sentence comprehension under each condition also explicitly required analysis of two different thematic roles, i.e., who initiates the action, and who is affected by it. In Japanese syntax, the grammatical relations are first marked by case markers (nominative, dative, or accusative), which in turn allow the assignment of thematic roles (*agent*, *experiencer*, or *patient*), whereas passiveness is also marked in the verb morphology (*-areru*). More specifically, the canonical/subject-initial active sentences, noncanonical/subject-initial passive sentences, and noncanonical/object-initial active sentences correspond to S-DO-V (*agent* and *patient*), S-IO-V (*experiencer* and *agent*), and DO-S-V (*patient* and *agent*) types, respectively. Therefore, these syntactic analyses for the two-argument relationships were critically required in our paradigm. The patients preoperatively underwent a

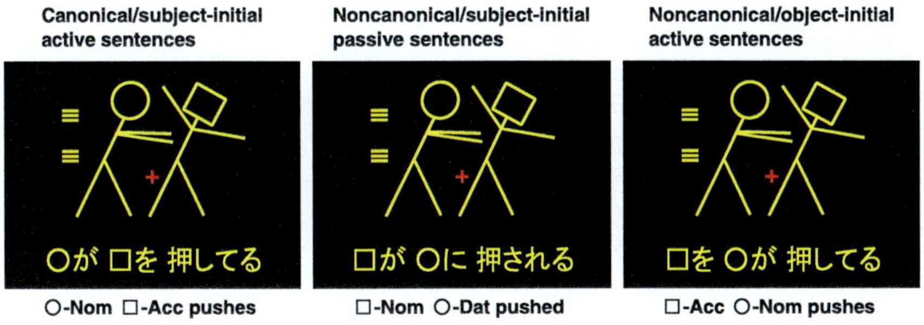

Fig. 10.1 The three main conditions used in the picture-sentence verification task. Each stimulus consisted of one picture (top) and one sentence (bottom). Pictures depicting actions consisted of two stick figures; each stick figure was distinguished by one of three "head" symbols: a circle (●), square (■), or triangle (▲). The participants indicated whether or not the meaning of each sentence matched the action depicted in the corresponding picture by pressing one of two buttons. Below each example, a word-by-word translation in English is shown. *Nom* nominative case, *Acc* accusative case, *Dat* dative case. An identical picture set was used under these three conditions. The sentence stimuli were all grammatical and commonly used in Japanese

high-resolution 3D-MRI, and voxel-based lesion-symptom mapping (VLSM; [38]) was employed for the error rates data.

This study showed that patients with a glioma in the left lateral premotor cortex had a profound deficit in the comprehension of noncanonical/object-initial active sentences. In contrast, patients with a glioma in the left pars opercularis and triangularis had a profound deficit in the comprehension of noncanonical/subject-initial passive sentences, and noncanonical/object-initial active sentences. These condition-selective deficits indicated the patients' deficits in syntactic analyses for the two-argument relationships.

10.3.1 Importance of Functional Connectivity for Preserving Syntactic Ability of Patient with a Glioma

A glioma has been generally considered to cause hyperexcitability throughout the entire brain, leading to epileptic seizures [39]. However, a magnetoencephalography study of the resting-state showed that a glioma disrupted functional connectivity across distant regions in both hemispheres [40]. Therefore, it was supposed that the agrammatic comprehension in patients with a glioma in the left IFG or left lateral premotor cortex was due to abnormal functional connectivity related syntax-related networks. In a functional MRI (fMRI) study, glioma patients who exhibited agrammatic comprehension showed abnormal overactivity and/or underactivity in the 14 regions during syntactic processing when compared to the healthy controls [41]. These 14 regions were grouped into three syntax-related networks (Fig. 10.2): Network I consists of the left pars opercularis and triangularis, left intraparietal sulcus, right frontal regions, pre-supplementary motor area, and right temporal regions. Network II consists of the left lateral premotor cortex, left angular gyrus, lingual gyrus, and cerebellar nuclei. Network III consists of the left ventral frontal and posterior temporal regions. When focusing on the functional connectivity among the three networks, the left fronto-parietal regions and the left pars triangularis and pars orbitalis are most important for preserving syntactic abilities of patients with a glioma in the left frontal cortex [42]. These findings led us to conclude that the disruption of connectivity between the left IFG and other brain regions is related to the deficits in syntactic abilities for patients with a glioma rather than the damage of brain region.

The importance for language processing of the connectivity between the left IFG and other brain regions in patients with a glioma has also been demonstrated in another study with fMRI and diffusion tensor imaging [43]. This study demonstrated that patients with lesion extension to the arcuate fasciculus connecting frontal to parietal and temporal regions are likely to show profound deficits in language processing. The selectivity for syntax remained unclear, but this study suggested the importance of functional connectivity for patients with a glioma. Other studies using VLSM for patients with a glioma showed that deficits in syntactic processing are significantly associated with a glioma in the left fronto-temporal regions, including the arcuate fasciculus [44], as well as a Broca-striatum tract linking pars

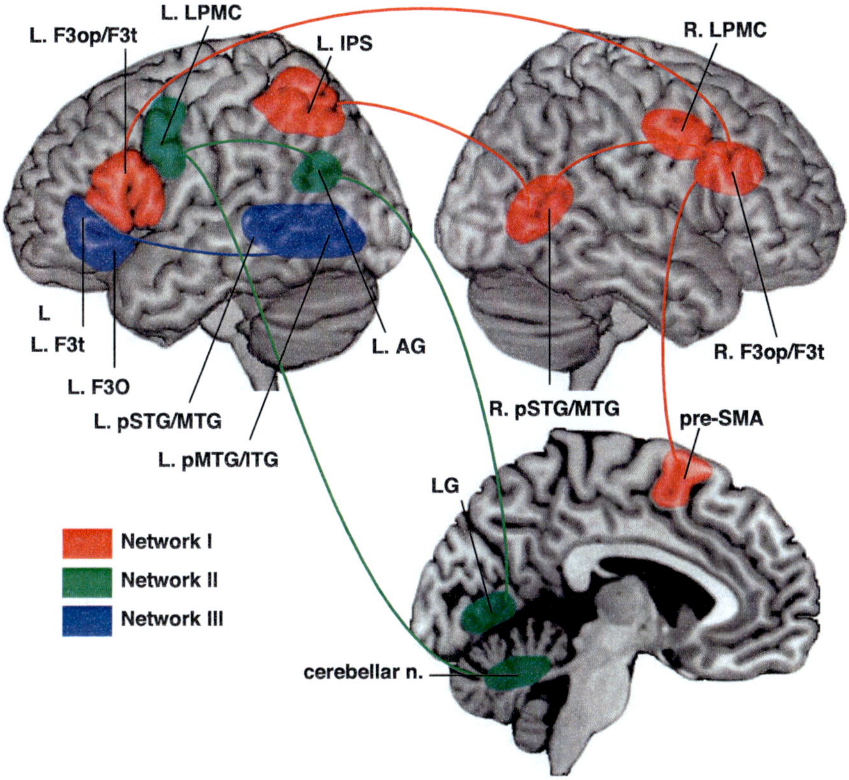

Fig. 10.2 Schematic of the three syntax-related networks in the normal brain. The brain regions for Networks I, II, and III are shown in red, green, and blue, respectively. Note that these three networks involve the left pars opercularis, left LPMC, and pars triangularis, respectively. Connections within individual networks are shown with colored lines. *AG* angular gyrus, *F3O* pars orbitalis, *F3op/F3t* pars opercularis and triangularis, *F3t* pars triangularis, *IPS* intraparietal sulcus, *L* left, *LG* lingual gyrus, *n.* nuclei, *pMTG/ITG* posterior middle/inferior temporal gyri, *pre-SMA* pre-supplementary motor area, *pSTG/MTG* posterior superior/middle temporal gyri, *R* right

triangularis with the left caudate head [45]. In addition to the syntactic ability to comprehend sentences, an intraoperative cortical stimulation study has shown the importance of connectivity between the left IFG and other brain regions for syntactic gender processing [46]. Taking these findings together, the authors concluded that a glioma in the left IFG disrupts the functional connectivity between the left IFG and other syntax-related regions, which results in deficits in syntactic processing. The deficits in syntactic ability of patients with a glioma may be subtle and therefore preoperative deficits in syntactic ability are difficult to detect by using a standard aphasia battery. Indeed, a recent study showed that most patients with presumed low-grade glioma had normal or nearly normal language function prior to surgical treatment [47]. These authors recommend conducting a thorough assessment of patients' language ability before surgery to identify possible subtle language deficits such as agrammatic comprehension and to establish a baseline against which to compare language functioning at post-treatment follow-ups. Further study will be required for better understanding of presurgical deficits in syntactic processing of patients with a glioma.

10.4 Review of the Different Tasks Newly Designed to Monitor Syntax Intraoperatively

Given the constraints on tasks that can be used intraoperatively due to time restrictions and the situation in the operation room, tasks to test syntactic abilities have to be considered with care.

Rofes and Miceli [22] in their review discussed the task used in the intraoperative setting. They suggest that the tasks should be based on current knowledge of the neuroscience of language, and that tasks should be language-specific. The present short review of the lesion studies across the different languages support this view. It is not that syntax per se is localized differently in the different languages, but it is the way the stimulus material is constructed. Languages differ with respect to fixed/free word order, presence/absence of case marking, amount of inflectional morphology, presence/absence of tonal parameters and their function. Thus, it is difficult to design a standardized test across the different languages.

Rather there seems to be the need to construct language-specific tests, which guarantee that syntactic structure building is tested independent of semantic cues preventing strategic processes that allow to circumvent syntactic structure building. The stimuli of these tests could require phrase structure building at the phrase level (determiner phrase, prepositional phrase, verb phrase) or the sentence level.

Also, specific behavioral tasks have to be defined that can be applied in the production domain and the comprehension domain. Fortunately, both domains can be investigated using line drawings, either for phrase/sentence generation during production or for phrase/sentence picture matching tasks during comprehension.

10.4.1 Possible Intraoperative Tests

Structure building can be investigated at the phrase and at the sentence level. Both structures can be realized in two-word sequences: for example, in a determiner phrase consisting of a determiner and a noun */a singer/* or a sentence consisting of a pronoun and a verb */he sings/*.

However, just asking which determiner goes together with what noun as in the study by Vidorreta et al. [46] is not a syntactic operation, since the grammatical gender is a property of the individual lexical item and stored in the lexicon. Thus, it is not surprising that during cortical stimulus mapping some patients showed elicited effects in the middle temporal gyrus.

In order to test syntactic processes, the task has to trigger phrase structure building while keeping the variation in the lexical items low. In principle phrases */a* *singer*/ and short sentences /*he sings*/ could be used a stimulus material. Such items have been successfully used during comprehension in a grammaticality judgment task for correct and incorrect combinations of these elements [48–50]. Ideally, an intraoperative test would not require grammaticality judgment, but rather production and comprehension performance triggered by line drawing pictures.

10.5 Review of Studies Evidencing a Functional Improvement in Series of Patients Operated on with Versus Without Syntax Monitoring

Diffuse grade II and III gliomas are considered as generally less aggressive tumors [51]. Modern neurosurgical oncology for these gliomas has the goal of maximal tumor resection while at the same time maintaining the patient's functional integrity, which ultimately defines the so-called onco-functional balance [52]. Operation with function monitoring has been shown to increase the extent of resection within eloquent areas, while lowering the number of late severe neurological deficits. Saito et al. [53] stated that continuous observation of the patient's intraoperative condition under awake craniotomy is the most reliable and direct method for monitoring their neurological function. This technique can be used to detect early deficits in language function. In addition, continuous direct observation under awake conditions may help the clinician to recognize unexpected neurological complications (e.g., disturbed consciousness due to hemorrhage outside the operative field in rare cases, thus leading to further imaging studies [e.g., intraoperative MRI or computed tomography]), which is useful from the viewpoint of risk management. Importantly, the direct clinical assessments with awake craniotomy do not show false negative results, which prevent suboptimal resection in patients undergoing glioma surgery. Consequently, the parallel use of awake craniotomy and intraoperative neurophysiological monitoring results in more accurate evaluations of the language functions. There was no study that provided direct evidence for the usefulness of function monitoring for preserving syntactic ability. We will thus review the studies that focused on the operation with monitoring of the language function of glioma patients in left IFG, which is one of the most important regions for syntactic abilities.

10.5.1 Functional Intraoperative Monitoring for the Left IFG

It is well known that the left pars opercularis and triangularis and its connection to other language areas are important for syntactic processing [13, 41]. A previous study examined 14 patients with suspected low-grade astrocytoma in the left pars opercularis [54]. In this study, degree and duration of postoperative deficits were retrospectively evaluated according to tumor location and boundaries on MR, intraoperative functional monitoring results, and extent of tumor resection. They found that 8 of 14 patients postoperatively showed speech or language disturbances. Among 6 patients who underwent neuropsychological evaluation, 3 patients exhibited speech apraxia while the other 3 patients had a true aphasic syndrome. The severity and duration of postoperative deficits correlated well with the distance from the resection margin to the next positive stimulation points, and a distance of more than 0.5 cm proved to avoid major impairments. Based on these findings, the authors concluded that surgery for WHO grade II and III gliomas in the left pars opercularis can result in speech apraxia or an aphasic syndrome, and therefore functional monitoring with intraoperative cortical electrical stimulation is essential in resecting tumors in the opercular region to avoid permanent morbidity.

Another study for patients with a glioma in the left pars opercularis and triangularis had found language reorganization with recruitment of the ventral and dorsal premotor cortices, orbitofrontal cortex, and insula, whereas no or few language sites were detected within the left IFG [55]. All patients recovered and returned to a normal social and professional life. Based on these findings, the authors concluded that, in patients with a glioma within the opercular and triangular parts of the left IFG who showed no apparent language deficits, thanks to brain plasticity, the tumor can be removed without inducing sequelae and even improving the quality of life.

The usefulness of functional monitoring may be enhanced in the case of patients with a glioma including the left pars triangularis. The left pars triangularis is also supposed to contribute to syntactic processing [37, 41, 56]. A previous study has demonstrated that identification of the frontal language area can be difficult in patients with frontal gliomas involving the left pars triangularis, but the positive mapping rate of the frontal language area was 95% in patients without involvement of the left pars triangularis [57]. These findings suggested that more careful continuous neurological monitoring combined with subcortical electrical stimulation is needed when removing the left frontal gliomas that involve the left pars triangularis. Taken together, functional monitoring for patients with a glioma in the left pars opercularis and triangularis may be effective at preventing postoperative deficits in syntactic processing.

10.5.2 Functional Intraoperative Monitoring for Subcortical Fibers Related to the Left IFG

For patients with a glioma in the left frontal gyrus, electrical stimulation is useful not only in cortical regions but also on the subcortical fibers. The first report for intraoperative mapping of the subcortical fibers using direct electrical stimulation was published in 2002 [58]. In this study, the arcuate fasciculus was successfully identified by eliciting transient language deficits, particularly anomia, and the patients showed no apparent postoperative deficits in language. Although this research did not extensively examine the syntactic ability of the patients, considering the importance for syntactic processing of connection between the left pars opercularis and temporal regions via the arcuate fasciculus [13], it is possible that functional intraoperative monitoring for the arcuate fasciculus is useful for preventing intraoperative deficits in syntactic processing.

Some studies investigating subcortical fibers described the frontal aslant tract (FAT) as a frontal white matter fiber connecting the supplementary motor area proper and/or the pre-supplementary motor area in the medial frontal regions of the superior frontal gyrus to the posterior IFG, especially the left pars opercularis [59]. A recent study with awake surgery reported that permanent speech disturbance was not observed in patients with a left frontal glioma after tumor removal with functional monitoring [60]. However, this study did not include a control group without functional monitoring. A recent study compared the functional outcome of glioma patients with functional monitoring to that without functional monitoring [61]. This study showed that there was no significant difference in functional outcome between patients with intraoperative functional monitoring and those without intraoperative functional monitoring. Rather, patients who were operated on with intraoperative functional monitoring performed slightly worse after surgery than patients without intraoperative functional monitoring.

It is currently still unclear whether or not operation with functional monitoring can help preserve syntactic abilities for patients with a glioma. Nevertheless, we assumed that the functional monitoring of not only syntactic processing but also other domain-general cognitive processes such as attention and memory is crucial for preserving the ability of syntactic processing, because language networks are interconnected to the domain-general cognitive control system [62]. Although there are no ideal intraoperative tests available today, specific tests should be added to address the interaction between syntax and other cognitive functions and prevent deficits in syntactic processing.

10.6 Which Additional Anatomo-Functional Knowledge Has Been Gained from Intraoperative Mapping Studies

Applications of electrocortical stimulation (ECS) towards mapping syntax in the human brain are the least understood of all language domains. Studying syntax requires stringing multiple words together in phrases or sentences, which has historically rarely been done with ECS mapping.

Ojemann and Mateer [63] found several sites resulting in syntactic errors during stimulation of peri-Sylvian cortex, across frontal, temporal, and parietal lobes. The authors stimulated cortex while having patients read a sentence with a portion near the end of the sentence omitted, requiring the patient to complete it correctly with specific syntactic form. Grammatical reading errors were highly variable and distributed in location across patients, but interestingly focal in individuals.

Previous lesion-deficit studies have suggested that action naming (i.e., verbs), which is more pivotal for correct syntactic structure than object naming (i.e., nouns), are located in different regions of the brain. Work from Corina et al. [64] found support for this observation, with more anterior regions in the dominant temporal lobe specific for object naming and more posterior sites specific for action naming.

In a different approach, Chang et al. [65] were interested to discover which brain regions where cortical stimulation interferes with sentence production, but not with single word or automatic speech tasks. They applied ECS while asking patients to describe a picture of transitive actions using a complete sentence, and also perform counting, repetition, and picture naming tasks as controls to ensure stimulation induced errors were specific to syntax encoding. Each picture depicted a boy and a girl engaged in a simple transitive action (e.g., push, pull, hug, kick, chase, wash, and kiss), with either the boy or the girl acting as the agent of the action. Errors following stimulation to a particular brain region during sentence production, but not repetition or single word speech tasks were specific for the syntactic encoding of sentence production.

The authors found syntactic encoding errors at sites in the left IFG in 50% of patients that specifically did not result in speech arrest, automatic speech, or word-level language function (Fig. 10.3). This frequency of syntactic encoding errors (50%) is similar to the rate of encountering anomia (33%) and speech arrest (58%) found during standard ECS. Interference with syntactic encoding took several different forms, including misassignment of arguments to grammatical roles, misassignment of nouns to verb slots, omission of function words and inflectional morphology, and various paragrammatic constructions.

Specifically, stimulation of the left IFG was more likely to create syntactic errors, perseverations (e.g., previous trial action was used to describe the current trial's verb), and retracings (e.g., complete words uttered more than once in a row), which may also represent interferences with syntactic encoding in the left STG or MTG. The IFG sites were located in the pars triangularis and opercularis and were not identified during counting, naming, or repetition tasks with ECS, suggesting the specificity of these areas to sentence production.

A key methodological difference between the Ojemann and Mateer [63] and Chang [65] studies is the use of sentence completion in the former study, and sentence generation from pictures in the latter study. Tasks involving sentence comprehension presumably recruit an additional receptive language component from the larger, distributed language processing network compared to picture description.

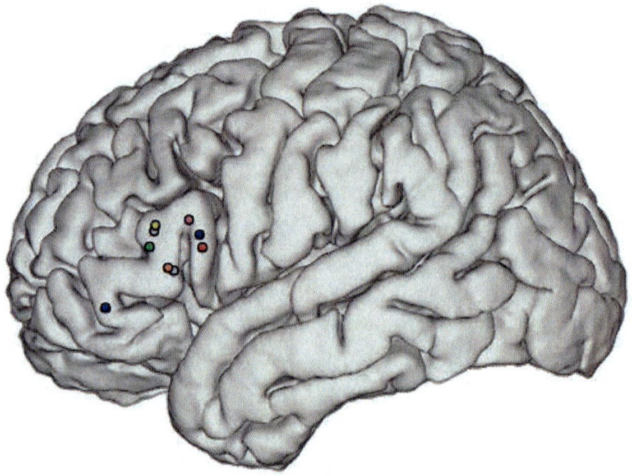

Fig. 10.3 Syntactic encoding sites. Colors denote the seven out of fourteen patients in whom sites were observed. Note that most sites localize to posterior pars triangularis and opercularis

Future research will need to determine which discrepancies in methodologies can reconcile differences in our understanding of syntactic encoding.

Although some lesion-deficit studies support the role of the left IFG in syntactic encoding, seminal work from the stroke literature has demonstrated that infarcts restricted to the left IFG rarely produce agrammatism and permanent deficits are quite rare. Moreover, surgical resection of the frontal operculum has repeatedly been shown to not result in significant postoperative aphasia based on assessment during clinical follow-up visits: for example, Teichmann et al. [45] has reported that only 15% of patients with a glioma did not fully recover, and these patients showed the deficits in syntactic processing only for harder syntactic structures. Preserved syntactic abilities after the tumor resection in the left IFG may be due to the postoperative reorganization through the three syntax-related networks (Fig. 10.2). The contributions of the other regions to syntactic processing may be enhanced in the postoperative period. Among these networks, the bilateral topography of Network I might be a key element of the postoperative reorganization. It could allow to understand why patients can have immediate postoperative syntactic difficulties after removal of the posterior left IFG, while recovering in the long term for many of them. Further evidences regarding functional and anatomical reorganization induced by gliomas will be required for a better understanding of the syntactic ability of patients with glioma.

References

1. Chomsky N. Aspects of the theory of syntax. Cambridge: MIT Press; 1965.
2. Chomsky N. The minimalist program. Cambridge: MIT Press; 1995.
3. Friederici AD, Chomsky N, Berwick RC, Moro A, Bolhuis JJ. Language, mind and brain. Nat Hum Behav. 2017;1:713–22.
4. Demonét JF, Chollet F, Ramsay S, Cardebat D, Nespoulous JL, Wise R, et al. The anatomy of phonological and semantic processing in normal subjects. Brain. 1992;115(6):1753–68.
5. Fiez JA. Phonology, semantics, and the role of the left inferior prefrontal cortex. Hum Brain Mapp. 1997;5(2):79–83.
6. Poldrack RA, et al. Functional specialization for semantic and phonological processing in the left inferior prefrontal cortex. NeuroImage. 1999;10:15–35.
7. Price CJ, Moore CJ, Humphreys GW, Wise RJ. Segregating semantic from phonological processes during reading. J Cogn Neurosci. 1997;9(6):727–33.
8. Thompson-Schill SL, et al. Role of left inferior prefrontal cortex in retrieval of semantic knowledge: a re-evaluation. Proc Natl Acad Sci U S A. 1997;94:14792–7.
9. Dapretto M, Bookheimer SY. Form and content: dissociating syntax and semantics in sentence comprehension. Neuron. 1999;24:427–32.
10. Friederici AD, Meyer M, von Cramon DY. Auditory language comprehension: an event-related fMRI study on the processing of syntactic and lexical information. Brain Lang. 2000;74:289–300.
11. Kuperberg GR, et al. Common and distinct neural substrates for pragmatic, semantic, and syntactic processing of spoken sentences: an fMRI study. J Cogn Neurosci. 2000;12:321–41.
12. Stromswold K, et al. Localization of syntactic comprehension by positron emission tomography. Brain Lang. 1996;10:132–44.
13. Friederici AD. The brain basis of language processing: from structure to function. Physiol Rev. 2011;91(4):1357–92. https://doi.org/10.1152/physrev.00006.2011.

14. Menenti L, Gierhan SME, Segaert K, Hagoort P. Shared language: overlap and segregation of the neuronal infrastructure for speaking and listening revealed by functional MRI. Psychol Sci. 2011;22(9):1173–82.
15. Moro A, Tettamanti M, Perani D, Donati C, Cappa SF, Fazio F. Syntax and the brain: disentangling grammar by selective anomalies. NeuroImage. 2001;13(1):110–8.
16. Pallier C, Devauchelle AD, Dehaene S. Cortical representation of the constituent structure of sentences. Proc Natl Acad Sci U S A. 2011;108:2522–7.
17. Wu C-Y, Zaccarella E, Friederici AD. Universal neural basis of structure building evidenced by network modulations emerging from Broca's area: the case of Chinese. Hum Brain Mapp. 2019;40(6):1705–17.
18. Friederici AD, Fiebach CJ, Schlesewsky M, Bornkessel I, von Cramon DY. Processing linguistic complexity and grammaticality in the left frontal cortex. Cereb Cortex. 2006;16:1709–17.
19. Friederici AD, Makuuchi M, Bahlmann J. The role of the posterior superior temporal cortex in sentence comprehension. Neuroreport. 2009;20:563–8.
20. den Ouden DB, Saur D, Mader W, Schelter B, Lukic S, Wali E, Timmer J, Thompson CK. Network modulation during complex syntactic processing. NeuroImage. 2012;59(1):815–23.
21. Makuuchi M, Friederici AD. Hierarchical functional connectivity between the core language system and the working memory system. Cortex. 2013;49(9):2416–23.
22. Rofes A, Miceli G. Language mapping with verbs and sentences in awake surgery: a review. Neuropsychol Rev. 2014;24:185–99.
23. Zaccarella E, Friederici AD. Merge in the human brain: a sub-region based functional investigation in the left pars opercularis. Front Psychol. 2015;6:1818. https://doi.org/10.3389/fpsyg.2015.01818.
24. Schell M, Zaccarella E, Friederici AD. Differential cortical contribution of syntax and semantics: an fMRI study on two-word phrasal processing. Cortex. 2017;96:105–20.
25. Zaccarella E, Friederici AD. The neurobiological nature of syntactic hierarchies. Neurosci Biobehav Rev. 2017;81(Part B):205–12.
26. Makuuchi M, Bahlmann J, Anwander A, Friederici AD. Segregating the core computational faculty of human language from working memory. Proc Natl Acad Sci U S A. 2009;106:8362–7.
27. Broca P. Remarques sur le siège de la faculté du langage articulé, suivies d'une observation d'aphémie (parte de la parole). Bull Soc Anatom Paris. 1861;6:330–57.
28. Wernicke C. Der aphasische Symptomencomplex. Berlin: Springer; 1874.
29. Caramazza A, Zurif EB. Dissociation of algorithmic and heuristic processes in language comprehension—evidence from aphasia. Brain Lang. 1976;3(4):572–82.
30. Zurif EB, Caramazza A, Myerson R. Grammatical judgments of agrammatic aphasics. Neuropsychologia. 1972;10(4):405–17.
31. Berndt RS, Mitchum CC, Haendiges AN. Comprehension of reversible sentences in "agrammatism": a meta-analysis. Cognition. 1996;58:289–308.
32. Friederici AD, Graetz PAM. Processing passive sentences in aphasia: deficits and strategies. Brain Lang. 1987;30:93–105.
33. Heeschen C. Strategies of decoding actor-object-relations by aphasic patients. Cortex. 1980;16:5–19.
34. Kinno R, Muragaki Y, Hori T, Maruyama T, Kawamura M, Sakai KL. Agrammatic comprehension caused by a glioma in the left frontal cortex. Brain Lang. 2009;110:71–80.
35. Hirotani M, Makuuchi M, Rüschemeyer S-A, Friederici AD. Who was the agent? The neural correlates of reanalysis processes during sentence comprehension. Hum Brain Mapp. 2011;32:1775–87.
36. Rolston JD, Englot DJ, Benet A, Li J, Cha S, Berger MS. Frontal operculum gliomas: language outcome following resection. J Neurosurg. 2015;122(4):725–34.
37. Kinno R, Kawamura M, Shioda S, Sakai KL. Neural correlates of noncanonical syntactic processing revealed by a picture-sentence matching task. Hum Brain Mapp. 2008;29:1015–27.
38. Bates E, Wilson SM, Saygin AP, Dick F, Sereno MI, Knight RT, Dronkers NF. Voxel-based lesion-symptom mapping. Nat Neurosci. 2003;6(5):448–50. https://doi.org/10.1038/nn1050.

39. de Groot M, Reijneveld JC, Aronica E, Heimans JJ. Epilepsy in patients with a brain tumour: focal epilepsy requires focused treatment. Brain. 2012;135(4):1002–16. https://doi.org/10.1093/brain/awr310.
40. Bartolomei F, Bosma I, Klein M, Baayen JC, Reijneveld JC, Postma TJ, et al. How do brain tumors alter functional connectivity? A magnetoencephalography study. Ann Neurol. 2006;59(1):128–38.
41. Kinno R, Ohta S, Muragaki Y, Maruyama T, Sakai KL. Differential reorganization of three syntax-related networks induced by a left frontal glioma. Brain. 2014;137(4):1193–212. https://doi.org/10.1093/brain/awu013.
42. Kinno R, Ohta S, Muragaki Y, Maruyama T, Sakai KL. Left frontal glioma induces functional connectivity changes in syntax-related networks. Springerplus. 2015;4(1):317. https://doi.org/10.1186/s40064-015-1104-6.
43. Bizzi A, Nava S, Ferre F, Castelli G, Aquino D, Ciaraffa F, et al. Aphasia induced by gliomas growing in the ventrolateral frontal region: assessment with diffusion MR tractography, functional MR imaging and neuropsychology. Cortex. 2012;48(2):255–72. https://doi.org/10.1016/j.cortex.2011.11.015.
44. Banerjee P, Leu K, Harris RJ, Cloughesy TF, Lai A, Nghiemphu PL, et al. Association between lesion location and language function in adult glioma using voxel-based lesion-symptom mapping. NeuroImage Clin. 2015;9:617–24.
45. Teichmann M, Rosso C, Martini J-B, Bloch I, Brugières P, Duffau H, et al. A cortical–subcortical syntax pathway linking Broca's area and the striatum. Hum Brain Mapp. 2015;36(6):2270–83.
46. Vidorreta JG, Garcia R, Moritz-Gasser S, Duffau H. Double dissociation between syntactic gender and picture naming processing: a brain stimulation mapping study. Hum Brain Mapp. 2011;32(3):331–40.
47. Antonsson M, Longoni F, Jakola A, Tisell M, Thordstein M, Hartelius L. Pre-operative language ability in patients with presumed low-grade glioma. J Neurooncol. 2018;137(1):93–102. https://doi.org/10.1007/s11060-017-2699-y.
48. Hasting AS, Kotz SA. Speeding up syntax: on the relative timing and automaticity of local phrase structure and morphosyntactic processing as reflected in event-related brain potentials. J Cogn Neurosci. 2008;20(7):1207–19.
49. Hasting AS, Kotz SA, Friederici AD. Setting the stage for automatic syntax processing: the mismatch negativity as an indicator of syntactic priming. J Cogn Neurosci. 2007;19:386–400.
50. Herrmann B, Obleser J, Kalberlah C, Haynes J-D, Friederici AD. Dissociable neural imprints of perception and grammar in auditory functional imaging. Hum Brain Mapp. 2012;33:584–95.
51. Suzuki H, Aoki K, Chiba K, Sato Y, Shiozawa Y, Shiraishi Y, et al. Mutational landscape and clonal architecture in grade II and III gliomas. Nat Genet. 2015;47(5):458–68. https://doi.org/10.1038/ng.3273.
52. Rossi M, Nibali MC, Torregrossa F, Bello L, Grasso G. Innovation in neurosurgery: the concept of cognitive mapping. World Neurosurg. 2019;131:364–70. https://doi.org/10.1016/j.wneu.2019.06.177.
53. Saito T, Muragaki Y, Maruyama T, Tamura M, Nitta M, Okada Y. Intraoperative functional mapping and monitoring during glioma surgery. Neurol Med Chir. 2015;55(1):1–13.
54. Peraud A, Ilmberger J, Reulen HJ. Surgical resection of gliomas WHO grade II and III located in the opercular region. Acta Neurochir. 2004;146(1):9–17; discussion 17–8. https://doi.org/10.1007/s00701-003-0165-4.
55. Benzagmout M, Gatignol P, Duffau H. Resection of World Health Organization Grade II gliomas involving Broca's area: methodological and functional considerations. Neurosurgery. 2007;61(4):741–752; discussion 752–43. https://doi.org/10.1227/01.NEU.0000298902.69473.77.
56. Musso M, Moro A, Glauche V, Rijntjes M, Reichenbach J, Buchel C, Weiller C. Broca's area and the language instinct. Nat Neurosci. 2003;6(7):774–81. https://doi.org/10.1038/nn1077.
57. Saito T, Muragaki Y, Maruyama T, Tamura M, Nitta M, Tsuzuki S, et al. Difficulty in identification of the frontal language area in patients with dominant frontal gliomas that involve the pars triangularis. J Neurosurg. 2016;125(4):803–11.

58. Duffau H, Capelle L, Sichez N, Denvil D, Lopes M, Sichez JP, et al. Intraoperative mapping of the subcortical language pathways using direct stimulations: an anatomo-functional study. Brain. 2002;125(1):199–214.
59. Kinoshita M, de Champfleur NM, Deverdun J, Moritz-Gasser S, Herbet G, Duffau H. Role of fronto-striatal tract and frontal aslant tract in movement and speech: an axonal mapping study. Brain Struct Funct. 2015;220(6):3399–412. https://doi.org/10.1007/s00429-014-0863-0.
60. Motomura K, Chalise L, Ohka F, Aoki K, Tanahashi K, Hirano M, et al. Neurocognitive and functional outcomes in patients with diffuse frontal lower-grade gliomas undergoing intraoperative awake brain mapping. J Neurosurg. 2019;132(6):1683–91. https://doi.org/10.3171/2019.3.JNS19211.
61. Rijnen SJM, Kaya G, Gehring K, Verheul JB, Wallis OC, Sitskoorn MM, Rutten, GM. Cognitive functioning in patients with low-grade glioma: effects of hemispheric tumor location and surgical procedure. J Neurosurg. 2019;1–12. https://doi.org/10.3171/2019.8.JNS191667.
62. Mandonnet E. A surgical approach to the anatomo-functional structure of language. Neurochirurgie. 2017;63(3):122–8. https://doi.org/10.1016/j.neuchi.2016.10.004.
63. Ojemann G, Mateer C. Human language cortex: localization of memory, syntax, and sequential motor-phoneme identification systems. Science. 1979;205(4413):1401–3.
64. Corina DP, Loudermilk BC, Detwiler L, Martin RF, Brinkley JF, Ojemann G. Analysis of naming errors during cortical stimulation mapping: implications for models of language representation. Brain Lang. 2010;115(2):101–12.
65. Chang EF, Kurteff G, Wilson SM. Selective interference with syntactic encoding during sentence production by direct electrocortical stimulation of the inferior frontal gyrus. J Cogn Neurosci. 2018;30(3):411–20.

11 Naming: Nouns and Verbs

Adrià Rofes and Bradford Z. Mahon

11.1 Introduction

Nouns and verbs are word categories that refer to different aspects of human experience (e.g., people, places, things, states, events, actions, goals, experiences). Nouns and verbs are also categories core to the basic structure of human language (e.g., subject, predicate, argument, temporal reference). Within the scope of language mapping in a neurosurgical context, noun and verb production is typically operationalized through object and action naming tasks, respectively [1, 2]. In a typical object naming task, sometimes referred to as noun naming, participants are asked to say the name of an object by using a noun (e.g., "book"). The noun can be preceded by a lead-in sentence or preamble (e.g., "This," "This is," or "Here is"), which is arguably included to disentangle articulatory from lexical-semantic processing [3]. In some languages (e.g., French), the lead-in sentence engages the production of a determiner that agrees in number and gender with the noun (e.g., *Ceci est un livre* → *"This is a book,"* where the determiner "*un*" and "*livre*" are masculine and singular), adding a lexical-syntactic component [4]. For reviews of peri- and intraoperative tasks with nouns see [5–7].

As noted, the naming task with verbs that has been most widely adopted in an intraoperative context is action naming. In this task, participants are asked to say the

A. Rofes (✉)
Faculty of Arts—Neurolinguistics and Language Development, Center for Language and Cognition, University of Groningen, Groningen, The Netherlands
e-mail: a.rofes@rug.nl

B. Z. Mahon
Department of Psychology, Dietrich College of Humanities and Social Sciences, Carnegie Mellon University, Pittsburgh, PA, USA

Neuroscience Institute, Carnegie Mellon University, Pittsburgh, PA, USA

Department of Neurosurgery, University of Rochester Medical School, Rochester, NY, USA
e-mail: bmahon@andrew.cmu.edu

E. Mandonnet, G. Herbet (eds.), *Intraoperative Mapping of Cognitive Networks*,
https://doi.org/10.1007/978-3-030-75071-8_11

name of an action using a nonfinite verb form (e.g., "reading," "to read"). Alternatively, participants may be asked to produce a finite form preceded by the subject of the sentence (e.g., "she reads" or "the woman reads"), in which case the task can also be referred to as finite verb naming or naming with finite verbs. In the latter case, the task also includes a lead-in sentence, which is typically a pronoun (e.g., "he," "she") or a noun phrase (e.g., "the woman," "the boy"). Action naming should be distinguished from the related task of verb generation, in which people are shown or told the name of an object and then asked to produce the first verb that comes to mind (e.g., for a picture of a book, someone may say "reading" or "to read"). Action naming should also be distinguished from verbal fluency, where participants are asked to say as many words as possible starting with a specific letter (e.g., "F") or belonging to a specific category or nouns or actions (e.g., animals, "things you do in the kitchen"). For a broader review of tasks with verbs see [8].

Language mapping using naming tasks with nouns and verbs is often constrained by the need to elicit an overt oral response or judgment. In that sense, tasks have been emphasized that are easy to administer and score, aiding real-time decision-making in the service of supporting a maximal safe resection: maximize tumor resection and minimize postoperative deficits (e.g., [9]). By contrast, research on nouns and verbs in healthy individuals and people with chronic lesions, typically patients with post-stroke aphasia, has fewer constraints and thus a broader range of issues have been addressed over the past several decades, including theoretical work on specific characteristics of nouns and verbs and the degree to which the two word classes depend on dissociable or (partially) shared neural substrates (e.g., [10–12]).

In this chapter, we sketch a neurocognitive framework motivated by a broader range of neuropsychological, neurophysiological, and neuroimaging evidence. Our goal is to inform future investigations and clinical interventions in people undergoing awake surgery. A central theme is that in order to effectively map nouns and verbs in the brain it is important to be explicit about the (1) function(s) or nature of the computations engaged by any given task (e.g., object recognition, semantic access, lexical retrieval, articulation); (2) the cortical and subcortical representation of those functions; and on the basis of that information, to (3) chose tasks and items that are most appropriate for mapping a given brain region. For instance, to map speech motor cortex, it matters little what type of linguistic output the patient is engaged in producing (counting, picture naming, spontaneous speech); by contrast, to map regions that support word retrieval from meaning representations for instance in temporal lobe regions, tasks that emphasize fine-grained semantic processing, such as picture naming or auditory definition naming, are likely to be required.

11.2 The Neural Basis of Nouns and Verbs

Lesion studies of people with post-stroke aphasia and other neurological pathologies have shown greater involvement of left temporal lobe structures in the production and comprehension of nouns, and greater involvement of left prefrontal and inferior parietal structures in the production and comprehension of verbs (e.g., [10, 13–15]; for contrasting evidence see [16, 17]). Neuroimaging studies including positron emission tomography (PET), functional magnetic resonance imaging (fMRI), electro- and magnetoencephalography (EEG, MEG), and navigated transcranial magnetic stimulation (nTMS) have provided a more intricate picture of the neural basis of naming tasks with nouns and verbs. Studies with those methods also implicate a dominant role for perisylvian areas in the left hemisphere and an involvement of similar areas in the right hemisphere (e.g., [11, 18]). At the subcortical level, direct electrical stimulation (DES) studies in people with brain tumors have stressed the role of white-matter pathways such as the arcuate fasciculus, inferior-frontal occipital fasciculus, superior and inferior longitudinal fasciculi, uncinate fasciculus, and periventricular white matter during both object and action naming (e.g., [19–22]).

Importantly, there are aspects of the representation of nouns and verbs that have been little explored in the peri- and intraoperative literature. Here we suggest that, by examining some of these aspects carefully, future studies may enhance the sensitivity and specificity of techniques for intraoperative mapping. Such future studies will also help to build a clearer picture of perioperative language impairments—which is relevant to tailor prehabilitation regimens, intraoperative tasks, and eventual language therapy to the needs of the patient. Below, we approach this broad goal from four perspectives: (1) manipulable objects such as tools and utensils, (2) biological entities, (3) action recognition and naming, and (4) verb argument structure.

Graspable and manipulable objects Graspable and manipulable objects (hereafter "tools") such as "hammer" and "cup" are tools/utensils with strongly associated and often stereotyped actions involving one or both hands. Recognizing and naming tools engages left hemisphere regions in the posterior lateral temporal cortex, posterior parietal and premotor cortex (reviews in [23, 24], see Fig. 11.1). Those areas are automatically activated when viewing or naming tools and utensils, compared to various baseline categories that are not graspable or manipulable (e.g., faces, vehicles, houses). Furthermore, tools also activate parietal and premotor areas that are engaged by action planning and production [26–29]. This observation is supported as well by neurophysiological studies of so-called "canonical neurons" [30]. That is, neurons that are active both during first person object-directed action and during (mere) perception of the object. What is interesting about this network of regions is that it represents cortical regions where representations of objects and actions are integrated at post-perceptual and pre-linguistic levels of processing. In other words, it would not be interesting or surprising that naming tools and actions should both engage, for instance, early visual processes (to process the contrast and luminance gradients of an image) or late-stage articulatory processes (to produce speech sounds); what is interesting is the engagement of common neural mechanisms for higher-level semantic and cognitive representations, that is integrated representations of tools and the actions associated with their use. The question relevant to present

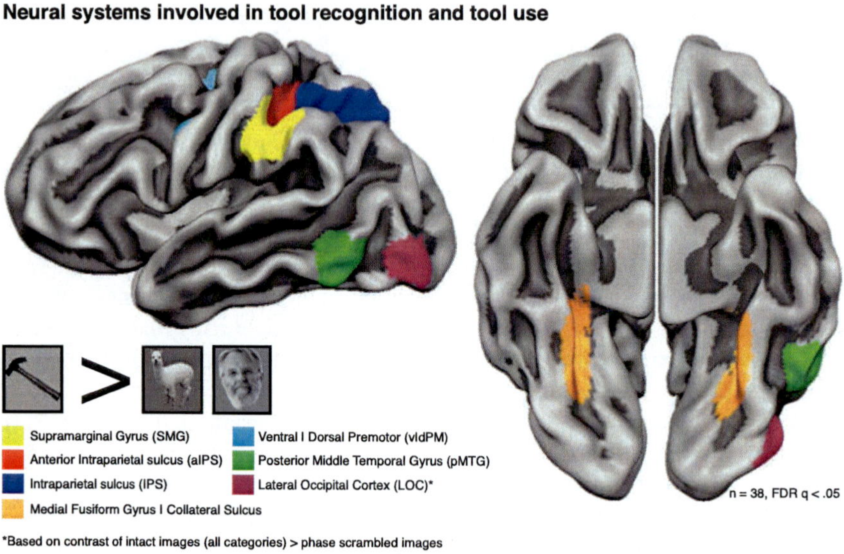

Fig. 11.1 Functional MRI has been used to delineate the neural substrates of the neural regions that support recognition and use of tools. The data shown in the figure were obtained while participants viewed tool stimuli compared to images of animals and faces. Regions are color-coded to distinguish what are functionally dissociable regions, as documented in the neuropsychological literature. (Figure reproduced, in part, from Mahon [25], with permissions)

purposes is whether (and if so, how) this broader network of action areas figures causally in visual confrontation naming of tools and other manipulable objects.

While the neuroimaging evidence is clear in that motor and motor-relevant areas in left parietal and frontal areas are automatically engaged during naming of tools, the available neuropsychological data indicate that tool naming can be preserved in the setting of damage to the same areas [31–33]. People with lesions to left parietal or premotor areas can present with limb apraxia (among other, nonaction, impairments), but can still be able to name the same objects they are unable to use correctly (provided the lesion does not involve the speech production systems) [31–33]. The dissociation between impaired action production and spared naming indicates that the ability to conceptually individuate an object does not require implicit motor simulation of the action associated with the use of the object. This frames the need for hypothesis-driven direct electrical stimulation mapping to evaluate whether transient disruption of those fronto-parietal structures specifically affects naming of graspable objects. By contrast, there is compelling evidence from both activation and lesion studies that the left posterior middle temporal gyrus plays a decisive role in supporting recognition and understanding of actions, and objects that are associated with actions [34–36]. Lesions involving the left posterior middle temporal gyrus can lead to naming impairments that are differentially profound for tools compared to other categories (e.g., animals, vehicles), and for action concepts [15, 29, 37–39].

Biological entities There is a rich neuropsychological tradition of studying dissociations by semantic category within the broad category "nouns" [40–42]. About 150 well-studied neuropsychological cases have been described with conceptual level deficits that are differential or selective for one of the categories of *fruit/vegetables, animals, nonliving things,* or *conspecifics* (i.e., *familiar faces and people)* [43]. The evidence that the deficit in such patients is to conceptual knowledge (e.g., word and object meanings), as opposed to perceptual input (e.g., early visual/auditory processes) or linguistic output representations (e.g., word retrieval, phonological encoding), is provided by the boundaries of the impairment. Patients with category-specific *semantic* impairments have problems accessing knowledge about the impaired category independent of the format of the stimulus or the required response. For instance, such patients may be impaired at naming, but also at identification tasks that do not require a naming response, such as matching tasks like the Pyramids and Palm Trees test (see Chap. 15 and reviews in [23, 44]). Similarly, such patients can be impaired for knowledge about the impaired category regardless of whether that knowledge is cued through a picture or a spoken or written word. This is in contrast to, for example, a category-specific visual agnosia, such as prosopagnosia, for which patients have a category-specific deficit specifically for *visual* recognition but have not otherwise lost knowledge about the same category [45, 46].

While it is far from a universal generalization [47, 48], one pattern that emerges is that impairments with biological entities are often associated with damage to temporal lobe areas, in particular anterior basal and medial structures such as are affected in semantic dementia and herpes simplex encephalitis [49, 50]. This includes patients with impairments affecting animals [51], plants, and fruit/vegetables [52], as well as loss of knowledge of other people which is generally associated with right anterior temporal lobe injury [53–58]. In partial agreement with these studies, Papagno and colleagues [59] report DES positive sites in the temporal lobe and inferior frontal gyrus for naming living objects, while stimulation to other areas in the posterior third of the supramarginal gyrus and possibly the arcuate fasciculus induced more errors for nonliving things.

A related topic is the involvement of nouns referring to *names of famous people* in the anterior temporal lobe and subcortical structures, particularly, the uncinate fasciculus [59]. A topic that seems interesting to explore is whether the role of this subcortical structure is specific to names of famous people or includes other proper name categories, including individual-specific person name knowledge (e.g., surnames, first names, nicknames), geographical names (e.g., cities, countries, rivers), and names of commercial brands, books, paintings, and events (e.g., [53–57, 60]).

Action recognition and naming A critical aspect of the neural basis of action naming is the neural circuitry involved in action recognition and understanding. At the broadest level, actions are intentional movements of the body that satisfy a goal (e.g., we move the hand "to peel" a pear, or move the leg "to kick" a football). Both noninvasive and invasive neural and/or neuronal recording techniques demonstrate automatic engagement of perceptual areas, and pre- and supplemental motor areas during perception and recognition of actions [61–63]. In a similar vein, reading verbs related to different parts of the body such as the hand (e.g., "peel"), the mouth (e.g., "bite"), or the feet (e.g., "kick") drive activity in motor and motor-relevant areas [61–63]. The question is what functional role do motor production processes play in recognition and naming of actions. A currently popular interpretation of such findings [64] derives from the idea of "analysis by synthesis" [65, 66]—in order to recognize an action, the processes involved in production of the same action are internally (implicitly and automatically) simulated. For example, when naming the action "to cut," the motor areas that support the action of "cutting" at the level of the hand are active.

There has been a lot of interest in the concept of motor resonance and motor simulation, including critical discussions of the proposal [67–71]. Neuropsychological data can play a decisive role in evaluating the role(s) of action/motor processes in frontal and parietal areas in supporting action recognition and, more broadly, processing of words referring to actions. On the one hand, TMS studies [72, 73] and some patient studies [74, 75] have indicated action recognition impairments subsequent to (transient or chronic) lesions involving motor areas. On the other hand, patients can be impaired at action production but spared for action recognition. This has been observed in the setting of arm actions [32, 76, 77] and speech processing [78, 79]. Those types of patient-based findings indicate that even when motor output processes are damaged and patients are unable to produce actions in the first person, they can still recognize the same actions (for reviews, see [80–83]). In simpler terms, a person may be unable "to cut a piece of paper" but would understand the meaning of "cutting" when seeing a picture or reading a word. The implication is that while motor and motor-relevant structures are active during naming, it seems that those motor processes are not strictly necessary in order to name actions. This motivates hypothesis-driven DES studies to evaluate whether disruption of fronto-parietal structures specifically affects action naming compared to (a) nonaction events, and (b) actions outside the human action repertoire (e.g., "she jumps" vs. "the window breaks" vs. "the bug bites").

Verb argument structure Another issue to consider when assessing the integrity of verb knowledge is verb argument structure. *Transitive verbs* like "eating" take an object (e.g., Mary eats an apple, where "an apple" is the object) and are different from *intransitive verbs* such as "sleeping" which do not take such an argument (e.g., Mary sleeps). Neuroimaging studies have suggested that transitive verbs have further representation in the posterior part of the left superior temporal gyrus (e.g., [84–86]) This evidence is reinforced by lesion studies where people with post-stroke aphasia typically have more difficulties producing verbs that have more arguments (See Fig. 11.2) [87–89].

Arguments for the difference between these two types of verbs often note that transitive verbs require more complex computations than intransitive verbs in order to be expressed. Different theories emphasize different aspects of transitive and intransitive verbs. If we take a sentence with a transitive verb like "Mary eats an apple" and a sentence with an intransitive verb like "Mary sleeps," the differences

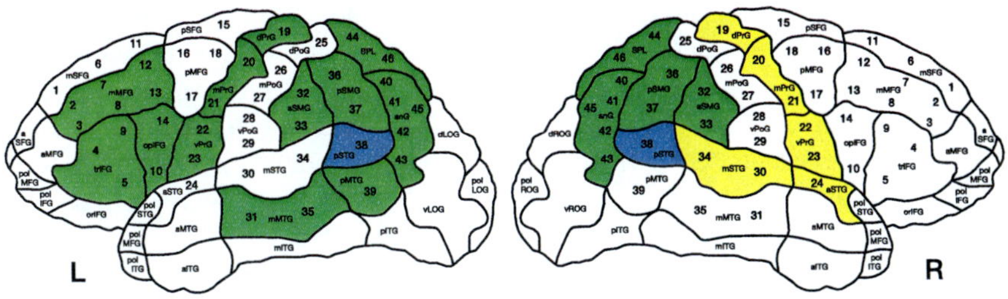

Fig. 11.2 Cortical representation of transitive and intransitive verbs in the left and right hemisphere. **Green**: Areas reported to be significantly more activated with transitive verbs. **Yellow**: Areas that have been reported to be significantly more activated with intransitive verbs. **Blue**: Areas that have been reported to be significantly more activated with both verb types

include: the amount of specified arguments (e.g., having an object like "apple" or not having an object); thematic roles (e.g., "Mary" as the agent or doer of the action of eating, and "apple" as the theme or entity that is affected by the action; compared to "Mary" as the experiencer or entity undergoing the action of sleeping); and the subcategorization frame (e.g., the lexical entry of the verb "to eat" takes two arguments with a noun phrase that functions as a subject, i.e., "Mary," and a noun phrase that functions as an object "an apple"; the lexical entry of the verb "to sleep" which can express only one event which involves one participant, namely, a noun phrase that functions as a subject, i.e., "Mary") [90, 91].

With respect to neural correlates of verb argument structure, it has been argued that there is a positive relation between the number of regions recruited and argument structure complexity. That is, further tissue is recruited to integrate the verb and its arguments into the syntactic structure of the sentence. In that sense, it may be hypothesized that transitive verbs should rely more heavily on posterior regions, as opposed to intransitive verbs [86, 92].

To summarize our arguments on the neural basis of nouns and verbs, studies indicate a general tendency for partial overlapping between cortical areas and less evidence for differentiation at the subcortical level. The partial consistency between lesion and neuroimaging studies may relate to factors such as the spatial and temporal resolution of each of the methods, the varieties of tasks/paradigms that can be used to assess object naming, and detecting areas that support and/or are essential for each of its functions (e.g., object recognition, semantic access, lexical retrieval, articulation). In this section, we argued for the use of potential differences between nouns and verbs. This emphasizes the differences within types or characteristics of nouns and verbs in order to gain new leverage on approaches for intraoperative mapping. These differences can advance understanding of how nouns and verbs are processed in the brain, while also increasing the sensitivity and specificity of language mapping, in line with the goals of the brain mapping in a neurosurgical setting.

Two of the topics we reviewed indicate that words with strong sensorimotor associations (e.g., graspable objects and actions) automatically activate sensorimotor areas during a naming task. In the same vein, a related constellation of findings points to this being a relatively broad phenomenon and not limited only to the action domain: nouns with strong gustatory ("salt"), olfactory ("jasmine"), and auditory associations ("telephone") drive activity in sensory brain regions related to taste (e.g., anterior insula, frontal operculum, lateral orbitofrontal gyrus, thalamus), smell (e.g., piriform cortex and amygdala), and audition (Heschl's gyrus) (for the original theoretical precedent, see [93]; for recent empirical studies, see [94–98]). And similarly, nouns with strong motion properties (e.g., car) differentially drive activity in the vicinity of motion sensitive area MT/V5 in posterior-lateral temporal cortex [99]. However, the available neuropsychological evidence forms a pattern in that disruption of the same structures that are automatically engaged does not necessarily disrupt naming performance—thus it remains an open question whether DES to sensory- and motor-specific structures may disrupt naming of the corresponding word types.

11.3 Evidence of Long-Term Deficits in People Who Did Not Benefit from Intraoperative Language Mapping with Naming Tasks with Nouns and/or Verbs

Here we highlight four studies in which patients were operated on with intraoperative object naming but not action naming (nonfinite forms, e.g., "jumping"), and three studies where patients were operated on with intraoperative mapping that involved both object and action naming. To the best of our knowledge, there are no studies in which only action naming, or only tasks with verbs, have been used for intraoperative mapping.

With respect to studies for which only object naming was administered, Santini and colleagues [100] studied the perioperative results of 22 people with low- and high-grade gliomas and reported a decline in naming scores immediately after surgery (within a week after surgery), with recovery at follow-up (3–6 months after surgery). The authors indicated the same pattern for other language tasks. Unfortunately, both object and action naming scores were combined as one measure of naming; hence, it is not possible to assess whether action naming was more impaired than object naming. Nonetheless, the authors showed scores below the normal level on word fluency, verbal working memory, and immediate recall of words—all of these being tasks that require language processing (along with other cognitive functions).

Satoer and colleagues [101] looked at 45 people with low- and high-grade gliomas, mostly in the perisylvian regions of the left hemisphere. The authors studied the scores of people who underwent surgery without action naming, before surgery, 3 months after surgery, and 1 year after surgery. Similar to Santini and colleagues [100], the authors reported issues in word fluency and immediate recall of words. Also, they reported problems in attention, executive functions, and object naming—the latter resolving 1 year after surgery. In this study, action naming scores were not reported. In another longitudinal study by the same group, Satoer and colleagues [102] reported spontaneous speech impairments in 18 people with low- and high-grade gliomas, also 3 months and 1 year after surgery. The majority of those patients were assessed intraoperatively with object naming and repetition, not necessarily with action naming. Interestingly, the authors reported issues with spontaneous speech that relate to lexical-semantic and morphosyntactic impairments; these aspects of linguistic computation would arguably be well mapped with action naming and, particularly, action naming with finite verbs.

Norrelgen and colleagues [103] reported findings from 27 people with a low-grade glioma or cavernoma in the left hemisphere. All patients underwent surgery with object naming but not action naming. Relative to preoperative scores, patients declined in animal and verb fluency at 3 and 12 months after surgery. Five people had impairments on object naming before surgery, but none of the patients had below-normal scores on object naming or sentence comprehension at follow-up.

With respect to studies where both object naming and action naming were used, Papagno and colleagues [104] reported preoperative data from 226 people operated on for a low- or high-grade glioma. Of those, 117 were assessed 3 months after surgery. The data are presented as percentages and participants are divided by brain area. Higher percentages of people were impaired for object naming and action naming before surgery than at follow-up. A number that is particularly striking is that 40% of people with lesions in the left parietal lobe were impaired for action naming before surgery, but only one participant presented with below-normal scores 3 months after surgery. Other than that, there is an increase of about 20% in the percentage of people with lesions in the left frontal lobe whose scores are impaired for phonemic fluency after surgery. Similar results were reported in a recent study that used a similar testing protocol and included 102 people with high-grade gliomas [105]. In contrast, Pisoni and colleagues [106] reported the perioperative results of 102 people with a high- or a low-grade glioma in either the left or right hemisphere. Interestingly, postoperative results 1–7 days after surgery revealed new action naming impairments in nearly 30% of the people, the majority of which had tumors in the left hemisphere.

In summary, while the literature remains sparse at present, postoperative testing in people with brain tumors who underwent intraoperative mapping with object naming, or with both object and action naming, do contain some language impairments, particularly, in tasks that tap into lexical-semantic and morphosyntactic processes. Fluency tasks have been shown to be impaired, along with object naming, and sometimes action naming. When both object and action naming tasks have been used intraoperatively, two studies report an increase in new impairments in action naming and a third a decrease, at least for lesions in the left parietal lobe, an area known to be involved in the processing of action verbs (see Sect. 11.1 above).

Further work is needed to understand for how long after surgery such impairments remain, if the incidence is higher when object naming alone is used during intraoperative language mapping, and how these impairments impact in quality of life. With respect to the latter point, a study examining both accuracy and response times would be valuable, similar to the report on object naming latencies and return-to-work by Moritz-Gasser and colleagues [107]. Further work on spontaneous speech could also be valuable, given the correspondence between formal testing and spontaneous speech in people with brain tumors (see Chap. 6 and [102, 108]).

11.4 Knowledge Gained from Lesion-Symptom Mapping

To our knowledge, only two studies have carried out lesion-symptom mapping with both object and action naming in people with brain tumors. Both studies included nearly one hundred Italian-speaking people with either a low- or a high-grade glioma. Pisoni and colleagues [106] looked at pre- and early postoperative results (1–7 before/days after surgery) in individuals with tumors in the left and right hemisphere, while Tomasino and colleagues [109] only considered preoperative results (1 week before surgery) and people with tumors in the left hemisphere. The results of both studies stress the role of the left hemisphere. With respect to the representation of objects, Pisoni and colleagues [106] stress the role of the anterior temporal lobe, whereas Tomasino and colleagues [109] discuss the role of basal temporo-occipital regions (see also Fig. 11.1). As discussed above (Sect. 11.1), both of these regions are known to support dissociable components of object knowledge that is accessed during naming. With respect to actions, both studies agree on a role of left parietal cortex for the production of action verbs. What is less clear is the involvement of the left frontal lobe (reported only in Tomasino et al. [109]) and the temporal cortex (only posterior aspects are reported in Pisoni and colleagues [106], while broader areas are reported in Tomasino and colleagues [109]). The involvement of subcortical pathways is also unclear, in that one study specifically reported finding no pathways [106]. However, Tomasino and colleagues reported involvement of the superior and posterior corona radiata and the inferior fronto-occipital fasciculus for actions, while the inferior longitudinal fasciculus, corpus callosum, thalamic radiation, internal capsule, and fornix were implicated in processing of objects [109].

These results for people with brain tumors are not entirely in agreement with a similarly powered study of people with left-hemisphere stroke [110]. In that study, impairment in object naming was associated with the anterior and posterior middle temporal gyrus, superior temporal gyrus, and inferior parietal cortex. Interestingly, when controlling for impairments in articulation and visual recognition, the left middle posterior temporal gyrus and underlying white matter appeared to play a critical role in object naming (see also [29]). Adding to this literature, an earlier less powered study in individuals with left-hemisphere stroke found that the inferior frontal gyrus and the anterior part of the temporal lobe were relevant for action naming [111]. In a similar study that considered different neurological populations (mostly stroke) and a variety of tasks tapping on verb processing [15], the role of the inferior frontal gyrus was also stressed. However, the anterior part of the temporal lobe was argued to not be essential for representing or processing action concepts, since a number of patients they studied who underwent anterior temporal lobe surgery for epilepsy were not impaired for tasks involving actions.

Findings with lesion-symptom mapping in people with brain tumors warrant replication in other languages, as currently available studies were conducted in Italian. For example, it would be interesting to cross-validate the results in typologically similar languages, such as French, Spanish, and Catalan, as well as to look for potential differences in languages that are rich in morphology such as Korean and Turkish, and languages with impoverished morphological markers such as English or Chinese. This is because, differences could emerge between languages that have verbs that engage more or less in morphosyntactic processes (e.g., [112]). Nonetheless, we expect action naming to be, on average, more impaired than object naming, as this is the case even in languages with poor morphological inflection (e.g., [113]). This is possibly because, even when we disregard morphological processes, verbs are key elements for structuring sentences (e.g., they specify arguments, thematic roles, have a subcategorization frame, are useful to refer to the time when the event happened), while nouns refer to concepts and are dependent on verbs to "make sense" in a sentence (e.g., "John ate pasta" vs. "John is eating/cooking pasta").

Future work could also consider running similar analyses for naming actions with finite verbs (e.g., she runs), as the use of finite verbs taps into morphosyntactic processes, which may index a broader set of linguistic computations than non-finite verbs (e.g., to run, running) or nouns [114]. Finally, the studies we reported include behavioral data at a preoperative stage or at an acute stage early after surgery (~1 week). In this sense, the performance of people at a more chronic stage such as three to six or even more months after surgery could contextualize early postoperative deficits that may not be as specifically related to the location of the surgical resection per se, but to more general consequences of neurosurgical interventions (e.g., early presence of edema, decompression of tissue around the surgical cavity [115]).

There are also important limitations associated with lesion-symptom mapping that should be considered:

First, whereas the lesion, at least defined for analytic purposes, is a static variable for any given individual, performance levels are dynamically changing along the timeline from preoperative assessment to subacute to chronic assessment; thus, for the same lesions in a group of patients, the lesion-behavioral correlates can change quite dramatically depending on when patients are tested over the trajectory of their recovery [116–118].

Second, the effect of the lesion on behavior is due not only to the tissue that is physically lost to the lesion but also to tissue that was part of a functional network with the lesioned area [119]. Lesions to one region will disrupt information processing for computations in other regions that depend(ed) on the lesioned area for inputs or outputs [120]. In a recent study of preoperative tumor patients [121], it was found that functional MRI responses in basal temporal structure (fusiform gyrus, collateral sulcus) were modulated by the presence of lesions to parietal cortex. This relation was category-specific, in that fMRI responses in the fusiform gyrus were modulated only for tools by lesions to parietal cortex, while responses to places, faces, and animals were unaffected. That finding was interpreted in terms of the need for tools (compared to places, faces, and animals) to integrate visual representations of surface structure and texture (processed by medial basal temporal lobe structures) with motor-relevant properties of the use of the objects (parietal cortex).

Third, these issues are compounded in the setting of tumor patients, as there could be reorganization of function during the period when the tumor was growing. The result is that the behavioral performance level for a given task may not be what would be predicted were an otherwise typically developed individual to have a sudden onset of a lesion in the same location as the tumor. Herbet and colleagues [122] reported a case series in which some of the patients had a low-grade glioma in the left anterior temporal lobe, while in others, this brain area was not involved with tumor. All of the patients underwent an awake craniotomy with language mapping, and specifically DES of the inferior longitudinal fasciculus (ILF) in the dominant hemisphere. The authors found that stimulation of the ILF caused anomic errors, but only in patients who did not have long-standing pathology in the anterior temporal lobe. The implications of these findings are that (1) the ILF does play a critical role in language processing, and specifically naming; and (2) if tumors have infiltrated the left anterior temporal lobe, there is reorganization of the language network (such that stimulation of the ILF no longer disrupts naming). Future systematic investigations such as reported by Herbet and colleagues will be critical for understanding plasticity, reorganization of function, and redundancy of functional pathways.

11.5 Tasks Newly Designed to Map Language

Marla Hamberger and colleagues [123–128] explored a different paradigm within noun production that does not depend on the targets being picturable—the authors refer to this paradigm as "*auditory naming*"; more generally, it is a form of *definition naming or naming to description*. For instance, the patient listens to a short description: "The yellow part of an egg" (answer: yolk) with stimulation being applied during the period that the patient is presented with the definition. Those authors found that auditory definition naming, and not visual/picture naming, identified essential language sites in the anterior temporal lobe [123]. A subsequent study by the same group investigated language outcome in people undergoing temporal lobe surgery in whom both picture naming and auditory naming were used to define essential language sites intraoperatively [126]. The key point of comparison concerned resections that avoided essential language sites identified with picture naming (i.e., the clinical standard), but did not avoid essential language sites identified with auditory naming. The authors found increased word finding difficulties in people who had auditory-naming-defined essential language sites resected, compared to people without resection of auditory naming sites. For ethical reasons, there was no comparison group where visual/picture naming-defined essential language sites were resected. Interestingly, the postoperative deficits observed in people with auditory-defined language sites resected were observed both in auditory naming and in picture naming.

The discussion about the most effective tasks for identifying essential language sites in the anterior temporal lobe continues [8, 9, 123, 126, 129–132]. Hamberger et al. [123, 126] emphasized the *auditory* nature of the stimuli and suggested an auditory representational code in the anterior temporal lobe. Subsequent research and theoretical proposals argued that the anterior temporal lobes represent amodal conceptual information [133–138]—in which case the modality of the cueing stimuli (auditory, visual) would be expected to matter less [69, 139–143].

Another important issue is that experimental paradigms in which pictures, as opposed to auditorily presented definitions, are used to cue word retrieval may allow for additional and parallel pathways to a target name from the stimulus (picture). Anatomically, such redundant pathways could be (1) right hemisphere identification processes that bypass left anterior temporal semantic representations, and access words via callosal projections (for evidence from split brain patients, see [144, 145]), and/or (2) projections that connect occipital and frontal naming sites and bypass the anterior temporal lobe (e.g., the inferior frontal occipital fasciculus [116, 146–148]).

Following the aforementioned work on naming to definition, a novel way to administer verb naming could be by providing participants a short description of the verb (e.g., what do we do with a book, "reading"). This version of the task may engage auditory processes to segment strings of sounds into words as well as understand grammatical information. This is distinct from using line drawings, as picture naming requires visual perceptual analysis and other perceptual processes (e.g., [149, 150]). To the best of our knowledge action naming to description has not been used intraoperatively.

Clinicians and researchers implement action naming and naming tasks with finite verbs with the help of line drawings, color pictures, or short vignettes [151–154]. The most common approach uses line drawings, following the tradition of intraoperative mapping with object naming [154]. The way in which the tasks are administered seems relevant, as different methods engage different language functions. For surgical mapping, it has been argued that vignettes (e.g., a person peeling a banana or cracking an egg) are more natural depictions of actions and, hence, more ecologically valid than line drawings [151]. However, this study did not compare the two types of stimuli but rather used vignettes instead of drawings.

Further inspiration for the type of stimuli that could prove useful for intraoperative mapping may be found in the psycholinguistic and post-stroke literature. For example, Salmon and colleagues [155] found that manipulable objects (e.g., "banana," "hammer") are named faster by healthy individuals when presented as photographs compared to black-and-white line drawings. Interestingly, the authors reported no difference between photographs and black-and-white drawings, when the items were non-manipulable objects (e.g., "pigeon," "staircase"). Consequently, if the amount of visual detail in photographs facilitates the retrieval of nouns that require "bodily movement," it may also be argued that action verbs (e.g., "cutting" vs. "sleeping") may be produced faster and more accurately when presented as pictures, as opposed to black-and-white drawings. The extent to which this type of work may affect peri- and intraoperative results in people with brain tumors is unknown. However, it seems relevant to consider, as it could help minimize intraoperative false positives.

A key issue, when considering how to generalize observations to broader groups of patients, is whether the group of patients in question is homogenous in terms of the neurocognitive processes affected by the lesion. For instance, the picture-naming performance of people with impairments to earlier levels of processing (e.g., picture recognition, due to posterior temporal or occipital lesions) will be affected by manipulations to the format of the visual stimuli. However, people with impairments to other levels of processing, such as peripheral phonological problems or lexical-semantic impairments, may perform the same regardless of manipulations to the input, but may be affected by output dimensions (e.g., word length). This emphasizes the need to develop explicit hypotheses, up front, about the nature of computations believed to be supported by a brain region. Therefore, it is critical to not interpret clinical categories such as "post-stroke" aphasia too seriously without further examination, as the patients subsumed under that label will be heterogenous in terms of the underlying mechanisms affected by the injury [156]. Similar arguments should also hold when considering postsurgical cases.

It should be noted that even though for action naming the final output is a verb, there exist significant differences between producing a verb in a nonfinite form (e.g., "reading," "to read") and producing a verb in its finite form (e.g., "she reads"). When producing a verb in the finite form, there is agreement over the fact that a subset of the processes necessary to produce a sentence are needed, thus engaging the retrieval of the word (lexical retrieval) as well as grammatical processing (e.g., subject-verb agreement, reference to time, use of tense). However, when producing a nonfinite form, while it is clear that lexical retrieval is involved, it is not as clear whether the same grammatical processes are obligatorily engaged [11, 157]. The engagement of those grammatical processes is consequential for the regions that will be recruited (e.g., [112, 157]), and also renders the task sensitive to processes that are involved in the use of language on an everyday basis (i.e., spontaneous speech, see Chap. 6 and [114]). A study comparing pre-, intra-, and postoperative mapping of action naming with nonfinite verbs and finite verbs, as well as more general measures of language, would shed light on these issues.

Finally, action naming tasks were discussed in early reviews of tasks to be used for intraoperative language mapping [158], and are currently included in protocols in numerous languages including English [159], German [159], Russian [160], Dutch/Flemish [159, 161], and Italian [162, 163]. Some of these versions are particularly interesting, as they include ratings for a number of word properties such as frequency, imageability, age of acquisition, and other variables [149, 150, 164]. Controlling the items for such properties may be relevant at the preoperative level, to have a better understanding of which language functions may be impaired, as well as to understand whether specific subsets within word types are differentially affected (e.g., low frequency items). All of this is also relevant to tailor the tasks to the capacities of each individual patient; for example, instead of removing single words that a person may have problems with, it may be possible to remove a whole word type (e.g., intransitive verbs). This approach could also help diminish the number of intraoperative false positives.

11.6 Functional Improvement in Patients Engaged in Intraoperative Naming Task with Nouns and/or Verbs Compared to Patients Not Studied with Those Tasks

The administration of action naming and naming finite verbs has been argued to provide intraoperative maps with more and different positive cortico-subcortical areas, particularly when compared with object naming (e.g., [19, 20, 130, 151–153]). To our knowledge, there are no studies providing evidence in favor of the unique administration of action naming or finite verbs for intraoperative language mapping. Rather, researchers and clinicians advocate for an approach with both action naming and object naming. It could be that the combination of the two tasks allows for more reliable mapping of cortico-subcortical areas and language processes that are engaged in everyday language abilities—particularly when using finite verbs [114]. However, this hypothesis has not been directly tested by prospectively manipulating the inclusion (versus not) of finite verb naming.

It is difficult to find reports stating that there is a functional improvement in patients mapped intraoperatively with action naming only, as opposed to other mapping approaches such as object naming alone. Indeed, at this stage, it seems unethical to assess patients only with action naming, particularly when many teams advocate for a combination of tasks and when the current gold standard is object naming (e.g., [130]). In this regard, if the goal is to understand functional improvement, it could be relevant to study the perioperative relation between different tasks used in awake surgery and scores on functional tasks (e.g., such as spontaneous speech, everyday communication scales, questionnaires, or quality of life measures). This is relevant to assess whether a task used during surgery engages processes required for everyday communication (e.g., [114]).

Likewise, in the domain of language, we are unaware of studies that have assessed postoperative performance when other tasks were used instead of object naming. However, it seems evident that operating on the patient awake with object naming is preferable to an asleep surgery without language testing [165].

11.7 Additional Anatomo-Functional Knowledge Gained from Intraoperative Mapping Studies

At the cortical level, intraoperative mapping studies have provided information that is not much different from lesion studies or studies with neuroimaging techniques. That is, there exist a number of brain areas in left perisylvian areas that are involved in naming tasks with objects and verbs, with substantial variability across participants (for reviews of intraoperative results, see [8, 22]). Important in this context, future intraoperative mapping studies can provide unique insight regarding the role of subcortical structures in supporting these tasks.

An example of the types of inferences about subcortical pathways that are afforded by stimulation mapping is provided by two case studies that focused on the recently described Frontal Aslant Tract, which connects the inferior frontal gyrus with pre-supplementary motor cortex [166]. One study used subcortical stimulation of the Frontal Aslant Tract while the patient was engaged in a controlled sentence production task designed to have sensitivity to subtle disruptions to sentence planning [167]. The patient was engaged in producing sentences such as "The red triangle is above the yellow circle" where the color and shapes varied from trial to trial and were cued via a visual stimulus. It was found that stimulation of the Frontal Aslant Tract disrupted sentence production specifically at the boundaries of grammatical phrases (i.e., in the example above, after the determiner phrase "the red triangle," or before the determiner phrase "the yellow circle"). Those intraoperative findings were in agreement with a prior case report of a patient, whose left middle frontal gyrus tumor required partial resection of the Frontal Aslant Tract, and for whom postoperative spontaneous speech was marked by substantial hesitations at the boundaries of grammatical phrases [168]. The authors suggested findings from those two studies frame the hypothesis that the Frontal Aslant Tract supports mapping from the grammatical structure of sentences (inferior frontal gyrus) to linearized surface forms required for motor planning (anterior supplementary motor cortex)—referred to as the Syntagmatic Constraints on Positional Elements (SCOPE) hypothesis [167, 168]. For instance, in the sentence "The boy ate the apple," the representations of the subject (boy) and object (apple) are processed together within the overall thematic structure of the sentence at a semantic and grammatical level; however, at the level at which the sentence is articulated, "boy" and "apple" are computationally separated in time. The idea is that the FAT maps between the structural form of the sentence and its surface form.

With respect to tasks with verbs, Lorenzo Bello's group [19, 20] reported involvement of different portions of long association fiber pathways (e.g., arcuate fasciculus, superior longitudinal fasciculus, uncinate fasciculus, inferior fronto-occipital fasciculus) in action naming (with nonfinite verbs). Rofes and colleagues [130] also reported the involvement of subcortical pathways in action naming with finite verbs, particularly the anterior part of the arcuate fasciculus and the inferior fronto-occipital fasciculus [19, 20].

Further work is needed to understand the cortical and subcortical representation of currently used tasks via intraoperative mapping, including in patients with lesions in the right hemisphere [11]. Looking forward, there are many exciting questions to be pursued using action naming in an intraoperative context, and the clinical preparation afforded by awake language mapping holds tremendous potential to disclose new insights about the neural basis of nouns and verbs.

Acknowledgments We thank Drs. Barbara Zarino, Djaina Satoer, Gabriele Miceli, Marla Hamberger, Costanza Papagno, and Effrosyni Ntemou for answering questions regarding specific action naming paradigms and for clarifications of their studies. We thank Ann-Katrin Ohlerth and Effrosyni Ntemou for providing the image used in Fig. 11.2. We are grateful to Drs. Emmanuel Mandonnet, Guillaume Herbet, and Webster Pilcher for comments on an earlier draft, and to Dr. Srdjan Popov for clarifying some aspects of linguistic theory. Preparation of this article was supported, in part, by NIH grants R01NS089069 and R01EY028535 to BZM.

References

1. Duffau H, Capelle L, Sichez J, Faillot T, Abdennour L, Law Koune JD, et al. Intra-operative direct electrical stimulations of the central nervous system: the Salpetriere experience with 60 patients. Acta Neurochir (Wien). 1999;141(11):1157–67.
2. Ojemann G, Mateer C. Human language cortex: localization of memory, syntax, and sequential motor-phoneme identification systems. Science. 1979;205(4413):1401–3.
3. Rofes A, Mandonnet E, de Aguiar V, Rapp B, Tsapkini K, Miceli G. Language processing from the perspective of electrical stimulation mapping. Cogn Neuropsychol. 2019;36(3–4): 117–39.
4. Vidorreta J, Garcia R, Moritz-Gasser S, Duffau H. Double dissociation between syntactic gender and picture naming processing: a brain stimulation mapping study. Hum Brain Mapp. 2011;32(3):331–40.
5. De Witte E, Marien P. The neurolinguistic approach to awake surgery reviewed. Clin Neurol Neurosurg. 2013;115(2):127–45.
6. Ruis C. Monitoring cognition during awake brain surgery in adults: a systematic review. J Clin Exp Neuropsychol. 2018;40(10):1081–104.
7. Wager M, Rigoard P, Bouyer C, Baudiffier V, Stal V, Bataille B, et al. Operating environment for awake brain surgery—choice of tests. Neurochirurgie. 2017;63(3):150–7.
8. Rofes A, Miceli G. Language mapping with verbs and sentences in awake surgery: a review. Neuropsychol Rev. 2014;24(2):185–99.
9. Rofes A, Spena G, Miozzo A, Fontanella MM, Miceli G. Advantages and disadvantages of intraoperative language tasks in awake surgery: a three-task approach for prefrontal tumors. J Neurosurg Sci. 2015;59(4):337–49.
10. Matzig S, Druks J, Masterson J, Vigliocco G. Noun and verb differences in picture naming: past studies and new evidence. Cortex. 2009;45(6):738–58.
11. Vigliocco G, Vinson D, Druks J, Barber H, Cappa S. Nouns and verbs in the brain: a review of behavioural, electrophysiological, neuropsychological and imaging studies. Neurosci Biobehav Rev. 2011;35(3):407–26.
12. Kemmerer D, Eggleston A. Nouns and verbs in the brain: implications of linguistic typology for cognitive neuroscience. Lingua. 2010;120(12):2686–90.
13. Damasio AR, Tranel D. Nouns and verbs are retrieved with differently distributed neural systems. Proc Natl Acad Sci U S A. 1993;90(11):4957–60.
14. Daniele A, Barbier A, Di Giuda D, Vita MG, Piccininni C, Spinelli P, et al. Selective impairment of action-verb naming and comprehension in progressive supranuclear palsy. Cortex. 2013;49(4):948–60.
15. Kemmerer D, Rudrauf D, Manzel K, Tranel D. Behavioral patterns and lesion sites associated with impaired processing of lexical and conceptual knowledge of actions. Cortex. 2012;48(7):826–48.
16. De Renzi E, di Pellegrino G. Sparing of verbs and preserved, but ineffectual reading in a patient with impaired word production. Cortex. 1995;31(4):619–36.
17. Silveri M, Di Betta A. Noun-verb dissociation in brain-damaged patients: further evidence. Neurocase. 1997;3:477–88.
18. Crepaldi D, Berlingeri M, Cattinelli I, Borghese NA, Luzzatti C, Paulesu E. Clustering the lexicon in the brain: a meta-analysis of the neurofunctional evidence on noun and verb processing. Front Hum Neurosci. 2013;7:303.
19. Bello L, Acerbi F, Giussani C, Baratta P, Taccone P, Songa V, et al. Intraoperative language localization in multilingual patients with gliomas. Neurosurgery. 2006;59(1):115–25; discussion 115–25.
20. Bello L, Gallucci M, Fava M, Carrabba G, Giussani C, Acerbi F, et al. Intraoperative subcortical language tract mapping guides surgical removal of gliomas involving speech areas. Neurosurgery. 2007;60(1):67–80; discussion 80–2.

21. Bello L, Gambini A, Castellano A, Carraba G, Acerbi F, Fava E, et al. Motor and language DTI fiber tracking combined with intraoperative subcortical mapping for surgical removal of gliomas. Neuroimage. 2008;39(1):369–82.
22. Sarubbo S, Tate M, De Benedictis A, Merler S, Moritz-Gasser S, Herbet G, et al. Mapping critical cortical hubs and white matter pathways by direct electrical stimulation: an original functional atlas of the human brain. Neuroimage. 2020;205:116237.
23. Mahon BZ, Caramazza A. Concepts and categories: a cognitive neuropsychological perspective. Annu Rev Psychol. 2009;60:27–51.
24. Martin A. The representation of object concepts in the brain. Annu Rev Psychol. 2007;58:25–45.
25. Mahon BZ. The representation of tools in the human brain. In: Poeppel D, Mangun GR, Gazzaniga MS, editors. The cognitive neurosciences. 6th ed. Cambridge: MIT Press; 2020.
26. Chao LL, Haxby JV, Martin A. Attribute-based neural substrates in temporal cortex for perceiving and knowing about objects. Nat Neurosci. 1999;2(10):913–9.
27. Chao LL, Martin A. Representation of manipulable man-made objects in the dorsal stream. Neuroimage. 2000;12(4):478–84.
28. Noppeney U, Price CJ, Penny WD, Friston KJ. Two distinct neural mechanisms for category-selective responses. Cereb Cortex. 2006;16(3):437–45.
29. Mahon BZ, Milleville SC, Negri GA, Rumiati RI, Caramazza A, Martin A. Action-related properties shape object representations in the ventral stream. Neuron. 2007;55(3): 507–20.
30. Rizzolatti G, Umiltà M. Canonical neurons. In: RALCaO L, editor. Encyclopedia of sciences and religions. Dordrecht: Springer; 2013.
31. Garcea FE, Dombovy M, Mahon BZ. Preserved tool knowledge in the context of impaired action knowledge: implications for models of semantic memory. Front Hum Neurosci. 2013;7:120.
32. Negri GA, Rumiati RI, Zadini A, Ukmar M, Mahon BZ, Caramazza A. What is the role of motor simulation in action and object recognition? Evidence from apraxia. Cogn Neuropsychol. 2007;24(8):795–816.
33. Ochipa C, Rothi L, Heilman K. Ideational apraxia: a deficit in tool selection and use. Ann Neurol. 1989;25(2):190–3.
34. Buxbaum LJ, Shapiro AD, Coslett HB. Critical brain regions for tool-related and imitative actions: a componential analysis. Brain. 2014;137(Pt 7):1971–85.
35. Wurm MF, Ariani G, Greenlee MW, Lingnau A. Decoding concrete and abstract action representations during explicit and implicit conceptual processing. Cereb Cortex. 2016;26(8):3390–401.
36. Wurm MF, Caramazza A, Lingnau A. Action categories in lateral occipitotemporal cortex are organized along sociality and transitivity. J Neurosci. 2017;37(3):562–75.
37. Tranel D, Damasio H, Damasio AR. A neural basis for the retrieval of conceptual knowledge. Neuropsychologia. 1997;35(10):1319–27.
38. Tranel D, Kemmerer D, Adolphs R, Damasio H, Damasio AR. Neural correlates of conceptual knowledge for actions. Cogn Neuropsychol. 2003;20(3):409–32.
39. Brambati SM, Myers D, Wilson A, Rankin KP, Allison SC, Rosen HJ, et al. The anatomy of category-specific object naming in neurodegenerative diseases. J Cogn Neurosci. 2006;18(10):1644–53.
40. Warrington EK, McCarthy R. Category specific access dysphasia. Brain. 1983;106(Pt 4):859–78.
41. Warrington EK, Shallice T. Category specific semantic impairments. Brain. 1984;107(Pt 3):829–54.
42. Warrington EK, McCarthy RA. Categories of knowledge. Further fractionations and an attempted integration. Brain. 1987;110(Pt 5):1273–96.
43. Capitani E, Laiacona M, Mahon B, Caramazza A. What are the facts of category-specific deficits? A critical review of the clinical evidence. Cogn Neuropsychol. 2003;20: 213–61.

44. Humphreys GW, Forde EM. Hierarchies, similarity, and interactivity in object recognition: "category-specific" neuropsychological deficits. Behav Brain Sci. 2001;24(3):453–76; discussion 476–509.
45. Corrow SL, Dalrymple KA, Barton JJ. Prosopagnosia: current perspectives. Eye Brain. 2016;8:165–75.
46. Geskin J, Behrmann M. Congenital prosopagnosia without object agnosia? A literature review. Cogn Neuropsychol. 2018;35(1–2):4–54.
47. Bruffaerts R, De Weer AS, De Grauwe S, Thys M, Dries E, Thijs V, et al. Noun and knowledge retrieval for biological and non-biological entities following right occipitotemporal lesions. Neuropsychologia. 2014;62:163–74.
48. Caramazza A, Shelton JR. Domain-specific knowledge systems in the brain the animate-inanimate distinction. J Cogn Neurosci. 1998;10(1):1–34.
49. Gainotti G. What the locus of brain lesion tells us about the nature of the cognitive defect underlying category-specific disorders: a review. Cortex. 2000;36(4):539–59.
50. Gainotti G. Representional and connectivity-based accounts of the cognitive consequences of atrophy of the right and left anterior temporal lobes. Cogn Neuropsychol. 2020;37(7–8):466–81.
51. Blundo C, Ricci M, Miller L. Category-specific knowledge deficit for animals in a patient with herpes simplex encephalitis. Cogn Neuropsychol. 2006;23(8):1248–68.
52. Samson D, Pillon A. A case of impaired knowledge for fruit and vegetables. Cogn Neuropsychol. 2003;20(3):373–400.
53. Haslam C, Kay J, Hanley JR. Selective loss and preservation of biographical knowledge: implications for representation. Neurocase. 2002;8(3):169–93.
54. Haslam C, Kay J, Hanley JR, Lyons F. Biographical knowledge: modality-specific or modality-neutral? Cortex. 2004;40(3):451–66.
55. Kay J, Hanley JR. Preservation of memory for people in semantic memory disorder: further category-specific semantic dissociation. Cogn Neuropsychol. 2002;19(2):113–33.
56. Lyons F, Hanley JR, Kay J. Anomia for common names and geographical names with preserved retrieval of names of people: a semantic memory disorder. Cortex. 2002;38(1):23–35.
57. Lyons F, Kay J, Hanley JR, Haslam C. Selective preservation of memory for people in the context of semantic memory disorder: patterns of association and dissociation. Neuropsychologia. 2006;44(14):2887–98.
58. Miceli G, Capasso R, Daniele A, Esposito T, Magarelli M, Tomaiuolo F. Selective deficit for people's names following left temporal damage: an impairment of domain-specific conceptual knowledge. Cogn Neuropsychol. 2000;17(6):489–516.
59. Papagno C, Miracapillo C, Casarotti A, Romero Lauro L, Castellano A, Falini A, et al. What is the role of the uncinate fasciculus? Surgical removal and proper name retrieval. Brain. 2011;134(2):405–14.
60. Semenza C. Naming with proper names: the left temporal pole theory. Behav Neurol. 2011;24(4):277–84.
61. Gallese V, Fadiga L, Fogassi L, Rizzolatti G. Action recognition in the premotor cortex. Brain. 1996;119:593–609.
62. di Pellegrino G, Fadiga L, Fogassi L, Gallese V, Rizzolatti G. Understanding motor events: a neurophysiological study. Exp Brain Res. 1992;91:176–80.
63. Calvo-Merino B, Grezes J, Glaser DE, Passingham RE, Haggard P. Seeing or doing? Influence of visual and motor familiarity in action observation. Curr Biol. 2006;16(19):1905–10.
64. Rizzolatti G, Craighero L. The mirror-neuron system. Annu Rev Neurosci. 2004;27:169–92.
65. Liberman AM, Mattingly IG. The motor theory of speech perception revised. Cognition. 1985;21(1):1–36.
66. Liberman A, Cooper F, Shankweiler D, Studdert-Kennedy M. Perception of the speech code. Psychol Rev. 1967;74(6):431–61.
67. Dinstein I, Thomas C, Behrmann M, Heeger DJ. A mirror up to nature. Curr Biol. 2008;18(1):R13–8.
68. Caramazza A, Anzellotti S, Strnad L, Lingnau A. Embodied cognition and mirror neurons: a critical assessment. Annu Rev Neurosci. 2014;37:1–15.

69. Mahon BZ, Caramazza A. A critical look at the embodied cognition hypothesis and a new proposal for grounding conceptual content. J Physiol Paris. 2008;102(1–3):59–70.
70. Hickok G. Eight problems for the mirror neuron theory of action understanding in monkeys and humans. J Cogn Neurosci. 2009;21:1229–43.
71. Hickok G. The myth of mirror neurons: the real neuroscience of communication and cognition. New York: W.W. Norton; 2014.
72. Meister IG, Wilson SM, Deblieck C, Wu AD, Iacoboni M. The essential role of premotor cortex in speech perception. Curr Biol. 2007;17(19):1692–6.
73. Möttönen R, Watkins K. Using TMS to study the role of the articulatory motor system in speech perception. Aphasiology. 2012;26(9):1103–18.
74. Pazzaglia M, Pizzamiglio L, Pes E, Aglioti SM. The sound of actions in apraxia. Curr Biol. 2008;18(22):1766–72.
75. Pazzaglia M, Smania N, Corato E, Aglioti SM. Neural underpinnings of gesture discrimination in patients with limb apraxia. J Neurosci. 2008;28(12):3030–41.
76. Rapcsak S, Ochipa C, Anderson K, Poizner H. Progressive ideomotor apraxia: evidence for a selective impairment in the action production system. Brain Cogn. 1995;27: 213–36.
77. Rumiati R, Zanini S, Vorano L. A form of ideational apraxia as a selective deficit of contention scheduling. Cogn Neuropsychol. 2001;18:617–42.
78. Rogalsky C, Love T, Driscoll D, Anderson S, Hickok G. Are mirror neurons the basis of speech perception? Evidence from five cases with damage to the purported human mirror system. Neurocase. 2011;17:178–87.
79. Stasenko A, Bonn C, Teghipco A, Garcea FE, Sweet C, Dombovy M, et al. A causal test of the motor theory of speech perception: a case of impaired speech production and spared speech perception. Cogn Neuropsychol. 2015;32(2):38–57.
80. Mahon BZ, Caramazza A. The orchestration of the sensory-motor systems: Clues from Neuropsychology. Cogn Neuropsychol. 2005;22(3):480–94.
81. Rothi L, Ochipa C, Heilman K. A cognitive neuropsychological model of limb praxis. Cogn Neuropsychol. 1991;8:443–58.
82. Stasenko A, Garcea FE, Mahon BZ. What happens to the motor theory of perception when the motor system is damaged? Lang Cogn. 2013;5(2–3):225–38.
83. Rech F, Wassermann D, Duffau H. New insights into the neural foundations mediating movement/language interactions gained from intrasurgical direct electrostimulations. Brain Cogn. 2020;142:105583.
84. den Ouden DB, Fix S, Parrish TB, Thompson CK. Argument structure effects in action verb naming in static and dynamic conditions. J Neurolinguistics. 2009;22(2):196–215.
85. Friederici AD. The cortical language circuit: from auditory perception to sentence comprehension. Trends Cogn Sci. 2012;16(5):262–8.
86. Thompson C, Meltzer-Asscher A. Neurocognitive mechanisms of verb argument structure processing. In: Bachrach A, Roy I, Stockall I, editors. Structuring the argument. Amsterdam: John Benjamins; 2014. p. 141–68.
87. Jonkers R, Bastiaanse R. The influence of instrumentality and transitivity on action naming in Broca's and anomic aphasia. Brain Lang. 1996;55:37–9.
88. Kim M, Thompson CK. Verb deficits in Alzheimer's disease and agrammatism: implications for lexical organization. Brain Lang. 2004;88(1):1–20.
89. De Bleser R, Kauschke C. Acquisition and loss of nouns and verbs: parallel or divergent patterns? J Neurolinguistics. 2003;16:213–29.
90. Bock K, Levelt W. Grammatical encoding. In: Altmann GT, editor. Psycholinguistics: critical concepts in psychology, vol. 2. New York: Taylor & Francis; 1994.
91. Chang F. Symbolically speaking: a connectionist model of sentence production. Cogn Sci. 2002;26(5):609–51.
92. Thompson CK, Bonakdarpour B, Fix SC, Blumenfeld HK, Parrish TB, Gitelman DR, et al. Neural correlates of verb argument structure processing. J Cogn Neurosci. 2007;19(11):1753–67.

93. Allport D. Distributed memory, modular subsystems and dysphasia. In: Newman SP, Epstein R, editors. Current perspectives in dysphasia. Edinburgh: Churchill Livingstone; 1985. p. 32–60.
94. Barros-Loscertales A, Gonzalez J, Pulvermuller F, Ventura-Campos N, Bustamante JC, Costumero V, et al. Reading salt activates gustatory brain regions: fMRI evidence for semantic grounding in a novel sensory modality. Cereb Cortex. 2012;22(11):2554–63.
95. Gonzalez J, Barros-Loscertales A, Pulvermuller F, Meseguer V, Sanjuan A, Belloch V, et al. Reading cinnamon activates olfactory brain regions. Neuroimage. 2006;32(2):906–12.
96. Kiefer M, Sim E, Herrnberger B, Grothe J, Hoenig K. The sound of concepts: four markers for a link between auditory and conceptual brain systems. J Neurosci. 2008;28(47):12224–30.
97. Bonner M, Grossman M. Gray matter density of auditory association cortex relates to knowledge of sound concepts in primary progressive aphasia. J Neurosci. 2012;32:7986–91.
98. Simmons WK, Martin A, Barsalou LW. Pictures of appetizing foods activate gustatory cortices for taste and reward. Cereb Cortex. 2005;15(10):1602–8.
99. Revill KP, Aslin RN, Tanenhaus MK, Bavelier D. Neural correlates of partial lexical activation. Proc Natl Acad Sci U S A. 2008;105(35):13111–5.
100. Santini B, Talacchi A, Squintani G, Casagrande F, Capasso R, Miceli G. Cognitive outcome after awake surgery for tumors in language areas. J Neurooncol. 2012;108(2):319–26.
101. Satoer D, Visch-Brink E, Smits M, Kloet A, Looman C, Dirven C, et al. Long-term evaluation of cognition after glioma surgery in eloquent areas. J Neurooncol. 2014;116(1):153–60.
102. Satoer D, Vincent A, Ruhaak L, Smits M, Dirven C, Visch-Brink E. Spontaneous speech in patients with gliomas in eloquent areas: evaluation until 1 year after surgery. Clin Neurol Neurosurg. 2018;167:112–6.
103. Norrelgen F, Jensdottir M, Ostberg P. High-level language outcomes three and twelve months after awake surgery in low grade glioma and cavernoma patients. Clin Neurol Neurosurg. 2020;195:105946.
104. Papagno C, Casarotti A, Comi A, Gallucci M, Riva M, Bello L. Measuring clinical outcomes in neuro-oncology. A battery to evaluate low-grade gliomas (LGG). J Neurooncol. 2012;108(2):269–75.
105. Zarino B, Di Cristofori A, Fornara G, Bertani G, Locatelli M, Caroli M, et al. Long-term follow-up of neuropsychological functions in patients with high grade gliomas: can cognitive status predict patient's outcome after surgery? Acta Neurochir (Wien). 2020;162(4):803–12.
106. Pisoni A, Mattavelli G, Casarotti A, Comi A, Riva M, Bello L, et al. Object-action dissociation: a voxel-based lesion-symptom mapping study on 102 patients after glioma removal. Neuroimage Clin. 2018;18:986–95.
107. Moritz-Gasser S, Herbet G, Maldonado I, Duffau H. Lexical access speed is significantly correlated with the return to professional activities after awake surgery for low-grade gliomas. J Neurooncol. 2012;107(3):633–41.
108. Rofes A, Talacchi A, Santini B, Pinna G, Nickels L, Bastiaanse R, et al. Language in individuals with left hemisphere tumors: is spontaneous speech analysis comparable to formal testing? J Clin Exp Neuropsychol. 2018;40(7):722–32.
109. Tomasino B, Tronchin G, Marin D, Maieron M, Fabbro F, Cubelli R, et al. Noun–verb naming dissociation in neurosurgical patients. Aphasiology. 2019;33(12):1418–40.
110. Baldo JV, Arevalo A, Patterson JP, Dronkers NF. Grey and white matter correlates of picture naming: evidence from a voxel-based lesion analysis of the Boston Naming Test. Cortex. 2013;49(3):658–67.
111. Piras F, Marangolo P. Noun-verb naming in aphasia: a voxel-based lesion-symptom mapping study. Neuroreport. 2007;18(14):1455–8.
112. Finocchiaro C, Basso G, Giovenzana A, Caramazza A. Morphological complexity reveals verb-specific prefrontal engagement. J Neurolinguistics. 2010;23(6):553–63.
113. Arevalo AL, Lu CC, Huang LB, Bates EA, Dronkers NF. Action and object processing in brain-injured speakers of Chinese. Neuropsychology. 2011;25(6):792–805.
114. Rofes A, Capasso R, Miceli G. Verb production tasks in the measurement of communicative abilities in aphasia. J Clin Exp Neuropsychol. 2015;37(5):483–502.

115. Gerard IJ, Kersten-Oertel M, Petrecca K, Sirhan D, Hall JA, Collins DL. Brain shift in neuronavigation of brain tumors: a review. Med Image Anal. 2017;35:403–20.
116. Duffau H, Herbet G, Moritz-Gasser S. Toward a pluri-component, multimodal, and dynamic organization of the ventral semantic stream in humans: lessons from stimulation mapping in awake patients. Front Syst Neurosci. 2013;7:1–4.
117. Herbet G, Maheu M, Costi E, Lafargue G, Duffau H. Mapping neuroplastic potential in brain-damaged patients. Brain. 2016;139(Pt 3):829–44.
118. Crinion J, Holland A, Copland D, Thompson C, Hillis A. Neuroimaging in aphasia treatment research: quantifying brain lesions after stroke. Neuroimage. 2013;73:208–14.
119. Carrera E, Tononi G. Diaschisis: past, present, future. Brain. 2014;137(Pt 9):2408–22.
120. Price CJ, Warburton EA, Moore CJ, Frackowiak RS, Friston KJ. Dynamic diaschisis: anatomically remote and context-sensitive human brain lesions. J Cogn Neurosci. 2001;13(4):419–29.
121. Garcea FE, Almeida J, Sims MH, Nunno A, Meyers SP, Li YM, et al. Domain-specific diaschisis: lesions to parietal action areas modulate neural responses to tools in the ventral stream. Cereb Cortex. 2019;29(7):3168–81.
122. Herbet G, Moritz-Gasser S, Lemaitre AL, Almairac F, Duffau H. Functional compensation of the left inferior longitudinal fasciculus for picture naming. Cogn Neuropsychol. 2019;36(3–4):140–57.
123. Hamberger MJ, Goodman RR, Perrine K, Tamny T. Anatomic dissociation of auditory and visual naming in the lateral temporal cortex. Neurology. 2001;56(1):56–61.
124. Hamberger MJ, Seidel WT. Auditory and visual naming tests: normative and patient data for accuracy, response time, and tip-of-the-tongue. J Int Neuropsychol Soc. 2003;9(3):479–89.
125. Hamberger MJ, Seidel WT, Goodman RR, Perrine K, McKhann GM. Temporal lobe stimulation reveals anatomic distinction between auditory naming processes. Neurology. 2003;60(9):1478–83.
126. Hamberger MJ, Seidel WT, McKhann GM, Perrine K, Goodman RR. Brain stimulation reveals critical auditory naming cortex. Brain. 2005;128:2742–9.
127. McClelland S, Hamberger MJ, McKhann GM, Goodman RR. Distribution of auditory and visual naming sites in patients with and without temporal lobe lesions. Epilepsia. 2005;46:531–8.
128. Hamberger MJ, Miozzo M, Schevon CA, Morrison C, Carlson C, Mehta AD, Klein GE, McKhann GM, Williams AC, et al. Epilepsy Behav. 2016;60:124–9.
129. Impairment TCoMRoP. Guides to the evaluation of permanent impairment; the visual system. J Am Med Assoc. 1958;168(4):475–88.
130. Rofes A, Spena G, Talacchi A, Santini B, Miozzo A, Miceli G. Mapping nouns and finite verbs in left hemisphere tumors: a direct electrical stimulation study. Neurocase. 2017;23(2):105–13.
131. Hamberger MJ, McClelland S, McKhann GM, Williams AC, Goodman RR. Distribution of auditory and visual naming sites in nonlesional temporal lobe epilepsy patients and patients with space-occupying temporal lobe lesions. Epilepsia. 2007;48(3):531–8.
132. Coello AF, Moritz-Gasser S, Martino J, Martinoni M, Matsuda R, Duffau H. Selection of intraoperative tasks for awake mapping based on relationships between tumor location and functional networks. J Neurosurg. 2013;119(6):1380–94.
133. Rogers TT, Lambon Ralph MA, Garrard P, Bozeat S, McClelland JL, Hodges JR, Patterson K. Structure and deterioration of semantic memory: a neuropsychological and computational investigation. Psychol Rev. 2004;111(1):205–35.
134. Patterson K, Nestor PJ, Rogers TT. Where do you know what you know? The representation of semantic knowledge in the human brain. Nat Rev Neurosci. 2007;8(12):976–87.
135. Ralph MA, Jefferies E, Patterson K, Rogers TT. The neural and computational bases of semantic cognition. Nat Rev Neurosci. 2017;18(1):42–55.
136. Binder JR, Desai RH, Graves WW, Conant LL. Where is the semantic system? A critical review and meta-analysis of 120 functional neuroimaging studies. Cereb Cortex. 2009;19(12):2767–96.

137. Fernandino L, Binder JR, Desai RH, Pendl SL, Humphries CJ, Gross WL, Conant LL, Seidenberg MS. Concept representation reflects multimodal abstraction: a framework for embodied semantics. Cereb Cortex. 2016;26(5):2018–34.
138. Binder JR. In defense of abstract conceptual representations. Psychon Bull Rev. 2016;23(4):1096–108.
139. Mahon BZ. The burden of embodied cognition. Can J Exp Psychol. 2015;69(2):172–8.
140. Mahon BZ. Response to glenberg: conceptual content does not constrain the representational format of concepts. Can J Exp Psychol. 2015;69(2):179–80.
141. Mahon BZ. What is embodied about cognition? Lang Cogn Neurosci. 2015;30(4):420–9.
142. Mahon BZ. Missed connections: a connectivity-constrained account of the representation and organization of object concepts. In: Conceptual mind: new directions in the study of concepts. 2015. p. 79–115.
143. Mahon BZ, Hickok G. Arguments about the nature of concepts: symbols, embodiment, and beyond. Psychon Bull Rev. 2016;23(4):941–58.
144. Suzuki K, Yamadori A, Endo K, Fujii T, Ezura M, Takahashi A. Dissociation of letter and picture naming resulting from callosal disconnection. Neurology. 1998;51(5):1390–4.
145. Gazzaniga MS. Principles of human brain organization derived from split-brain studies. Neuron. 1995;14(2):217–28.
146. Forkel SJ, Thiebaut de Schotten M, Kawadler JM, Dell'Acqua F, Danek A, Catani M. The anatomy of fronto-occipital connections from early blunt dissections to contemporary tractography. Cortex. 2014;56:73–84.
147. Sarubbo S, De Benedictis A, Maldonado IL, Basso G, Duffau H. Frontal terminations for the inferior fronto-occipital fascicle: anatomical dissection, DTI study and functional considerations on a multi-component bundle. Brain Struct Funct. 2013;218(1):21–37.
148. Duffau H, Gatignol P, Mandonnet E, Peruzzi P, Tzourio-Mazoyer N, Capelle L. New insights into the anatomo-functional connectivity of the semantic system: a study using cortico-subcortical electrostimulations. Brain. 2005;128(4):797–810.
149. Alyahya RSW, Halai AD, Conroy P, Lambon Ralph MA. Mapping psycholinguistic features to the neuropsychological and lesion profiles in aphasia. Cortex. 2020;124:260–73.
150. Rofes A, de Aguiar V, Ficek B, Wendt H, Webster K, Tsapkini K. The role of word properties in performance on fluency tasks in people with primary progressive aphasia. J Alzheimers Dis. 2019;68(4):1521–34.
151. Corina DP, Gibson EK, Martin R, Poliakov A, Brinkley J, Ojemann GA. Dissociation of action and object naming: evidence from cortical stimulation mapping. Hum Brain Mapp. 2005;24(1):1–10.
152. Havas V, Gabarros A, Juncadella M, Rifa-Ros X, Plans G, Acebes JJ, et al. Electrical stimulation mapping of nouns and verbs in Broca's area. Brain Lang. 2015;145–146: 53–63.
153. Lubrano V, Filleron T, Demonet JF, Roux FE. Anatomical correlates for category-specific naming of objects and actions: a brain stimulation mapping study. Hum Brain Mapp. 2014;35(2):429–43.
154. Rofes A, Mandonnet E, Godden J, Baron M, Colle H, Darlix A, et al. Survey on current cognitive practices within the European Low-Grade Glioma Network: towards a European assessment protocol. Acta Neurochir. 2017;159(7):1167–78.
155. Salmon JP, Matheson HE, McMullen PA. Photographs of manipulable objects are named more quickly than the same objects depicted as line-drawings: evidence that photographs engage embodiment more than line-drawings. Front Psychol. 2014;5:1187.
156. Caramazza A. The logic of neuropsychological research and the problem of patient classification in aphasia. Brain Lang. 1984;21(1):9–20.
157. Shapiro K, Caramazza A. The representation of grammatical categories in the brain. Trends Cogn Sci. 2003;7(5):201–6.
158. Połczyńska M. New tests for language mapping with intraoperative electrical stimulation of the brain to preserve language in individuals with tumors and epilepsy: a preliminary follow-up study. Poznań Stud Contemp Linguist. 2009;45(2):261–79.

159. Ohlerth AK, Valentin A, Vergani F, Ashkan K, Bastiaanse R. The verb and noun test for peri-operative testing (VAN-POP): standardized language tests for navigated transcranial magnetic stimulation and direct electrical stimulation. Acta Neurochir (Wien). 2020;162(2):397–406.
160. Akinina Y, Malyutina S, Ivanova M, Iskra E, Mannova E, Dragoy O. Russian normative data for 375 action pictures and verbs. Behav Res Methods. 2015;47(3):691–707.
161. De Witte E, Satoer D, Robert E, Colle H, Verheyen S, Visch-Brink E, et al. The Dutch Linguistic Intraoperative Protocol: a valid linguistic approach to awake brain surgery. Brain Lang. 2015;140:35–48.
162. Papagno C, Casarotti A, Zarino B, Crepaldi D. A new test of action verb naming: normative data from 290 Italian adults. Neurol Sci. 2020;41(10):2811–7.
163. Rofes A, de Aguiar V, Miceli G. A minimal standardization setting for language mapping tests: an Italian example. Neurol Sci. 2015;36(7):1113–9.
164. Rofes A, de Aguiar V, Jonkers R, Oh S, Dede G, Sung J. What drives task performance during animal fluency in people with Alzheimer's disease? Front Psychol. 2020;11:1485.
165. De Witt Hamer PC, Robles SG, Zwinderman AH, Duffau H, Berger MS. Impact of intraoperative stimulation brain mapping on glioma surgery outcome: a meta-analysis. J Clin Oncol. 2012;30(20):2559–65.
166. Catani M, Mesulam MM, Jakobsen E, Malik F, Martersteck A, Wieneke C, et al. A novel frontal pathway underlies verbal fluency in primary progressive aphasia. Brain. 2013;136(Pt 8):2619–28.
167. Chernoff BL, Sims MH, Smith SO, Pilcher WH, Mahon BZ. Direct electrical stimulation of the left frontal aslant tract disrupts sentence planning without affecting articulation. Cogn Neuropsychol. 2019;36(3–4):178–92.
168. Chernoff BL, Teghipco A, Garcea FE, Sims MH, Paul DA, Tivarus ME, et al. A role for the frontal aslant tract in speech planning: a neurosurgical case study. J Cogn Neurosci. 2018;30(5):752–69.

Verbal Short-Term Memory

12

Costanza Papagno and Juan Martino

12.1 Introduction

Short-term memory (STM) is the capacity to keep a small amount of information in mind in an active, readily available state for a brief period of time (several seconds to minutes), in the absence of sensory input [1]. STM should be distinguished from working memory [2], which adds processes that support manipulation of the information, providing a basis for goal-directed behaviors [3–5]. Therefore, the difference between STM and working memory is in terms of operativity. In other words, the concept of working memory includes the manipulation of information. Working memory consists of two so-called slave systems, the phonological loop and the visuo-spatial sketchpad, which are coordinated by a control system, the central executive. More recently, Baddeley [6] has added a fourth component, the episodic buffer, that holds multidimensional stimuli from semantic and episodic long-term memory in addition to information from the other subsystems of working memory, combining them into multidimensional episodes (see also [7]). Deficits in working memory are so frequently associated with executive function disorders that some neuropsychologists classify working memory with executive functions.

Imagine you move through an airport to reach the boarding gate, you have to memorize the gate, the departure time, the time in advance by which you have to reach the gate, the time it takes to reach the gate, etc. You have to do several mental calculations to estimate if you have to change terminals, if you have to take a train, if there will be a lot of queue at the luggage control, etc. You weigh alternatives, make decisions, and order your thoughts until you think the plan achieves your

C. Papagno (✉)
Neurocognitive Rehabilitation Center (CeRiN), CIMeC (Center for Mind/Brain Sciences), University of Trento, Rovereto, Italy
e-mail: costanza.papagno@unimib.it, costanza.papagno@unitn.it

J. Martino
Department of Neurosurgery, Hospital Universitario Marques de Valdecilla, Santander, Spain

E. Mandonnet, G. Herbet (eds.), *Intraoperative Mapping of Cognitive Networks*,
https://doi.org/10.1007/978-3-030-75071-8_12

objectives. Working memory stores information in an online fashion, allowing its contents to be easily accessed by other cognitive processes. Consequently, working memory is considered to be one of the most crucial components in the execution of many complex cognitive tasks that require holding and manipulating information for short periods of time, such as general fluid intelligence, reasoning ability, language, learning, mathematical ability, and spatial ability [8, 9, 10–13].

Verbal STM includes the activity of interrelated components. The most popular psychological model of verbal STM distinguishes a component devoted to the storage of verbal information (phonological short-term store—STS—or buffer), and a process (articulatory rehearsal), which revives the memory trace held in the phonological store, preventing its decay. The rehearsal process recirculates verbal information between the phonological STS and a component, the phonological output buffer, or assembly system, participating in speech production. Auditory-verbal input has direct access, after acoustic analysis, to the phonological store, while a written verbal information undergoes a process of recoding in a phonological form and accesses the phonological store by means of rehearsal (see [14]).

The main problem with this topic is that different authors not always use in a correct way the term and consequently they test differently (and not always properly) this faculty. Moreover, they use interchangeably working memory and STM, which are in fact two different concepts. Finally, verbal STM includes two distinct information: one concerning the item and the other the order, namely the position of an item in the sequence (see [15]). All tests of simple recognition involve only the item information and not the order one; consequently, they only partially test STM.

For the sake of clarity, we will discuss issues concerning verbal STM, which corresponds to the phonological loop of the Baddeley and Hitch's [2] working memory model. There are indeed other models that are not the focus of this chapter (see [16] for a review). We will also briefly mention some studies on working memory, both verbal and spatial.

12.2 The Neural Basis of Verbal STM

Distinct anatomical correlates subserve the different components of verbal STM, as demonstrated by various studies using different methodologies. Indeed, this evidence derives from anatomo-clinical studies in brain-damaged patients (see [17], for reviews), neuroimaging studies with positron emission tomography ([18, 19]; but see [20]) and fMRI [21], and, finally, studies using repetitive transcranial magnetic stimulation [22, 23]. Such different methodologies converge in showing that the phonological short-term store depends on the activity of the inferior parietal lobule (more specifically, the supramarginal gyrus, Brodmann's area BA 40, but also the angular gyrus, BA 39, see [24–26]), while the rehearsal process depends on the activity of the inferior frontal operculum (BA 44 and BA 6, but also BA 45). Further evidence is provided by direct electrical stimulation studies [27]. Recently, in a voxel-based lesion-symptom mapping study on 103 patients after glioma removal [28], the role of the supramarginal gyrus in phonological storage has been confirmed.

Verbal STM has been demonstrated to be involved in learning a new language [29] and in sentence comprehension, in particular when word order is crucial for comprehension (like "put the small red square over the big black circle") or when the sentence is syntactically complex and loads on memory (like "the cat, that the boy is watching, is drinking milk") (see [16] for a review). In addition, being a component of working memory, its damage impairs functions related to it. Therefore, it is crucial to preserve the phonological loop function during surgery in these areas of the brain.

12.3 Long-Term Deficits in Patients Who Did Not Benefit from Intraoperative Monitoring of Verbal STM

As already mentioned, a serious problem in the memory domain is that clinicians do not use the correct terms in defining the different memory subsystems. In fact, they often name STM what is episodic learning, namely anterograde amnesia. So, they define as STM impairment, the problems reported by patients with anterograde memory/learning deficits. This is particularly evident in the neurosurgical literature.

Intraoperative electrical stimulation mapping is an indispensable tool to guide the resection of gliomas within eloquent areas, as it enables to identify and preserve the functional margins, and maximize the tumoral resection [30, 31]. Regarding language mapping, object naming has been the preferred task for identifying cortical and subcortical eloquent sites [32]. The object naming areas identified with this technique are considered essential, as language decline has been observed after removal of these sites [33]. On the other hand, memory areas are generally not considered as part of the "eloquent" brain in neurosurgical practice, and they are currently not localized during brain mapping. However, several glioma series with intraoperative evaluation of picture naming task demonstrated high rates (up to 73.3% in the long term) of postoperative memory impairment, raising the question regarding the efficacy of this approach to preserve memory function [34–39]. Moreover, memory deficits seem to represent one of the main sources of dysfunction in glioma patients affecting their quality of life [40, 41].

Racine et al. [37] evaluated the postoperative neurocognitive function in a cohort of 22 newly diagnosed low-grade gliomas. All patients were operated awake with IES mapping, and evaluation of language with a picture naming task. Memory was not tested intraoperatively. Six months after surgery, seven patients underwent repeated neuropsychological testing, revealing a decline in what the authors call STM tests in 40–60% of cases. However, the effective decline was observed in immediate story recall (which assesses episodic buffer integrity) and backward digit span (assessing verbal working memory) but forward digit span did not decrease.

Similarly, the effect of surgery in specific tumor locations like the insula has also been analyzed. Wu et al. [39] studied 35 patients with insular low-grade and anaplastic gliomas operated awake with language IES. The authors report that 3 months after surgery, the rate of STM decline was higher than 50%. However, the impaired test was a learning one, as well as a delayed recall test, while verbal STM, as assessed by means of a span task, was not impaired.

Teixidor et al. [38] evaluated 23 low-grade gliomas operated with the same methodology of language mapping. Immediately after surgery, 96% of patients showed verbal working memory worsening. Only nine patients had long-term follow-up, but all of them recovered 3 months after surgery with intensive rehabilitation.

Martino et al. [36] studied the long-term deficits in a series of 16 patients operated with intraoperative evaluation of language. They reported at 6 months after surgery a 73.3% of STM decline, which was tested with a recognition task and not with serial recall, therefore assessing only item information.

In contrast, a single case has been reported [42] who underwent awake surgery for removal of an oligodendroglioma involving Broca's area and the insula. This patient showed a severe decrease in her auditory-verbal span due to a deficit in rehearsal, coupled with a sentence comprehension deficit. This patient represents a "true" case of STM impairment demonstrated by appropriate testing.

12.4 Locations at Risk of Long-Term Deficits in Verbal STM

The identification of specific anatomical hotspots that are critical for adequate STM functioning would be crucial for surgeons. Indeed, it allows knowing which specific brain regions are to be considered "eloquent" for memory.

Previous studies demonstrated that intraoperative damage to memory areas is associated with a long-term decline in memory function. Ojemman et al. [43] evaluated language and verbal memory organization by electrical stimulation mapping in 14 adults undergoing left temporal lobectomy for epilepsy. Memory sites were identified at the lateral temporal cortex in 13 cases. At the temporo-parietal cortex, language sites were mainly located in the posterior portion of the superior temporal gyrus, while memory sites were located in the middle and anterior portion of the superior and middle temporal gyri, and in the inferior parietal lobule. Therefore, the authors describe a lateral cortical temporal memory system separated, although adjacent to the posterior language areas. The authors also assessed memory deficits 1 month and 1 year after temporal lobectomy with the Wechsler Verbal Memory Scale. They reported a 22% of verbal memory decrease at 1 month, and 11% at 1 year after surgery. Unfortunately, the previous version of this scale (now accurately revised) evaluated different forms of memory and did not provide a pure measure of verbal STM. In order to evaluate the risk of memory impairment if functional areas were damaged, cases were divided into those with resections that were close or even including language or memory areas, and those with resections far from these functional areas. The resection close or within language and memory areas was associated to an 83% risk of verbal memory impairment 1 year after surgery. On the other hand, when resection was far from language or memory areas, the risk decreased to 25. Unfortunately, the authors combine language and memory sites in the resection zone, and the exact number of cases in which memory sites were damaged is not reported. Therefore, based on this report, it is not possible to calculate the exact risk of memory decline when memory sites are damaged. In addition, the authors do not exclusively refer to STM.

Campanella et al. [35] evaluated memory sequelae in a series of 75 operated low-grade gliomas. Verbal STM was evaluated preoperatively and 4 months after surgery with the Digit Span Forward. A voxel-based lesion-symptom mapping technique was used in order to identify specific hubs which appeared to be particularly susceptible of causing verbal STM disturbances. Regarding the Digit Span Forward Test, two specific hotspots were identified: the conjunction between the left superior and the middle temporal gyri, and the white matter area involving the intersection between the left inferior longitudinal fasciculus, inferior fronto-occipital fasciculus, and posterior arcuate fasciculus.

In the neurosurgical literature there are other studies concerning both verbal and spatial working memory and not specifically verbal STM. We will briefly mention these studies on both, verbal and spatial, working memory.

Kho et al. [44] described a single case of a patient with a left frontal desmoplastic gangliocytoma and medically intractable epilepsy that was operated awake with IES. Working memory was evaluated intraoperatively with a backward digit span test. IES identified a working memory area at the left dorsolateral prefrontal cortex. The memory site identified was included in the resection as it was part of the epileptogenic region, and was far from language areas. The authors conclude that this area was critically involved in memory, as neuropsychological evaluation 2 years after surgery revealed a selective impairment in working memory tasks. However, an improvement was observed, suggesting that compensatory mechanism took place. This case emphasizes the important role of the dorsolateral prefrontal cortex in working memory.

Spatial working memory decline was evaluated in 24 patients with frontal gliomas, who underwent awake surgery, while performing a spatial two-back task; 14 healthy volunteers were also tested [45]. A significant correlation between spatial working memory deficits and injury to the dorsal frontoparietal subcortical white matter pathways, i.e., the first and second portions of the superior longitudinal fasciculus, was found.

Nakajima et al. [46] evaluated intraoperatively working memory in two patients with gliomas in the supplementary motor area using a two-back task. In one of the two cases, the authors decided to resect the positive memory site due to the infiltration of the glioma. The patient presented with an impairment of working memory immediately after surgery, but fully recovered 1 month later. This rapid recovery may be explained by an unmasking of an extensive neurological network involved in working memory.

12.5 How to Monitor STM Intraoperatively

Ojemann et al. ([43], see also [33]) in 1985 designed a task to evaluate verbal STM intraoperatively. This task has been recently used by another group [36]. Each verbal memory trial consists in a sequence of four slides (Fig. 12.1). The first and second slides are black-and-white pictures with a common name with the phrase "This is a" above it. The third slide consists in a 4–8 word sentence that is read. The fourth slide, shown for 4 s, has a black-and-white picture with the word "recall" on it. The patient has to recall if this picture was present or not at the first or second slides with a response type Yes/No. As reported above, this task investigates only the item component of STM, but not the position one, which is also a crucial aspect and can be selectively impaired (see [27]). Each cortical area was stimulated under each test condition. Language sites with interference in object naming or reading tasks were excluded from the memory analysis in order to ensure that the information committed to memory had been processed correctly. A positive verbal memory site was defined with a patient's inability to recall the pictures during 2 out of 3 of the stimulation trials [47]. One of the main advantages of this task is that, in addition to verbal memory, it evaluates the most important aspects of language with the picture naming and reading tests. The specific aspects of how the tasks are performed intraoperatively are described in Fig. 12.2.

Brandlin-Bennet et al. [48] reported the case of a patient with a tumor in the posterior third ventricle undergoing awake surgery to test memory during fornix manipulation. They used a similar task to the previous one. In this case, the distractor task between picture naming and recall consisted in three simple mathematical addition and subtraction problems. However, it is not clear whether the fornix is involved in short-term or long-term memory network.

A complete evaluation of verbal STM requires the use of digit span. Papagno et al. [27] evaluated STM intraoperatively by means of this task, which provides both an item and an order information, in a series of 29 patients. Participants heard

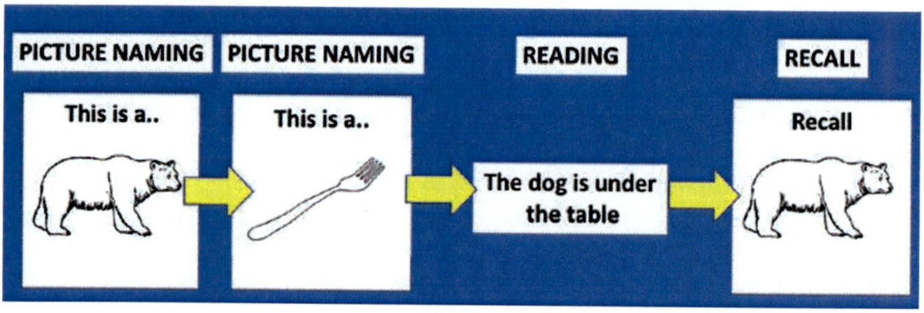

Fig. 12.1 Verbal STM task. Each verbal memory trial consists in a sequence of four slides (this figure). The first and second slides are black-and-white pictures representing animate and inanimate items with the phrase "This is a" written above. The third slide consists in a 4–8 words sentence that has to be read. The fourth slide, shown for 4 s, has a black-and-white picture, with the word "recall" written above it. The patient has to recall if this picture was present or not on the first or second slides, and a binary response (Yes/No) is expected

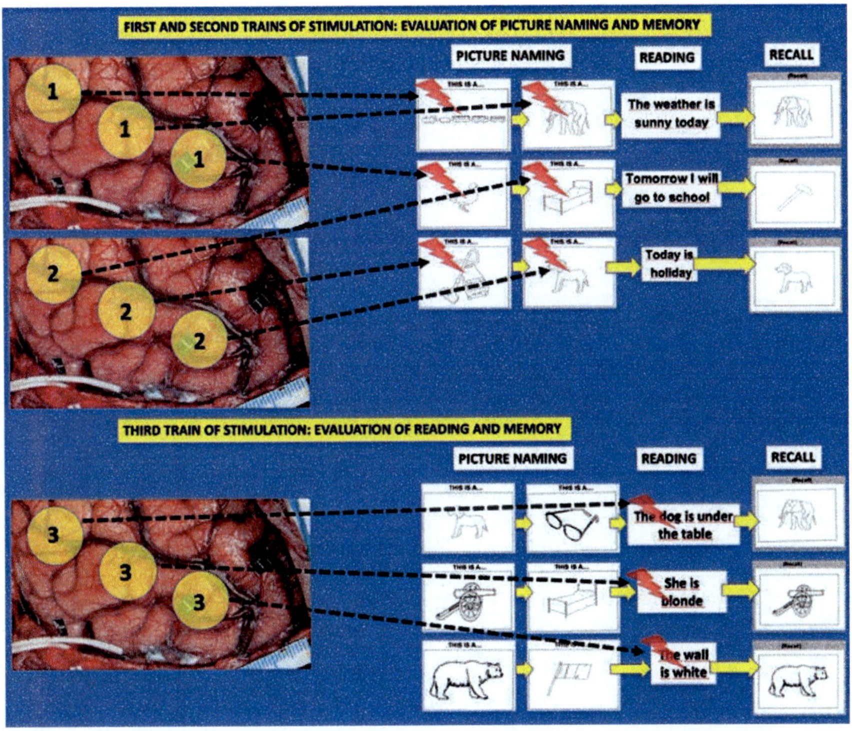

Fig. 12.2 Verbal STM task. Three different cortical sites are tested with the verbal STM task. In the first and second trains of stimulation, each site is only stimulated during the picture naming part of the task. Therefore, in this stage, picture naming and memory are evaluated. If the stimulation of a specific site induces picture naming errors, then this area is classified as a language-naming area. If the stimulation of a specific site induces memory errors without picture naming errors, then it is classified as a verbal memory area. In the third train of stimulation, each site is only stimulated during the reading part of the task. Therefore, in this stage, reading and (encoding) memory are evaluated. If the stimulation of a specific site induces reading errors, then this area is classified as a language-reading area. If the stimulation of a specific site induces memory errors without reading errors, then it is classified as a (retrieval) verbal memory area

a sequence of digits and were asked to repeat the sequence in the same order. Stimulation of Broca's area induced more item errors than order errors, indicating that this area is crucial in maintaining item information. On the other hand, stimulation of the supramarginal gyrus induced significantly more order than item errors, indicating its role in serial order information storage (see Fig. 12.3). Similarly, stimulation of the anterior segment of the arcuate fascicle produced more order than item errors, suggesting that it is involved in transferring order information from Geschwind's area to Broca's area.

In contrast, two studies evaluated verbal working memory during awake surgery, one by using a verbal N-back task and the other a backward letter span. In the former [46], an occupational therapist read Kana (Japanese syllabogram) at a speed of

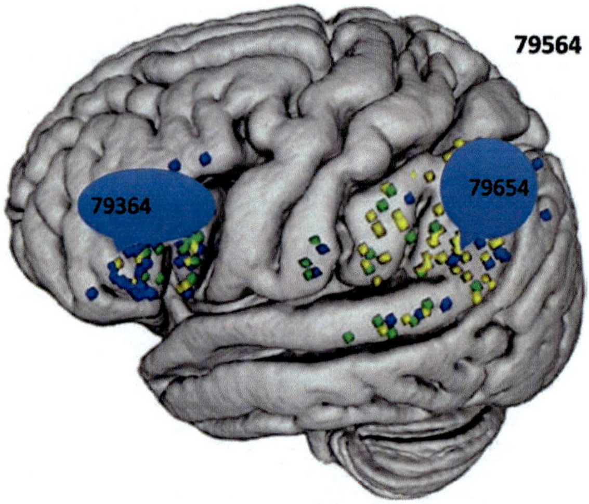

Fig. 12.3 Positive sites during intraoperative brain mapping using digit span. The yellow dots indicate sites where stimulation produced an order error, while blue dots indicate site where item errors were produced. In green sites where both errors appeared. The example show the digit span presented by the examiner (79564) and the two uncorrect responses (left parietal inferior lobule: 79654, order error; Broca's area: 79364, item error) (modified from [27])

1 sound per second. The patient then repeated the Kana which had been heard 2 sounds before. If the patient provided an incorrect response during stimulation, then a positive mapping site was defined.

The backward letter span test was applied by Kho et al. [44] to evaluate working memory in an awake surgery. The stimulation of the dorsolateral prefrontal cortex interfered with this task.

There are a number of limiting factors to consider in conducting intraoperative memory testing. Working memory tasks are cognitively demanding; therefore, they may be interfered by multiple factors such as low attention or concentration, pain, discomfort, and recovery from anesthesia. There is a limited time to conduct the testing as the patient quickly becomes tired during intraoperative cognitive testing. Careful attention and a close interaction between the neuropsychologist and the surgeon is necessary in order to distinguish between random errors and significant, repeatable errors.

12.6 Functional Improvement in Series of Patients Operated on with Versus Without Verbal STM Monitoring

Short-term and working memory areas are not considered by most neurosurgeons as part of the "eloquent" brain and are thus not localized by intraoperative electrical stimulation. The series evaluating long-term deficits when memory areas have been identified and preserved are scarce.

Martino et al. [36] in a matched paired cohort study compared the memory decline in a cohort of 16 subjects with gliomas that were operated with intraoperative evaluation of language and verbal memory (cohort A), with a cohort of 16 subjects that were operated with intraoperative evaluation of language (cohort B). Verbal memory was evaluated intraoperatively with a picture naming-reading-memory task that has been previously described. Detailed neuropsychological assessment was performed before and 6 months after surgery. Intraoperative memory mapping was a strong predictor of verbal memory prognosis. Memory decline was significatively reduced from 73.3 to 26.7% by adapting the resection to avoid those memory areas.

In a VLSM study performed on 103 patients undergoing resection in general without STM monitoring [28], postoperative digit span scores were linked to lesions in both the left supramarginal gyrus and superior-posterior temporal areas, as reported in the literature on patients with a selective deficit of auditory-verbal STM.

12.7 Additional Anatomo-Functional Knowledge Gained from Intraoperative Mapping Studies

The use of STM tasks in intraoperative mapping studies has produced relevant information on current models of STM and it has prompted new research. For example, a more detailed mapping of the phonological loop has been provided, including pathways connecting the different buffers (see Fig. 12.4). In addition, since a specific site for order information was found during awake surgery [27], Guidali et al. [15] conducted a series of TMS experiments, in which participants

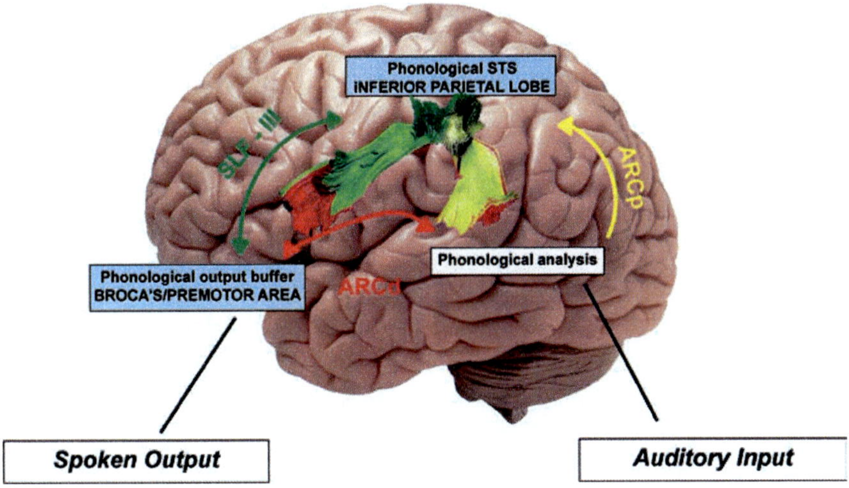

Fig. 12.4 The anatomical correlates of verbal STM. Cortical areas and subcortical pathways. *ARCd* direct segment of the arcuate fasciculus (in red), *ARCp* posterior branch of the arcuate fasciculus (in yellow), *SLF-III* third branch of the superior longitudinal fasciculus, or anterior branch of the arcuate fasciculus (in green) (from [28], Brain Structure and Function)

performed different STM tasks, requiring maintenance of an ordered sequence in three distinct modalities (verbal, spatial, motor), and they demonstrated that the left supramarginal gyrus is one key node of the STM network involved in retaining an abstract representation of serial order information, independently from the content information, namely the nature of the item to be remembered, which instead is stored separately. This is very relevant from the point of view of rehabilitation, since many human tasks require serial order as Lashley pointed out in 1951 [49]: "Temporal integration is not found exclusively in language; …the architect designing a house, and the carpenter sawing a board present a problem of sequences of action." Sequencing would depend from a single structure.

References

1. Brodziak A, Brewczynski A, Bajor G. Clinical significance of knowledge about the structure, function, and impairments of working memory. Med Sci Monit. 2013;19:327–38.
2. Baddeley AD, Hitch G. Working memory. In: Bower GA, editor. Recent advances in learning and motivation, vol. 8. New York: Academic; 1974. p. 47–90.
3. Baddeley A. Working memory: looking back and looking forward. Nat Rev Neurosci. 2003;4(10):829–39.
4. Baddeley A. Working memory: theories, models, and controversies. Annu Rev Psychol. 2012;63:1–29.
5. D'Esposito M, Postle BR. The cognitive neuroscience of working memory. Annu Rev Psychol. 2015;66:115–42.
6. Baddeley AD. The episodic buffer: a new component of working memory? Trends Cogn Sci. 2000;4(11):417–23.
7. Baddeley AD, Hitch GJ. The phonological loop as a buffer store: an update. Cortex. 2019;112:91–106.
8. Ashcraft MH, Krause JA. Working memory, math performance, and math anxiety. Psychon Bull Rev. 2007;14:243–8.
9. Linck JA, Osthus P, Koeth JT, Bunting MF. Working memory and second language comprehension and production: a meta-analysis. Psychon Bull Rev. 2014;21(4):861–83.
10. Christophel TB, Klink PC, Spitzer B, Roelfsema PR, Haynes JD. The distributed nature of working memory. Trends Cogn Sci. 2017;21(2):111–24.
11. Courtney SM, Ungerleider LG, Keil K, Haxby JV. Transient and sustained activity in a distributed neural system for human working memory. Nature. 1997;386(6625):608–11.
12. Eriksson J, Vogel EK, Lansner A, Bergstrom F, Nyberg L. Neurocognitive architecture of working memory. Neuron. 2015;88(1):33–46.
13. Funahashi S, Bruce CJ, Goldman-Rakic PS. Mnemonic coding of visual space in the monkey's dorsolateral prefrontal cortex. J Neurophysiol. 1989;61(2):331–49.
14. Papagno C, Lucchelli F, Vallar G. Phonological recoding, visual short-term store and the effect of unattended speech: evidence from a case of slowly progressive anarthria. Cortex. 2008;44:312–24.
15. Guidali G, Pisoni A, Bolognini N, Papagno C. Keeping order in the brain: the supramarginal gyrus and serial order in short-term memory. Cortex. 2019;119:89–99.
16. Papagno C, Cecchetto C. Is STM involved in sentence comprehension? Cortex. 2019;112:80–90. https://doi.org/10.1016/j.cortex.2018.08.028.
17. Shallice T, Papagno C. Impairments of auditory-verbal short-term memory: do selective deficits of the input phonological buffer exist? Cortex. 2019;112:107–21.

18. Awh E, Smith EE, Jonides ANDJ. Human rehearsal processes and the frontal Lobes: PET evidence. In: Grafman J, editor. Structure and functions of the human prefrontal cortex. New York: New York Academy of Science; 1995. p. 97–117.
19. Paulesu E, Frith CD, Frackowiak RSJ. The neural correlates of the verbal component of working memory. Nature. 1993;362:342–5.
20. Poeppel D. A critical review of PET studies of phonological processing. Brain Lang. 1996;55(3):317–51.
21. Henson RNA, Burgess N, Frith CD. Recoding, storage, rehersal, and grouping in verbal short-term memory: an fMRI study. Neuropsychologia. 2000;38:426–40.
22. Romero Lauro L, Reis J, Cohen LG, Cecchetto C, Papagno C. A case for the involvement of phonological loop in sentence comprehension. Neuropsychologia. 2010;48(14):4003–11.
23. Romero Lauro L, Walsh V, Papagno C. The neural correlates of phonological short-term memory: a repetitive transcranial magnetic stimulation study. J Cogn Neurosci. 2006;18(7):1147–55.
24. Newhart M, Trupe LA, Gomez Y, Cloutman L, Molitoris JJ, Davis C, Leigh R, Gottesman RF, Race D, Hillis AE. Asyntactic comprehension, working memory, and acute ischemia in Broca's area versus angular gyrus. Cortex. 2012;48(10):1288–97.
25. Vallar G, Di Betta AM, Silveri MC. The phonological short-term store-rehearsal system: patterns of impairment and neural correlates. Neuropsychologia. 1997;35:795–812.
26. Warrington EK, Logue V, Pratt RTC. The anatomical localisation of selective impairment of auditory verbal short-term memory. Neuropsychologia. 1971;9:377–87.
27. Papagno C, Comi A, Riva M, Bizzi A, Vernice M, Casarotti A, Fava E, Bello L. Mapping the brain network of the phonological loop. Hum Brain Mapp. 2017;38(6):3011–24.
28. Pisoni A, Mattavelli G, Casarotti A, Comi A, Riva M, Bello L, Papagno C. The neural correlates of auditory-verbal short-term memory: a voxel-based lesion symptom mapping study on 103 patients after glioma removal. Brain Struct Funct. 2019;224(6):2199–211.
29. Baddeley AD, Gathercole S, Papagno C. The phonological loop as a language learning device. Psychol Rev. 1998;105(1):158–73.
30. De Witt Hamer PC, Gil Robles S, Zwinderman AH, Duffau H, Berger MS. Impact of intraoperative stimulation brain mapping on glioma surgery outcome: a meta-analysis. J Clin Oncol. 2012;30(20):2559–65.
31. Martino J, Taillandier L, Moritz-Gasser S, Gatignol P, Duffau H. Re-operation is a safe and effective therapeutic strategy in recurrent WHO grade II gliomas within eloquent areas. Acta Neurochir. 2009;151(5):427–36; discussion 436.
32. Ojemann G, Ojemann J, Lettich E, Berger M. Cortical language localization in left, dominant hemisphere. An electrical stimulation mapping investigation in 117 patients. J Neurosurg. 1989;71(3):316–26.
33. Haglund MM, Berger MS, Shamseldin M, Lettich E, Ojemann GA. Cortical localization of temporal lobe language sites in patients with gliomas. Neurosurgery. 1994;34(4):567–76; discussion 576.
34. Alpherts WC, Vermeulen J, van Rijen PC, da Silva FH, van Veelen CW, Dutch P, Collaborative Epilepsy Surgery. Standard versus tailored left temporal lobe resections: differences in cognitive outcome? Neuropsychologia. 2008;46:455–60.
35. Campanella F, Del Missier F, Shallice T, Skrap M. Localizing memory functions in brain tumor patients: anatomical hotspots over 260 patients. World Neurosurg. 2018;120:e690–709.
36. Martino J, Gomez E, de Lucas EM, Mato D, Vazquez-Bourgon J. Intraoperative identification and preservation of verbal memory in diffuse gliomas: a matched-pair cohort study. Neurosurgery. 2018;83(6):1209–18.
37. Racine CA, Li J, Molinaro AM, Butowski N, Berger MS. Neurocognitive function in newly diagnosed low-grade glioma patients undergoing surgical resection with awake mapping techniques. Neurosurgery. 2015;77(3):371–9; discussion 379.
38. Teixidor P, Gatignol P, Leroy M, Masuet-Aumatell C, Capelle L, Duffau H. Assessment of verbal working memory before and after surgery for low-grade glioma. J Neurooncol. 2007;81(3):305–13.

39. Wu AS, Witgert ME, Lang FF, Xiao L, Bekele BN, Meyers CA, Ferson D, Wefel JS. Neurocognitive function before and after surgery for insular gliomas. J Neurosurg. 2011;115:1115–25.
40. Boele FW, Zant M, Heine EC, Aaronson NK, Taphoorn MJ, Reijneveld JC, Postma TJ, Heimans JJ, Klein M. The association between cognitive functioning and health-related quality of life in low-grade glioma patients. Neurooncol Pract. 2014;1(2):40–6.
41. Gehring K, Sitskoorn MM, Gundy CM, Sikkes SA, Klein M, Postma TJ, van den Bent MJ, Beute GN, Enting RH, Kappelle AC, Boogerd W, Veninga T, Twijnstra A, Boerman DH, Taphoorn MJ, Aaronson NK. Cognitive rehabilitation in patients with gliomas: a randomized, controlled trial. J Clin Oncol. 2009;27(22):3712–22.
42. Papagno C, Cecchetto C, Reati F, Bello L. Processing of syntactically complex sentences relies on verbal short-term memory. Evidence from a STM patient. Cogn Neuropsychol. 2007;24(3):292–311.
43. Ojemann GA, Dodrill CB. Verbal memory deficits after left temporal lobectomy for epilepsy. Mechanism and intraoperative prediction. J Neurosurg. 1985;62(1):101–7.
44. Kho KH, Rutten GJ, Leijten FS, van der Schaaf A, van Rijen PC, Ramsey NF. Working memory deficits after resection of the dorsolateral prefrontal cortex predicted by functional magnetic resonance imaging and electrocortical stimulation mapping. Case report. J Neurosurg. 2007;106(6 Suppl):501–5.
45. Kinoshita M, Nakajima R, Shinohara H, Miyashita K, Tanaka S, Okita H, Nakada M, Hayashi Y. Chronic spatial working memory deficit associated with the superior longitudinal fasciculus: a study using voxel-based lesion-symptom mapping and intraoperative direct stimulation in right prefrontal glioma surgery. J Neurosurg. 2016;125(4):1024–32.
46. Nakajima R, Okita H, Kinoshita M, Miyashita K, Nakada M, Yahata T, Hamada J, Hayashi Y. Direct evidence for the causal role of the left supplementary motor area in working memory: a preliminary study. Clin Neurol Neurosurg. 2014;126:201–4.
47. Tarapore PE, Martino J, Guggisberg AG, Owen J, Honma SM, Findlay A, Berger MS, Kirsch HE, Nagarajan SS. Magnetoencephalographic imaging of resting-state functional connectivity predicts postsurgical neurological outcome in brain gliomas. Neurosurgery. 2012;71(5):1012–22.
48. Brandling-Bennett EM, Bookheimer YS, Horsfall JL, Moftakhar P, Sedrak M, Barkulis CT, Gertsch JH, MacDougall MG, Boucharel W, Nuwer MR, Bergsneider M. A paradigm for awake intraoperative working memory mapping during forniceal stimulation. Neurocase. 2012;18(1):26–38.
49. Lashley K. The problem of serial order in behavior. Bobbs-Merrill; 1951. https://doi.org/10.1093/rfs/hhq153.

Proper Names Retrieval

13

Costanza Papagno and Carlo Giussani

13.1 Introduction

Naming familiar people has a fundamental role in human social life [1]. It is a more demanding task than naming objects [2], and, therefore, more vulnerable when cognitive resources are globally reduced. Indeed, proper name retrieval is one of the most common difficulties in the aging population [3]. It is reported that 30% of people above age 65 complain of difficulties in word retrieval, and among them, 64% have problems in retrieval of proper names. Accordingly, James [4] found that older adults show greater impairment in learning proper names than other biographical information in association with a new face, possibly because proper names establish a single, direct link with one correct exemplar [2]. Unlike common names, exemplars with the same proper name do not in general share the same characteristics (not all people named "Sharon" have the same hair color).

Proper nouns are considered pure referring expressions [5] without sense, defining individual entities, while common nouns refer to anyone of a class of beings or things. However, the deficit in proper name retrieval cannot be explained with the above reported fact that proper nouns are more difficult to retrieve than common ones. In fact, there are cases of double dissociations suggesting that proper name retrieval engages different functional processes with respect to common nouns. Indeed, neurological damage can result in a proper name deficit, while common names are unaffected, and the opposite condition, namely sparing of proper nouns with anomia for common nouns, has also been observed, although less frequently

C. Papagno (✉)
Neurocognitive Rehabilitation Center (CeRiN), CIMeC (Center for Mind/Brain Sciences), University of Trento, Rovereto, Italy
e-mail: costanza.papagno@unimib.it, costanza.papagno@unitn.it

C. Giussani
School of Medicine and Surgery, San Gerardo Hospital, Monza, Italy
e-mail: carlo.giussani@unimib.it

E. Mandonnet, G. Herbet (eds.), *Intraoperative Mapping of Cognitive Networks*,
https://doi.org/10.1007/978-3-030-75071-8_13

[6]. Other examples are preservation of people's names despite severe jargon [7], and preservation of the ability to write famous people's and geographical names [8] despite impaired ability to write common names. Semenza [2] suggested that at least four different varieties of proper name anomia exist, namely (1) pure proper name anomia, in which the deficit is at a post-semantic level, consisting in a failure to access the name's phonological form from an intact semantic system; (2) anomia from damage at the semantic level, in which the information about people is selectively lost; (3) isolation of individual semantics, in which the information is available but only when the patient is given the proper name itself; (4) prosopanomia, i.e., anomia for faces, in which the patient is unable to retrieve the name from face but can do it on definition. In all these cases, the processing of common names is virtually intact.

This reported distinction is drawn referring to an information processing model [9], which considers the input from different sources, i.e., names, definitions, faces, and voices, activating individual semantics, while names, definitions, and visual images of objects activating general semantics. In other words, the name George Clooney, his voice, or the definition "a North American handsome actor playing the role of a pediatrician in a famous TV series" activate semantics of a specific individual, while the word "dog" or the barking of a dog or the definition of an animal with four legs that barks activate a general semantic which is not specific for a single dog. Both individual and general semantics, in turn, independently activate the phonological forms in the lexicon. The activating mechanisms are thus separate.

More frequently, the proper name impairment is *a post-semantic deficit* (see [2] for a review). Accordingly, patients are in general able to retrieve biographical information about people they could not name, suggesting normal recognition of them.

13.2 The Neural Basis of Proper Name Retrieval

Converging evidence from semantic dementia, lesion and functional imaging studies have shown that the most anterior portion of the temporal lobe (ATL), namely BA 38 and possibly the adjacent enthorinal cortex, is certainly involved in the retrieval of proper names. Indeed, its damage is associated to it, leaving intact the access to names of entities at categorical level, i.e., common nouns (see, for example, [10–13]). This area is also crucial for learning new proper name-person relationships [14]. In addition, the ventral anterior portion of the thalamus may be involved in the retrieval of names by activating and coordinating the left temporal lobe (where proper names may be stored) and the left frontal language area, which is crucial to the production of any verbal output [15, 16].

According to Damasio and Tranel [17], the ATLs are converging or intermediating [10] zones for the different components of a distributed representation of people in order to retrieve a name [10]. However, Semenza [18] highlighted that the left temporal pole only provides some resources to the naming process and its involvement is not mandatory.

Cases of near global proper-name anomia have occurred in patients with left parieto-occipital [19–22] and left fronto-temporal lesions [23], suggesting that both anterior and posterior cortical regions are engaged in proper name retrieval. The mechanism underlying proper names impairment in these posterior lesions is not clear.

In fact, in a 4% of patients with lesion in the left ATL there is a normal proper name retrieval, while an abnormal performance has been found in 12% of subjects with lesions outside the ATL. For example, Otsuka et al. [24] described a patient with a proper name retrieval deficit, showing a rostro-caudal elongated high intensity area in the subcortical region along the upper bank of the superior temporal sulcus, sparing Heschl's gyrus and adjacent parts of Wernicke's area, but including the caudal ¾ of the STG, SMG, MTG, and parts of the optic radiation, tapetum, and inferior longitudinal fasciculus. Additional small bilateral, frontal parietal, temporal lesions in the deep white matter were found. The anterior part of the temporal lobe, the uncus, and hippocampus were not affected.

People's name anomia has been also caused by lesions in the left basal ganglia (amygdala included) [19, 25, 26], as reported by Yasuda et al. [27].

The deficit in retrieving proper names can extend to other unique entities, such as famous places [28, 29]. This deficit seems modality-aspecific, involving name retrieval on visual and auditory stimuli, as well as on verbal description [30].

A further structure that seems to be involved in proper name retrieval is the uncinate fasciculus (UF). In a study on 44 patients submitted to awake surgery for removal of a left frontal or temporal glioma, Papagno et al. [31] found that 18 patients, in whom the removal included the UF, showed a significant impairment in naming of famous faces as compared to patients without removal. The percentage of patients without UF removal but long-lasting deficits was negligible. Crucially, the two groups did not differ before surgery. When patients were further divided according to the site of the tumor (either frontal or temporal), those with a temporal glioma who underwent UF removal had the worst performance in famous face naming at 3 months after surgery. In addition, on the same task, the group with a frontal glioma that underwent resection of the frontal part of the UF performed significantly worse than the group with a frontal glioma but without UF removal. In conclusion, the resection of the UF, in its frontal or temporal segment, produces long-lasting consequences for famous face naming. Therefore, this fiber tract seems to be part of a circuitry involved in the retrieval of word form for proper names. Retrieval of conceptual knowledge was intact.

In a subsequent follow-up study of 17 patients at 9–12 months who did not suffer any tumor recurrence, Papagno et al. [32] showed that proper naming remained significantly impaired with no improvement after 12 months in patients with UF removal.

However, naming was not always affected following UF resection. Normal performance in naming persons despite temporal lobe lesions was found by Damasio et al. [33]; Semenza [9] concluded that a dedicated module dealing with proper name retrieval is either distributed in a large portion of the left hemisphere or subject to great interindividual variation. Therefore, one cannot predict that nearly equal lesions (and of course lesions cannot be absolutely identical) would be associated with precisely the same deficits.

Naming unique faces also requires regions related to the processing of emotions, such as the ventromedial prefrontal cortices [33], the UF being also a crucial structure in emotion.

Age of lesion is another important variable. Indeed, anterior temporal lobectomy to manage pharmaco-resistant temporal lobe epilepsy produced no postsurgical impairment in proper name retrieval in patients with an early onset of seizures that probably produced a reorganization outside the left ATL [34].

Neuroimaging studies confirmed this role of the left ATL [10].

In conclusion, we suggest that the left anterior temporal regions contain zones acting as intermediaries between retrieval of conceptual knowledge and retrieval of names. Therefore, at least three types of neural structures would be involved in the network for naming people, namely those supporting conceptual knowledge, those supporting the implementation of word forms in eventual vocalization, and the intermediate ones, which are engaged by the structures supporting conceptual knowledge to trigger and guide the implementation of a word form [35]. The UF could connect the intermediary structures to those involved in the retrieval of word form for proper names.

13.3 Long-Term Deficits in Patients Who Did Not Benefit from Intraoperative Monitoring of Proper Name Retrieval

Unfortunately, the follow-up of neurosurgical patients is difficult to relate directly to the intervention. Many of them undergo radiotherapy or chemotherapy, which introduce possible side effects on cognition [36]. In several cases tumors show an aggressive behavior and progress quickly affecting the neuropsychological performance of patients [37], and some patients can die during the follow-up period. Patients may suffer tumor recurrence, requiring repeated surgical procedures [38] that can cause further deficits or worsen previous ones.

In this view, stable findings at follow-up can be sought after surgery for epilepsy. In this situation, resection of ATL has been associated with proper name retrieval deficit especially when the resection is performed on the dominant side. Such finding has been commonly experienced by several epilepsy surgeons and some strategies have been put in place in order to elude the risk of a permanent deficit. In a report by Kendall and colleagues, a presurgical training for famous faces, famous places, and personally relevant faces was able to increase the maintenance of those skills after surgery or to increase the performances after surgery [39]. These results suggest that circuits involved in name retrieval have some plasticity and it is possible to speculate that this feature might be related with the fact that multiple brain regions (cortical and subcortical) are involved in object and proper name retrieval. This fact justifies how complex is to define both the function of name retrieval and the location of this function in a circumscribed area of the brain.

In addition, proper name retrieval is not considered a first-choice function to be preserved by neurosurgeons. Consequently, there is little concern about the presence of this deficit and it is not often monitored intraoperatively or checked in follow-up studies.

In the previous paragraph we have reported the follow-up at 1-year of a group of patients who continued to show deficits in proper naming [32], suggesting that left ATL and UF removal produces a permanent deficit of this ability.

Similarly, a patient was described with a severe deficit in retrieving proper names after a left anterior temporal lobectomy [40]. He was unable to retrieve proper names in conversation or when shown photographs or given verbal descriptions of people, despite being able to provide semantic information about the person he could not name. Comprehension of names was preserved, since he could point to his relatives' photographs and famous people's pictures when the name was produced by the examiner. His ability to retrieve common nouns was relatively intact.

A more recent study [41] reported that patients with language-dominant temporal lobectomy were impaired in retrieval of familiar and newly learned people's names, while in nondominant lobectomy the difficulty only concerned newly learned people's names.

Finally, Moran et al. [42] described a deficit in acquiring face and person identity information following anterior temporal lobectomy.

13.4 Locations at Risk of Long-Term Deficits in Proper Name Retrieval

Observations from neurodegenerative diseases and surgery represent the most important evidence about long-term deficits in proper name retrieval. As depicted above, name retrieval represents a complex brain function performed by the interaction of more than one cerebral structure. In particular, proper name retrieval seems to have the main core structure in the ATL. Around this part of the brain, connections with the surrounding structures like fusiform gyrus, amygdala, thalamus, frontal cortex, etc. contribute to realize proper name retrieval. As a consequence, lesions of one of such areas can produce a deficit in this function which might be disabling [43]. Given the extended network behind proper name retrieval, it has always been difficult to establish and map a specific and circumscribed area of the brain devoted to this function.

However, all the reported evidence suggests that face naming can be mostly impaired in case of dominant temporal pole removal, with a permanent deficit when subcortical fibers are included; but, in some cases, it can appear also after nondominant temporal pole resection, eventually secondary to impaired face recognition.

Studies from neuro-oncological patients have contributed to the description of neuropsychological brain functions as a consequence of a lesional surgery but, on the other hand, surgery usually interferes with a pre-existing neoplastic brain damage. Moreover, patients can be very heterogeneous with different brain areas simultaneously affected by the same tumor. So far, studies on these patients might deliver indirect or incorrect information about the neuropsychological functions of the brain. Studies from brain mapping performed during surgical removal of brain tumors allowed to recognize a brain area more extended than the temporal pole that encompasses the lateral aspect of the frontal lobe (superior, middle, and inferior frontal gyri) and the anterior part of the superior and middle temporal gyri [44]. Such areas showed that there is also an overlapping between famous face naming and object naming which renders the study of name retrieval quite challenging. In the study by Giussani et al., most interferences (50%) were typical face anomia with patients able to recognize the face or to evoke related biographic information but without being able to name the corresponding person. Interestingly, semantic paraphasias (patients attributing repeatedly a wrong name to a famous face) were found mainly in the frontal gyri and the superior temporal gyrus [44]. This result is in line with a tDCS study [45] in which anodal tDCS over the left ATL decreased naming accuracy compared to sham stimulation because participants produced significantly more intrusions. Apparently, stimulation increased interference among arising competitors when retrieving the correct name associated to the presented face. Anodal tDCS over the left IFG led to a significant decrease in intrusions compared to sham stimulation, possibly improving the selection mechanism.

Although knowledge of the cortex and its functions has increased over time, that of white matter connections and their functions is still a matter of study and debate. Indeed, face naming can be affected also by resection of white matter tracts despite sparing the ATL. This fact has been enlightened in the study by Papagno et al. [31], as reported above.

13.5 How to Monitor Proper Name Retrieval Intraoperatively

Brain mapping procedure consists of a general assessment of naming, namely an object naming (animate and inanimate objects) and an action-naming task because it is easily reproducible and effective in searching for standard anomia. A famous face naming should be added, especially when surgery concerns tumors involving the left ATL. Before concluding the direct brain mapping procedure, essential naming sites are routinely confirmed by repeating the naming task. Findings on different tasks may be affected or biased by the frequency or familiarity of the items presented. The object-naming task and the famous face-naming task are not equivalent in terms of lexical frequency and complexity. This lack of comparability could be explained by the differences existing between these two categories, as reported above. The face-naming stimuli are colored or black-and-white photographs of celebrities taken from different categories of public life (actors, politicians, sportsmen/women, etc.) balanced for gender, when possible by nationality (half from the patient's same country and half foreigner people), alive or dead. Faces are presented in a prototypical pose and appearance. A correct response is defined as the complete and exact famous person name or only the surname when this unequivocally defines the celebrity.

Ability in naming people is variable also in healthy individuals. Therefore, the best procedure to adopt is to evaluate face naming before surgery, during the baseline assessment. For intraoperative testing, only items produced correctly three times out of three without delay should be selected for intraoperative monitoring. Therefore, each patient is submitted to a specific, ad hoc intraoperative protocol designed according to his/her presurgical performance; also, each patient serves as a control for him/herself. Items are presented by means of a computer screen and 3 s are allowed for response.

A different way to assess proper name retrieval could be through voice, thus confirming that the problem is not one of face recognition, but typically a naming one. A short fragment not containing any element that could allow the direct recognition of the person (neutral discourses) can be presented to the patient who has to name the person's voice. This task has been submitted to 15 patients with a left temporal lobectomy and 13 patients with a right lobectomy and only left patients were impaired in naming [46].

Although cortical and subcortical mapping during brain tumor resection are becoming common practice in neurosurgery, some limitations in awake surgery have been enlightened through the years. First of all, awake surgery requires the patient's collaboration which needs to be optimal under conditions of high stress. This means that some of the results might be altered because of lack of compliance by the patient. Second, as reported in 2019 by Roux et al., in order to have a sure and reliable finding at least three trials are needed. So far, the need of more than one positive confirmation might increase the stress on the patient and the reliability about its collaboration [47]. This is particularly relevant considering that face naming in general is performed after object and, eventually, action naming. Finally, the patient's pathology might influence the results of testing. In fact, patients undergoing surgical resection for epilepsy are different from patients undergoing tumor resection. Patients with drug-resistant epilepsy might have altered brain networks due to long-standing epilepsy while patients with brain tumors might have altered cerebral networks due to white matter dislocation or infiltration or due to perilesional edema. Among these patients, those with high-grade gliomas (HGGs) and those with low-grade gliomas (LGGs) can present several differences: patients with HGGs might be impaired in face naming due to associated edema or mass effect while patients with LGGs might be impaired because of white matter infiltration. These two different patterns of impairment definitely affect the surgical outcome in terms of safe resection on functional structures like the cortex or white matter bundles. In case of HGGs, white matter bundles might be spared due to the displacing behavior of the tumor during its growing; in the case of LGGs, white matter bundles are not spared by the tumor due to its infiltrative nature. As a consequence, resection of HGGs might interfere with object and face naming mainly due to a cortical damage, while resection of LGGs can affect them because of a cortical and subcortical damage. In the same way, cortical and subcortical mapping might be influenced by the behavior of the tumor [48].

A further limitation is that the possibility exists that the patient cannot retrieve the name because he/she does not recognize the face. In other words, a problem of recognition cannot be excluded. However, in general they spontaneously report semantic information (see above, as reported in Giussani et al.'s paper), suggesting that recognition is unimpaired; in addition, there is an increasing literature confirming that face recognition depends on the nondominant hemisphere, while naming is related to the dominant one (see [49, 50] for reviews, [51]). Additionally, the same problem, namely a lack of recognition, would concern object naming. Finally, a voice-naming task, as reported above, can help in the diagnosis.

A similar procedure has been used by Kurimoto et al. [52]. The picture-naming task for famous people's faces was undertaken, after object naming, on the exposed areas of the superior and middle temporal gyri but no positive sites were found. However, postoperatively, their patient showed marked difficulty in retrieving famous people's names that extended to his friends and coworkers making impossible for him to return to work; the deficit remained stable for 15 months, despite speech therapy. The authors suggest that the crucial aspect, apart from the resection of the anterior temporal lobe and temporal base (areas 20, 28, and 36), was the removal of subcortical pathways. Accordingly, stimulation of a subcortical area, underlying the temporal pole and probably corresponding to the UF (although DTI was not available), produced proper name anomia (see Fig. 13.1 and [44]).

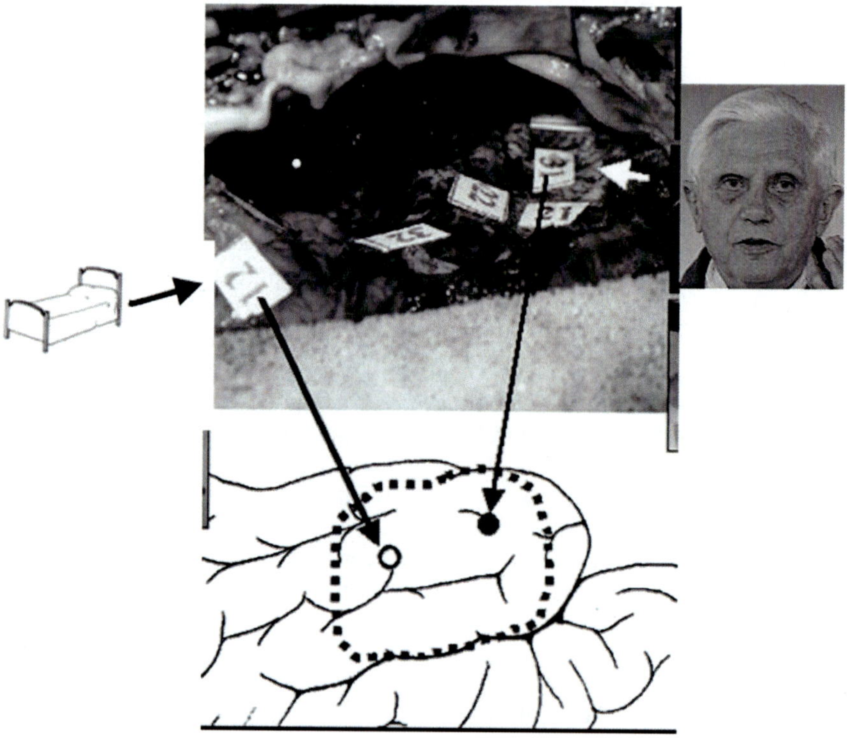

Fig. 13.1 Subcortical intraoperative mapping of famous faces, showing a dissociation between proper (Joseph Ratzinger) and common (bed) nouns in the left temporal lobe. Site (12) is a cortical area involved in naming things, while (31) corresponds to a subcortical site whose stimulation produces disruption of proper names. The schematic drawing of the temporal lobe depicts the position of the two sites. Note that the black dot reported on the cortex corresponds to the underlying white matter (Modified from [44]).

13.6 Functional Improvement in Series of Patients Operated with Versus Without Proper Name Retrieval Monitoring

Monitoring patients for proper name retrieval is not easy, because of the multiple areas involved in this function, but it should be considered each time the temporal pole is involved.

In any case, the intraoperative mapping of proper names is limited to a few cases. Surgeons try to preserve language in general, without considering such specific aspect of language. In fact, extension of resection is considered a critical prognostic factor for delaying the progression and increasing survival. Considering the proved benefit of a radical surgical approach, a major criterion in selecting the surgical strategy should be the preservation of the neurocognitive profile and, as a consequence, the quality of life. Therefore, extension of resection is considered the priority, and proper name is "sacrificed," since it is not considered a crucial ability, as already reported.

Although in the literature few preliminary experiences about the potential long-term compensatory mechanisms that patients can train in order to overcome the acquired name retrieval deficit are reported, present experience shows that such a deficit in proper naming is permanent and not solved by speech therapy, especially when the subcortical pathways have been resected [32, 52]. Deficit in proper names retrieval might preclude return to work. This aspect should be carefully considered at least in those cases in which ability with proper names is a fundamental function for the professional life of that specific patient.

13.7 Additional Anatomo-Functional Knowledge Has Been Gained from Intraoperative Mapping Studies

As repeatedly reported in this chapter, intraoperative mapping on proper names, though performed very seldom, has produced important outcomes from an anatomical point of view. It has confirmed that proper name retrieval is based on a complex network involving several structures in the brain, the core one being the left ATL; it has also shown that white matter pathways are crucial in producing permanent deficits, and a fundamental bundle of fibers is represented by the UF. Therefore, researchers have pointed their attention on this structure and an increasing number of investigations has focused on the property of the UF. Finally, an important information that has been acquired is that despite the complex circuit involved in proper name retrieval, some of its components are unique, so that, despite the potential plasticity that has been described in brain tumors, especially in LGGs, no recovery seems possible in the case of damage of subcortical fibers. An example is represented by four patients in Giussani et al.'s [44] series who, when tested preoperatively, had a partially selective famous and relative's face anomia. All of them had tumors in the anterior part, cortical and subcortical, of the left temporal lobe, so that face-naming mapping was impossible.

References

1. Brédart S. The cognitive psychology and neuroscience of naming people. Neurosci Biobehav Rev. 2017;83:145–54.
2. Semenza C. The neuropsychology of proper names. Mind Lang. 2009;24(4):347–69.
3. Evrard M. Ageing and lexical access to common and proper names in picture naming. Brain Lang. 2002;81:174–9.
4. James LE. Meeting mister farmer versus meeting a farmer: specific effects of aging in learning proper names. Psychol Aging. 2004;19:512–22.
5. Kripke S. Naming and necessity. Oxford: Basil Blackwell; 1980.
6. Lyons F, Hanley JR, Kay J. Anomia for common names and geographical names with preserved retrieval of names of people: a semantic memory disorder. Cortex. 2002;38:23–35.
7. Semenza C, Sgaramella TM. Production of proper names: a clinical case study of the effects of phonemic cueing. Memory. 1993;1:265–80.
8. Cipolotti L, McNeil JE, Warrington EK. Spared written naming of proper nouns: a case report. Memory. 1993;1:289–311.
9. Semenza C. Retrieval pathways for common and proper names. Cortex. 2006;42:884–91.
10. Damasio H, Grabowsky TJ, Tranel D, Hichwa RD, Damasio AR. A neural basis for lexical retrieval. Nature. 1996;380:499–505.
11. Papagno C, Capitani E. Proper name anomia: a case with sparing of the first-letter knowledge. Neuropsychologia. 1998;36(7):669–79.
12. Saetti MC, Marangolo P, De Renzi E, Rinaldi MC, Lattanzi E. The nature of the disorder underlying the inability to retrieve proper names. Cortex. 1999;35(5):675–85.
13. Tranel D, Damasio H, Damasio AR. A neural basis for the retrieval of conceptual knowledge. Neuropsychologia. 1997;35:1319–27.
14. Sperling R, Chua E, Cocchiarella A, Rand-Giovannetti E, Poldrack R, Schacter DL, Albert M. Putting names to faces: successful encoding of associative memories activates the anterior hippocampal formation. Neuroimage. 2003;20:1400–10.
15. Cohen L, Bolgert F, Timsit S, Chermann JF. Anomia for proper names after left thalamic infarct. J Neurol Neurosurg Psychiatry. 1994;57:1283–4.
16. Lucchelli F, De Renzi E. Proper name anomia. Cortex. 1992;28:221–30.
17. Damasio A, Tranel D. Nouns and verbs are retrieved with differently distributed neural systems. Proc Natl Acad Sci U S A. 1993;90:4957–60.
18. Semenza C. Naming with proper names: the left temporal pole theory. Behav Neurol. 2011;24(4):277–84.
19. Fukuhara M, Tagawa K, Nakano M, Iino K. Anomia for proper names: report of two cases with cerebrovascular disease. Nossotyu [Japanese Journal of Stroke]. 1992;14:666–70.
20. McKenna P, Warrington EK. Testing for nominal dysphasia. J Neurol Neurosurg Psychiatry. 1980;43:781–8. https://doi.org/10.1136/jnnp.43.9.781.
21. Reinkemeier M, Markowitsch HJ, Rauch M, Kessler J. Differential impairments in recalling people's names: a case study in search of neuroanatomical correlates. Neuropsychologia. 1997;35:677–84.
22. Semenza C, Zettin M. Generating proper names: a case of selective inability. Cogn Neuropsychol. 1988;5:711–21.
23. Semenza C, Zettin M. Evidence from aphasia for proper names as pure referring expressions. Nature. 1989;342:678–9.
24. Otsuka Y, Suzuki K, Fujii T, Miura R, Endo K, Kondo H, Yamadori A. Proper name anomia after left temporal subcortical hemorrhage. Cortex. 2005;41:39–47.
25. Fery P, Vincent E, Brédart S. Personal name anomia: a single case study. Cortex. 1995;31:191–8.
26. Hittmair-Delazer M, Denes G, Semenza C, Mantovan MC. Anomia for people's names. Neuropsychologia. 1994;86:345–58.
27. Yasuda K, Beckmann B, Nakamura T. Brain processing of proper names. Aphasiology. 2000;14:1067–89.

28. Grabowski TJ, Damasio H, Tranel D, Boles Ponto LL, Hichwa RD, Damasio AR. A role for left temporal pole in the retrieval of words for unique entities. Hum Brain Mapp. 2001;13:199–212.
29. Tranel D. The left temporal pole is important for retrieving words for unique concrete entities. Aphasiology. 2009;23:867–84.
30. Belfi AM, Tranel D. Impaired naming of famous musical melodies is associated with left temporal polar damage. Neuropsychology. 2014;28:429–35.
31. Papagno C, Miracapillo C, Casarotti A, Romero Lauro LJ, Castellano A, Falini A, et al. What is the role of the uncinate fasciculus? Surgical removal and proper name retrieval. Brain. 2011;134:405–14.
32. Papagno C, Casarotti A, Comi A, Pisoni A, Lucchelli F, Bizzi A, Riva M, Bello L. Long-term proper name anomia after removal of the uncinate fasciculus. Brain Struct Funct. 2016;221:687–94. https://doi.org/10.1007/s00429-014-0920-8.
33. Damasio H, Tranel D, Grabowski T, Adolphs R, Damasio A. Neural systems behind word and concept retrieval. Cognition. 2004;92:179–229.
34. Yucus CJ, Tranel D. Preserved proper naming following left anterior temporal lobectomy is associated with early age of seizure onset. Epilepsia. 2007;48:2241–52.
35. Tranel D. Impaired naming of unique landmarks is associated with left temporal polar damage. Neuropsychology. 2006;20:1–10.
36. Klein M, Heimans JJ, Aaronson NK, van der Ploeg HM, et al. Effect of radiotherapy and other treatment-related factors on mid-term to long-term cognitive sequelae in low-grade gliomas: a comparative study. Lancet. 2002;360:1361–8.
37. Zarino B, Di Cristofori A, Abete Fornara G, Bertani GA, Locatelli M, Caroli M, Rampini P, Cogiamanian F, Crepaldi D, Carrabba G. Long-term follow-up of neuropsychological functions in patients with high grade gliomas: can cognitive status predict patient's outcome after surgery? Acta Neurochir. 2020;162:803–12.
38. Shaw EG, Berkey B, Coons SW, Bullard D, Brachman D, et al. Recurrence following neurosurgeon-determined gross-total resection of adult supratentorial low-grade glioma: results of a prospective clinical trial. J Neurosurg. 2008;109(10):3171.
39. Kendall DL, Minkina I, Bislick L, Grabowski TJ, Phatak V, Silkes JAP, Ojemann JG. Language treatment prior to anterior temporal lobe surgery: can naming skills be preserved? J Rehabil Res Dev. 2016;53:813–26.
40. Fukatsu R, Fujii T, Tsukiura T, Yamadori A, Otsuki T. Proper name anomia after left temporal lobectomy: a patient study. Neurology. 1999;52:1096–9.
41. Tsukiura T, Fujii T, Fukatsu R, Otsuki T, Okuda J, Umetsu A, et al. Neural basis of the retrieval of people's names: evidence from brain-damaged patients and fMRI. J Cogn Neurosci. 2002;14(6):922–37.
42. Moran M, Seidenberg M, Sabesevits D, Swanson S, Hermann B. The acquisition of face and person identity information following anterior temporal lobectomy. J Int Neuropsychol Soc. 2005;11:237–48.
43. Abel TJ, Rhone AE, Nourski KV, Kawasaki H, Oya H, Griffiths TD, Howard MA, Tranel D. Direct physiological evidence of a heteromodal convergence region for proper naming in human left anterior temporal lobe. J Neurosci. 2015;35(4):1513–20. https://doi.org/10.1523/JNEUROSCI.3387-14.2015.
44. Giussani C, Bello L, Démonet JF, Lauwers-Cances V, Papagno C, Gaini SM, et al. Who is who? Famous face naming areas. J Neurosurg. 2009;110:289–99.
45. Pisoni A, Vernice M, Iasevoli L, Cattaneo Z, Papagno C. Guess who? Investigating the proper name processing network by means of tDCS. Neuropsychologia. 2015;66:267–78.
46. Papagno C, Mattavelli G, Casarotti A, Bello L, Gainotti G. Defective recognition and naming of famous people from voice in patients with unilateral temporal lobe tumors. Neuropsychologia. 2018;116:194–204. https://doi.org/10.1016/j.neuropsychologia.2017.07.021.
47. Roux FE, Djidjeli I, Quéhan R, Réhault E, Giussani C, Durand JB. Intraoperative electrostimulation for awake brain mapping: how many positive interference responses are required for reliability? J Neurosurg. 2019. https://doi.org/10.3171/2019.6.JNS19925.

48. Bello L, Gambini A, Castellano A, Carrabba G, Acerbi F, Fava E, et al. Motor and language DTI fiber tracking combined with intraoperative subcortical mapping for surgical removal of gliomas. Neuroimage. 2008;39:369–82.
49. Gainotti G. Different patterns of famous people recognition disorders in patients with right and left anterior temporal lesions: a systematic review. Neuropsychologia. 2007;45(8):1591–607.
50. Gainotti G. Laterality effects in normal subjects' recognition of familiar faces, voices and names. Perceptual and representational components. Neuropsychologia. 2013;51:1151–60.
51. Piccininni C, Gainotti G, Carlesimo GA, Luzzi S, Papagno C, Trojano L, Ferrara A, Marra C, Quaranta D. Naming famous people through face and voice: a normative study. Neurol Sci. 2020;41(7):1859–64. https://doi.org/10.1007/s10072-020-04272-1.
52. Kurimoto M, Takaiwa A, Nagai S, Hayashi N, Endo S. Anomia for people's names after left anterior temporal lobe resection. Neurol Med Chir. 2010;50:36–40.

Multilingual Naming

14

Alejandro Fernandez-Coello, Santiago Gil-Robles,
and Manuel Carreiras

14.1 Introduction: Neural Basis of Bilingualism

The neural bases of language processing in bilinguals have been extensively investigated with the advent of neuroimaging techniques, such as the functional magnetic resonance imaging (fMRI) and the electrical stimulation mapping (ESM). However, there are still many unanswered questions and live debates on (1) which cortical and subcortical areas of the language circuit show common and specific activation for the two languages; (2) to which extent overlap in the language circuit depends on the age of acquisition, proficiency, or language exposure; (3) which language control mechanism allows to manage two languages in one brain so that we can speak only in one language at a time while avoiding intrusions from the other language; and (4) the brain plasticity associated to tumor growth and tumor resection in a bilingual brain.

A. Fernandez-Coello
Hospital Universitari de Bellvitge (HUB), Neurosurgery Section, Campus Bellvitge, University of Barcelona e IDIBELL, L'Hospitalet de Llobregat, Barcelona, Spain

CIBER de Bioingeniería, Biomateriales y Nanomedicina (CIBER-BBN), Barcelona, Spain

University of Barcelona, Barcelona, Spain
e-mail: afernandezc@bellvitgehospital.cat, fernandezcoello@ub.edu

S. Gil-Robles
Department of Neurosurgery, Hospital Quiron, Madrid, Spain

BioCruces Research Institute, Bilbao, Spain

M. Carreiras (✉)
BCBL, Basque Center on Cognition, Brain and Language, Donostia-San Sebastián, Spain

Ikerbasque, Basque Foundation for Science, Bilbao, Spain

University of the Basque Country, UPV/EHU, Bilbao, Spain
e-mail: m.carreiras@bcbl.eu

E. Mandonnet, G. Herbet (eds.), *Intraoperative Mapping of Cognitive Networks*,
https://doi.org/10.1007/978-3-030-75071-8_14

ESM studies on bilinguals [1–4] have shown the co-existence of common brain regions for the two languages through language-specific areas. In particular, they reported disruptions during stimulations in sites where speech arrest arose for both languages and sites where speech arrest arose for one language but not for the other. Thus, language circuits are crafted with common and specific pathways. In addition, studies using ESM have revealed remarkable differences in language areas between individuals, rendering the overlapping range of sites very variable [1, 2, 5].

Ojemann and Whitaker [3] already noticed this variability when reporting, for the first time, different cortical-functional sites (frontal and parietal) in two bilingual patients, using a picture naming task under ESM. More recently, the same team reported frequent but variable overlap in temporoparietal areas for L2 and L1. However, none of the 22 patients had complete overlapping of L1 and L2 and 8 of them had no overlap at all [1]. Similar results have also been reported in bilingual pediatric population using several tasks [6]. Serafini et al. tested bilingual patients with reading and naming tasks; they reported the existence of overlapping "multitask" cortical areas in the frontotemporal regions and single language task sites more located in the postcentral areas. These data align with the previous results supporting the idea of a specific functional network for multilinguals with variable overlapping. Not surprisingly, European and Asian teams using ESM in multilinguals have found results that are also very similar to those summarized in 2007 [2] in a review by Giussani and, more recently, in 2019 by Teo et al. [7] and Roux and Tremoulet [4]. For example, Roux and Tremoulet stimulated cortical areas of 12 right-handed bilingual patients during surgery, using counting and reading, besides naming tasks, and found strict overlapping of both languages in only 5 of them, which implies that differences in the networks subserving each language are general and not task-specific.

Similarly, neuroimaging studies have revealed common and specific activation for the two languages in a bilingual brain [8]. In a seminal work using fMRI with bilinguals, Kim et al. [9] reported overlap of activation for L1 and L2 in the left inferior frontal gyrus if both languages were acquired early, but different spots of activation if the L2 was acquired later in life. However, overlap of activation was found in the left superior temporal gyrus both for early and for late bilinguals. Many other teams have reported different networks subserving the organization of multilingual brains, with variable overlapping. In fact, current evidence suggests that languages are represented mostly in overlapping networks, including areas within the left perisylvian cortex and frontal, temporal, and parietal regions as well as subcortical structures. In short, similar activation has been found for the processing of the L1 and L2 in the so-called language network [10–13]. Nonetheless, some studies have also reported language specificity in several brain regions attributed to age of acquisition (AoA) and proficiency differences [14, 15].

Whether the same or different brain areas get activated for each language seems to be modulated by age of acquisition, proficiency, usage, and exposure, among other variables. Though controversial, ESM evidence supports the idea that the languages acquired earlier in life may have a larger cortical representation [16–20]. However, others have found that the number of distinct cortical sites for L2 was much higher than for L1, suggesting that the use of L2 implies a wider functional network [21]. On the other hand, regarding similarity between languages, it is noteworthy that a recent fMRI study [22] with native speakers of four very different languages (Chinese, English, Hebrew, and Spanish) showed mostly brain activation overlap for the four languages, together with some specific activations during speech and reading. It is important to note that these four languages differ in many linguistic and orthographic dimensions (e.g., logographic vs. alphabetic Chinese vs. the three others; opaque vs. transparent orthographies: English and Hebrew vs. Spanish.), and the main result is a high overlap of activation for print and speech.

The fact that similar neural networks get activated during the processing of two different languages brings up to the table another interesting question: how bilinguals are able to manage the two co-activated languages so that they can speak in one of them without interference from the other. Bilinguals need to focus on the target language while inhibiting the nontarget language or ignoring it. To do so, and to account for the lack of interference between languages, a language control mechanism responsible for language switching has been proposed. This control circuit would be different from the language circuit. In fact, some researchers [23, 24] suggested that cortical areas outside the language circuit such as the right dorsolateral prefrontal cortex, and subcortical areas like the caudate, should be involved in language control. Specifically, the language control mechanism recruits neural regions involved in the control of action in general [25], including the dorsal anterior cingulate cortex (dACC)/pre-supplementary motor (pre-SMA) area, the left prefrontal cortex, the left caudate, and the inferior parietal lobules, bilaterally together with control input from the right prefrontal cortex, the thalamus and the putamen of the basal ganglia, and the cerebellum [24].

Finally, low-grade gliomas may induce plastic changes in the topography of brain functions [26]. In most of the cases, the slow growth of the tumors promotes neural reorganization so that patients are often neurologically normal or only slightly impaired. Eloquent functions can be redistributed in neighbor areas around the tumor, and/or recruited by a distributed network within the lesioned hemisphere and/or in the contralateral hemisphere [26], and this can change also after surgery. Some previous studies on patients with LGGs in eloquent brain areas suggested that post-surgery functional compensation occurred mainly in peritumoral and in contratumoral regions [27–31]. However, Lizarazu et al. (2020) [32], using magnetoencephalography (MEG), found that functional connectivity in peritumoral regions was higher 3 months after surgery than before surgery. In contrast, alpha functional connectivity values in contratumoral areas did not differ between sessions. Interestingly, this enhancement of functional connectivity that emerged in the alpha frequency band was observed in all patients regardless of the LGG location. Thus, post-surgery functional reorganization in peritumoral regions may be a general mechanism of brain plasticity that plays a major role in the recovery of brain function through compensatory mechanisms. Importantly, the preservation of white matter tracts (long-distance connectivity and U-fiber white tracts) may be critical for plasticity in these regions [33]. The risk of inducing permanent deficits without functional recovery is very high in cases of white matter injury [34]. It remains to be seen whether the same compensatory mechanisms work for L1 and L2 in bilingual brains.

14.2 Intraoperative Language Monitoring in Bilingual Patients

Comparative data between selective impairment of one specific language in patients operated on and brain mapping and those undergoing brain surgery without are scarce. One possible explanation may be the fact that this specific language and cognitive evaluation in multilinguals, which is needed to monitor these potential sequelae, is only performed in patients undergoing mapping and awake brain surgery, with the precise purpose of reducing this kind of deficit.

Multilingual patients undergoing brain surgery without mapping are simply not tested for language in most series. Then, the specific rate of selective language impairment in this last population is widely unknown. Some limited data are available in the literature about long-term impairment of a selective language in multilinguals. One of these cases of selective language impairment has been reported after stroke and left frontal brain tumor by Ibrahim [35, 36] in Arabic-Hebrew bilinguals. The patient showed selective difficulty for the lexical access in one of the languages after lesioning. Others have noticed selective aphasia of one language during the Wada test [37, 38] or after perisylvian surgery of MAV [39]. However, none of these data of selective language deficit in bilinguals who did not benefit from intraoperative monitoring are strong enough to compare with data from the mapped population. In any case, several considerations can be made.

To date, ESM has been established as the best way to avoid permanent deficits in brain tumor surgery [2, 18, 40]. Thus, there are no phase-three randomized control trials in the field comparing postoperative deficits after surgery in eloquent areas with and without ESM. Nonetheless, there is a recent meta-analysis of 10 years of published studies comparing the short- and long-term neurological deficits of series of patients having undergone surgery for supratentorial gliomas with and without intraoperative mapping [40]. This meta-analysis showed a rate of permanent deficits in the unmapped population of 8.3% vs. 3.4% in the mapped population, with a median resection volume of 78% in the mapped vs. 58% in the unmapped. This means that the unmapped population has almost three times more risk of developing a long-lasting neurological deficit.

The results of this meta-analysis have important implications for the intraoperative mapping in bilinguals. Considering that they have at least the same risk as monolinguals, bilinguals should be mapped. In fact, they could be tested only in one of the languages if the neural circuits underpinning the two languages overlapped. However, the empirical evidence shows that, while there is some overlap, multilinguals seem to have specific networks also not shared for all the languages. Therefore, performing multilingual intraoperative tests is probably the best way to avoid a selective language deficit, testing separately not only all the languages but also the ability to switch between them, as switching is crucial in patients using at least two languages in daily life. Not performing these tasks may result in a loss of quality of life [7], as shown for other neurological functions [40].

14.3 Cortical and Subcortical Key Networks for Bilinguals

The evidence from research on bilingualism studies using ESM has shown that most of the functional points are within the perisylvian classic language areas (namely the inferior frontal gyrus—pars triangularis, orbitalis, and opercularis—, superior temporal gyrus, supramarginal gyrus, angular gyrus, etc.: IFG, STG, SMG, AG). However, a significant percentage of them are still located outside of the perisylvian areas, recruiting cortical regions not traditionally regarded as subserving language functions, such as the mid-frontal gyrus (MFG).

On the other hand, it is well established nowadays that intraoperative testing of language networks implies subcortical stimulation of language-related tracts. Data on subcortical stimulation have helped to define the brain connectivity and build models of language organization [41, 42]. Subcortical tracts were also reported in bilinguals. Using naming and counting tasks together with stimulation of subcortical tracts in seven high proficiency multilingual patients, Bello et al. reported specific subcortical tracts for L1 in four patients and L2 in three patients; however, authors did not specify which tracts were differentially involved [18].

Subcortical connectivity is of critical relevance to investigate the portrayal of two languages, but also to understand the ability of bilinguals to switch between languages. At the cortical level, dominant dorsolateral prefrontal cortex in the middle frontal gyrus seems to be highly specified in this shifting mechanism, as recently demonstrated by Sierpowska and Fernandez Coello [42]. These results align with those reported by Duffau and colleagues during subcortical stimulation of the superior longitudinal fasciculus, which generated intraoperative and post-surgery involuntary language switching in bilinguals. Stimulation of this bundle generated a transitory "disconnection" of the speech areas, which need to be functional in order to avoid switching impairment [43, 44]. Some other studies agree with the left dorsolateral prefrontal region as a fundamental piece in the executive control of language switching (LS). Lubrano et al. reported the participation of the left dorsolateral prefrontal region in LS in a case study in which the ESM caused involuntary LS when this region was stimulated [19]. However, other regions seem to contribute to language control. For instance, Sierpowska et al. [45] identified the posterior middle frontal gyrus as being involved in the process of controlling language because, when it was stimulated, patients showed control language difficulties in LS. In addition, Tomasino et al. [46] describe an involuntary LS after stimulation during a mapping procedure in the superior temporal region. Wang et al. [47] provided new evidence of basal ganglia involvement in LS. Using ESM during the performance of LS tasks, their results showed a participation of the head of the left caudate nucleus.

Taking into account the information about cortical and subcortical connectivity, Duffau and collaborators proposed an ESM-based model of LS that involves a large cortical-subcortical neural network. The model would include an executive system (prefrontal cortex, anterior cingulum, caudate nucleus), controlling a more dedicated language subcircuit, which involves posterotemporal areas, supramarginal and angular gyri, Broca's area, and the superior longitudinal fasciculus [48].

To sum up, in the case of bilinguals, it is important to test both languages and language switching not only on cortical sites but also in subcortical units and white matter tracts for cortical and subcortical connectivity.

14.4 Newly Designed Tasks for Monitoring Multilingualism Intraoperatively

Picture naming tasks are currently the gold standard for identifying eloquent areas during awake brain surgery [49–51]. With multilingual populations increasing worldwide, patients frequently need to be tested in more than one language. In addition, a detailed and precise language mapping procedure requires picture naming of objects and actions. Some previous studies using ESM reported a dissociation between temporal and frontal regions when stimulating objects and actions [52–55]. This dissociation between nouns and verbs has been demonstrated at the behavioral, electrophysiological, and brain activation levels (see Chap. 11 and [56]). Therefore, testing object and action naming in the two languages of a bilingual patient with comparable stimuli is desirable for a comprehensive mapping.

MULTIMAP [57] is an open-source battery that entails a multilingual picture naming of objects and actions for mapping eloquent areas during awake brain surgery. Pictures included in the MULTIMAP test are colored drawings of objects and actions that have been standardized in nine different languages (Spanish, Basque, Catalan, Italian, French, English, German, Modern Standard Arabic, and Mandarin Chinese), controlling for name agreement, frequency, length, and neighbors across objects and verbs in nine languages and their combinations. Thus, the database was designed for allowing direct comparisons between objects and actions within and across languages (i.e., Spanish-Basque, Spanish-Catalan, Spanish-Italian, Spanish-French, Spanish-English, Spanish-German, Spanish-Modern Standard Arabic, and Spanish-Chinese).

MULTIMAP will improve language mapping in multilingual patients, testing objects and actions, and facilitating the identification of areas that show interference in all or only one of their languages that would not be detected by a monolingual test. Moreover, although the use of object naming tasks is widespread across surgical teams in many different geographical locations, heterogeneity in the stimuli selection criteria of pictures across different studies hinders comparison and generalization of results. The MULTIMAP battery allows for direct comparison between objects and actions as well as between pairs of languages in awake surgery.

The use of single picture naming tasks to test the different languages is mandatory but it is not fully comprehensive to capture the complexity of language. This is why, depending on the tumor, other tasks such as Counting, Reading, and Translation [58–60], to name a few, have also been used in order to preserve an optimal quality of life according to the patient's specific language requirements. Additional tasks at the sentence/discourse level are needed in the field.

Finally, to keep effective communication in bilinguals, a correct capacity for change (language switching) and control (language inhibition) of the different languages is necessary. Most of the studies to monitor language function in bilinguals used the picture naming task. This task seems to tap into single word production. In addition, picture naming has been also used to investigate LS. Participants can be instructed to name the picture in one language (e.g., Spanish) or another language (e.g., English) depending on a specific cue (i.e., the color of the picture frame or a flag, etc.). This way we can compare the responses to trials in which participants have to change the language to name the next picture (switching trials: Picture 1 in Spanish, *libro*, Picture 2 in English, *table*) with those in which the same language is used to name two consecutive pictures (repeat trials: Picture 1 in English, *book*, and Picture 2 in English: *table*). Error rates and/or reaction times are larger for switching trials as compared to repeat trials.

Interestingly, this LS task has been used intraoperatively by the group from Bellvitge, who implemented a LS-electrical stimulation mapping (ESM) paradigm assessment. Their results showed different functional distributions when comparing single-language naming to the LS. Within the frontal lobe, the single language naming sites were found significantly more frequently within the inferior frontal gyrus as compared to the middle frontal gyrus. Contrarily, switching naming sites were distributed across the middle frontal gyrus significantly more often than within the inferior frontal gyrus. These findings support the notion that non-domain-specific cognitive control prefrontal regions (posterior MFG), together with language frontal-related sites (IFG), mediate LS processing in bilinguals [42] (see Fig. 14.1).

14.5 Functional Improvement in Patients Operated on with Versus Without Function Monitoring

ESM studies in bilinguals have yielded heterogeneous results, ranging from a greater spatial representation for L1 [2] or for L2 [21] to an equivalent total cortical surface area involved in L1 and L2 processing, with partially overlapping regions [4] or significantly different anatomical distribution [1]. This spatial separability could imply that testing only one language would put the second language abilities at risk in the postoperative period.

There is only one series of bilingual patients operated under LS monitoring using a newly developed LS task that allowed a systematic evaluation of externally triggered LS synchronously with ESM [42]. Based on previous proposals [45], the authors evidenced that the postsurgical neuropsychological scores did not differ significantly from the presurgical ones, and patients did no report involuntary LS in their daily life conversations; however there is no evidence of improvement in comparative cohorts. On the other hand, we are not aware of any study describing a long-lasting deficit for the intraoperatively non-tested language. Nonetheless, as we mentioned in point 2, there are consistent data on global permanent deficits being

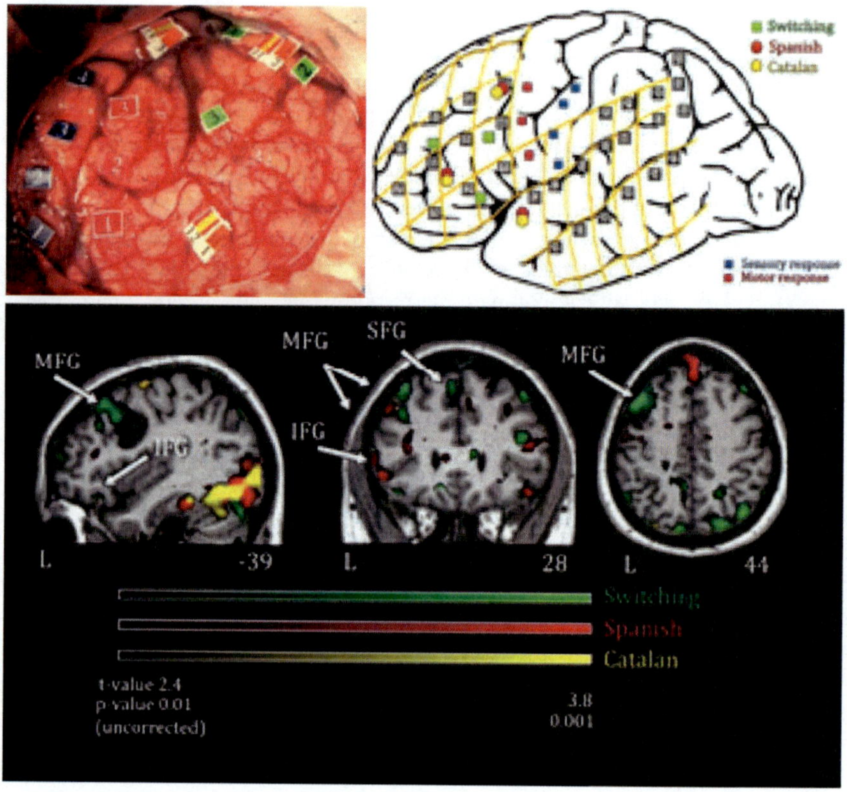

Fig. 14.1 Language functional maps reconstructed on the basis of intraoperative ESM in comparison with neuroimaging results from fMRI in a bilingual patient. Image from the LS-patient series from Sierpowska and Fernandez-Coello [42]

twice more frequent in the unmapped patients undergoing brain surgery for supratentorial gliomas.

Numerous papers in the field of ESM in glioma surgery have reported its usefulness to minimize neurological permanent deficits and, at the same time, to improve oncological outcome [40]. It now seems well established that neuro-oncological surgery needs to get to the best balance of quality of life and survival at the same time. Identifying the "connectome" intraoperatively by means of subcortical stimulation has been consolidated as the best tool for this purpose, in a clear new surgical oncofunctional brain surgery philosophy [41, 61–63], but what about not only preserving but improving?

As mentioned previously, there are no objective data in the specific field of multilingualism, unlike in the field of global neurocognition. There are no reasons to believe that bilinguals should behave differently. Actually, Duffau already reported a 10% improvement in language skills after surgery of supratentorial LGG in his early series of 103 patients in 2003 [64]. This improvement in language skills is even reported for the insular lobe, probably the most challenging area for glioma surgery in awake patients. Duffau reported language improvements in 6 out of 24 patients after insular surgery [65]. These conclusions are shared by other teams, as Pallud et al., who are also reporting up to 30% of language improvement after glioma surgery with ESM [66].

Another neurocognitive aspect of language that is crucial for multilinguals is working memory (see Chap. 12). In particular, working memory capabilities are crucial for daily living, for instance, for a correct and fluid language switching. Recent data from ESM testing working memory before and after oncofunctional surgery preserving the connectome showed that, although 91% of 45 patients experienced working memory loss in the first 3 months, after that time, all 42 patients recovered their preoperative status and 3 of them experienced improvement [67]. Interestingly, these improvements are not only within the neurocognitive sphere; they also have an impact on the patients' daily life, according to recently published data focusing on returning to their work status, which show that a 97% of them were able to resume their professional practice [68].

The lack of specific comparative series of a possible improvement of multilinguals that had surgery undercover of ESM implies that we cannot conclude that using this technique will improve their language skills. Nonetheless, the data for selective improvement in some patients in all the other neurocognitive aspects mentioned before, and the robust data sustaining the existence of specific functional networks for each language mentioned in the first paragraph of this chapter, partially suggest that oncofunctional surgery may also improve at least one of the languages in some selected patients. In this sense, the increase of functional connectivity observed in peritumoral regions when comparing it 3 months after surgery and before surgery [32] is very promising.

14.6 Closing Remarks

The contradictory results in ESM studies testing multiple languages, ranging from a complete overlap among the different languages to spatially distinct and separate areas for each language, lead us to individualize and tailor a neuropsychological protocol testing all the languages the patient fluently speaks or test only their native language, depending on daily needs.

The results of ESM-LS studies suggest an executive control functional network that takes advantage both from language-specific areas and non-language cognitive control regions, working together to maintain effective communication. Therefore, testing LS also involves testing non-domain-specific cognitive control networks, resulting in a patient-relevant medical benefit.

Finally, the gained evidence from cognitive psychology, neuroimaging studies, and ESM teaches us that the localizationist approach of trying to segregate languages topographically has not yielded conclusive results. Answers possibly lie beyond the cortex, understanding the brain as a dynamic network involving white matter tracts and subcortical structures.

Acknowledgments This research is supported by the Basque Government through the BERC 2018-2021 program, and by the Agencia Estatal de Investigación through BCBL Severo Ochoa excellence accreditation SEV-2015-0490 and project RTI2018-093547-B-I00.

References

1. Lucas TH 2nd, McKhann GM 2nd, Ojemann GA. Functional separation of languages in the bilingual brain: a comparison of electrical stimulation language mapping in 25 bilingual patients and 117 monolingual control patients. J Neurosurg. 2004;101:449–57.
2. Giussani C, Roux F-EF-E, Lubrano V, Gaini SM, Bello L. Review of language organisation in bilingual patients: what can we learn from direct brain mapping? Acta Neurochir (Wien). 2007;149:1109–16; discussion 1116.
3. Ojemann GA, Whitaker HA. The bilingual brain. Arch Neurol. 1978;35:409–12.
4. Roux F-E, Trémoulet M. Organization of language areas in bilingual patients: a cortical stimulation study. J Neurosurg. 2002;97:857–64.
5. Gao H, et al. Brain cancer surgery in the language areas of Mandarin-Cantonese bilinguals. J Cancer Res Ther. 2015;11:415.
6. Serafini S, Gururangan S, Friedman A, Haglund M. Identification of distinct and overlapping cortical areas for bilingual naming and reading using cortical stimulation. Case report. J Neurosurg Pediatr. 2008;1:247–54.
7. Ann CTK, Satoer D, Chan HM, Rossi M, Yeo TT, Guo YTE, Loh NHW, Witte ED, Teo K. Language localization in multilingual patients—evidence from direct electrical stimulation: a systematic review and single institution case series. Neurosurgery. 2019;66(1):310–509. https://doi.org/10.1093/neuros/nyz310_509.
8. Perani D, Abutalebi J. The neural basis of first and second language processing. Curr Opin Neurobiol. 2005;15(2):202–6.
9. Kim KH, Relkin NR, Lee KM, Hirsch J. Distinct cortical areas associated with native and second languages. Nature. 1997;388:171–4.
10. Cao F, Tao R, Liu L, Perfetti CA, Booth JR. High proficiency in a second language is characterized by greater involvement of the first language network: evidence from Chinese learners of English. J Cogn Neurosci. 2013;25(10):1649–63. https://doi.org/10.1162/jocn_a_00414.
11. Chee MWL, Tan EWL, Thiel T. Mandarin and English single word processing studied with functional magnetic resonance imaging. J Neurosci. 1999;19(8):3050–6. https://doi.org/10.1523/jneurosci.19-08-03050.1999.
12. Kim SY, et al. How does language distance between L1 and L2 affect the L2 brain network? An fMRI study of Korean–Chinese–English trilinguals. Neuroimage. 2016;129:25–39.
13. Van de Putte E, De Baene W, Brass M, Duyck W. Neural overlap of L1 and L2 semantic representations in speech: a decoding approach. Neuroimage. 2017;162:106–16. https://doi.org/10.1016/j.neuroimage.2017.08.082.
14. Jamal NI, Piche AW, Napoliello EM, Perfetti CA, Eden GF. Neural basis of single-word reading in Spanish-English bilinguals. Hum Brain Mapp. 2012;33(1):235–45. https://doi.org/10.1002/hbm.21208.
15. Liu H, Cao F. L1 and L2 processing in the bilingual brain: a meta-analysis of neuroimaging studies. Brain Lang. 2016;159:60–73. https://doi.org/10.1016/j.bandl.2016.05.013.
16. Chan HM, Loh WNH, Yeo TT, Teo K. Awake craniotomy and excision of a diffuse low-grade glioma in a multilingual patient: neuropsychology and language. World Neurosurg. 2019;128:91–7.
17. Fernandez-Coello A, et al. Age of language acquisition and cortical language organization in multilingual patients undergoing awake brain mapping. J Neurosurg. 2017;126(6):1912–23.
18. Bello L, et al. Intraoperative language localization in multilingual patients with gliomas. Neurosurgery. 2006;59:115–25.

19. Lubrano V, Prod'homme K, Démonet JF. Language monitoring in multilingual patients undergoing awake craniotomy: a case study of a German–English–French trilingual patient with a WHO grade II glioma. J Neurolinguist. 2012;25(6):567–78.
20. Połczyńska MM, Benjamin CFA, Japardi K, Frew A, Bookheimer SY. Language system organization in a quadrilingual with a brain tumor: implications for understanding of the language network. Neuropsychologia. 2016;86:167–75.
21. Cervenka MC, Boatman-Reich DF, Ward J, Franaszczuk PJ, Crone NE. Language mapping in multilingual patients: electrocorticography and cortical stimulation during naming. Front Hum Neurosci. 2011;5:13.
22. Rueckl JG, et al. Universal brain signature of proficient reading: evidence from four contrasting languages. Proc Natl Acad Sci. 2015;112:15510–5.
23. Hernandez AE, Dapretto M, Mazziotta J, Bookheimer S. Language switching and language representation in Spanish–English bilinguals: an fMRI study. Neuroimage. 2001;14:510–20.
24. Green DW, Abutalebi J. Language control in bilinguals: the adaptive control hypothesis. J Cogn Psychol. 2013;25:515–30.
25. De Baene W, Duyck W, Brass M, Carreiras M. Brain circuit for cognitive control is shared by task and language switching. J Cogn Neurosci. 2015;27:1752–65.
26. Robles SG, Gatignol P, Lehéricy S, Duffau H. Long-term brain plasticity allowing a multistage surgical approach to World Health Organization Grade II gliomas in eloquent areas. J Neurosurg. 2008;109:615–24.
27. Thiel A, et al. Plasticity of language networks in patients with brain tumors: a positron emission tomography activation study. Ann Neurol. 2001;50:620–9.
28. Duffau H, et al. Functional recovery after surgical resection of low grade gliomas in eloquent brain: hypothesis of brain compensation. J Neurol Neurosurg Psychiatry. 2003;74(7):901–7. https://doi.org/10.1136/jnnp.74.7.901.
29. Krainik A, et al. Role of the healthy hemisphere in recovery after resection of the supplementary motor area. Neurology. 2004;62(8):1323–32. https://doi.org/10.1212/01.WNL.0000120547.83482.B1.
30. Noppeney U, Price CJ, Duncan JS, Koepp MJ. Reading skills after left anterior temporal lobe resection: an fMRI study. Brain. 2005;128(Pt 6):1377–85. https://doi.org/10.1093/brain/awh414.
31. Sarubbo S, Le Bars E, Sylvie MG, Duffau H, Sarubbo S. Complete recovery after surgical resection of left Wernicke's area in awake patient: a brain stimulation and functional MRI study. Neurosurg Rev. 2012;35(2):287–92. https://doi.org/10.1007/s10143-011-0351-4.
32. Lizarazu M, et al. Spatiotemporal dynamics of postoperative functional plasticity in patients with brain tumors in language areas. Brain Lang. 2020;202:104741. https://doi.org/10.1016/j.bandl.2019.104741.
33. Gil-Robles S, Duffau H. Surgical management of World Health Organization Grade II gliomas in eloquent areas: the necessity of preserving a margin around functional structures. Neurosurg Focus. 2010;28(2):E8. https://doi.org/10.3171/2009.12.FOCUS09236.
34. Duffau H. Does post-lesional subcortical plasticity exist in the human brain? Neurosci Res. 2009;65:131–5.
35. Ibrahim R. Performance in L1 and L2 observed in Arabic-Hebrew bilingual aphasic following brain tumor: a case constitutes double dissociation. Psychol Res Behav Manag. 2008;1:11–9. https://doi.org/10.2147/PRBM.S4125.
36. Ibrahim R. Selective deficit of second language: a case study of a brain-damaged Arabic-Hebrew bilingual patient. Behav Brain Funct. 2009;5:17. https://doi.org/10.1186/1744-9081-5-17.
37. Berthier ML, Starkstein SE, Lylyk P, Leiguarda R. Differential recovery of languages in a bilingual patient: a case study using selective amytal test. Brain Lang. 1990;38:449–53.
38. Kho KH, et al. Involuntary language switching in two bilingual patients during the Wada test and intraoperative electrocortical stimulation. Brain Lang. 2007;101:31–7.
39. Gomeztortosa E, Martin EM, Gaviria M, Charbel F, Ausman JI. Selective deficit of one language in a bilingual patient following surgery in the left perisylvian area. Brain Lang. 1995;48(3):320–5. https://doi.org/10.1006/brln.1995.1014.

40. De Witt Hamer PC, Robles SG, Zwinderman AH, Duffau H, Berger MS. Impact of intraoperative stimulation brain mapping on glioma surgery outcome: a meta-analysis. J Clin Oncol. 2012;30:2559–65.
41. Duffau H, Moritz-Gasser S, Mandonnet E. A re-examination of neural basis of language processing: proposal of a dynamic hodotopical model from data provided by brain stimulation mapping during picture naming. Brain Lang. 2014;131:1–10.
42. Sierpowska J, Fernandez-Coello A, et al. Involvement of the middle frontal gyrus in language switching as revealed by electrical stimulation mapping and functional magnetic resonance imaging in bilingual brain tumor patients. Cortex. 2018;99:78–92.
43. Gatignol P, Duffau H, Capelle L, Plaza M. Naming performance in two bilinguals with frontal vs. temporal glioma. Neurocase. 2009;15:466–77.
44. Moritz-Gasser S, Duffau H. Evidence of a large-scale network underlying language switching: a brain stimulation study. J Neurosurg. 2009;111:729–32.
45. Sierpowska J, et al. Intraoperative electrical stimulation of language switching in two bilingual patients. Neuropsychologia. 2013;51:2882–92.
46. Tomasino B, et al. Involuntary switching into the native language induced by electrocortical stimulation of the superior temporal gyrus: a multimodal mapping study. Neuropsychologia. 2014;62:87–100.
47. Wang X, Wang Y-Y, Jiang T, Wang Y-Z, Wu C-X. Direct evidence of the left caudate's role in bilingual control: an intra-operative electrical stimulation study. Neurocase. 2013;19:462–9.
48. Moritz-Gasser S, Duffau H. Cognitive processes and neural basis of language switching: proposal of a new model. Neuroreport. 2009;20:1577–80.
49. De Benedictis A, Moritz-Gasser S, Duffau H. Awake mapping optimizes the extent of resection for low-grade gliomas in eloquent areas. Neurosurgery. 2010;66:1074–84; discussion 1084.
50. De Witte E, Mariën P. The neurolinguistic approach to awake surgery reviewed. Clin Neurol Neurosurg. 2013;115:127–45.
51. Miceli G, Capasso R, Monti A, Santini B, Talacchi A. Language testing in brain tumor patients. J Neurooncol. 2012;108(2):247–52. https://doi.org/10.1007/s11060-012-0810-y.
52. Corina DP, et al. Dissociation of action and object naming: evidence from cortical stimulation mapping. Hum Brain Mapp. 2005;24:1–10.
53. Crepaldi D, Berlingeri M, Paulesu E, Luzzatti C. A place for nouns and a place for verbs? A critical review of neurocognitive data on grammatical-class effects. Brain Lang. 2011;116(1):33–49. https://doi.org/10.1016/j.bandl.2010.09.005.
54. Lubrano V, Filleron T, Démonet JF, Roux FE. Anatomical correlates for category-specific naming of objects and actions: a brain stimulation mapping study. Hum Brain Mapp. 2014;35(2):429–43. https://doi.org/10.1002/hbm.22189.
55. Rofes A, et al. Mapping nouns and finite verbs in left hemisphere tumors: a direct electrical stimulation study. Neurocase. 2017;23:105–13.
56. Vigliocco G, Vinson DP, Druks J, Barber H, Cappa SF. Nouns and verbs in the brain: a review of behavioural, electrophysiological, neuropsychological and imaging studies. Neurosci Biobehav Rev. 2011;35(3):407–26. https://doi.org/10.1016/j.neubiorev.2010.04.007.
57. Gisbert-Muñoz S, et al. MULTIMAP: multilingual visual naming test for the mapping of eloquent areas during awake surgeries. bioRxiv. 2020. https://doi.org/10.1101/2020.02.20.957282.
58. Roux F-E, et al. Intra-operative mapping of cortical areas involved in reading in mono- and bilingual patients. Brain. 2004;127:1796–810.
59. Roux F-E, et al. The graphemic/motor frontal area Exner's area revisited. Ann Neurol. 2009;66:537–45.
60. Borius P-Y, Giussani C, Draper L, Roux F-E. Sentence translation in proficient bilinguals: a direct electrostimulation brain mapping. Cortex. 2011;48:614–22.
61. Duffau H. Mapping the connectome in awake surgery for gliomas: an update. J Neurosurg Sci. 2017;61(6):612–30. https://doi.org/10.23736/S0390-5616.17.04017-6.

62. Duffau H. Surgery of low-grade gliomas: towards a 'functional neurooncology'. Curr Opin Oncol. 2009;21:543–9.
63. Ferracci FX, Duffau H. Improving surgical outcome for gliomas with intraoperative mapping. Expert Rev Neurother. 2018;18(4):333–41. https://doi.org/10.1080/14737175.2018.1451329.
64. Duffau H, Capelle L, Denvil D, Sichez N. Usefulness of intraoperative electrical subcortical mapping during surgery for low-grade gliomas located within eloquent brain regions: functional results in a consecutive series of 103 patients. J Neurosurg. 2003;98(4):764–78.
65. Duffau H, Moritz-Gasser S, Gatignol P. Functional outcome after language mapping for insular World Health Organization Grade II gliomas in the dominant hemisphere: experience with 24 patients. Neurosurg Focus. 2009;27:E7.
66. Pallud J, Dezamis E. Functional and oncological outcomes following awake surgical resection using intraoperative cortico-subcortical functional mapping for supratentorial gliomas located in eloquent areas. Neurochirurgie. 2017;63:208–18.
67. Duffau H. Diffuse low-grade glioma, oncological outcome and quality of life: a surgical perspective. Curr Opin Oncol. 2018;30(6):383–9. https://doi.org/10.1097/CCO.0000000000000483.
68. Ng S, Herbet G, Moritz-Gasser S, Duffau H. Return to work following surgery for incidental diffuse low-grade glioma: a prospective series with 74 patients. Neurosurgery. 2020;87(4):720–9. https://doi.org/10.1093/neuros/nyz513.

Part III

Higher-Order Functions

Semantic Cognition

15

Sylvie Moritz-Gasser and Guillaume Herbet

15.1 Introduction

The meaning assigned to words, objects, pictures, sounds, faces, and facts is stored in semantic memory [1, 2]. Stored concepts are thus associated with a number of shared or defining/distinctive features, corresponding to categorical, functional, visual, cultural, and emotional attributes (for instance: *the trout is an aquatic animal, living in fresh water, I don't know how to fish trout, I like its taste, Schubert composed a quintet named the trout*). Semantic knowledge then supports many everyday activities, and is critical for both verbal and nonverbal behaviors. However, an efficient semantic processing not only requires to access this store of conceptual knowledge, but also to activate adequately relevant stored information, in a goal-directed manner. Semantic cognition designs these neurocognitive processes enabling to organize, generalize, and manipulate efficiently semantic representations, thanks to the involvement of control mechanisms [2–4].

Current neuro-computational models of semantic cognition arise from nearly five decades of studies on acquired semantic impairments among which pioneering works highlighted notably the phenomenon of modality-specific and category-specific semantic deficits [5, 6], generating by the way different assumptions about the organization of conceptual knowledge in the brain, suggesting either that different semantic categories are represented or not in dissociable brain areas, depending or not on modality-specific input/output (for a review, see [7]). A number of questions in this topic are still a matter of striking debate, the most controversial being thus probably whether semantic knowledge is represented in distributed isolable—even if connected—brain areas or in a unified amodal hub. A convincing and

S. Moritz-Gasser (✉) · G. Herbet
Institute of Functional Genomics, INSERM U1191, Team "Plasticity, Stem Cells and Glial Tumors", University of Montpellier, Montpellier, France

Gui de Chauliac Hospital, Montpellier, France
e-mail: sylvie.gasser@umontpellier.fr

E. Mandonnet, G. Herbet (eds.), *Intraoperative Mapping of Cognitive Networks*,
https://doi.org/10.1007/978-3-030-75071-8_15

reconciling answer is brought by the "distributed-plus-hub" view [1], described by the *hub-and-spoke model* in which modality-specific aspects of conceptual knowledge shaping the organization of semantic memory in distributed brain areas are integrated in a transmodal anterior temporal hub encoding generalizable higher-order conceptual representations by mediating cross-modal interactions between these sources of information [3]. In the setting of the hub-and-spoke model, the controlled semantic cognition (CSC) framework refers to how this conceptual knowledge is adequately activated, in a goal-directed manner, thanks to the interaction of a semantic control system relying on executive mechanisms, which constrains semantic representation activations depending on the task at hand, whether verbal or nonverbal (for example, different semantic attributes associated with the concept "trout" will have to be activated depending on the situation: accessing the name of this fish, preparing a meal, fishing, painting, or listening to Schubert's work). CSC framework further accounts for different patterns of semantic impairments observed in various neurological conditions such as loss of semantic knowledge reported in semantic dementia (SD), related to a degradation of the semantic system itself, or semantic access deficit reported in stroke aphasia, likely reflecting impairments of the semantic control system [8–11]. Studies aiming to compare patterns of semantic impairments between SD and stroke aphasia patients have indeed provided a number of differences in both verbal and nonverbal domains, patients with stroke-induced semantic impairments exhibiting notably, in contrast with SD-induced semantic impairments, inconsistent results across tests, no effect of frequency or familiarity of stimuli, and strong effect of cueing on task performance [12, 13].

By bringing meaning to most of everyday situations, semantic cognition is then critical for verbal and nonverbal human behaviors, and disorders in semantic processing have thus extremely debilitating consequences. Needless to say, semantic cognition, as a defining feature of human being, should imperiously be thoroughly monitored during intraoperative awake surgery mapping, with full up-to-date knowledge of its neural bases, in order to avoid long-lasting verbal and/or nonverbal semantic impairments.

15.2 Neural Bases of Semantic Cognition: State of Knowledge

Neural bases of semantic cognition have been addressed in a large number of clinical studies analyzing patterns of brain damage in patients and functional neuroimaging-based studies, in patients and healthy volunteers (e.g., [14–20]), suggesting a broad distributed neural representation, mostly but not exclusively left lateralized. A recent meta-analysis of 120 functional neuroimaging studies reported a network of 7 left-sided loci involved in semantic processing [21], namely the posterior inferior parietal lobe, especially the angular gyrus (post IPL, AG), the middle and posterior inferior temporal gyri (MTG and ITG), the mid-fusiform and parahippocampal gyri, the dorsomedial prefrontal cortex (DMPFC), the inferior frontal gyrus (IFG), the ventromedial prefrontal cortex (VMPFC), and the posterior cingulate gyrus. It is worth noting here that, because the goal of this meta-analysis was to identify brain regions involved *specifically* in semantic processing, the authors excluded studies employing contrasting tasks that differed in terms of difficulty, in order to identify only semantic areas and not regions involved in more general cognitive processes required in any goal-directed task. However, some studies show that a number of control processes mediated by the left inferior prefrontal cortex (LIPC) and temporo-parietal cortices (notably pMTG and AG) are specifically engaged in goal-directed retrieval of semantic knowledge per se [4, 22–27], indicating that these regions should be identified as belonging to the semantic network.

Furthermore, semantic dementia (SD), a neurodegenerative disease marked by a progressive loss of semantic knowledge in all modalities with well-preserved other aspects of cognition, that is a selective impairment of semantic abilities [28, 29], is associated with a bilateral—albeit often asymmetrical—degeneration of the anterior temporal lobes (ATLs), especially in their ventral portion [30–34], suggesting that these regions act as semantic hubs, supporting the formation of amodal semantic representations [1, 35, 36]. Conceptual knowledge would then be represented in an amodal fashion *bilaterally* in the ATLs, explaining why unilateral ATL damage due to stroke or resection typically does not result in such profound semantic impairments as those encountered in SD patients [37, 38]. This bilateral representation of course does not mean that the two ATLs are equipotent in semantic processing, but rather that they work jointly to process semantic information and that the effects of unilateral damage might be at least partially compensated by the contralateral system, with however slowing of reaction times and poorer performance in particularly demanding semantic tasks [39]. Further studies suggest besides that activations are more likely to be left lateralized to process verbal input or when word retrieval is required and for the processing of distinctive vs. shared semantic features [40, 41], and that pictorial semantic processing is less affected than verbal semantic processing following unilateral ATL resection, because it draws on a bilateral network [42].

Finally, it is now well established that this widely distributed semantic network is underlain by a bilateral ventral white matter connectivity involving the inferior fronto-occipital, inferior longitudinal, and uncinate fasciculi (IFOF, ILF, and UF) [43–51]. In this setting, some authors (e.g., [52]) suggest that this ventral semantic stream would consist of a critical direct route sub-served by the IFOF, connecting occipito-temporo-parietal cortices to inferior frontal and dorsolateral prefrontal cortices [53], and an indirect route, likely to be compensable in case of unilateral damage, sub-served by the anterior part of the ILF and the UF, connecting respectively the posterior temporo-basal cortex to the temporal pole, and the temporal pole to the pars orbitalis of the IFG [54]. Indeed, left IFOF has been shown to crucially support verbal as well as nonverbal semantic processes, since intraoperative direct electrical stimulation (DES) of this fasciculus entails both transient verbal semantic impairments (production of semantic paraphasia during naming task) and nonverbal semantic deficits (inability to associate two visually presented concepts) [47], whereas the indirect pathway (ILF/UF) can be functionally compensated when unilaterally damaged, as demonstrated following anterior temporal and orbitofrontal glioma resections [55, 56].

Of note, given its connections with components of the limbic system, namely amygdala and para hippocampal gyrus [57], this parallel indirect pathway has further been suggested to be involved in emotional-valued semantic processing [58, 59]. Interestingly, studies based on the Klingler fiber dissection technique identified in the IFOF a superficial dorsal subcomponent, connecting the superior and middle occipital gyri, the superior parietal lobule, and the posterior part of the STG to the IFG, and a deep ventral subcomponent, connecting the inferior occipital gyrus, the posterior temporal-basal area and the posterior part of the MTG to the orbitofrontal cortex, middle frontal gyrus, and dorsolateral prefrontal cortex [60], suggesting a possible anatomo-functional segregation of this fasciculus, the superficial layer being involved in verbal semantics and the deep one in amodal and control semantic processes, and possibly in the awareness of semantic knowledge [47, 61].

Studies based on intraoperative mapping, as detailed in subsequent parts of this chapter, contribute highly to shed light on the neural bases of semantic processing, emphasizing especially, in addition to the above-described left-lateralized semantic network, the implication of a right-lateralized network.

15.3 Semantic Impairments in Brain Tumor Patients

Crucial for language production and comprehension as well as nonverbal human behaviors, semantic cognition is supported by a broad distributed neural representation. As a defining feature of human being, verbal and nonverbal semantic cognition should then be thoroughly assessed perioperatively and monitored during intraoperative awake surgery mapping, in order to avoid long-lasting dramatically debilitating impairments. Yet, because semantic processing is so far not routinely fully assessed [62–64], it should be acknowledged that studies reporting semantic disorders in brain-damaged patients in general and in brain tumor patients in particular are scarce, and focus mainly on verbal semantics. Thereon, a recent study aiming to characterize language impairments in brain tumor patients thanks to a specific language assessment based on the analysis of cognitive processes involved in language processing (*BLAST: Brief Language Assessment for Surgical Tumour Patients*) highlighted the existence of preoperative disorders in accessing semantic knowledge (assessed notably through picture naming, picture-word verification, and verb generation) in these patients compared to healthy controls [65]. Interestingly, these disorders were present mostly in patients with left-lateralized frontal, temporal, and parietal tumors, but also, although in a lesser extent, in patients with right-lateralized tumors. A case series study, aiming to validate the *Dutch Linguistic Intraoperative Protocol (DuLIP)*, suggested further that by monitoring lexical-semantic processes intraoperatively, especially by the means of a semantic odd word/picture out task and a semantic association task, lexical-semantic disorders potentially observed during the immediate postoperative period (e.g., [66]) may resolve 6 months postoperatively [67]. Furthermore, a study aiming to distinguish semantic access disorders from semantic memory degradation in patients with brain tumor located to the temporal lobe showed that whenever (pre- and/or postoperatively) semantic deficits emerged, they were clearly of access type (i.e., inconsistency of concept activation and performance weakly affected by word frequency) and that high-grade tumors regularly impaired access to semantic representations, whereas low-grade tumors did not [68]. Importantly, the same type of semantic access disorders has been reported after surgical resection of a glioma infiltrating the left dorsal and ventral prefrontal cortices and underlying white matter, thus sparing the temporal lobe but disrupting efficient access to semantic representations [66].

15.4 Networks at Risk for Semantic Cognition in Glioma Surgery

While the study of semantic cognition has been the target of numerous works in certain neuropathological conditions, attempts to determine which cortical or subcortical structures might be especially vulnerable to resective surgery have been very limited in the context of glioma. Yet this knowledge is absolutely vital for the care of patients since results from lesion studies are not completely transposable from one brain condition to another due to differing physiopathological mechanisms (and associated neuroplasticity potential). To the best of your knowledge, only two studies employing voxelwise brain-behavioral analyses are available in the current literature.

The first of them [43] focused on the behavioral performances obtained on a task assessing semantic and phonological fluency. In this study, 31 patients with a histologically proven diffuse low-grade glioma infiltrating the left hemisphere were included. Patients were examined before surgery, 4–5 days after and then 3 months after surgery. Mass-univariate voxel-based lesion-symptom (VLSM) mapping analyses were conducted on the behavioral performances gained at each time point. Interestingly, before patients had been operated on, the performance on the semantic fluency task was associated with a large amount of voxels mainly situated in the white matter underlying the ventral system. Further analyses showed that these correlated voxels greatly overlapped with the typical course of the left IFOF. As a matter of fact, a significant correlation was obtained between semantic fluency score and the amount of tumor infiltration into the IFOF. No significant results were obtained with the phonological fluency task. After surgery, no brain-behavior relationships were identified for both tasks and for the two postoperative periods, suggesting that the surgery in itself did not lead to additional and permanent difficulties. Note that all patients were operated on under awake conditions with a mapping of semantic processes allowing the IFOF to be spared from the surgical procedure. In sum, progressive tumor infiltration of the left IFOF is associated with declining performances in terms of semantic fluency but, in turn, sparing the IFOF during surgery helps to maintain the level of performance after surgery. This general finding cannot be, however, generalized as only one specific aspect of semantic cognition was assessed.

In the second study [69], 66 patients operated on in awake surgery but with different etiologies (including WHO II, III, and IV grade glioma, arteriovenous malformation and cavernous angioma, lymphoma and metastasis) were assessed preoperatively with a range of neuropsychological tasks, including tasks tapping into the processes of semantic cognition (i.e., a naming task, a synonym judgment task, and a semantic matching task). Standard VLSM and tract-oriented lesion-symptom analyses were performed. First, VLSM failed to identify any relationships between the location of lesions and performances obtained on the synonym judgement and the semantic association task. However, a large bulk of significant voxels was found for the naming task, mainly in the ITG and the MTG and their underlying white matter connectivity—thus widely replicating the findings from Herbet et al. [70] (see also Chap. 5). Second, trackwise analyses indicated that naming performances in general were correlated with the amount of damage of the three ventral white matter tracts (i.e., the IFOF, the ILF, and the UF), but only the number of semantic paraphasias correlated with the IFOF. Furthermore, scores of the association semantic task specifically correlated with the left IFOF. Taken together, the results confirmed that left IFOF damage is especially deleterious for both verbal and nonverbal semantic cognition, as demonstrated in a previous work using electrostimulation mapping [47].

It is worth mentioning here that, to date, no study has been performed to assess semantic cognition in a comprehensive manner using a longitudinal experimental design. As a consequence, it is unknown whether damage to the cortical structures classically belonging to the semantic network (such as, for example, the IFG and the MTG) may cause permanent deficits in specific or multiple aspects of semantic cognition. In the same way, it remains unknown whether surgically related damage to the UF, ILF, or IFOF is associated with marked semantic deficits. This lack of data should prompt us to plan studies to ascertain the extent to which the processes of semantic cognition may be impaired despite a mapping of some of them. This is the only way to decide whether or not other behavior tasks than those usually employed (see the next section) should be envisioned for the intraoperative mapping [71].

15.5 Intraoperative Monitoring of Semantic Cognition

As mentioned above, whereas semantic cognition supports verbal as well as non-verbal behaviors, it is still not routinely fully assessed and when it is, solely through verbal tasks. In this regard, a number of authors proposed intraoperative examinations of language including lexical semantics (e.g., [64, 65, 67, 72–74]), which proved their value by highlighting broadly their sensitivity in detecting lexical-semantic transient disorders intraoperatively induced by DES, and consequently the absence of long-lasting postsurgical lexical-semantic disorders. These batteries assess verbal semantic processing by means of different tasks such as picture naming, semantic odd word/picture out, picture-word verification, verb generation, word-to-picture matching, or synonym judgement. However, intraoperative monitoring of semantic cognition cannot be limited to verbal semantics and a broader assessment of conceptual knowledge is needed, as emphasized in a recent electrical stimulation and lesion-symptom mapping study [69], as well as in previous works on SD, stressing the importance of assessing semantic knowledge in both verbal and nonverbal modalities of input/output [75, 76]. Finally, a few studies described besides a dissociation between naming and comprehension (notably preserved naming despite poor comprehension assessed by means of word-picture matching or semantic association tasks, the reverse situation being largely more common), emphasizing the necessity to assess conceptual knowledge in addition to naming, in order to detect a possible impairment in the former especially when the latter is preserved [77–79], and to specify the nature of the semantic impairment underlying the production of semantic paraphasias during intraoperative naming [47].

In sum, intraoperative monitoring of semantic cognition should include at least, in addition to pointing out semantic errors in picture naming, a nonverbal semantic association task (e.g., pictures version of the *Pyramids and Palm Trees Test—PPTT*, [80]) enabling to assess the ability for the patient to retrieve semantic and conceptual information from pictures, and then to indicate whether a given semantic impairment is dependent or not on the modality of processing. Given that neural bases of semantic processing are broadly distributed, this intraoperative assessment of nonverbal conceptual knowledge should be performed whatever the location of a tumor invading the left and right ventral routes, cortically and subcortically, especially at the level of the IFOF and its cortical terminations [53, 60]. Pre- and postoperatively, a more comprehensive battery of semantic cognition assessment should be used, including verbal and nonverbal tasks varying in complexity (that is requiring various levels of semantic control) such as, in addition to picture naming and word/picture semantic association, word-to-picture matching, picture/word sorting, semantic feature verification, sound recognition, verb generation, synonym judgement, and category fluency (compared to letter fluency), in order to build up thoroughly and as accurately as possible the semantic profile of the patient at both times of evaluation, and to design consequently specific and individualized rehabilitation programs if needed. Of note, some existing batteries propose a number of these tasks using the same items across them, controlled for category, frequency, and imageability, allowing a fine-grained analysis of semantic impairments in verbal and nonverbal modalities (e.g., *CSM battery*, [75]; *BETL*, [81]; *BECS*, [82]). These extensive evaluations, confronted with a standard neuropsychological assessment, could allow to implement longitudinal studies addressing long-term outcomes concerning semantic cognition and subsequently the clinical relevance of adding adapted new intraoperative semantic tasks, guided by the onco-functional balance, that is the challenging goal of maximizing the extent of resection while preserving the quality of life [83].

15.6 Which Additional Anatomo-Functional Knowledge Has Been Gained from Intraoperative Mapping Studies?

As mapping the language system with an object naming task has been the "gold standard" in awake surgery for a long while, data on the cortical organization of the verbal semantic system gained from electrostimulation mapping has accumulated over time, with the advantage of revealing the interindividual differences into the neural implementation of this system—contrary to other imaging modalities such as activation MRI. For example, in two successive stimulation-based probabilistic atlases [84, 85], sites for verbal semantic cognition (i.e., anatomical loci associated with semantic paraphasia) were identified in the anterior-to-posterior part of the STG and the most posterior portion of the MTG posteriorly, and in the pars triangularis and opercularis of the IFG, and the posterior dorsolateral prefrontal cortex anteriorly (Fig. 15.1). In the same way, based on the stimulation data of patients with diffuse low-grade glioma in whom semantic loci were found in the prefrontal cortex (left and right hemisphere), Herbet et al. [86] identified 45 verbal semantic sites that were equally distributed in pars opercularis and pars triangularis of the IFG as well as in the posteriormost portion of the dorsolateral prefrontal cortex (Fig. 15.2a, b). The entire cortical surface of these areas was covered, demonstrating a large interindividual variability. Interestingly, in this work, nonverbal semantic sites, as identified with the PPTT, were also processed. The analysis revealed this time a bilateral representation mainly involving the posterior dorsolateral prefrontal cortex with minor engagement of the IFG (Fig. 15.2c, d). Once again, there was a certain degree of interindividual variation in the location of sites, as they differed topologically along both a rostro-caudal and a dorsoventral axis.

At the subcortical level, critical insights into the white matter connections that might be involved in broadcasting semantic-related signals have been gained from electrostimulation mapping, this technique being the sole to allow direct inferences into the functions of white matter tracts [87]. In a first work by Duffau et al. [44], white matter sites associated with verbal semantic processing (obtained from 17 patients operated on under local anesthesia for left low-grade glioma) were considered conjointly. They were distributed in the white matter under the depth of the superior temporal sulcus, in the anterior floor of the external capsule and in the white matter deep in lateral orbitofrontal and dorsolateral prefrontal regions, a distribution that widely overlaps with the spatial course of the IFOF. This was the first demonstration that the IFOF may constitute the white matter connectivity underlying the ventral stream for semantic processing [46].

This finding was replicated by the same group a few years later but a new result was also provided [47]. The authors showed that transitory inactivation of the left IFOF not only disrupted verbal semantic processing but also nonverbal semantic processing as assessed by the PPTT. Furthermore, some sites were associated with both verbal and nonverbal semantic impairments, whereas other ones were uniquely associated with verbal semantic impairments, suggesting a bipartite functional organization of the IFOF. More specifically, in view of the multilayered structure of the IFOF evidenced by diffusion MRI and dissection studies (e.g., [60, 88, 89]), the

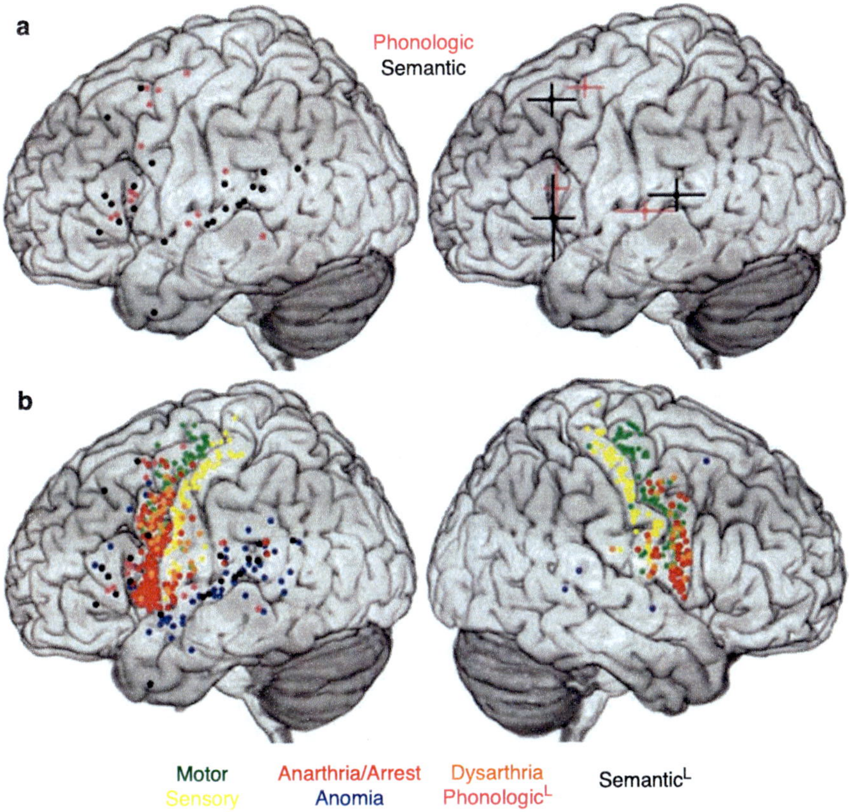

Fig. 15.1 Linguistic components of naming and summary map of cortical stimulation data. (**a**) Raw stimulation data and corresponding clusters for phonological (pink) and semantic (black) aspects of naming in right-handed patients. Phonological epicenters were located in the middle superior temporal gyrus, pars opercularis, and junction of precentral/dorsolateral prefrontal cortex. Three semantic nodes were identified: junction of posterior superior temporal gyrus and supramarginal gyrus, pars triangularis/opercularis, and dorsolateral prefrontal cortex. (**b**) Compilation of all stimulation data ($n = 771$ stimulation sites) in the right and left hemisphere demonstrating the wide distribution of cortical representation within and between critical functions of the human brain: motor (green), sensory (yellow), anarthria/arrest (red), anomia (blue), dysarthria (orange), phonological (pink), semantic (black). *L* left hemisphere only. Reused with permission from Tate et al. [85]

authors postulated that the superficial layer of the IFOF may be involved in verbal, modality-specific semantic processing, whereas the deep one may be rather involved in multimodal semantic processing [61]. This hypothesis needs, however, to be firmly supported by further experimental evidence.

In another study by Herbet et al. [90], direct evidence for the role of the right IFOF in nonverbal semantic cognition, assessed by means of the PPTT, was provided. In particular, 13 patients having undergone an awake surgery for a right

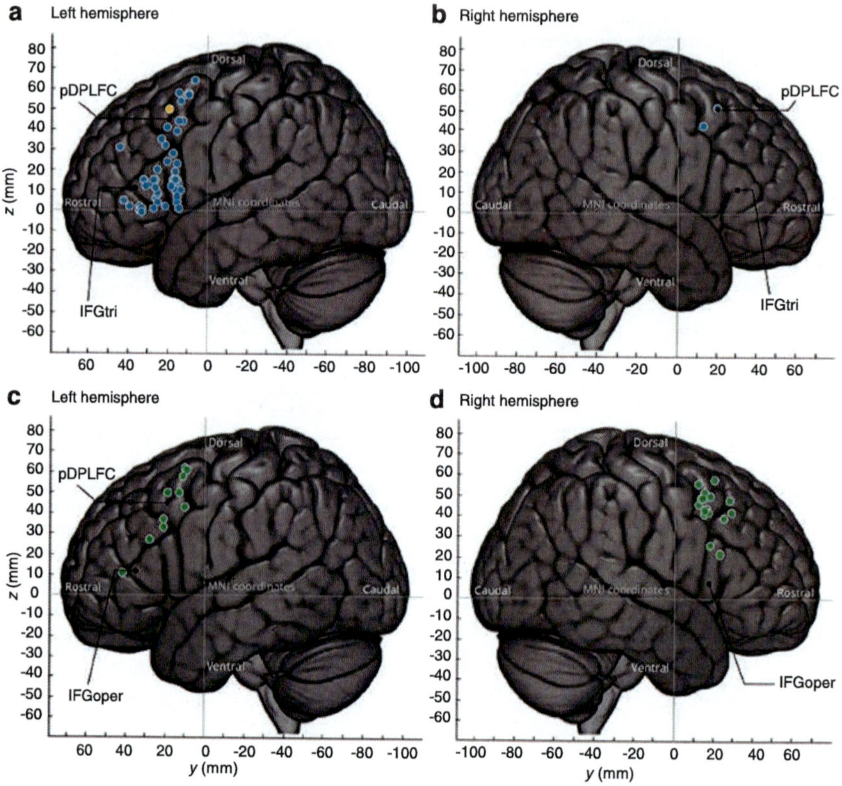

Fig. 15.2 Anatomical sites associated with (**a**) semantic paraphasia in the left frontal lobe, (**b**) semantic paraphasia in the right frontal lobe, (**c**) a disturbance of nonverbal semantic cognition in the left frontal lobe, and (**d**) a disturbance of nonverbal semantic cognition in the right frontal lobe. Blue circles: sites associated with semantic paraphasia; green circles: sites associated with nonverbal semantic disturbances; yellow circles: amodal site (i.e., associated with both semantic paraphasia and nonverbal semantic sites). *IFGoper* pars opercularis of the inferior frontal gyrus, *IFGtri* pars triangularis of the inferior frontal gyrus, *MNI* Montreal Neurological Institute, *pDLPFC* posterior dorsolateral prefrontal cortex. Reused with permission from Herbet et al. [86]

diffuse low-grade glioma were included. Positive sites were observed in the white matter of the angular gyrus and of the middle and superior temporal gyri, in the temporal stem, and in the white matter of the dorsolateral prefrontal cortex—a distribution that widely overlaps with the IFOF according to most of the anatomical studies (Fig. 15.3). This finding confirms that the nonverbal semantic network has a homotypic organization at the white matter level, as suggested by Herbet et al. [86] at the cortical level.

Finally, Sierpowska et al. [69] used conjointly a naming task, a semantic pair task, and a semantic association task to map white matter tracts involved in some

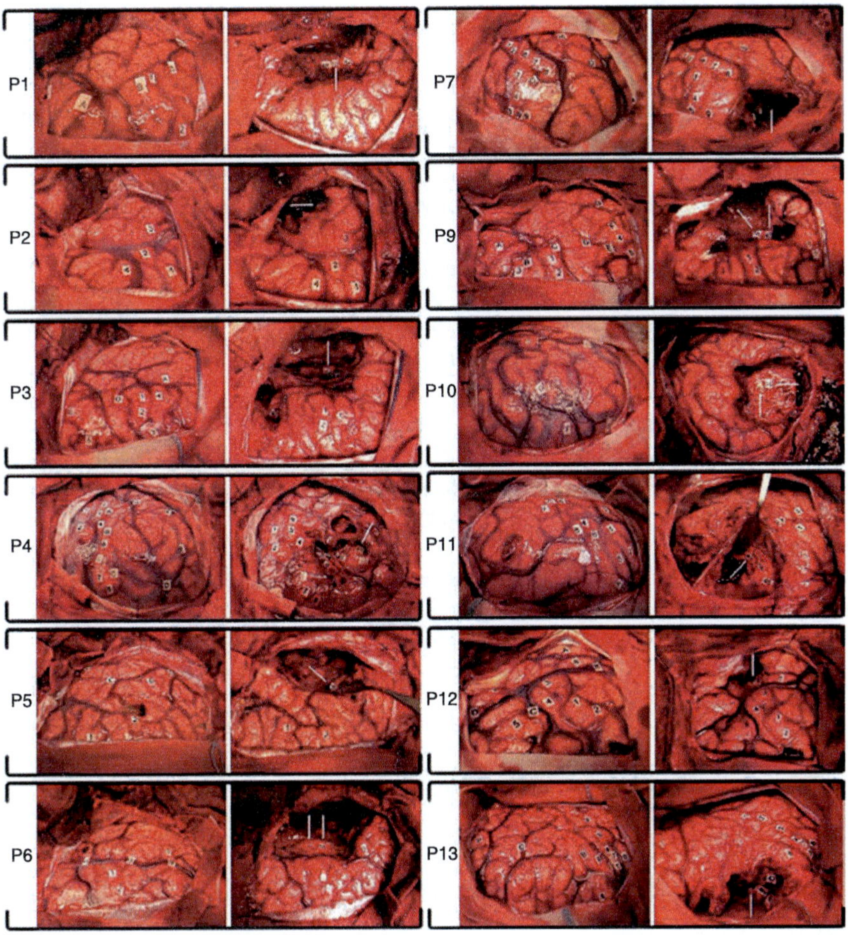

Fig. 15.3 Intraoperative mappings of nonverbal semantic cognition. The white lines indicate the subcortical anatomical sites for which a nonverbal semantic impairment was elicited during electrostimulation. Reused with permission from Herbet et al. [90]

aspects of semantic cognition. Globally, the authors found an involvement of both the left IFOF and the left ILF in the three tasks, but no precise anatomo-functional correlation analyses were performed on the intraoperative data.

In sum, electrostimulation mapping studies in awake patients were the first to allow to characterize the white matter pathways of the semantic network, in particular the central involvement of the IFOF in the left and the right cerebral hemispheres, a finding that has been now strengthened in neuropsychological studies using voxelwise lesion-symptom analyses (e.g., [91]).

15.7 Conclusion

Semantic cognition is a defining feature of human being, essential for verbal and nonverbal behaviors, involving numerous sub-processes supported by a broad distributed neural representation. As such, verbal and nonverbal semantic cognition should then be thoroughly assessed perioperatively and monitored during intraoperative awake surgery mapping, cortically and subcortically along the ventral route, especially at the level of the IFOF and its cortical terminations, in both hemispheres, in order to avoid long-lasting debilitating impairments. Intraoperative monitoring of semantic cognition should thus include at least, in addition to pointing out semantic errors in picture naming, a nonverbal semantic association task. Pre- and postoperatively, a more comprehensive battery of semantic cognition assessment should be used, including existing verbal and nonverbal tasks varying in complexity. These extensive evaluations, by drawing up the semantic profile of the patient at both times of evaluation, would allow, on the one hand, to design individualized rehabilitation programs, and, on the other hand, to implement longitudinal studies addressing long-term outcomes concerning semantic cognition and subsequently the clinical relevance of adding adapted new intraoperative semantic tasks, guided by the onco-functional balance aiming at maximizing the extent of resection while preserving the quality of life.

References

1. Patterson K, Nestor PJ, Rogers TT. Where do you know what you know? The representation of semantic knowledge in the human brain. Nat Rev Neurosci. 2007;8:976–87.
2. Rogers TT, McClelland JL. Semantic cognition: a parallel distributed processing approach. Cambridge: MIT Press; 2004.
3. Lambon Ralph MA, Jefferies E, Patterson K, Rogers TT. The neural and computational bases of semantic cognition. Nat Rev Neurosci. 2017;18(1):42–55.
4. Whitney C, Kirk M, O'Sullivan J, Lambon Ralph MA, Jefferies E. The neural organization of semantic control: TMS evidence for a distributed network in left inferior frontal and posterior middle temporal gyrus. Cereb Cortex. 2011;21:1066–75.
5. Lhermitte F, Beauvois MF. A visual speech disconnection syndrome: report of a case with optic aphasia, agnosic alexia and color agnosia. Brain. 1973;96:695–714.
6. Warrington EK, Shallice T. Category specific semantic impairments. Brain. 1984;107:829–54.
7. Caramazza A, Mahon BZ. The organisation of conceptual knowledge in the brain: the future's past and some future directions. Cogn Neuropsychol. 2006;23(1):13–38.
8. Jefferies E, Lambon Ralph MA. Semantic impairment in stroke aphasia versus semantic dementia: a case-series comparison. Brain. 2006;129:2132–47.
9. Jefferies E, Baker SS, Doran M, Lambon Ralph MA. Refractory effects in stroke aphasia: a consequence of poor semantic control. Neuropsychologia. 2007;45:1065–79.
10. Warrington EK, McCarthy R. Category specific access dysphasia. Brain. 1983;106:859–78.
11. Warrington EK, Cipolotti L. Word comprehension. The distinction between refractory and storage impairments. Brain. 1996;119(Pt 2):611–25.
12. Corbett F, Jefferies E, Ehsan S, Lambon Ralph MA. Different impairments of semantic cognition in semantic dementia and semantic aphasia: evidence from the non-verbal domain. Brain. 2009;132:2593–608.

13. Rogers TT, Patterson K, Jefferies E, Lambon Ralph MA. Disorders of representation and control in semantic cognition: effects of familiarity, typicality, and specificity. Neuropsychologia. 2015;76:220–39.
14. Chertkow H, Bub D, Deaudon C, Whitehead V. On the status of object concepts in aphasia. Brain Lang. 1997;58:203–32.
15. Damasio H, Tranel D, Grabowski T, Adolphs R, Damasio A. Neural systems behind word and concept retrieval. Cognition. 2004;92:179–229.
16. Dronkers NF, Wilkins DP, Van Valin RD, Redfern BB, Jaeger JJ. Lesion analysis of the brain areas involved in language comprehension. Cognition. 2004;92:145–77.
17. Gainotti G. What the locus of brain lesion tells us about the nature of the cognitive defect underlying category-specific disorders: a review. Cortex. 2000;36:539–59.
18. Martin A, Chao LL. Semantic memory in the brain: structure and processes. Curr Opin Neurobiol. 2001;11:194–201.
19. Mummery CJ, Patterson K, Wise RJ, Vandenberghe R, Price CJ, Hodges JR. Disrupted temporal lobe connections in semantic dementia. Brain. 1999;122(Pt 1):61–73.
20. Thompson-Schill SL. Neuroimaging studies of semantic memory: inferring "how" from "where". Neuropsychologia. 2003;41:280–92.
21. Binder JR, Desai RH, Graves WW, Conant LL. Where is the semantic system? A critical review and meta-analysis of 120 functional neuroimaging studies. Cereb Cortex. 2009;19(12):2767–96.
22. Badre D, Poldrack RA, Paré-Blagoev EJ, Insler RZ, Wagner AD. Dissociable controlled retrieval and generalized selection mechanisms in ventrolateral prefrontal cortex. Neuron. 2005;47:907–18.
23. Gardner HE, Lambon Ralph MA, Dodds N, Jones T, Ehsan S, Jefferies E. The differential contributions of pFC and temporo-parietal cortex to multimodal semantic control: exploring refractory effects in semantic aphasia. J Cogn Neurosci. 2012;24:778–93.
24. Noonan KA, Jefferies E, Corbett F, Lambon Ralph MA. Elucidating the nature of deregulated semantic cognition in semantic aphasia: evidence for the roles of prefrontal and temporo-parietal cortices. J Cogn Neurosci. 2010;22:1597–613.
25. Noonan KA, Jefferies E, Visser M, Lambon Ralph MA. Going beyond inferior prefrontal involvement in semantic control: evidence for the additional contribution of dorsal angular gyrus and posterior middle temporal cortex. J Cogn Neurosci. 2013;25:1824–50.
26. Thompson-Schill SL, Desposito M, Aguirre GK, Farah MJ. Role of left inferior prefrontal cortex in retrieval of semantic knowledge: a reevaluation. Proc Natl Acad Sci U S A. 1997;94:14792–7.
27. Wagner AD, Pare-Blagoev EJ, Clark J, Poldrack RA. Recovering meaning: left prefrontal cortex guides controlled semantic retrieval. Neuron. 2001;31:329–38.
28. Snowden JS, Goulding PJ, Neary D. Semantic dementia: a form of circumscribed cerebral atrophy. Behav Neurol. 1989;2:111–38.
29. Warrington EK. The selective impairment of semantic memory. Q J Exp Psychol. 1975;27:635–57.
30. Acosta-Cabronero J, Patterson K, Fryer TD, Hodges JR, Pengas G, Williams GB, et al. Atrophy, hypometabolism and white matter abnormalities in semantic dementia tell a coherent story. Brain. 2011;134:2025–35.
31. Agosta F, Henry RG, Migliaccio R, Neuhaus J, Miller BL, Dronkers NF, et al. Language networks in semantic dementia. Brain. 2010;133:286–99.
32. Desgranges B, Matuszewski V, Piolino P, Chetelat G, Mezenge F, Landeau B, et al. Anatomical and functional alterations in semantic dementia: a voxel-based MRI and PET study. Neurobiol Aging. 2007;28:1904–13.
33. Hodges JR, Patterson K. Semantic dementia: a unique clinicopathological syndrome. Lancet Neurol. 2007;6:1004–14.
34. Mesulam MM, Wieneke C, Hurley R, Rademaker A, Thompson CK, Weintraub S, et al. Words and objects at the tip of the left temporal lobe in primary progressive aphasia. Brain. 2013;136:601–18.

35. Lambon Ralph MA, Patterson K. Generalisation and differentiation in semantic memory: insights from semantic dementia. Ann N Y Acad Sci. 2008;1124:61–76.
36. Lambon Ralph MA, Pobric G, Jefferies E. Conceptual knowledge is underpinned by the temporal pole bilaterally: convergent evidence from rTMS. Cereb Cortex. 2009;19:832–8.
37. Lambon Ralph MA, Cipolotti L, Manes F, Patterson K. Taking both sides: do unilateral anterior temporal lobe lesions disrupt semantic memory? Brain. 2010;133:3243–55.
38. Schapiro AC, McClelland JL, Welbourne SR, Rogers TT, Lambon Ralph MA. Why bilateral damage is worse than unilateral damage to the brain. J Cogn Neurosci. 2013;25:2107–23.
39. Lambon Ralph MA, Ehsan S, Baker GA, Rogers TT. Semantic memory is impaired in patients with unilateral anterior temporal lobe resection for temporal lobe epilepsy. Brain. 2012;135(Pt 1):242–58.
40. Reilly M, Machado N, Blumstein SE. Hemispheric lateralization of semantic feature distinctiveness. Neuropsychologia. 2015;75:99–108.
41. Rice GE, Lambon Ralph MA, Hoffman P. The roles of left versus right anterior temporal lobes in conceptual knowledge: an ALE meta-analysis of 97 functional neuroimaging studies. Cereb Cortex. 2015;25(11):4374–91.
42. Rice GE, Caswell H, Moore P, Lambon Ralph MA, Hoffman P. Revealing the dynamic modulations that underpin a resilient neural network for semantic cognition: an fMRI investigation in patients with anterior temporal lobe resection. Cereb Cortex. 2018;28(8):3004–16.
43. Almairac F, Herbet G, Moritz-Gasser S, de Champfleur NM, Duffau H. The left inferior fronto-occipital fasciculus subserves language semantics: a multilevel lesion study. Brain Struct Funct. 2015;220(4):1983–95.
44. Duffau H, Gatignol P, Mandonnet E, Peruzzi P, Tzourio-Mazoyer N, Capelle L. New insights into the anatomo-functional connectivity of the semantic system: a study using cortico-subcortical electrostimulations. Brain. 2005;128(Pt 4):797–810.
45. Duffau H. The anatomo-functional connectivity of language revisited. New insights provided by electrostimulation and tractography. Neuropsychologia. 2008;46(4):927–34.
46. Hickok G, Poeppel D. Dorsal and ventral streams: a framework for understanding aspects of the functional anatomy of language. Cognition. 2004;92(1–2):67–99.
47. Moritz-Gasser S, Herbet G, Duffau H. Mapping the connectivity underlying multimodal (verbal and non-verbal) semantic processing: a brain electrostimulation study. Neuropsychologia. 2013;51(10):1814–22.
48. Papagno C, Miracapill C, Casarotti A, Lauro R, Leonor J, Castellano A, et al. What is the role of the uncinate fasciculus? Surgical removal and proper name retrieval. Brain. 2011;134(Pt 2):405–14.
49. Saur D, Kreher BW, Schnell S, Kümmerer D, Kellmeyer P, Vry MS, et al. Ventral and dorsal pathways for language. Proc Natl Acad Sci U S A. 2008;105(46):18035–40.
50. Tremblay P, Dick AS. Broca and Wernicke are dead, or moving past the classic model of language neurobiology. Brain Lang. 2016;162:60–71.
51. Turken AU, Dronkers NF. The neural architecture of the language comprehension network: converging evidence from lesion and connectivity analyses. Front Syst Neurosci. 2011;5:1.
52. Duffau H, Moritz-Gasser S, Mandonnet E. A re-examination of neural basis of language processing: proposal of a dynamic hodotopical model from data provided by brain stimulation mapping during picture naming. Brain Lang. 2014;131:1–10.
53. Martino J, Brogna C, Gil Robles S, Vergani F, Duffau H. Anatomic dissection of the inferior fronto-occipital fasciculus revisited in the lights of brain stimulation data. Cortex. 2010;46:691–9.
54. Catani M, Howard RJ, Pajevic S, Jones DK. Virtual in vivo interactive dissection of white matter fasciculi in the human brain. Neuroimage. 2002;17:77–94.
55. Duffau H, Gatignol P, Moritz-Gasser S, Mandonnet E. Is the left uncinate fasciculus essential for language? A cerebral stimulation study. J Neurol. 2009;256(3):382–9.
56. Mandonnet E, Nouet A, Gatignol P, Capelle L, Duffau H. Does the left inferior longitudinal fasciculus play a role in language? A brain stimulation study. Brain. 2007;130(Pt 3):623–9.

57. Martino J, de Lucas EM. Subcortical anatomy of the lateral association fascicles of the brain: a review. Clin Anat. 2014;27:563–9.
58. Catani M, Dell'acqua F, Thiebaut de Schotten M. A revised limbic system model for memory, emotion and behaviour. Neurosci Biobehav Rev. 2013;37(8):1724–37.
59. Moritz-Gasser S, Herbet G, Duffau H. Integrating emotional valence and semantics in the human ventral stream: a hodological account. Front Psychol. 2015;6:32.
60. Sarubbo S, de Benedictis A, Maldonado IL, Basso G, Duffau H. Frontal terminations for the inferior fronto-occipital fascicle: anatomical dissection, DTI study and functional considerations on a multi-component bundle. Brain Struct Funct. 2013;218(1):21–37.
61. Duffau H, Herbet G, Moritz-Gasser S. Toward a pluri-component, multimodal, and dynamic organization of the ventral semantic stream in humans: lessons from stimulation mapping in awake patients. Front Syst Neurosci. 2013;7:44.
62. De Witte E, Mariën P. The neurolinguistic approach to awake surgery reviewed. Clin Neurol Neurosurg. 2013;115(2):127–45.
63. Ruis C. Monitoring cognition during awake brain surgery in adults: a systematic review. J Clin Exp Neuropsychol. 2018;40(10):1081–104.
64. Skrap M, Marin D, Ius T, Fabbro F, Tomasino B. Brain mapping: a novel intraoperative neuropsychological approach. J Neurosurg. 2016;125(4):877–87.
65. Faulkner JW, Wilshire CE, Parker AJ, Cunningham K. An evaluation of language in brain tumor patients using a new cognitively motivated testing protocol. Neuropsychology. 2017;31(6):648–65.
66. Campanella F, Crescentini C, Mussoni A, Skrap M. Refractory semantic access dysphasia resulting from resection of a left frontal glioma. Neurocase. 2013;19(1):27–35.
67. De Witte E, Satoer D, Robert E, Colle H, Verheyen S, Visch-Brink E, Mariën P. The Dutch Linguistic Intraoperative Protocol: a valid linguistic approach to awake brain surgery. Brain Lang. 2015;140:35–48.
68. Campanella F, Mondani M, Skrap M, Shallice T. Semantic access dysphasia resulting from left temporal lobe tumours. Brain. 2009;132(1):87–102.
69. Sierpowska J, Gabarrós A, Fernández-Coello A, Camins À, Castañer S, Juncadella M, François C, Rodríguez-Fornells A. White-matter pathways and semantic processing: intrasurgical and lesion-symptom mapping evidence. Neuroimage Clin. 2019;22:101704.
70. Herbet G, Moritz-Gasser S, Boiseau M, Duvaux S, Cochereau J, Duffau H. Converging evidence for a cortico-subcortical network mediating lexical retrieval. Brain. 2016;139(11):3007–21.
71. Mandonnet E, Herbet G, Duffau H. Letter: introducing new tasks for intraoperative mapping in awake glioma surgery: clearing the line between patient care and scientific research. Neurosurgery. 2020;86(2):E256–7.
72. Fernández Coello A, Moritz-Gasser S, Martino J, Martinoni M, Matsuda R, Duffau H. Selection of intraoperative tasks for awake mapping based on relationships between tumor location and functional networks. J Neurosurg. 2013;119(6):1380–94.
73. Połczyńska M. New tests for language mapping with intraoperative electrical stimulation of the brain to preserve language in individuals with tumors and epilepsy: a preliminary follow-up study. In: Poznan studies in contemporary linguistics. 2009. p. 261–79.
74. Rofes A, Spena G, Miozzo A, Fontanella MM, Miceli G. Advantages and disadvantages of intraoperative language tasks in awake surgery: a three-task approach for prefrontal tumors. J Neurosurg Sci. 2015;59(4):337–49.
75. Adlam AL, Patterson K, Bozeat S, Hodges JR. The Cambridge Semantic Memory Test Battery: detection of semantic deficits in semantic dementia and Alzheimer's disease. Neurocase. 2010;16(3):193–207.
76. Bozeat S, Lambon Ralph MA, Patterson K, Garrard P, Hodges JR. Non-verbal semantic impairment in semantic dementia. Neuropsychologia. 2000;38(9):1207–15.
77. Gatignol P, Capelle L, Le Bihan R, Duffau H. Double dissociation between picture naming and comprehension: an electrostimulation study. Neuroreport. 2004;15(1):191–5.
78. Kremin H. Spared naming without comprehension. J Neurolinguistics. 1986;2(1–2):131–50.

79. Silveri MC, Colosimo C. Hypothesis on the nature of comprehension deficit in a patient with transcortical mixed aphasia with preserved naming. Brain Lang. 1995;49(1):1–26.
80. Howard D, Patterson KE. The Pyramids and Palm Trees Test: a test of semantic access from words and pictures. St. Edmunds: Thames Valley Test Company; 1992.
81. Tran TM, Godefroy O. La Batterie d'Évaluation des Troubles Lexicaux: effet des variables démographiques et linguistiques, reproductibilité et seuils préliminaires. Rev Neuropsychol. 2011;1(3):52–69.
82. Merck C, Charnallet A, Auriacombe S, Belliard S, Hahn-Barma V, Kremin H, et al. La batterie d'évaluation des connaissances sémantiques du GRECO (BECS-GRECO): validation et données normatives. Rev Neuropsychol. 2011;4(3):235–55.
83. Duffau H, Mandonnet E. The "onco-functional balance" in surgery for diffuse low-grade glioma: integrating the extent of resection with quality of life. Acta Neurochir (Wien). 2013;155(6):951–7.
84. Sarubbo S, Tate M, De Benedictis A, Merler S, Moritz-Gasser S, Herbet G, Duffau H. Mapping critical cortical hubs and white matter pathways by direct electrical stimulation: an original functional atlas of the human brain. Neuroimage. 2020;205:116237.
85. Tate MC, Herbet G, Moritz-Gasser S, Tate JE, Duffau H. Probabilistic map of critical functional regions of the human cerebral cortex: Broca's area revisited. Brain. 2014;137(Pt 10):2773–82.
86. Herbet G, Moritz-Gasser S, Duffau H. Electrical stimulation of the dorsolateral prefrontal cortex impairs semantic cognition. Neurology. 2018;90(12):e1077–84.
87. Duffau H. Stimulation mapping of white matter tracts to study brain functional connectivity. Nat Rev Neurol. 2015;11(5):255–65.
88. Hau J, Sarubbo S, Perchey G, Crivello F, Zago L, Mellet E, Jobard G, Joliot M, Mazoyer BM, Tzourio-Mazoyer N, Petit L. Cortical terminations of the inferior fronto-occipital and uncinate fasciculi: anatomical stem-based virtual dissection. Front Neuroanat. 2016;10:58.
89. Wu Y, Sun D, Wang Y, Wang Y. Subcomponents and connectivity of the inferior fronto-occipital fasciculus revealed by diffusion spectrum imaging fiber tracking. Front Neuroanat. 2016;10:88.
90. Herbet G, Moritz-Gasser S, Duffau H. Direct evidence for the contributive role of the right inferior fronto-occipital fasciculus in non-verbal semantic cognition. Brain Struct Funct. 2017;222(4):1597–610.
91. Mirman D, Chen Q, Zhang Y, Wang Z, Faseyitan OK, Coslett HB, Schwartz MF. Neural organization of spoken language revealed by lesion-symptom mapping. Nat Commun. 2015;6:6762.

Inhibition

16

Jérôme Cochereau, Michel Wager, Marco Rossi, Antonella Leonetti, Tommaso Sciortino, Lorenzo Bello, and Guglielmo Puglisi

16.1 Introduction

Awake surgery of brain tumors has led to a paradigmatic shift consisting of an increased interest in assessing the functional consequences of surgical procedures. It has clearly demonstrated its great effectiveness in preserving functions supported by primary or unimodal cortex. However, only a few studies have focused on the value of awake surgery to preserve higher order functions such as executive functions. Inhibition is a pervasive cognitive control process, needed in many everyday life situations, and particularly when threatening events occur, such as holding back the suction device while operating a patient who starts producing errors to peroperative tests during an awake surgery. Subjects with impaired inhibitory control can present with impulsivity, perseverative behavior, and distractibility [1–4]. It has been implicated in multiple psychopathological conditions such as attention deficit hyperactivity disorder and obsessive compulsive disorder [5]. The purpose of this chapter is to provide the reader a comprehensive understanding of inhibitory control

J. Cochereau · M. Wager (✉)
Neurosurgery Department, Poitiers University Hospital, Poitiers, France
e-mail: Jerome.COCHEREAU@chu-poitiers.fr; Michel.WAGER@chu-poitiers.fr

M. Rossi · T. Sciortino · L. Bello
Department of Oncology and Hemato-Oncology, Università degli studi di Milano, Milan, Italy

Neurosurgical Oncological Unit, IRCCS Istituto Ortopedico Galeazzi, Milan, Italy
e-mail: marco.rossi2@unimi.it; lorenzo.bello@unimi.it

A. Leonetti · G. Puglisi
Neurosurgical Oncological Unit, IRCCS Istituto Ortopedico Galeazzi, Milan, Italy

MOCA Lab, Department of Medical Biotechnologies and Translational Medicine, Università degli Studi di Milano, Milan, Italy
e-mail: antonella.leonetti@unimi.it

E. Mandonnet, G. Herbet (eds.), *Intraoperative Mapping of Cognitive Networks*,
https://doi.org/10.1007/978-3-030-75071-8_16

processes applied to neurosurgical patients and to initiate a discussion on the relevance of peroperative inhibition monitoring during awake surgery.

16.2 Neural Basis of Inhibition

16.2.1 Definition

Inhibitory control, as part of the three core executive functions (EF), i.e., cognitive flexibility, inhibition, and working memory [1, 2], corresponds to multiple taxonomies. However, one commonly admitted segregation of this multifaceted concept is to consider inhibition as a twofold concept comprising behavioral and cognitive inhibition [2, 3]. The former refers to response inhibition, deferred gratification, and reversal learning while the latter relates to the inhibition of prepotent memories, perceptions, thoughts, and emotions. Response inhibition is by far the most studied phenomenon as it can be easily experimentally implemented in motor response inhibition paradigms that involve the inhibition of prepotent and automatic motor responses. According to the taxonomy we employ, interference control, i.e., the cognitive control needed to prevent irrelevant stimuli to interfere with a goal-directed behavior, can be part of both types of inhibitory control described above or considered as a separate type of inhibitory control process [4].

16.2.2 Inhibition Tests

In clinical settings, diverse tests address inhibitory mechanisms, though whether such tasks isolate processes of response inhibition remain controversial, as opposed to related processes such as response selection, conflict resolution, attention, and working memory [5].

For the purpose of our chapter, we briefly recall the main features of some of the commonly used tests. Motor response inhibition is frequently assessed by the go-no-go and the stop-signal reaction-time tasks. Interference control can be evaluated by the Stroop color-word interference test and the Eriksen flanker task.

In a **go-no-go task**, a cue tells participants to respond or withhold responding to "go" and "no-go" stimuli, respectively. The more frequent the go trials, the higher the prepotency of the response and the errors likelihood.

In the **stop-signal reaction-time task**, go trials require responding to arrows pointing right or left. In some of the trials, the go signal is followed after a variable delay by a "stop" signal that requires participants hold their response [6]. It is a measure of speed of inhibition. Task variations—including changing the probability of stop signals, influencing the participant's certainty of go trials, or using selective-stopping trials—alter the balance of engagement of proactive versus reactive strategies.

In the **Stroop color-word interference test**, participants name the ink colors of color words that are printed in concordant or discordant ink. The delay in reaction time between congruent and incongruent stimuli, namely the Stroop effect, is influenced by the process of inhibition of the prepotent response [7].

During an **Eriksen flanker task**, the subject is asked to indicate the direction the center arrow is pointing as quickly as possible, while ignoring flanking arrows that, on some trials, point in the opposite direction. Reaction times are faster when the response indicated by the central stimulus is consistent with the response indicated by the flanking stimuli than when these are incompatible [8]. It reflects the process of interference inhibition.

16.2.3 Neural Substrates of Inhibition

16.2.3.1 Neural Processes in Behavioral and Cognitive Inhibition. Same or Different?

There has been much debate in the field of inhibitory control neuroscience about the very existence of inhibitory processes in what is called cognitive inhibition [9, 10] whereas behavioral inhibition is readily accepted as an inhibitory process, and as a consequence, the generalizability of behavioral inhibition models to cognitive inhibition is not straightforward [11, 12]. To challenge that question, although cognitive inhibition is not as readily studied as motor inhibition due to the absence of overt behavioral measures, several studies have assessed the differences and similarities between these two phenomena thanks to the design of "cognitive" versions of the go-no-go test. For example, based on a "Think/no think" procedure [13], Anderson et al. *evidenced a bilaterally* increased activation of a cognitive control network, and especially the dorsolateral prefrontal cortex (DLPFC), a region formally known to participate to response inhibition [14], along with a deactivation of the hippocampus during trials where the subjects were asked to inhibit thoughts [15]. In their review, although they mention different prefrontal areas specifically implicated in diverse types of cognitive inhibition processes (namely the orbitofrontal cortex and the ventromedial prefrontal cortex, respectively associated with inhibition of cognitive sets and fear extinction), Dillon and Pizzagalli underline the implication of the right ventrolateral prefrontal cortex (VLPFC) in all types of inhibition processes [16]. In line with that observation, a more recent experience carried out by Tabibnia et al. using voxel-based morphometry on patients suffering from methamphetamine dependence compared to controls showed first that motor and affective inhibitory control in these patients were correlated and second that inhibitory control scores correlated to the right pars opercularis gray matter intensity [17].

To conclude, it would appear that cognitive and behavioral inhibition share overlapping processes distributed in the same cortical areas, i.e., the DLPFC and the right VLPFC, but also involve various additional cortical regions according to the inhibited cognitive function at hand [3]. Consequently, the study of response inhibition can shed a light on the key neural processes at play in inhibition. Moreover, as response inhibition can be rather easily implemented in an awake surgery paradigm [18, 19], the rest of that subchapter will focus on experimental results emanating from studies of response inhibition.

16.2.3.2 Neural Basis of Response Inhibition

The Modular Theory of Inhibition

The go-no-go and the stop-signal reaction-time tasks are both widely represented in response inhibition studies. These tasks, applied to patients with prefrontal cortex damage, drew attention on two regions correlated with delayed reaction time or errors in no-go trials, i.e., the right VLPFC [20] and the dorsomedial prefrontal cortex, namely the pre-supplementary motor area (pre-SMA) [21, 22]. These lesion studies have been supplemented by neuroimaging and neurodisruption experiments that confirmed the implication of both cortical areas in response inhibition [14, 23–26]. Together with those two key regions, premotor cortex, DLPFC, parietal cortex, insula, and basal ganglia seem to all be implicated in inhibitory control [22, 26–30]. The inhibitory subprocess carried by the right inferior frontal cortex (IFC) is equivocal and Aron stipulated that the right IFC could suppress basal ganglia outputs, probably via the subthalamic nucleus [12]. Rather than the sole activity of the IFC, a more elaborated theory suggested that the interplay between the right IFC and the pre-SMA leads to the suppression of ongoing motor plans via their mutual and respective connectivity with the subthalamic nucleus (STN) [31]. Interestingly, Duann et al. showed, using Granger causality, that the IFC, as part of the ventral attention system, could respond to stop signals and subsequently synchronize with the pre-SMA, involved in goal-directed behavior, that exerts its modulatory effect on the STN to pause a prepotent response [32]. Parietal cortex is naturally involved in response inhibition as visuospatial attention is constantly requested and modulated by the top-down effects of the prefrontal cortex [28]. The DLPFC has been identified as a pivotal hub of the cognitive control network [33], and its participation to response inhibition can be likened to maintenance of task rules in working memory as its level of activation has been related to increased working memory load [14, 29]. Activations of the insular cortex are also observed and can be related to interference resolution processes when conflicting responses are activated [34, 35].

The Role of the Left Hemisphere in Inhibitory Control

As defective response inhibition can be observed after a left hemisphere damage [36], the lateralization of response inhibition is strongly debated [3]. Indeed, the left IFC has been implicated in rule maintenance and retrieval [37] which is necessary for response inhibition efficiency, as demonstrated by Hirose et al. who correlated brain activity with the subjects' performances in go-no-go trials, revealing a left-sided cortical network encompassing notably the IFC and the inferior parietal cortex [38].

The Network Perspective on Inhibitory Control

More recently, the theory of inhibitory modules in the prefrontal cortex has been challenged. More specifically, the right IFC is no longer considered as a region involved in inhibitory control but rather an area belonging to the multiple demand system [39] with no specificity for inhibition. In that respect, inhibition would just be an example of the cognitive control processes supported by the same set of "domain general" functional networks [40]; hence inhibition would not rely on a dedicated network. Cortical regions that are "domain general" have the ability to rapidly adapt to support a variety of novel or demanding tasks [41]. In their review, by concatenating results of researches on various forms of cognitive control, Hampshire and Sharp make the assumption that domain general networks exert control by modulating local inhibitory connections (known as lateral inhibition) [42]. Neurons from the multiple demand system have the specific capability to rapidly switch in multiple states and subsequently settle into a stable low-activity state which adapts in function of the current task-relevant rule [43]. According to their theory, in the face of a nonroutine task, the multiple demand system is warned, resulting in a temporary program coding for top-down signals that will potentiate task-relevant processes in visual and motor areas according to the current task-relevant rule. Competing processes, including routine automatic motor responses, are then downregulated via lateral inhibition. This theory accounts well with the fact that right IFC/anterior insula activations during a stop-signal task attenuate sharply as the task becomes more familiar [41].

White Matter Correlates of Inhibition Processes

As discussed above, inhibition is a component of cognitive control processes that relies on widely distributed networks; hence a well-organized long range structural connectivity subserving those networks is mandatory to ensure efficient control. This white matter connectivity is not yet well described though this knowledge is crucial to anyone who aims to preserve those functions per operatively. In Aron's modular framework, it has been hypothesized that the right IFC, pre-SMA, and subthalamic nucleus were one by one connected leading to a functional and structural core for inhibition [31]. By controlling for processing speed in a go-no-go task, Hinton et al. found a significant correlation between the right IFG and STN structural connectivity and task performance [44]. The tract that connects IFC and pre-SMA is consistent with the frontal aslant tract (FAT); hence it has been suggested that the right FAT could play a role in inhibitory control [45], but this hypothesis has been challenged by the results of white matter direct stimulations that have highlighted the role of fronto-striatal tracts rather than the FAT [46]. Finally, given the fact that inhibition is a bilaterally represented process and that it relies on frontoparietal top-down modulations, both the corpus callosum and frontoparietal tracts should be involved. As a matter of fact, a correlation has been evidenced between an inhibition and both the corpus callosum and cingulum bundle [19, 47]. Moreover, the superior longitudinal fasciculus that connects the lateral aspects of frontal and parietal lobes seems to contribute to interference resolution processes [48].

16.3 Evidence of Long-Term Deficits in Patients Who Did Not Benefit from Intraoperative Inhibition Monitoring

Except in some rare neurosurgical centers [18, 19], executive function monitoring is not routinely performed during awake surgery [49]; hence one may interrogate if patients frequently suffer from inhibition impairment following such surgeries. That is, of course, an important question because it determines the need for such a monitoring if inhibition deficits frequently occur.

Besides, determining the exact impact of surgery on inhibition performance is challenging as studies interested in neuropsychological outcome after brain surgery readily refer to "executive functions" in general rather than its specific subcomponents. The delay between surgery and neuropsychological assessment is another important factor as executive functioning may improve or worsen between two postoperative timepoints. Indeed, executive functions worsening can be expected early after surgery (3 months) and can recover, at least partially, 6 months after surgery [50]. On the contrary, *Satoer* et al. reported interference inhibition worsening 1 year after surgery compared to 3 months after surgery although no worsening at 3 months post-surgery compared to the preoperative status was reported [51]. Those inconsistent findings may account for cohort inhomogeneities in terms of surgical results, natural disease evolution, and evaluation timing.

Although awake surgery (without executive functions mapping) readily leads to less (though not avoiding) postoperative executive dysfunctions than asleep surgery according to a recent meta-analysis [52], some other authors argue that it is more prone to cause deficits (notably in the Stroop test) as awake surgery leads to more extensive resections blinded from the unscreened functions [53].

The rationale of inhibition monitoring has been explored as a tool to preserve executive functions by Puglisi et al. as at 3 months after surgery, in a subset of 45 patients operated from a frontal nondominant hemisphere glioma, they showed a raised prevalence of executive dysfunctions of 22% and 61% in the Stroop monitored and Stroop non-monitored groups, respectively (statistically significant difference) [18]. However, executive dysfunction also occurs when tumors are located in the dominant hemisphere and/or in non-frontal regions [54].

To conclude, the actual literature provides some evidences of long-lasting surgically related inhibition deficits, but the real impact of those deficits in terms of quality of life, though addressed in other clinical populations, remains to be addressed in brain tumor patients.

16.4 Review About Knowledge Gained from Lesion-Symptom Mapping

16.4.1 Eligibility Criteria of Publications for This Research

Studies of patients with ischemic stroke or head injury were excluded as they did not allow a sufficiently precise definition of the affected anatomical regions and structures, and therefore no pathophysiological inferences. We have also discarded studies that explicitly evaluated global executive functions—usually conducted in these same patients. Finally, animal studies were discarded for fear that the conclusions drawn in animals—even primates—would not lend themselves well to extrapolation to humans for the function at hand. As a result of these limitations, only eight studies in the literature were found to meet all of these criteria. Finally, one of these studies [55] is not precise enough in its description of the cortical areas concerned to integrate it into the discussion in hodological terms. It was therefore not taken into account in the discussion.

16.4.2 Studies Involving a Single Cortical Lesion Site per Patient

The main characteristics of the selected studies appear in Table 16.1. These studies document an initial finding, which is that a single cortical lesion may be associated with lasting impairment—up to several years—of at least one aspect of executive function, namely inhibition. However, according to Lashley's principle of mass action, a focal lesion of a non-primary cortex has no noticeable functional repercussion, and especially not a lasting one [56]. However, the areas cited in these studies are not primary areas. On the other hand, these studies establish associations, which is not causality. Thus, the lasting nature of the observed deficits raises the question of the effect not of the cortical lesion itself, but of an alternative explanation associated with the cortical lesion.

From a hodological perspective, the possibility of the associated disconnection of a white matter tract—like Broca's famous patient—can be evoked. Under this hypothesis, it is no longer the responsibility of a cortical lesion that would be considered, but that of the whole formed by this damaged cortical area and a white matter bundle associated with it. As an example, this approach seems to be quite congruent when it comes to the inferior frontal gyrus as identified by Aron [20, 57]. For each cortical lesion it is thus possible to propose candidate bundles. Finally, in view of the proven functional importance of each of the abovementioned bundles, it will be possible to examine which aspect of the executive functions could be affected: either directly (e.g., by impairment of working memory, or attention), or indirectly (e.g., a slower verbal flow, resulting in longer response times).

Alexander loops describe cortical-subcortical networks including frontal areas [58]. These five loops carry a variety of functional meanings, some of which are likely to find a place in the neurobiological bases of executive functions. This raises the question of which of the Alexander loops the cortical areas identified in these studies fall within. All the more so since, for example, the unique target of the "lateral fronto-orbital circuit" loop is precisely the lateral frontal-orbital cortex.

Table 16.1 Studies mapping inhibition deficits to brain lesions locations

First author Year	Lesions	Time from lesion to neuropsychological assessment (latest)	Number of patients	Tests	Brain areas involved
Cochereau 2020 [63]	Diffuse low-grade gliomas	Mean 6.5 months	238 patients	Stroop color naming test	Left frontal aslant tract Left superior longitudinal fasciculus (SLF II and SLF III)
Puglisi 2019 [46]	Right frontal gliomas	One month	63 patients	Stroop color naming test	Right inferior fronto-striatal tracts
Santillo 2016 [61]	Fronto temporal dementia and supra-nuclear palsy	Non-applicable	21 patients 25 control	Hayling test and frontal behavioral inventory Cortical thickness Anisotropy fraction	Right Temporo polar—Orbitofrontal cortex/insula/and Uncinate-anterior cingular cortex
Tsuchida, A Cortex 2012 [60]	Bleeding Tumors	Median: 4 years	45 patients 50 control	Stroop color naming task Attention shifting task	LEFT vlPFC damage led to impaired performance on both tasks
Picton 2007 [22]	"Focal lesions" Bleedings Tumors Traumas	More than 3.5 months	43 patients 38 control	Go-No-go	– Right anterior cingulate cortex (AB 24 and 32) – Prefrontal ventrolateral cortex (AB 44, 45, 47)
Aron 2004 [57]	Hematomas Resected meningiomas	Three years	Right-sided lesions: 19 patients and Left-sided lesions: 17 patients and 20 control	Task-switching Inhibition measured by stop-signal task	– Right IFG (pars opercularis) – Top-down control/left MFG

Table 16.1 (continued)

First author Year	Lesions	Time from lesion to neuropsychological assessment (latest)	Number of patients	Tests	Brain areas involved
Aron 2003 [20]	Hematomas Resected meningiomas	Three years	18 patients and 16 control	Stop-signal	– Right IFG (pars triangularis)
Drewe 1975 [55]	Various	Three years	48 patients: 12 FF only, 12 RF only, 12 Non-FR only, 12 Non-FL only	Go-No-Go	Worse when "frontal lesions"

At the end of these approaches, one may wonder for each fascicle and each loop whether they would be likely to participate in a "behavioral" (i.e., limbic) or rather "cognitive" (i.e., neocortical) component of inhibition.

16.4.2.1 Interest of These Studies

We consider these studies to be important for two reasons. Firstly, they draw the surgeon's attention to areas functionally at risk—whether this risk was subcortical more than cortical. Second, they stimulate discussion and guide future studies on the neural networks underlying these few epicenters that are flush with the cortical surface, because within a network it is highly likely that not all bundles are equally important.

16.4.2.2 Limitations of These Studies

According to the results of the studies by Miyake [1], then Stuss [59], and Tsuchida [60], the interdependence of executive functions does not allow them to be studied in isolation. This seems to us consistent with a hodological approach which, as we can see from the above, quickly leads to networks that necessarily have cortical areas and/or white matter tracts in common. Moreover, in the absence of persistent handicap documented in the literature, there would be, on the sole basis of the results of very specific tests, a surgical risk of "under-treatment." Another limitation of these studies is that they did not include an assessment of quality of life, as they focused on test performance.

16.4.3 Study Involving Several Cortical Sites per Patient

One study evaluated executive functions in patients with neurodegenerative diseases [61]. The authors observed that these patients exhibited simultaneous alterations in cortical thickness measured by MRI of several regions: right parahippocampal gyrus, right fronto-orbital cortex, right insula, as well as a decrease in the anisotropy fraction of the right uncinate and right anterior cingulum. And they observed the association of these findings with a loss of inhibition.

This unique observation raises several questions. The first is to examine whether the anatomical locations of the different atrophied regions, taken together, correspond to a known network, and whether this network would potentially be involved in a particular aspect of executive functions. If this were the case, this would be a strong argument in favor of the authors of this study's discovery of an executive-valence network undergoing involution—the alternative hypothesis of a chance association being very weak. The second would be to adopt the same approach for each site as has been proposed for single-site studies, i.e., which clusters are affected in terms of function by such atrophy.

16.4.3.1 Interest of This Study

It is striking that all the structures identified have a direct relationship with the "paralimbic belt." Three cortical structures—parahippocampal gyrus, insula, and fronto-orbital cortex—belong to it. The other two are very closely associated with it: the uncinate fascicle connects to the temporal pole (another paralimbic area) and the anterior cingulum (the cingulate cortex is also a paralimbic area). It can therefore be hypothesized to explain such an anatomical conjunction that these neurodegenerative diseases affect the paralimbic areas. On the other hand, if the "paralimbic belt" itself meets a cyto-architectonic and not a hodological definition, the fact remains that these structures are themselves involved in the limbic networks [62]. This association thus raises the question of the relationship between the limbic system and inhibition. This again refers to Alexander's loops, and particularly to the "anterior cingulate" loop. But also to the "lateral orbitofrontal circuit" loop, of which the lateral orbitofrontal cortex is the sole target.

16.4.3.2 Limitations of This Study

Given the plurality of structures involved in the disease, it is not possible to make a privileged hypothesis as to which epicenters are responsible for impaired inhibition—since, as we have seen, the paralimbic belt is not a network in itself. Moreover, given the neurodegenerative nature of this disease, it is not possible to identify the loss of autonomy specifically in relation to the function being studied.

16.4.4 Studies of Disconnection - Behavior mapping

Two studies to date have focused on the relationship between surgically induced structural disconnections in low-grade glioma patients and postoperative inhibition impairment. It turns out that certain subcortical rather than cortical disconnections give rise to permanent inhibition deficits [46, 63]. The former focused exclusively on patients operated from a right frontal low-grade glioma and outlined the implication of the right fronto-striatal connectivity in postoperative worsening in Stroop test performance which is consistent with Aron's model [31]. Figure 16.1 illustrates

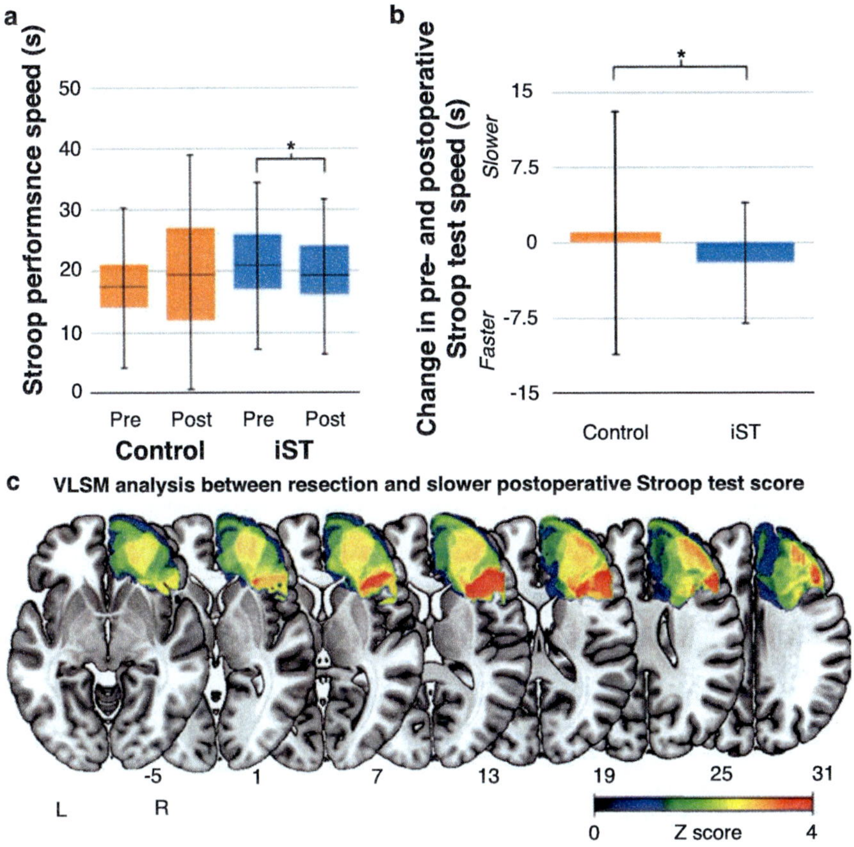

Fig. 16.1 The effect of resection on Stroop test performances. The effect of resection on behavioral outcome. (**a**) The change in Stroop performance time in the two groups (iST - intraoperative Stroop Test - and control group) at the different time points. $*p = 0.006$. (**b**) Change in performance on the Stroop test in the two groups measured as the difference between postoperative and preoperative test performance. Values >0 indicate postoperative test performance was slower and values <0 indicate postoperative test performance was higher; $*p = 0.03$. Both graphs are shown with 95% confidence intervals. (**c**) The resected brain regions identified by the voxel-based lesion-symptom analysis resulting in slower test performance on the Stroop test at 1 month in the entire group (63 patients). Only regions significant at $p < 0.05$ (corrected for multiple comparisons based on 5000 permutations) are presented. The MNI z-coordinates for each axial slice are displayed. (With permissions from Oxford University Press)

the main results of the study. The latter studied a cohort of diffuse low-grade glioma patients irrespective of the tumor location and found significant correlations between postoperative Stroop test performance worsening and both frontal intralobar (frontal aslant and fronto-striatal tracts) and frontoparietal connectivity, namely the second and third portions of the superior longitudinal fasciculus, which suggests the existence of a highly distributed network involved in inhibitory control (see Fig. 16.2).

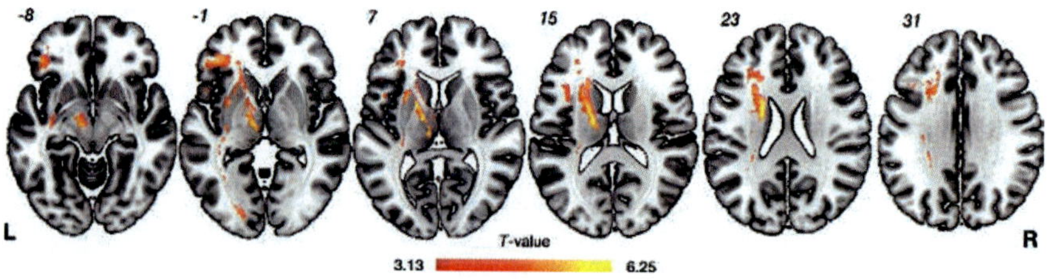

Fig. 16.2 Stroop test—white matter disconnections mapping. Stroop test (interference test, controlled for denomination impairment) disconnectome analysis in 238 patients operated from a diffuse low-grade glioma (both sides). Results are reported with an uncorrected p-value of 0.001 at the peak level and a FEW correction set at $p < 0.05$ at the cluster level. We notice disconnection hotspots in the left frontal, fronto-striatal, and frontoparietal white matter. (With permission from Springer)

16.4.5 The Issue of Right Lateralization

Right lesions are very generally encountered in works studying inhibition. The studies cited here are no exception (see Table 16.1). This finding is consistent with the association of inhibition with two other functions whose neurobiological bases are known to be strongly right lateralized: spatial cognition (SLF II and especially III) and working memory (SLF III) [1].

16.4.6 In Conclusion

Currently available studies document the association of certain frontal lesions with a persistent deficit of inhibition in clinical evaluations. Furthermore, the available data do not allow the exact nature of the underlying anatomical structures causing these deficits to be determined. On the clinical level, these studies therefore have the virtue of reminding the neurosurgeon that executive functions, although their neurobiological bases are widely distributed, are not invulnerable to the surgical gesture, and this message is important. However they do not make it possible today to establish recommendations regarding structures that would be surgical sanctuaries, at the risk of "under-treating" our patients. Further work is therefore necessary on this subject in order to design sound operating strategies in the future.

16.5 Review of the Different Tasks Newly Designed to Monitor Inhibitory Control Intraoperatively

Inhibitory control is a key construct in the domain of self-regulation and represents a very important target to preserve during brain tumor resection to maintain patients' quality of life. Basically, the measures of inhibitory control assess the ability to withhold or delay a prepotent/automatic response; an inhibitory control

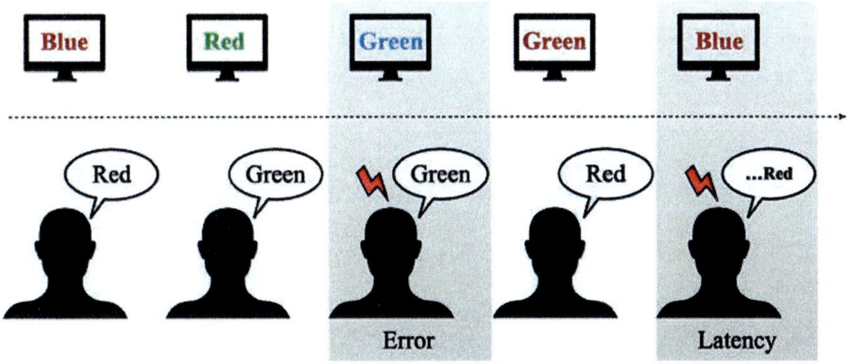

Fig. 16.3 Intraoperative Stroop task. The task consists of an adapted version of the Stroop task; one word at time was presented on a monitor and the patients are asked to name, as fast as they could, the color of the ink of the observed word presented on the monitor. The response of the patient is reported in the bubble below each illustrated monitor. The *red lightning* represents the time at which the direct electrical stimulation was applied

task usually requires (1) a stimulus (usually visual or auditory) eliciting an automatic or overlearned response (attentional redirection, thoughts, emotions, movement, or verbal output), (2) the inhibition of such a response, or (3) the inhibition of such a response in order to deliver a different and "correct" one. A classical test used to assess the inhibitory control in brain-damaged patients is the Stroop Color and Word test (see Fig. 16.3). In this task, subjects are required to look at a series of words describing colors (e.g., "green," "red," "blue" [stimuli]) and to report the color of the hue [task at hand to be accomplished]. Given that the words are written in an incongruent hue (e.g., the word "green" written in blue, "red" in green, etc.), the subject must suppress the prepotent and automatic tendency to read the word [inhibitory process], and, instead, name the color of the ink [correct response] [64]. Although inhibitory control deficits are often assessed [51, 65–68] during the pre- and postoperative evaluations, the intraoperative assessment of this function has been neglected for many years and only recently few groups started to develop intraoperative tools to this aim. To date, there are only three cohort studies reporting the use of a task specifically suited for the intraoperative assessment of inhibitory control process in adult patients, mainly operated for frontal nondominant tumors [18, 19, 46] and a single case study reporting the case of a young 16-year-old female patient operated on for a right fronto-insular tumor [69]. In all these studies, the tasks used during surgery are adapted versions of the classical Stroop test (see Fig. 16.3).

A relevant aspect in assessing intraoperatively the inhibitory processes is the definition of errors and of positive sites. In the setting of the Stroop task both the accuracy and the response time indicate a "failure" of inhibitory processes: a wrong response (patients read the colored word instead of saying the name of the color) or a delayed response (significantly longer than the average usual subject's response time, i.e., usually longer than 1 s) is considered as "errors." Generally, a stimulated site is considered as involved in a "function" (i.e., positive) when at least three non-consecutive stimulations stably produce the same function disruption (an error or a latency of response).

16.6 Review of Studies Documenting a Functional Improvement in Series of Brain Tumor Patients Operated on with or Without the Use of Inhibitory Control Mapping and Monitoring

Pre- or postoperative impairment of inhibitory processes has been repeatedly reported in brain tumor patients highlighting the importance to map and preserve this pivotal function [18, 46, 51, 65–68]. However, at now, there are only three cohort studies which reported the effectiveness and the feasibility of the use of an intraoperative task assessing the inhibitory control and only two of these studies compared the findings with those of a control group. Additionally, a single case report in a young patient is also available. In all these studies, the main aim was to develop an intraoperative task to improve the executive function focusing on the inhibitory control as one of its crucial components. Specifically, in his seminal work, Wager et al. [19] described the first intraoperative attempt to map the inhibitory process at cortical level by using an adapted version of the Stroop task in nine adult patients with frontal glioma, suggesting that mapping the inhibitory control during brain tumor surgery was feasible. The functional postoperative outcome showed a global preservation of executive functions: none of the nine patients had deficits in the postoperative assessment of inhibitory control process assessed by the extra-operative classical version of the Stroop test. However, two patients showed postoperative deficits in other executive domains (i.e., set shifting and divided attention) not documented in the preoperative assessment. More recently, the efficacy and feasibility of this task was assessed [18] at subcortical level in a larger sample of patients ($N = 27$ Stroop Group) operated for nondominant frontal lobe gliomas and compared to a retrospective control group of patients ($N = 18$ Control Group) who did not benefit from the task as they were operated before its introduction. While no significant difference in the incidence of executive function deficits (i.e., subnormal score in at least one test of the executive functions battery) between Stroop and control group were observed before surgery, the Stroop group patients had a statistically significant lower incidence of executive deficits compared to the control group patients at 1 and 3 months after surgery evaluation. Specifically, the analysis of the subcomponents of executive functions compromised in the long-term (3 months) showed that in the Stroop group, there are no patients developing postoperative inhibitory control deficits. However, other types of dysexecutive deficits were present in 22% of patients (i.e., verbal lexical speed/updating component of the executive functions). In contrast, 61% of the control group patients showed dysexecutive impairments in multiple domains (working memory, inhibitory control, lexical speed/updating). Notably, in a follow-up study on the use of the intraoperative Stroop task [46] the same authors showed that the group submitted to the intraoperative Stroop task performed better at follow-up in cognitive inhibition tests than in the preoperative phase, consistent with a well-described practice effect on Stroop performance [70–72]. Conversely, in the control group this effect was absent suggesting that the adapted intraoperative Stroop task is an effective tool for preserving inhibitory control of attention. In a recently published [69] single case report, a nonverbal variant (see NEPSI II inhibition sub-task) of the test was used to map inhibitory process in a 16-year-old female patient operated for fronto-insular tumor. Authors reported an improvement of inhibitory performances already in the immediate postoperative performances while a temporary impairment in lexical speed/updating. Taken together those studies suggest that the adapted versions of the Stroop test are an effective tool for preserving the inhibitory processes during brain tumor resection. However, since in all the above reported studies the analysis of postoperative outcome clearly showed that other components of executive functions (working memory, divided attention, lexical speed/updating) were still impaired, the intraoperative Stroop test cannot be considered as the tool able of mapping and preserving the global executive functioning, but should be implemented by the addition of other tools. A further issue raises from the fact that in all the studies in which the task was used intraoperatively, the resection was performed on right nondominant tumors. Future efforts should be put in implementing the assessment of inhibitory process also in patients with left hemisphere tumors. This is of importance to evaluate the role of a possible contralateral frontal lobe functional compensation in the post-surgical recovery.

16.6.1 Single Case

A 48-year-old subject was admitted to our Neuro-Oncological Surgery Unit after a generalized tonic–clonic seizure with morsus linguae and urinary incontinence. The MRI performed on admission displayed a right frontal lesion with no pathologic contrast enhancement compatible with a lower grade glioma (see Fig. 16.4). The tumor displayed no pathological methionine uptake at the 11C-methionine (Met) positron emission tomography (PET). The neurological and neuropsychological examinations at hospital admission were within normal ranges. Considering the radiological appearance, the optimal performance status and the absence of major comorbidities, after a multidisciplinary neuro-oncological evaluation, a surgical procedure under asleep-awake-asleep anesthesia was indicated and performed to achieve maximal safe tumor resection. Intraoperatively, cortical and subcortical mapping was performed to identify the morpho-functional boundaries for the resection: high-order functions mapped during the awake stage included haptic control (hand-manipulation test), language (semantic association task), and executive functions (Stroop test). The subcortical site where direct electrical stimulation determined a reliable interference with the Stroop Test is displayed below, overimposed to the postoperative MRI (black asterisk). Surgical resection was tailored according

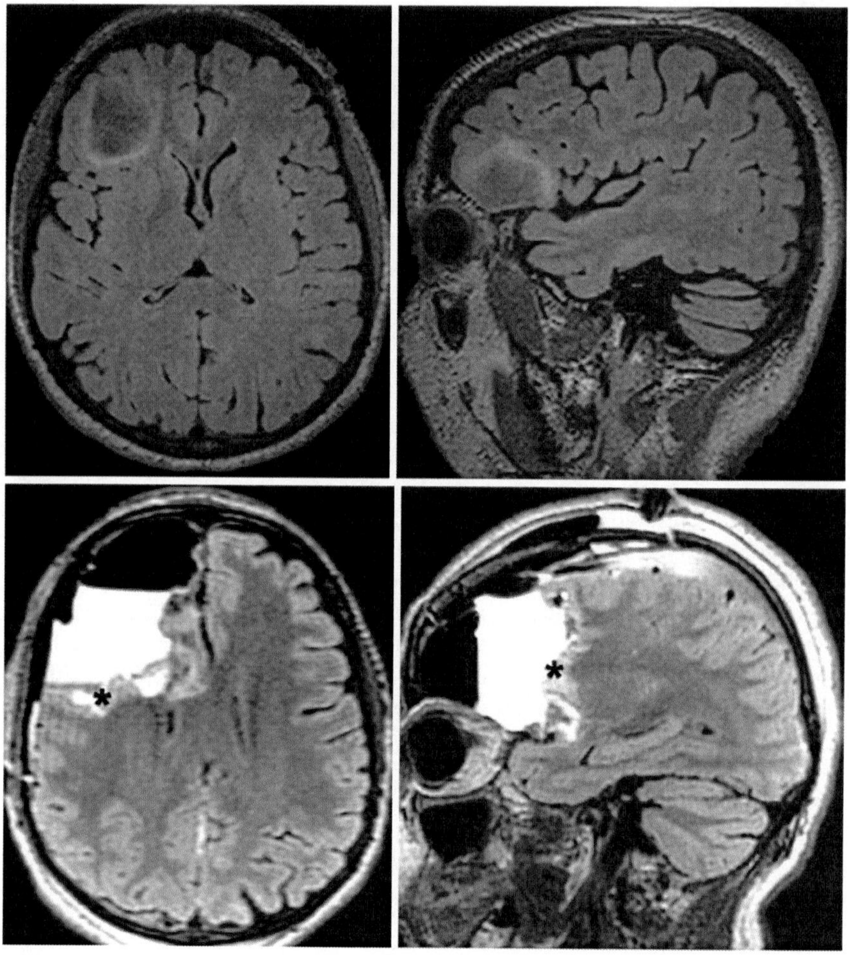

Fig. 16.4 Upper panel: preoperative MRI. Lower panel: postoperative MRI. Black asterisks represent the subcortical site where direct electrical stimulation determined a reliable interference with the Stroop Test

to this eloquent subcortical site, marking the posterior and deep functional limit of the surgical cavity. The postoperative course was regular, with no new-onset neurological deficit or irritative symptoms; the neuropsychological testing at the immediate postoperative phase (5 days) showed a mild deficit in processing speed and working memory. The neuropsychological status was normal 1 month after surgery. Pathological diagnosis was Anaplastic Astrocytoma (Grade III, WHO 2016), IDH-1 mutated. The patient was discharged 5 days after surgery and adjuvant therapies were initiated 1 month later.

16.7 Which Additional Anatomo-Functional Knowledge Has Been Gained from Intraoperative Mapping Studies

For many years, it has been presumed that the right hemisphere, except for motor or visual areas, was functionally "silent." Awake mapping is therefore usually restricted to tumors located in the language-dominant hemisphere or close to motor areas. However, in the last decade this view was significantly challenged by the identification of many higher order cognitive functions [73]. In fact, a growing body of evidence suggested that the right hemisphere plays a pivotal role in the inhibitory control [5]. Specifically, clinical and neuroimaging data described a right frontal network composed of cortico-cortical and cortico-subcortical regions, in the inferior frontal gyrus (IFG), dorsolateral prefrontal cortex, anterior cingulate and pre-supplementary motor area (pre-SMA), as well as the basal ganglia involved in the inhibitory control [74–80]. The awake neurosurgical setting offers the unique opportunity of testing these observations and offers new insights in the anatomo-functional organization of the inhibitory processes. Although at now few studies directly investigated with dedicated tools this function in the awake surgery setting, such initial results are intriguing. In the first study by Wager et al. [19] on nine patients underwent surgery for right hemisphere tumor, sites where stimulation interfered with the Stroop task execution were found in the posterior portion of anterior cingulate cortex (ACC) in both the right (ipsilesional) and left (contralateral) hemispheres. Interestingly, the resection of the right ACC did not impair the inhibitory processes as documented by the postoperative assessment with the extensive classic Stroop task. These results not only confirmed the role of ACC in inhibitory process showed in previous neuroimaging studies, but also suggested possible compensatory effects of the contralateral hemisphere in inhibitory functions. Other body of evidence reports the involvement of fronto-striatal connection in inhibitory control process [18, 46]. Different anatomical hypotheses have been proposed to explain the role of cortico-subcortical connectivity in cognitive inhibitory processes. Recent findings [31, 45] suggested a role of cortico-cortical connections between the IFG and pre-SMA, possibly mediated by the frontal aslant tract, in the right hemisphere. Other studies hypothesized the role of hyper-direct pathways connecting the IFG and the basal ganglia on inhibitory modulation of motor or verbal responses [81–83]. The evidence showed during the intraoperative awake surgery setting challenged the first hypothesis and supported the second one. In fact, in a recent report by Puglisi et al. [46], the disruption of Stroop task was mainly observed for stimulation of the inferior corticostriatal connections in comparison with superior corticostriatal connections. Interestingly, the superior fronto-striatal connection running from preSMA and IFG and the striatum are often removed without any postoperative impairment in Stroop performance evaluation. Such data suggested a role of the inferior fronto-striatal tracts in inhibitory control of attention, which is the aspect of cognitive control specifically assessed by the Stroop test. Globally considered, these data described the existence of a wide frontal network of inhibitory control that could be "easily" tested during awake procedures if suited tasks are applied. From a surgical point of view, the use of the Stroop test for mapping the inhibitory control network [46] is a safe and effective tool helping the surgeon in identifying the tumor's functional boundaries located in the deep and posterior margin of the resection in nondominant frontal lobe tumor. In the right hemisphere, by mapping the inhibitory process along with motor and praxis functions [84] add a further functional landmark where to stop the resection. Interestingly, the rate of complete resection was comparable in the group of patients in whom the Stroop task was delivered in comparison with the control. The oncological goal was accomplished along with the functional one.

Nevertheless, in light of the large connectivity between the frontal lobe and the parietal and temporal regions and considering other aspects of inhibitory control (attentional, perceptual, emotional, visuospatial), new tasks exploring additional "non-frontal" regions should be performed to get new insight on other unknown components of the inhibitory control.

16.8 Conclusion

Along with the improvements in awake surgery, neurosurgeons are more aware of the risk of damaging executive functions as they have become accustomed to testing patients more thoroughly before and after surgery. Then we are tempted to address the need and the feasibility of higher order cognitive functions preservation thanks to new peroperative monitoring paradigms. Preserving sufficient inhibitory control performances is mandatory to enjoy a satisfactory quality of life. New paradigms are being created and are efficient for such a preservation when dealing with gliomas located in specific regions, such as the right frontal lobe. However, the optimal use of an intraoperative test presupposes that it does not simply lead to satisfactory postoperative neuropsychological test results, but to the long-term preservation of functions that are essential for a good quality of life. In other words, before limiting a resection for functional reasons, one must be certain that the deficit observed cannot be recovered in the long term and that it will be disabling. Therefore, the next step would be to assess the balance between inhibition deficits and disability, eventually by the mean of more "ecological" tests before definitively validate the routine use of such tests. Finally, inhibition cannot be conceptualized separately from the other cognitive control functions because they are not independently implemented. Futures challenges will be to preserve executive functions as a whole rather than sparing each of these functions in isolation.

References

1. Miyake A, Friedman NP, Emerson MJ, Witzki AH, Howerter A, Wager TD. The unity and diversity of executive functions and their contributions to complex "frontal lobe" tasks: a latent variable analysis. Cogn Psychol. 2000;41(1):49–100.
2. Diamond A. Executive functions. Annu Rev Psychol. 2013;64:135–68.

3. Bari A, Robbins TW. Inhibition and impulsivity: behavioral and neural basis of response control. Prog Neurobiol [Internet]. 2013;108:44–79. https://doi.org/10.1016/j.pneurobio.2013.06.005.
4. Nigg JT. On inhibition/disinhibition in developmental psychopathology: views from cognitive and personality psychology and a working inhibition taxonomy. Psychol Bull. 2000;126(2):220–46.
5. Chambers CD, Garavan H, Bellgrove MA. Insights into the neural basis of response inhibition from cognitive and clinical neuroscience. Neurosci Biobehav Rev. 2009;33:631–46.
6. Lappin JS, Eriksen CW. Use of a delayed signal to stop a visual reaction-time response. J Exp Psychol [Internet]. 1966;72(6):805–11. http://content.apa.org/journals/xge/72/6/805.
7. Stroop J. Studies in interference in serial verbal reactions. J Exp Psychol. 1935;8(6):643–62.
8. Eriksen BA, Eriksen CW. Effects of noise letters upon the identification of a target letter in a nonsearch task. Percept Psychophys [Internet]. 1974;16(1):143–9. http://link.springer.com/10.3758/BF03203267.
9. MacLeod CM, Dodd MD, Sheard ED, Wilson DE, Bibi U. In opposition to inhibition. In: The psychology of learning and motivation: advances in research and theory. Vol. 43. 2003. p. 163–214.
10. Miller EK, Cohen JD. An integrate theory of PFC function. Annu Rev Neurosci. 2001;24:167–202.
11. Aron AR. The neural basis of inhibition in cognitive control. Neuroscientist. 2007;13(3):214–28.
12. Aron AR, Robbins TW, Poldrack RA. Inhibition and the right inferior frontal cortex. Trends Cogn Sci. 2004;8(4):170–7.
13. Anderson MC, Green C. Suppressing unwanted memories by executive control. Nature. 2001;410(6826):366–9.
14. Simmonds DJ, Pekar JJ, Mostofsky SH. Meta-analysis of Go/No-go tasks demonstrating that fMRI activation associated with response inhibition is task-dependent. Neuropsychologia. 2008;46(1):224–32.
15. Anderson MC, Ochsner KN, Kuhl B, Cooper J, Robertson E, Gabrieli SW, et al. Neural systems underlying the suppression of unwanted memories. Science. 2004;303(5655):232–5.
16. Dillon DG, Pizzagalli DA. Inhibition of action, thought, and emotion: a selective neurobiological review. Appl Prev Psychol. 2007;12(3):99–114.
17. Tabibnia G, Monterosso JR, Baicy K, Aron AR, Poldrack RA, Chakrapani S, et al. Different forms of self-control share a neurocognitive substrate. J Neurosci. 2011;31(13):4805–10.
18. Puglisi G, Sciortino T, Rossi M, Leonetti A, Fornia L, Conti Nibali M, et al. Preserving executive functions in nondominant frontal lobe glioma surgery: an intraoperative tool. J Neurosurg. 2018;131(2):474–80.
19. Wager M, Du Boisgueheneuc F, Pluchon C, Bouyer C, Stal V, Bataille B, et al. Intraoperative monitoring of an aspect of executive functions. Oper Neurosurg [Internet]. 2013;72:169–81. https://academic.oup.com/ons/article-lookup/doi/10.1227/NEU.0b013e31827bf1d6.
20. Aron AR, Fletcher PC, Bullmore ET, Sahakian BJ, Robbins TW. Stop-signal inhibition disrupted by damage to right inferior frontal gyrus in humans. Nat Neurosci. 2003;6(2):115–6.
21. Floden D, Stuss DT. Inhibitory control is slowed in patients with right superior medial frontal damage. J Cogn Neurosci. 2006;18(11):1843–9.
22. Picton TW, Stuss DT, Alexander MP, Shallice T, Binns MA, Gillingham S. Effects of focal frontal lesions on response inhibition. Cereb Cortex. 2007;17(4):826–38.
23. Chambers CD, Bellgrove MA, Stokes MG, Henderson TR, Garavan H, Robertson IH, et al. Executive "brake failure" following deactivation of human frontal lobe. J Cogn Neurosci. 2006;18(3):444–55.
24. Chambers CD, Bellgrove MA, Gould IC, English T, Garavan H, McNaught E, et al. Dissociable mechanisms of cognitive control in prefrontal and premotor cortex. J Neurophysiol. 2007;98(6):3638–47.

25. Rubia K, Smith AB, Brammer MJ, Taylor E. Right inferior prefrontal cortex mediates response inhibition while mesial prefrontal cortex is responsible for error detection. Neuroimage. 2003;20(1):351–8.
26. Boehler CN, Appelbaum LG, Krebs RM, Hopf JM, Woldorff MG. Pinning down response inhibition in the brain—conjunction analyses of the stop-signal task. Neuroimage [Internet]. 2010;52(4):1621–32. https://doi.org/10.1016/j.neuroimage.2010.04.276.
27. Menon V, Adleman NE, White CD, Glover GH, Reiss AL. Error-related brain activation during a Go/NoGo response inhibition task. Hum Brain Mapp [Internet]. 2001;12(3):131–43. http://doi.wiley.com/10.1002/1097-0193%28200103%2912%3A3%3C131%3A%3AAID-HBM1010%3E3.0.CO%3B2-C.
28. Rubia K, Russell T, Overmeyer S, Brammer MJ, Bullmore ET, Sharma T, et al. Mapping motor inhibition: conjunctive brain activations across different versions of go/no-go and stop tasks. Neuroimage. 2001;13(2):250–61.
29. Mostofsky SH, Schafer JGB, Abrams MT, Goldberg MC, Flower AA, Boyce A, et al. fMRI evidence that the neural basis of response inhibition is task-dependent. Cogn Brain Res. 2003;17(2):419–30.
30. Aron AR, Poldrack RA. Cortical and subcortical contributions to stop signal response inhibition: role of the subthalamic nucleus. J Neurosci. 2006;26(9):2424–33.
31. Aron AR, Behrens TE, Smith S, Frank MJ, Poldrack RA. Triangulating a cognitive control network using diffusion-weighted magnetic resonance imaging (MRI) and functional MRI. J Neurosci. 2007;27(14):3743–52.
32. Duann J-R, Ide JS, Luo X, Li C-sR. Functional connectivity delineates distinct roles of the inferior frontal cortex and presupplementary motor area in stop signal inhibition. J Neurosci. 2009;29(32):10171–9.
33. Gratton C, Sun H, Petersen SE. Control networks and hubs. Psychophysiology. 2018;55(3):1–18.
34. Bunge SA, Dudukovic NM, Thomason ME, Vaidya CJ, Gabrieli JDE. Immature frontal lobe contributions to cognitive control in children: evidence from fMRI. Neuron. 2002;33(2):301–11.
35. Wager TD, Sylvester CYC, Lacey SC, Nee DE, Franklin M, Jonides J. Common and unique components of response inhibition revealed by fMRI. Neuroimage. 2005;27(2):323–40.
36. Swick D, Ashley V, Turken AU. Left inferior frontal gyrus is critical for response inhibition. BMC Neurosci. 2008;9:1–11.
37. Bunge SA, Kahn I, Wallis JD, Miller EK, Wagner AD. Neural circuits subserving the retrieval and maintenance of abstract rules. J Neurophysiol. 2003;90(5):3419–28.
38. Hirose S, Chikazoe J, Watanabe T, Jimura K, Kunimatsu A, Abe O, et al. Efficiency of Go/No-Go task performance implemented in the left Hemisphere. J Neurosci. 2012;32(26):9059–65.
39. Duncan J. The multiple-demand (MD) system of the primate brain: mental programs for intelligent behaviour. Trends Cogn Sci [Internet]. 2010;14(4):172–9. https://doi.org/10.1016/j.tics.2010.01.004.
40. Hampshire A. Putting the brakes on inhibitory models of frontal lobe function. Neuroimage [Internet]. 2015;113:340–55. https://doi.org/10.1016/j.neuroimage.2015.03.053.
41. Erika-Florence M, Leech R, Hampshire A. A functional network perspective on response inhibition and attentional control. Nat Commun. 2014;5:4073.
42. Hampshire A, Sharp DJ. Contrasting network and modular perspectives on inhibitory control. Trends Cogn Sci [Internet]. 2015;19(8):445–52. https://doi.org/10.1016/j.tics.2015.06.006.
43. Stokes MG, Kusunoki M, Sigala N, Nili H, Gaffan D, Duncan J. Dynamic coding for cognitive control in prefrontal cortex. Neuron [Internet]. 2013;78(2):364–75. https://doi.org/10.1016/j.neuron.2013.01.039.
44. Hinton KE, Lahey BB, Villalta-Gil V, Boyd BD, Yvernault BC, Werts KB, et al. Right fronto-subcortical white matter microstructure predicts cognitive control ability on the Go/No-go task in a community sample. Front Hum Neurosci. 2018;12:1–11.
45. Dick AS, Garic D, Graziano P, Tremblay P. The frontal aslant tract (FAT) and its role in speech, language and executive function. Cortex. 2019;111:148–63.
46. Puglisi G, Howells H, Sciortino T, Leonetti A, Rossi M, Nibali MC, et al. Frontal pathways in cognitive control: direct evidence from intraoperative stimulation and diffusion tractog-

raphy. Brain [Internet]. 2019;142:2451–65. http://fdslive.oup.com/www.oup.com/pdf/production_in_progress.pdf.
47. Bettcher BM, Mungas D, Patel N, Elofson J, Dutt S, Wynn M, et al. Neuroanatomical substrates of executive functions: beyond prefrontal structures. Neuropsychologia [Internet]. 2016;85:100–9. https://doi.org/10.1016/j.neuropsychologia.2016.03.001.
48. Gao S, Liu P, Guo J, Zhu Y, Liu P, Sun J, et al. White matter microstructure within the superior longitudinal fasciculus modulates the degree of response conflict indexed by N2 in healthy adults. Brain Res [Internet]. 2017;1676:1–8. https://doi.org/10.1016/j.brainres.2017.09.008.
49. Rofes A, Mandonnet E, Godden J, Baron MH, Colle H, Darlix A, et al. Survey on current cognitive practices within the European Low-Grade Glioma Network: towards a European assessment protocol. Acta Neurochir (Wien). 2017;159(7):1167–78.
50. Santini B, Talacchi A, Squintani G, Casagrande F, Capasso R, Miceli G. Cognitive outcome after awake surgery for tumors in language areas. J Neurooncol. 2012;108(2):319–26.
51. Satoer D, Visch-Brink E, Smits M, Kloet A, Looman C, Dirven C, et al. Long-term evaluation of cognition after glioma surgery in eloquent areas. J Neurooncol. 2014;116(1):153–60.
52. Ng JCH, See AAQ, Ang TY, Tan LYR, Ang BT, King NKK. Effects of surgery on neurocognitive function in patients with glioma: a meta-analysis of immediate post-operative and long-term follow-up neurocognitive outcomes. J Neurooncol [Internet]. 2019;141(1):167–82. https://doi.org/10.1007/s11060-018-03023-9.
53. Rijnen SJM, Kaya G, Gehring K, Verheul JB, Wallis OC, Sitskoorn MM, et al. Cognitive functioning in patients with low-grade glioma: effects of hemispheric tumor location and surgical procedure. J Neurosurg. 2019:1–12.
54. Habets EJJ, Hendriks EJ, Taphoorn MJB, Douw L, Zwinderman AH, Vandertop WP, et al. Association between tumor location and neurocognitive functioning using tumor localization maps. J Neurooncol [Internet]. 2019;144(3):573–82. http://link.springer.com/10.1007/s11060-019-03259-z.
55. Drewe EA. Go—no go learning after frontal lobe lesions in humans. Cortex. 1975;11(1):8–16.
56. Lashley KS. Mass action in cerebral function. Science [Internet]. 1931;73(1888):245–54. https://www.sciencemag.org/lookup/doi/10.1126/science.73.1888.245.
57. Aron AR, Monsell S, Sahakian BJ, Robbins TW. A componential analysis of task-switching deficits associated with lesions of left and right frontal cortex. Brain. 2004;127(7):1561–73.
58. Alexander G. Parallel organization of functionally segregated circuits linking basal ganglia and cortex. Annu Rev Neurosci. 1986;9(1):357–81.
59. Stuss DT, Alexander MP. Is there a dysexecutive syndrome? Philos Trans R Soc Lond B Biol Sci. 2007;362(1481):901–15.
60. Tsuchida A, Fellows LK. Are core component processes of executive function dissociable within the frontal lobes? Evidence from humans with focal prefrontal damage. Cortex [Internet]. 2013;49(7):1790–800. https://doi.org/10.1016/j.cortex.2012.10.014.
61. Santillo AF, Lundblad K, Nilsson M, Waldö ML, Van Westen D, Lätt J, et al. Grey and white matter clinico-anatomical correlates of disinhibition in neurodegenerative disease. PLoS One. 2016;11(10):1–19.
62. Mesulam M. Principles of behavioral and cognitive neurology. 2nd ed. New York: Oxford University Press; 2000. 540 p.
63. Cochereau J, Lemaitre AL, Wager M, Moritz-Gasser S, Duffau H, Herbet G. Network-behavior mapping of lasting executive impairments after low-grade glioma surgery. Brain Struct Funct [Internet]. 2020;225(8):2415–29. https://doi.org/10.1007/s00429-020-02131-5.
64. Stroop JR. Studies of interference in serial verbal reactions. J Exp Psychol. 1935;18(6):643–62.
65. Vendrell P, Junqué C, Pujol J, Jurado MA, Molet J, Grafman J. The role of prefrontal regions in the Stroop task. Neuropsychologia. 1995;33(3):341–52.
66. Habets EJJ, Kloet A, Walchenbach R, Vecht CJ, Klein M, Taphoorn MJB. Tumour and surgery effects on cognitive functioning in high-grade glioma patients. Acta Neurochir (Wien). 2014;156(8):1451–9.

67. Charras P, Herbet G, Deverdun J, de Champfleur NM, Duffau H, Bartolomeo P, et al. Functional reorganization of the attentional networks in low-grade glioma patients: a longitudinal study. Cortex. 2015;63:27–41.
68. Arbula S, Pacella V, De Pellegrin S, Rossetto M, Denaro L, D'Avella D, et al. Addressing the selective role of distinct prefrontal areas in response suppression: a study with brain tumor patients. Neuropsychologia. 2017;100:120–30.
69. Guarracino I, Ius T, Pauletto G, Maieron M, Skrap M, Tomasino B. Junior-Real Time neuropsychological testing (j-RTNT) for a young patient undergoing awake craniotomy. Brain Cogn. 2020;140:105535.
70. Dulaney CL, Rogers WA. Mechanisms underlying reduction in stroop interference with practice for young and old adults. J Exp Psychol Learn Mem Cogn. 1994;20(2):470–84.
71. Edwards S, Brice C, Craig C, Penri-Jones R. Effects of caffeine, practice, and mode of presentation on stroop task performance. Pharmacol Biochem Behav. 1996;54(2):309–15.
72. Davidson DJ, Zacks RT, Williams CC. Stroop interference, practice, and aging. Neuropsychol Dev Cogn B Aging Neuropsychol Cogn. 2003;10(2):85–98.
73. Vilasboas T, Herbet G, Duffau H. Challenging the myth of right nondominant hemisphere: lessons from corticosubcortical stimulation mapping in awake surgery and surgical implications. World Neurosurg. 2017;103:449–56.
74. Stuss DT, Toth JP, Franchi D, Alexander MP, Tipper S, Craik FIM. Dissociation of attentional processes in patients with focal frontal and posterior lesions. Neuropsychologia. 1999;37(9):1005–27.
75. Stuss DT, Bisschop SM, Alexander MP, Levine B, Katz D, Izukawa D. The Trail Making Test: a study in focal lesion patients. Psychol Assess. 2001;13(2):230–9.
76. McDonald CR, Bauer RM, Filoteo JV, Grande L, Roper SN, Gilmore R. Attentional inhibition in patients with focal frontal lobe lesions. J Clin Exp Neuropsychol. 2005;27(4):485–503.
77. Koechlin E, Ody C, Kouneiher F. The architecture of cognitive control in the human prefrontal cortex. Science. 2003;302(5648):1181–5.
78. Badre D. Cognitive control, hierarchy, and the rostro-caudal organization of the frontal lobes. Trends Cogn Sci. 2008;12(5):193–200.
79. MacDonald AW, Cohen JD, Andrew Stenger V, Carter CS. Dissociating the role of the dorsolateral prefrontal and anterior cingulate cortex in cognitive control. Science. 2000;288(5472):1835–8.
80. Kerns JG, Cohen JD, MacDonald AW, Cho RY, Stenger VA, Carter CS. Anterior cingulate conflict monitoring and adjustments in control. Science [Internet]. 2004;303(5660):1023–6. http://www.ncbi.nlm.nih.gov/pubmed/14963333.
81. Nambu A, Tokuno H, Takada M. Functional significance of the cortico-subthalamo-pallidal "hyperdirect" pathway. Neurosci Res. 2002;43(2):111–7.
82. Liston C, Watts R, Tottenham N, Davidson MC, Niogi S, Ulug AM, et al. Frontostriatal microstructure modulates efficient recruitment of cognitive control. Cereb Cortex. 2006;16(4):553–60.
83. Aron AR, Herz DM, Brown P, Forstmann BU, Zaghloul K. Frontosubthalamic circuits for control of action and cognition. J Neurosci [Internet]. 2016;36(45):11489–95. http://www.ncbi.nlm.nih.gov/pubmed/27911752.
84. Rossi M, Fornia L, Puglisi G, Leonetti A, Zuccon G, Fava E, et al. Assessment of the praxis circuit in glioma surgery to reduce the incidence of postoperative and long-term apraxia: a new intraoperative test. J Neurosurg. 2019;130(1):17–27.

Set Shifting

17

Jérôme Cochereau, Martine Zandvoort, Thomas Santarius, and Emmanuel Mandonnet

Abbreviations

(d,v)ACC	(dorsal, ventral) anterior cingulate cortex
DLPFC	Dorsolateral prefrontal cortex
IFJ	Inferior frontal junction
PMC	Premotor cortex
PPC	Posterior parietal cortex
Pre-SMA	Pre-supplementary motor area
SMA	Supplementary motor area
VLPFC	Ventrolateral prefrontal cortex

J. Cochereau (✉)
Department of Neurosurgery, CHU Poitiers, Poitiers, France

Université de Poitiers, Poitiers, France
e-mail: Jerome.COCHEREAU@chu-poitiers.fr

M. Zandvoort
Department of Neurology and Neurosurgery, University Medical Center Utrecht, Utrecht, The Netherlands

Department of Experimental Psychology, Utrecht University, Utrecht, The Netherlands

T. Santarius
Department of Physiology, Development and Neuroscience, University of Cambridge, Cambridge, UK

Department of Neurosurgery, Cambridge University Hospitals NHS Foundation Trust, Cambridge, UK

E. Mandonnet
Department of Neurosurgery, Lariboisière Hospital, Paris Brain Institute (ICM) and Université de Paris, Paris, France

Frontlab, Institut du Cerveau de la Moelle, CNRS UMR 7225, INSERM U1127, Paris, France
e-mail: emmanuel.mandonnet@aphp.fr

E. Mandonnet, G. Herbet (eds.), *Intraoperative Mapping of Cognitive Networks*,
https://doi.org/10.1007/978-3-030-75071-8_17

17.1 Introduction

Glioma patients survive longer, but at the same time their functional prognosis might be hampered by the onset of cognitive disturbances that go beyond the traditionally considered basic motor or speech functions. For example, an impairment in cognitive flexibility would interfere with daily life functioning, especially with decision-making, adapting to novel situations and maintaining autonomy.

This has highlighted the need to develop additional tests to explore more complex cognitive functions, such as executive functions. Task development builds upon neuropsychological models. Historically, neuropsychology studies the relations between brain function and behavior, and its knowledge draws on information from both experimental and theoretical brain research. Clarification of brain-behavior relationships is being achieved through close clinical observation, interpretation of experimental paradigms, conceptual models derived from cognitive psychology, and (double) dissociations in brain-behavior relationships from, for example, classical lesion studies.

In parallel, innovations in techniques by which we can image the brain and non-invasively estimate the location of critical functional networks and hubs have deeply renewed our knowledge of the neural basis of cognitive functions. In particular, there has been a paradigm shift from a localizationist perspective to a network-based approach of brain mapping [1, 2].

Experience from the neurosurgical field greatly contributed to this paradigm shift. The use of real-time anatomo-functional correlations permitted by direct electrostimulations, especially in glioma surgery, is shedding new light on brain-behavior relationships. It now appears to be possible to (near total) resect tumors in presumed eloquent areas (e.g., Broca's area), while preserving neurologic function. This provides convergent evidence that functions such as language are subserved by large, distributed, and resilient neural networks, and not solely by discrete and isolated cortical areas. Moreover, new tasks have been developed to intraoperatively monitor complex cognitive functions, in addition to basic motor and language functions. Intraoperative electrical stimulation has revealed some of the different networks sustaining these complex functions. This chapter will focus on set shifting, an essential component of one of the most important human cognitive abilities grouped under the general term "executive functions."

17.2 Neural Basis of Set Shifting

17.2.1 Definition

To accomplish basic daily living activities, we constantly switch from one action set to another. For example, when one drives a car, speed limit changes according to road signs and one must adapt his behavior (driving speed) as a function of those cues. Such a basic situation brings into play, according to the commonly admitted theories [3, 4], the three core executive components, i.e., mental set shifting (the road sign cues a change in the driving speed setting), information updating in working memory (one keeps in mind the new speed limit that has been updated), and prepotent response inhibition (the previous speed limit has to be discarded). Patients with set shifting deficits show deficiencies in multitasking and rigid thinking and difficulties to adapt to new situations [5, 6]. Set shifting abilities and, in a more general perspective, cognitive flexibility are essential for creative problem-solving and "out-of-the-box" thinking in an adaptive cognitive framework [5].

This process has been scientifically investigated using the task-switching paradigm. In that respect, subjects are asked to sequentially perform several tasks that can be either a repetition (non-switch trial) or a distinct (switch trial) task. In such experiments, task-switching compared to task repetition induces a performance cost, i.e., a slower response time and/or increased error rate, a phenomenon termed the "switch cost." It is deemed to reflect the duration of a set of cognitive control processes devoted to task-switching [7–9].

Of note, the terms "set shifting" and "task-switching" are regularly confounded, though the term set shifting is specifically used when attentional set changes whether or not the task changes. However, for the sake of clarity, we will employ in this chapter both terms to relate to the same concept because most studies do not differentiate between them.

17.2.2 Set Shifting Tests

A myriad of tests can be formulated to explore set shifting so the purpose of the following subsections is to review the most commonly used set shifting tests in neurosurgical practice.

The Trail Making Test (TMT) [10] consists of two parts (A and B). In TMT part A, the subject is asked to draw, as fast as possible, lines that connect numbers in an ascending order, thus mobilizing visuospatial abilities, whereas in TMT part B, the subject is told to draw, as fast as possible, lines that connect numbers and letters in alternating and ascending order (1-A, 2-B, 3-C, … and so on), hence mobilizing set shifting abilities but also planification, working memory, and inhibition. The time difference between part B and part A (TMT-B minus TMT-A) is a better proxy of set shifting abilities, as it allows to control for visuoperceptive or spatial working memory deficits [11].

The Wisconsin Card Sorting Test (WCST) consists of sorting cards according to changing rules and based on examiner feedback [12]. Briefly, the participant is asked to sort different presented cards in categories but is not told how to sort them. The examiner tells him if the sorting is right or wrong and changes the rule after several trials. Numbers of categories achieved, trials, errors, and perseverative errors are recorded.

The Cambridge Neuropsychological Test Automated Battery (CANTAB®) **Intra-Extra Dimensional (IED) Set Shift Test** is a computerized analog of the WCST in which the participant is asked to select which pair of stimuli is correct according to changing rules and based on examiner feedback [13].

17.2.3 Neural Substrates of Set Shifting

Please refer to Fig. 17.1 to visualize the location of the functional cortical regions mentioned in this subsection.

Neural underpinnings of set shifting can be approached from three different perspectives, though these are not exclusive: the prefrontal (mostly left lateralized), frontoparietal, and basal ganglia systems [14].

In a task-switching paradigm, several subprocesses are involved. Firstly, action sets must be selected according to their level of priority with respect to the representation of goals and the expected outcome of each action. Evidences support the role of the pre-supplementary motor area (pre-SMA) and anterior cingulate cortex (ACC) in that process [15, 16]. In parallel, representation of the two task sets are maintained and a top-down modulation proceeds to resolve that interference conflict, which subsequently bias the modulation and make the relevant task set more active than the irrelevant one [8]. The left dorsolateral prefrontal cortex (DLPFC) seems to play a central role in that modulation process, especially the middle frontal gyrus [16, 17]. Several meta-analysis of task-switching fMRI studies are consistent with the involvement of these two regions of the prefrontal cortex [18–20], but other prefrontal foci have also been linked to task-switching according to the type of switching. Kim et al. [21] showed, in a decreasing level of abstraction, that cognitive set shifting recruited anterior prefrontal cortex regions whereas response switches recruited the DLPFC and stimulus switches recruited the dorsal premotor cortex. Moreover, the left inferior frontal junction (IFJ), located in the vicinity of the junction of the inferior frontal and precentral sulci, shows an increased activity in fMRI experiments involving different domains of cognitive control (task-switching, interference resolution, working memory) [22–24]. IFJ activations may reflect a common process between these different cognitive control tasks that could correspond to tasks representation updating [24–26]. Interestingly, in their meta-analysis,

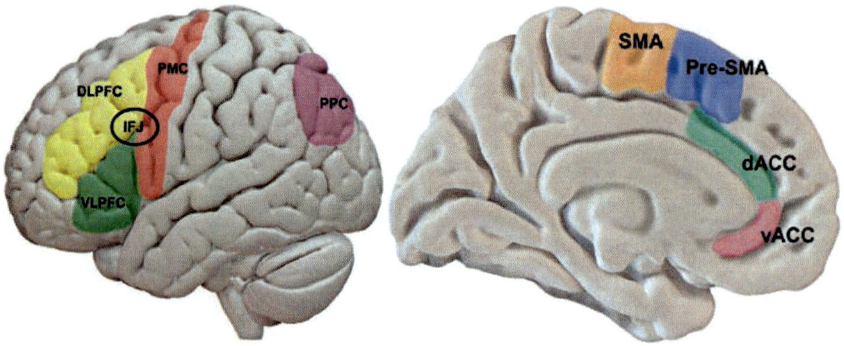

Fig. 17.1 Functional cortical regions implicated in set shifting. *dACC* dorsal anterior cingulate cortex, *DLPFC* dorsolateral prefrontal cortex, *IFJ* inferior frontal junction, *PMC* premotor cortex, *PPC* posterior parietal cortex, *vACC* ventral anterior cingulate cortex, *VLPFC* ventrolateral prefrontal cortex, *SMA* supplementary motor area

Kim et al [19] showed that the conjunction of context, response, and perceptual switching contrasts activated the left IFJ.

Within this framework of bottom-up and top-down control processes, prefrontal cortex exerts its control activity together with posterior regions, mainly the posterior parietal cortex (PPC) which is the site of visuo-attentional processing and visuomotor integration [27], constantly activated in conjunction with prefrontal cortex in task-switching fMRI studies [18–20]. Parietal regions are differently activated according to the switch type (rule or perceptual shift). Whereas rule switch (top-down) preferentially activates the DLPFC, perceptual switch (bottom-up) is specifically associated with an increase in parietal cortex activity [28].

Basal ganglia (BG) pathology such as Parkinson's disease displays, besides movement disorders, executive dysfunction because of BG's role in inhibiting competing action plans and filtering irrelevant information [29]. Specifically, the caudate nucleus and the lateral prefrontal cortex have been associated with cognitive functions [30], whereas the putamen and the premotor cortex have been associated with movement execution [31]. Monchi et al. [32] examined the basal ganglia's activation during two distinct shift processes, i.e., shifts requiring cognitive comparison and planning versus shifts with an implicit classification rule. They revealed that the caudate nucleus and the putamen activated respectively when a new task needed cognitive planning and during its execution, whereas the sub-thalamic nucleus activated in both shifting paradigms as a new motor program was solicited in both situations. These results have been replicated with a lexical set shifting experiment showing activations of a cortico-striatal loop including the ventrolateral prefrontal cortex and the caudate nucleus during the planning of a set-shift. During that planning phase, ventrolateral prefrontal cortex and caudate nucleus could be involved in the resolution of the uncertainty associated with a newly used rule [33].

These three brain systems are widely distributed across the brain and interconnected; hence set shifting may be impaired in multiple neurosurgical situations and is highly dependent on the underlying structural connectivity of those systems. Indeed, set shifting performances correlate to certain white matter bundles integrity measures. The superior longitudinal fasciculus that interconnects frontal and parietal cortices [34] has been identified as a key fascicle for set shifting in healthy aging and lesion studies [35–39] while other association and commissural tracts have been more scarcely mentioned. To go into more depth in the association between white matter disconnections and postoperative set shifting deficits, Cochereau et al. performed tract-wise lesion-symptom mapping on 270 patients operated on for a diffuse low-grade glioma and confirmed the association between frontoparietal connectivity disruption and set shifting deficits with a particular focus on the second portion of the left superior longitudinal fasciculus that connects the dorsolateral prefrontal cortex to the parietal cortex [40].

Finally, in a network perspective, more recent literature reports that at least five resting state networks (see Fig. 17.2) that reflect cognitive task activations [41] are involved in cognitive control (of which set shifting is an important part): the fronto-parieto-temporal network (FPTN), the cingulo-opercular network, the salience network, the dorsal attention network (DAN), and the ventral attention network (VAN)

[42]. Among them, the FPTN is the one that exhibits the most flexible functional connectivity patterns across various tasks. That flexibility could facilitate adaptive task performance in the face of a novel situation [43]. It is worth noting that in their case report of a patient with a postoperative drop in TMT-B performance, Mandonnet et al. showed a clear disorganization of the FPTN [38]. This leads to consider set shifting processes as emanating from multiple interacting hubs and functional networks as suggested by Dajani and Uddin [44]. In their speculative model of cognitive flexibility, FPTN would take a central role, as working memory continuously maintains and manipulates task representations, giving rise to DLPFC activity. In response to a novel situation, the DAN and the VAN would come online, where frontal eye field—posterior parietal cortex and ventrolateral prefrontal cortex—temporo-parietal junction activity would be expected, respectively. The salience network involving the anterior insula and anterior cingulate cortex may then trigger the switch to another neural network involving frontal regions, such as the right ventrolateral prefrontal cortex and inferior frontal junction, which are required to inhibit the previous task representation and employ the new rule.

17.3 Evidences of Long-Term Deficits in Patients Who Did Not Benefit from Set Shifting Intraoperative Monitoring

At present, awake intraoperative monitoring is mainly used to assess sensorimotor functions, vision, spatial cognition, and language [46]. In a systematic review, Ruis [47] described the published neuropsychological paradigms used to test cognitive functions during intraoperative cognitive monitoring in awake surgery procedures. From that, it became evident that paradigms to monitor set shifting have not been a part of the published test arsenal yet. Therefore, one can assume that preservation of

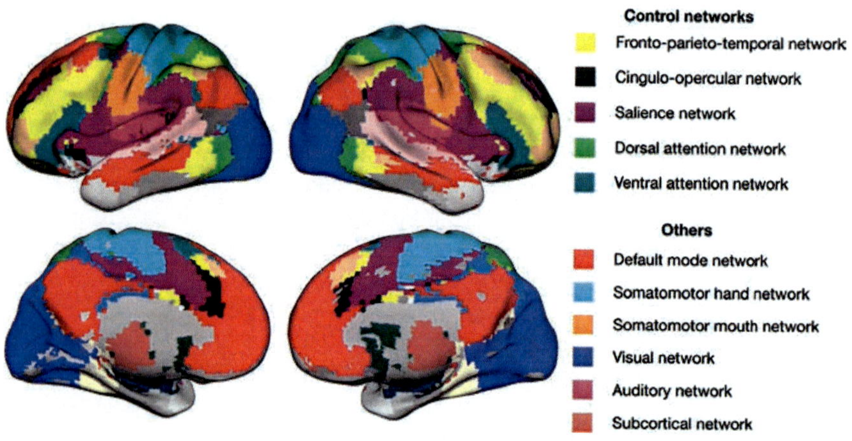

Fig. 17.2 Resting state networks defined by Power et al. [45]. Five of them are implicated in cognitive control

set shifting abilities is somewhat uncertain and highly dependent on the resilience of cognitive control networks and brain plasticity.

However, it should be mentioned that two teams reported the intraoperative monitoring of executive functions by relying on the Stroop task [48, 49], testifying the recent interest for the preservation of such functions.

As more attention has been paid on postoperative neuropsychological outcome in glioma surgery, several studies have thoroughly assessed patients pre- and postoperatively covering set shifting skills, generally by means of the Trail Making Test part B (TMT-B).

Given the relatively small number of participants in most single center studies and the inclusion criteria heterogeneity, results must be cautiously addressed. As an illustration, Talacchi et al. reported a TMT-B decline following glioma (17 high grade, 12 low grade) resection using a microsurgical technique whereas pre- versus postoperative performances in other neuropsychological tests taken independently remained nonsignificant [50]. In their meta-analysis, Ng et al. compared the postoperative (maximal follow-up of 6 months) neurocognitive functioning to the baseline in patient undergoing awake or asleep craniotomies for glioma and found an overall decline in executive functioning in both awake and asleep groups though with a smaller effect size in the awake group [51]. They nevertheless hypothesized that executive functions may take longer to recover than other neurocognitive functions, e.g., language or spatial awareness, that classically recover after a 1- to 3-month period [52]. Indeed, TMT-B can worsen at 3 months after glioma surgery and resume to the normal range at 1 year [53].

Aiming to compare neuropsychological outcome in 77 glioma patients undergoing awake (motor and language mapping) versus asleep surgery (42 and 35 patients, respectively), Rijnen et al. found a significantly worse performance at the 3 months postoperative follow-up compared to baseline on a set shifting attention test ($p = 0.018$) in the awake versus asleep group [54]. One explanation advanced by the authors to such results contrasting with Ng's meta-analysis is that executive functions were not monitored intraoperatively, and consequently the surgeon pushed the resection boundaries further than in the case of asleep surgery. However, no significant difference in the extent of resection was noted in that study. The fact remains that asleep and awake groups were not comparable, particularly in terms of lesion side: left lateralized glioma in 31/42 patients in the awake group and 8/35 patients in the asleep group.

In a recent paper dealing with a small series of insular glioma resections [55], Mandonnet reported that 6 patients out of 12 experienced impairments of the TMT-part B at the evaluation performed 4 months after the surgery, whatever the side of the tumor.

On the contrary, several studies did not reveal significant postoperative set shifting worsening. Focusing on right-sided frontal low-grade glioma patients undergoing awake craniotomy ($n = 10$), Herbet et al. [56] found no significant change on set shifting performances on the 3 months postoperative control. Likewise, working on patients with high-grade gliomas who have benefited from a supra-total resection either with awake (n = 16) or asleep (n = 17) surgery, Zigiotto et al. did not find significant TMT-B worsening after surgery in both groups [57].

Lastly, those papers suggest that set shifting abilities are inconstantly impaired after glioma surgery whether it was performed under awake condition or not, which is consistent with the fact that networks subserving set shifting abilities are widely distributed throughout the brain [44], and hence prediction of deficit occurrence after surgery remains challenging.

Before seeking to develop an intraoperative set shifting test, we should first elucidate the timeline factor influencing recovery from set shifting impairment, conditioning the need for such a test.

17.4 Preliminary Reports of Set Shifting Preservation by Means of Intraoperative Monitoring

In a proof-of-concept paper [58], Mandonnet et al. reported that it was possible to use a digital version of the TMT-B for intraoperative monitoring of set shifting abilities. No responsive sites were found at the cortical surface, but a functional site was found in the deep white matter: under stimulation, patient was unable to shift from numbers to letters. Importantly, the postoperative evaluation of this patient found unchanged scoring at TMT-B, demonstrating that intraoperative monitoring of TMT-B could help to preserve set shifting abilities. This first report awaits confirmation from larger series.

It should be emphasized that while there is now ample evidence that this monitoring should be used when operating in the right parietal lobe, it remains unclear where it should be used in other locations, like right and left frontal lobes.

17.5 Which Additional Anatomo-Functional Knowledge Has Been Gained from Neurosurgical Studies

As discussed in [38, 58], lesion studies have failed to produce concordant findings on the mechanisms supporting set shifting abilities and to reconcile these findings with fMRI reports in healthy controls.

Mandonnet and colleagues reported in [38] that from a hodotopic point of view, set shifting abilities may depend on an interaction between frontal, parietal, and temporal regions. This suggests a delocalized pattern and could explain the discrepancies that can be seen among the published reports, stemming from classical focal lesion studies. In their case report Mandonnet et al. described a marked deterioration of performance on TMT-B after the removal of a glioma located in the right temporo-parietal junction and demonstrated that resection of the white matter in the depth of the right supramarginal gyrus impacted locally the structural connectivity and remotely the functional connectivity of the right FTP network. Figure 17.3 gives an atlas view of this three-sites functional connectivity and its underlying structural connectivity.

In the case with intraoperative identification of a site whose electrical stimulation interfered with the shifting from numbers to letters at the TMT-B [58], it was found that the stimulated area comprised fibers belonging to the arcuate fasciculus, to the posterior transverse system (i.e., temporo-parietal fibers, commonly misnamed "indirect vertical portion of arcuate fasciculus," see [61] for nomenclature discussion), to the middle and basal longitudinal fasciculus, and to the corpus callosum. Introducing a new method estimating disconnection at the network level, they claimed that electrical stimulation impacted 3 out of the 17 resting state networks of Yeo et al. [59]: number 12, 13, and 16, respectively, known as cognitive control A and B and default A. Further studies are needed to confirm that any lesion that would result in a significant damage of these three networks would cause a permanent deficit of set shifting abilities.

In a recent international multicenter collaboration of pioneering neurosurgeons and neuropsychologists, a retrospective analysis was carried out on a series of patient operated on in the right parietal lobe [62]. This study confirmed that the right FTP network indeed contributed to impairments in set shifting as assessed by the TMT B/A. Especially the right posterior transvers system (previously named the posterior segment of the arcuate fasciculus) appeared more often associated with deficits in set shifting compared to involvement of SLF or the anterior and the long segment of the AF. However, this was not unequivocal and not based on

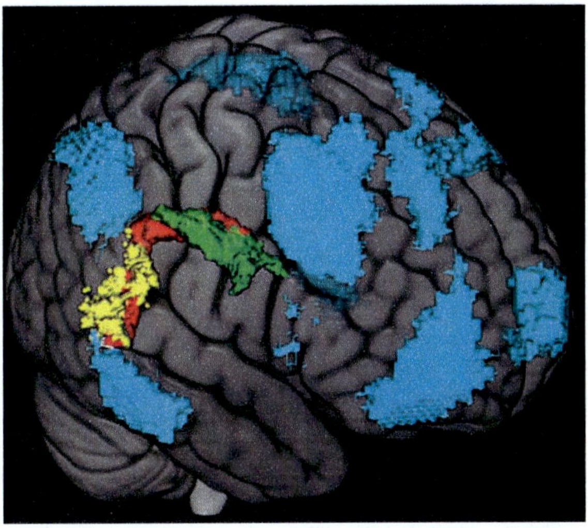

Fig. 17.3 Atlas view of the cognitive control network B. The cyan areas correspond to the cognitive control network B (the 13th resting state network of Yeo's parcellation [59], according to the nomenclature of Baker et al. [60]). The underlying structural connectivity has been extracted from the tracts of BCB toolkit (toolkit.bcblab.com): in yellow the posterior transverse system, in red the arcuate fasciculus, and in green the third branch of the superior longitudinal system. The white matter underlying the supramarginal gyrus is particularly at risk of damage for the control network B, as all the three tracts are in close neighborhood in this region. For clarity, callosal fibers are not represented, but important as well

intraoperative monitoring. Further studies involving protocolized intraoperative monitoring of set shifting are needed. This should be protocolized but with ample possibilities to adapt to individual patients. Tumor location, infiltration into subcortical networks, and possible pre-surgical impairments of the patient all need to be taken into account while monitoring.

Anecdotal report from another research group [63] also points towards involvement of the right Frontal Aslant Track (FAT); however, this was not yet tested in an intraoperative paradigm.

17.6 Conclusion

Convergent evidence from intraoperative DES during awake surgery to inform neurosurgical guidelines to preserve set shifting abilities from irreversible damage after tumor resection is still lacking. The FPTN in the right hemisphere, especially the posterior segment of the AF, should be respected as well as the right FAT. But based on current knowledge from lesion-symptom studies, and from both rsMRI and fMRI, set shifting is a delocalized function and should become part of the standard arsenal of perioperative neuropsychological tasks in order to better determine under which conditions (tumor location, preoperative network-level reshaping, and performance) this task should be monitored intraoperatively.

References

1. Catalino MP, Yao S, Green DL, Laws ER, Golby AJ, Tie Y. Mapping cognitive and emotional networks in neurosurgical patients using resting-state functional magnetic resonance imaging. Neurosurg Focus. 2020;48(2):E9.
2. Fox MD. Mapping symptoms to brain networks with the human connectome. N Engl J Med. 2018;379(23):2237–45.
3. Miyake A, Friedman NP, Emerson MJ, Witzki AH, Howerter A, Wager TD. The unity and diversity of executive functions and their contributions to complex "Frontal Lobe" tasks: a latent variable analysis. Cogn Psychol. 2000;41(1):49–100.
4. Diamond A. Executive functions. Annu Rev Psychol. 2013;64:135–68.
5. Grange J, Houghton G. In: Grange J, Houghton G, editors. Task switching and cognitive control. New York: Oxford University Press; 2014.
6. Rabinovici GD, Stephens ML, Possin KL. Executive dysfunction. Continuum: Lifelong Learning in Neurology. 2015;21:646–59.
7. Rogers RD, Monsell S. Costs of a predictible switch between simple cognitive tasks. J Exp Psychol Gen. 1995;124(2):207–31.
8. Meiran N, Chorev Z, Sapir A. Component processes in task switching. Cogn Psychol. 2000;41(3):211–53.
9. Altmann EM, Gray WD. An integrated model of cognitive control in task switching. Psychol Rev. 2008;115(3):602–39.
10. Reitan MR. Validity of the Trail Making test as an indicator of organic brain damage. Percept Mot Skills. 1958;8:271–6.
11. Sánchez-Cubillo I, Periáñez JA, Adrover-Roig D, Rodríguez-Sánchez JM, Ríos-Lago M, Tirapu J, et al. Construct validity of the Trail Making Test: role of task-switching, working

memory, inhibition/interference control, and visuomotor abilities. J Int Neuropsychol Soc. 2009;15(3):438–50.
12. Berg EA. A simple objective technique for measuring flexibility in thinking. J Gen Psychol. 1948;39(1):15–22.
13. Owen AM, Downes JJ, Sahakian BJ, Polkey CE, Robbins TW. Planning and spatial working memory following frontal lobe lesions in man. Neuropsychologia. 1990;28(10):1021–34.
14. Das A, Wylie GR. Task switching and executive dysfunction. In: Grange J, Houghton G, editors. Task switching and cognitive control. New York: Oxford University Press; 2015. p. 272–99.
15. Rushworth M, Walton M, Kennerley S, Bannerman D. Action sets and decisions in the medial frontal cortex. Trends Cogn Sci. 2004;8(9):410–7.
16. Hyafil A, Summerfield C, Koechlin E. Two mechanisms for task switching in the prefrontal cortex. J Neurosci. 2009;29(16):5135–42.
17. MacDonald AW, Cohen JD, Andrew Stenger V, Carter CS. Dissociating the role of the dorsolateral prefrontal and anterior cingulate cortex in cognitive control. Science. 2000;288(5472):1835–8.
18. Buchsbaum BR, Greer S, Chang WL, Berman KF. Meta-analysis of neuroimaging studies of the Wisconsin Card-Sorting Task and component processes. Hum Brain Mapp. 2005;25(1):35–45.
19. Kim C, Cilles SE, Johnson NF, Gold BT. Domain general and domain preferential brain regions associated with different types of task switching: a meta-analysis. Hum Brain Mapp. 2012;33(1):130–42.
20. Wager TD, Jonides J, Reading S. Neuroimaging studies of shifting attention: a meta-analysis. Neuroimage. 2004;22(4):1679–93.
21. Kim C, Johnson NF, Cilles SE, Gold BT. Common and distinct mechanisms of cognitive flexibility in prefrontal cortex. J Neurosci. 2011;31(13):4771–9.
22. Dove A, Pollmann S, Schubert T, Wiggins CJ, Yves Von Cramon D. Prefrontal cortex activation in task switching: an event-related fMRI study. Cogn Brain Res. 2000;9(1):103–9.
23. Milham MP, Banich MT, Webb A, Barad V, Cohen NJ, Wszalek T, et al. The relative involvement of anterior cingulate and prefrontal cortex in attentional control depends on nature of conflict. Cogn Brain Res. 2001;12(3):467–73.
24. Derrfuss J, Brass M, Yves Von Cramon D. Cognitive control in the posterior frontolateral cortex: evidence from common activations in task coordination, interference control, and working memory. Neuroimage. 2004;23(2):604–12.
25. Brass M. The role of the frontal cortex in task preparation. Cereb Cortex. 2002;12(9):908–14.
26. Brass M, Von Cramon DY. Decomposing components of task preparation with functional magnetic resonance imaging. J Cogn Neurosci. 2004;16(4):609–20.
27. Corbetta M, Shulman GL. Control of goal-directed and stimulus-driven attention in the brain. Nat Rev Neurosci. 2002;3(3):201–15.
28. Ravizza SM, Carter CS. Shifting set about task switching: behavioral and neural evidence for distinct forms of cognitive flexibility. Neuropsychologia. 2008;46(12):2924–35.
29. Filoteo JV, Maddox WT, Simmons AN, Ing AD, Cagigas XE, Matthews S, et al. Cortical and subcortical brain regions involved in rule-based category learning. Neuroreport. 2005;16(2):111–5.
30. Levy R, Friedman HR, Davachi L, Goldman-Rakic PS. Differential activation of the caudate nucleus in primates performing spatial and nonspatial working memory tasks. J Neurosci. 1997;17(10):3870–82.
31. Alexander G. Parallel organization of functionally segregated circuits linking basal ganglia and cortex. Annu Rev Neurosci. 1986;9(1):357–81.
32. Monchi O, Petrides M, Strafella AP, Worsley KJ, Doyon J. Functional role of the basal ganglia in the planning and execution of actions. Ann Neurol. 2006;59(2):257–64.
33. Provost JS, Petrides M, Simard F, Monchi O. Investigating the long-lasting residual effect of a set shift on frontostriatal activity. Cereb Cortex. 2012;22(12):2811–9.

34. Makris N, Kennedy DN, McInerney S, Sorensen AG, Wang R, Caviness VS, et al. Segmentation of subcomponents within the superior longitudinal fascicle in humans: a quantitative, in vivo, DT-MRI study. Cereb Cortex. 2005;15(6):854–69.
35. Perry ME, McDonald CR, Hagler DJ, Gharapetian L, Kuperman JM, Koyama AK, et al. White matter tracts associated with set-shifting in healthy aging. Neuropsychologia. 2009;47(13):2835–42.
36. Gold BT, Powell DK, Xuan L, Jicha GA, Smith CD. Age-related slowing of task switching is associated with decreased integrity of frontoparietal white matter. Neurobiol Aging. 2010;31(3):512–33.
37. Biesbroek JM, Kuijf HJ, van der Graaf Y, Vincken KL, Postma A, Mali WPTM, et al. Association between subcortical vascular lesion location and cognition: a voxel-based and tract-based lesion-symptom mapping study. The SMART-MR study. PLoS One. 2013;8(4):e60541.
38. Emmanuel M, Cerliani L, Siuda-Krzywicka K, Poisson I, Zhi N, Volle E, et al. A network-level approach of cognitive flexibility impairment after surgery of a right temporo-parietal glioma. Neurochirurgie. 2017;63(4):308–13.
39. Muir RT, Lam B, Honjo K, Harry RD, McNeely AA, Gao FQ, et al. Trail making test elucidates neural substrates of specific poststroke executive dysfunctions. Stroke. 2015;46(10):2755–61.
40. Cochereau J, Lemaitre A-L, Wager M, Moritz-Gasser S, Duffau H, Herbet G. Network-behavior mapping of lasting executive impairments after low-grade glioma surgery. Brain Struct Funct. 2020;225(8):2415–29.
41. Cole MW, Ito T, Bassett DS, Schultz DH. Activity flow over resting-state networks shapes cognitive task activations. Nat Neurosci. 2016;19(12):1718–26.
42. Power JD, Petersen SE. Control-related systems in the human brain. Curr Opin Neurobiol. 2013;23(2):223–8.
43. Cole MW, Reynolds JR, Power JD, Repovs G, Anticevic A, Braver TS. Multi-task connectivity reveals flexible hubs for adaptive task control. Nat Neurosci. 2013;16(9):1348–55.
44. Dajani DR, Uddin LQ. Demystifying cognitive flexibility: implications for clinical and developmental neuroscience. Trends Neurosci. 2015;38(9):571–8.
45. Power JD, Cohen AL, Nelson SM, Wig GS, Barnes KA, Church JA, et al. Functional network organization of the human brain. Neuron. 2011;72(4):665–78.
46. Rofes A, Mandonnet E, Godden J, Baron MH, Colle H, Darlix A, et al. Survey on current cognitive practices within the European Low-Grade Glioma Network: towards a European assessment protocol. Acta Neurochir. 2017;159(7):1167–78.
47. Ruis C. Monitoring cognition during awake brain surgery in adults: A systematic review. J Clin Exp Neuropsychol. 2018;40(10):1081–104. https://doi.org/10.1080/13803395.2018.1469602. Epub 2018 Aug 1.
48. Wager M, Du Boisgueheneuc F, Pluchon C, Bouyer C, Stal V, Bataille B, et al. Intraoperative monitoring of an aspect of executive functions. Oper Neurosurg. 2013;72:169–81.
49. Puglisi G, Howells H, Sciortino T, Leonetti A, Rossi M, Nibali MC, et al. Frontal pathways in cognitive control: direct evidence from intraoperative stimulation and diffusion tractography. Brain. 2019;142:2451–65.
50. Talacchi A, Santini B, Savazzi S, Gerosa M. Cognitive effects of tumour and surgical treatment in glioma patients. J Neurooncol. 2011;103(3):541–9.
51. Ng JCH, See AAQ, Ang TY, Tan LYR, Ang BT, King NKK. Effects of surgery on neurocognitive function in patients with glioma: a meta-analysis of immediate post-operative and long-term follow-up neurocognitive outcomes. J Neurooncol. 2019;141(1):167–82.
52. Duffau H, Capelle L, Denvil D, Sichez N, Gatignol P, Lopes M, et al. Functional recovery after surgical resection of low grade gliomas in eloquent brain: hypothesis of brain compensation. J Neurol Neurosurg Psychiatry. 2003;74(7):901–7.
53. Satoer D, Visch-Brink E, Smits M, Kloet A, Looman C, Dirven C, et al. Long-term evaluation of cognition after glioma surgery in eloquent areas. J Neurooncol. 2014;116(1):153–60.
54. Rijnen SJM, Kaya G, Gehring K, Verheul JB, Wallis OC, Sitskoorn MM, et al. Cognitive functioning in patients with low-grade glioma: effects of hemispheric tumor location and surgical procedure. J Neurosurg. 2019:1–12.

55. Mandonnet E. Transopercular resection of IDH-mutated insular glioma: a critical appraisal of an initial experience. World Neurosurg. 2019;132:e563–76.
56. Herbet G, Lafargue G, Bonnetblanc F, Moritz-Gasser S, Duffau H. Is the right frontal cortex really crucial in the mentalizing network? A longitudinal study in patients with a slow-growing lesion. Cortex. 2013;49(10):2711–27.
57. Zigiotto L, Annicchiarico L, Corsini F, Vitali L, Falchi R, Dalpiaz C, et al. Effects of supra-total resection in neurocognitive and oncological outcome of high-grade gliomas comparing asleep and awake surgery. J Neurooncol. 2020;148(1):97–108.
58. Mandonnet E, Vincent M, Valero-Cabre A, Facque V, Barberis M, Bonnetblanc F, et al. Network-level causal analysis of set-shifting during Trail Making Test part B: a multimodal analysis of a glioma surgery case. Cortex. 2020;132:238–49.
59. Yeo BTT, Krienen FM, Sepulcre J, Sabuncu MR, Lashkari D, Hollinshead M, et al. The organization of the human cerebral cortex estimated by intrinsic functional connectivity. J Neurophysiol. 2011;106(3):1125–65.
60. Baker JT, Holmes AJ, Masters GA, Thomas Yeo BT, Krienen F, Buckner RL, et al. Disruption of cortical association networks in schizophrenia and psychotic bipolar disorder. JAMA Psychiatry. 2014;71(2):109–18.
61. Mandonnet E, Sarubbo S, Petit L. The nomenclature of human white matter association pathways: proposal for a systematic taxonomic anatomical classification. Front Neuroanat. 2018;12:94.
62. Hartung S, Mandonnet E, De Witt Hamer P, Wager M, Rech F, Pallud J, et al. Connectivity correlates of impaired cognitive flexiblity after resection of a right parietal glioma. Cancers. Submitted.
63. Landers M, Meesters S, van Zandvoort MJE, De Baene W, Rutten GJ. The Frontal Aslant Tract and its role in executive functions: a lesion-symptom study in glioma patients. Hum Brain Mapp. Submitted.

Social Cognition

18

Riho Nakajima, Masashi Kinoshita, Mitsutoshi Nakada, and Guillaume Herbet

18.1 Neural Basis of Social Cognition: A Brief Review

Social cognition is defined as the ability to understand another person's behavior or mental state through the analysis of a wide range of perceptual cues, mainly including facial expression, eye gaze, body posture, and other sociolinguistic parameters [1, 2]. Social cognition is essential to produce appropriate behaviors in the context of interpersonal situations, and is unsurprisingly disrupted in a vast range of neurological or neurodevelopmental conditions marked by both communicational difficulties and abnormal behaviors such as, without being exhaustive, schizophrenia, autism spectrum disorders, or fronto-temporal dementia [3–5]. Social cognition is not a "monolithic" function but is rather shaped by various sociocognitive or socio-affective processes; among the most pivotal are empathy and theory of mind [6–9]. These processes are themselves under the dependency of hierarchically lower sub-processes, dynamic integration of which is required for an optimal mapping of the social environment [10, 11]. It is currently accepted that social cognition is underpinned by three anatomically segregated, but functionally interactive, networks: the

R. Nakajima
Department of Occupational Therapy, Faculty of Health Science, Institute of Medical, Pharmaceutical and Health Sciences, Kanazawa University, Kanazawa, Japan
e-mail: nakajima@mhs.mp.kanazawa-u.ac.jp

M. Kinoshita · M. Nakada
Department of Neurosurgery, Kanazawa University, Kanazawa, Japan
e-mail: m-kinoshita@med.kanazawa-u.ac.jp; mnakada@med.kanazawa-u.ac.jp

G. Herbet (✉)
Department of Neurosurgery, Gui de Chauliac Hospital, Montpellier & Institute of Functional Genomics, University of Montpellier, INSERM, CNRS, Montpellier, France
e-mail: guillaume.herbet@igf.cnrs.fr

E. Mandonnet, G. Herbet (eds.), *Intraoperative Mapping of Cognitive Networks*,
https://doi.org/10.1007/978-3-030-75071-8_18

face perception network, the "mirror" neuron network, and the mentalizing network [12–16].

The face perception network, which is lateralized in the right hemisphere, is fundamental to many aspects of social cognition, including face recognition, facial feature, and sex identification [17–19]; it is also dynamically modulated by face motion or eye gaze [20, 21]. Face perception and recognition is governed by a "core" network formed by the so-called "occipital face area" (OFA) and the "fusiform face area" (FFA), and a "peripheral" network composed of the posteriormost part of the superior temporal sulcus (STS), the anterior temporal pole, the amygdala, and areas of the prefrontal cortex (mainly including the inferior frontal gyrus and the orbito-frontal cortex) [19] (Fig. 18.1a). Unsurprisingly, current literature suggests that the face perception network is underpinned by at least two association fiber tracts that have cortical projections in associative occipital areas, namely the inferior fronto-occipital fasciculus (IFOF) and the inferior longitudinal fasciculus (ILF) (For a review, [22]). It has been, for example, shown that reduced integrity of the ILF, as estimated with diffusion parameters or number of streamlines, characterized patients with congenital or developmental prosopagnosia (i.e., the impaired ability to recognize familiar faces in the absence of primary visual defect, while recognition is possible with other sensory modalities) [22–24]. Prosopagnosia is frequently observed in the event of sudden lesions involving either the FFA or the OFA.

The "mirror" neuron network codes for cognitive and affective processes involved in the primate ability to access others' feelings automatically and effortlessly through observation of facial expression and actions [25]. Stated another way, this network is implicated in the reflexive aspect of empathy (termed also emotional empathy), but equally plays a role in other functionalities such as perceptive-based, low-level mentalizing, intention decoding, and the experiential understanding of agentive actions. In its more basic neuroanatomical formulation, the mirroring network comprises the posteriormost part of inferior frontal gyrus (i.e., pars opercularis) and the adjacent ventral premotor cortex, the anteriormost part of the inferior parietal lobe (i.e., supramarginal gyrus) and the posterior STS [26] (Fig. 18.1b). The latter area does not lodge neurons with mirror properties by itself but acts as a gateway by providing the mirror network visual representations with social content (i.e., STS neurons are well known to be modulated by biological motion) [27, 28]. From a physiological standpoint, mirror neurons are visuo-motor neurons which are equally fired by both the execution of a given action (or emotion) and the perception of the same action (or emotion) in others, a finding that has led to the hypothesis of a system of shared motor representations. Because other classes of neurons seem to possess mirror properties [29], the mirror network has been widely extended to other regions, including the anterior cingulate (empathy for pain), the amygdala (empathy for pain), the anterior insula (empathy for disgust), and somesthetic areas (empathy for touch) [29–32]. Currently, little is known about the anatomical connectivity broadcasting critical information for mirror network. It is however believed that the fronto-parietal network formed by the superior longitudinal fasciculus (SLF) and the arcuate fasciculus (AF) may significantly contribute [33], as well as,

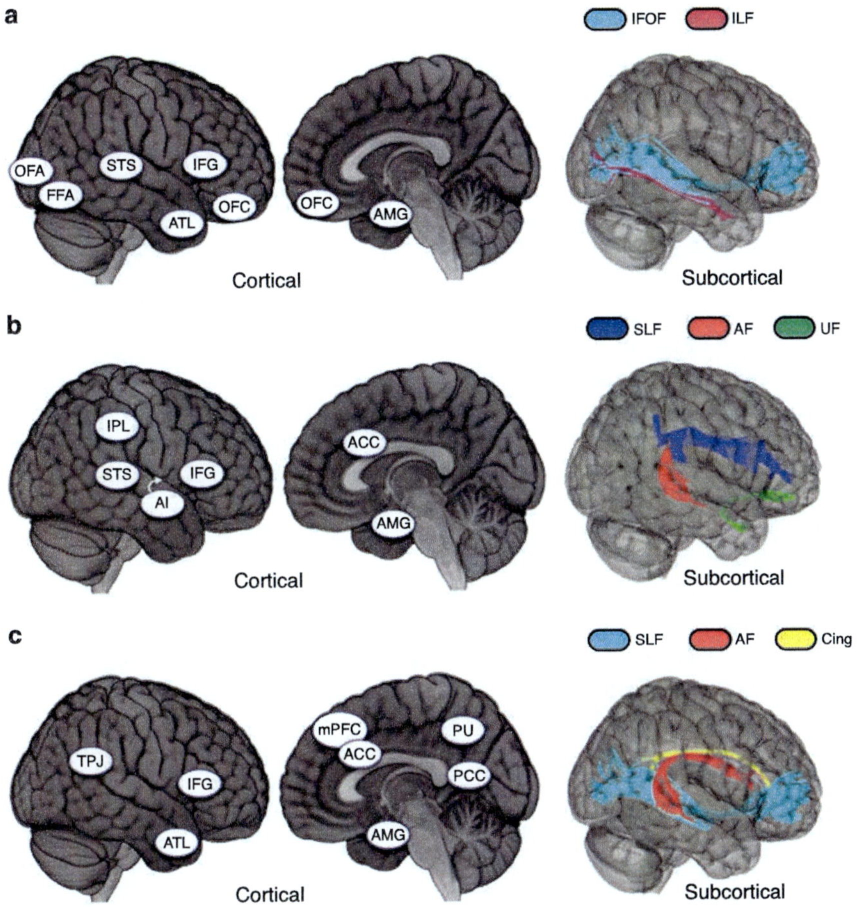

Fig. 18.1 Anatomo-functional organization of (**a**) the face perception network, (**b**) the mirror neuron network, and (**c**) the mentalizing network. *ACC* Anterior cingulate cortex, *AI* Anterior insula, *AMG* amygdala, *ATL* Anterior temporal lobe, *FFA* Fusiform face area, *IFG* Inferior frontal gyrus, *IPL* Inferior parietal lobe, *mPFC* Dorsal/ventral medial prefrontal cortex, *OFA* Occipital face area, *OFC* Orbito-frontal cortex, *PCC* Posterior cingulate cortex, *PU* Precuneus, *STS* Superior temporal sulcus, *TPJ* Temporo-parietal junction

albeit to a lesser extent, the uncinate fasciculus (UF), the anterior thalamic radiation, and the fornix, the latter of which constitutes the limbic white matter system.

Mentalizing (or theory of mind) is basically defined as the uniquely human propensity to attribute mental states (e.g., intentions, motives, believes) to others on the basis of observable behaviors and contextual information [2, 34]. Mentalizing allows to understand and anticipate others' behaviors and attitudes, and to adjust its own in return. Mentalizing is not a unitary process, but encompasses several subprocesses, the contribution of which is likely to be context-dependent as mentalizing situations are multi-faceted and diverse [11]. The mentalizing network has been the target of numerous functional MRI and lesion studies (for reviews, see [35–37]), so the cortical areas coding for mentalizing-related processes are today well understood. Basically, this includes, medially, the dorsal and ventral aspects of the medial prefrontal cortex and the posterior cingulate cortex along with the precuneus; laterally, the temporo-parietal junction along with the posterior STS, the inferior frontal gyrus, and less centrally, the temporal pole and its neighboring amygdala [35–39] (Fig. 18.1c). The anatomical connections of the mentalizing system is to date understudied. However, a handle of studies have suggested that three white matter tracts may play a central role, namely the cingulum, the SLF/AF, and the IFOF [40–45].

As social situations are especially various, these sociocognitive networks are likely to collaborate in a context-sensitive manner to allow individuals to flexibly adapt to novel intersubjective situations and to optimally understand the often fast-changing social environment, a kind of social metanetworking functioning [10]. Consequently, damage to these networks or to cortical regions allowing these networks to be functionally integrated is known to cause a decline in the way brain-damaged patients perceive and understand the social world; such impairments can sometimes be so marked that patients confine themselves in social recluse or behave in a way close to what is seen in acquired sociopathy. This is the reason why preserving social cognition in the context of glioma surgery has become a running theme in recent years. In the next part of this chapter, we review the literature evidencing social cognition deficits in glioma patients who did not benefit from a specific intraoperative procedure to map and spare aspects of social cognition.

18.2 Long-Lasting Impairments of Social Cognition in Unmapped Brain

Longitudinal studies assessing sociocognitive or socioaffective processes in tumor patients in whom no explicit mapping of social cognition was performed in the operating theater are actually scarce. Moreover, these studies concerned only a few aspects of sociocognitive functioning and typically included a small sample of patients. In a review by Pertz et al. [46], it is shown that, irrespective of the tumor histology, only emotion recognition appears to be affected but moderately. More specifically, high-grade glioma patients are more frequently impaired before the surgical procedure with no significant worsening after it. In contrast, low-grade glioma patients are relatively unaffected before the surgical treatment but show a decrease in performance in the acute postoperative phase. This worsening seems to recover over time (see also [47]). However, some individual studies do not always favor this general conclusion. For example, in a work by Goebel et al. [48], 30 patients were assessed preoperatively with a range of sociocognitive tasks. The authors found that 83% of them presented with impaired performance on at least one behavioral measure, whereas 77% of patients showed a combined deficit in two tasks measuring mentalizing abilities. In another work conducted by Herbet et al.

[49], ten patients with a low-grade glioma were assessed before, just after, and 3 months after surgery with two tasks gauging, respectively, the perceptual (low-level) and the attributional (high-level) aspect of mentalizing. Patients were divided in two groups according to where the tumors in the right prefrontal cortex were located (i.e., infero-ventral versus dorsomedial). Interestingly, patients with a resection centered on the dorsomedial prefrontal cortex were impaired in their ability to attribute intentions to others, but only just after surgery—the patient performance being no different to controls 3 months after surgery. Patients with a resection centered on the inferior frontal gyrus were specifically impaired in their low-level mentalizing abilities just after surgery but, contrary to the other group, they did not fully recover 3 months after surgery. Beyond the fundamental implications of this study revealing for the first time a double anatomo-functional dissociation in the prefrontal cortex for mentalizing, the results served as a basis for scientifically justifying the use of a mentalizing task in the operating theater to map the right inferior frontal gyrus, especially in the context of the trans-opercular approach of insular resections (see below) [50].

Other interesting works need to be discussed. For example, in Nakajima et al. [43], lasting impairments in the ability to identify complex mental states from the face (a prototypical task for assessing low-level mentalizing processes) were strongly predicted by the amount of surgically related damage into the right arcuate fasciculus, meaning that structural disconnection is one of the pathophysiological mechanisms accounting for the lack of complete recovery after surgery. According to another work by the same team [51], which will be further developed in another part of the chapter, decreased performance in a false-belief task a few months after surgery was partly associated with the resection of pars orbitalis of the right inferior frontal gyrus, showing again that neurosurgery can lead to permanent deficits in social cognition.

Taken as a whole, although neuro-oncological studies suggest that surgical resections have no strong and persistent detrimental effect on social cognition abilities, lesion mapping studies provide different results by showing that degraded performances in social cognition abilities a few months after surgery can be linked to identifiable neural correlates. This discrepancy in results can be explained by the fact that neuro-oncological studies generally do not use a comprehensive set of neuroanatomical analyses.

18.3 Cortical and Subcortical Structures at Risk: Evidence Gained from Lesion Mapping Studies Conducted with Glioma Patients

Unfortunately, anatomically unconstrained, whole-brain lesion mapping studies of social cognition in patients operating on for a diffuse glioma are scarce, and concerned only specific aspects of social cognition. However, they have provided critical results in full agreement with those obtained with electrostimulation mapping procedures performed a posteriori.

In a first work, Herbet and associates [52] assessed the mentalizing performances of a large series of 93 diffuse low-grade glioma patients with two behavioral tasks; the first one tapped the low-level, perceptive-based, and reflexive component of mentalizing whereas the second one evaluated the high-level, inference-based, reflective component of this sociocognitive function—according to the cognitive distinction made by several authors a few years ago (e.g., [53]). Three types of anatomo-functional analyses were conducted with the behavioral data, including standard mass-univariate voxelwise lesion-symptom mapping (VLSM, hereafter) [54], subtraction lesional analyses, and tract-oriented lesion-symptom analyses [55]. Although VLSM analyses did not provide significant results for the low-level task, the subtraction analyses revealed however that patients with a resection of the pars opercularis of the right inferior frontal gyrus were more frequently impaired in low-level mentalizing than others—in agreement with the results from Herbet et al. [49]. As regard to the high-level task, VLSM analyses found a significant brain-behavior relationship between resections of the supplementary motor area along with the neighboring posteriormost portion of the dorsolateral prefrontal cortex with impaired accuracy in inference-based mentalizing. This result was confirmed by subtraction analyses showing that patients with an impaired ability to infer intentions were more frequently resected than others in areas of both the posterior dorsolateral prefrontal cortex and the supplementary motor area, and to a lesser extent of the anteriormost portion of the inferior frontal gyrus. At the subcortical level, low-level mentalizing performance was correlated with the degree with which the AF/SLF was infiltrated whereas high-level mentalizing performance was rather associated with the amount of infiltration of the cingulum, still in the right hemisphere. Beyond the fundamental implications that will be discussed elsewhere in this chapter, this pattern of results indicates that damage to some structures is associated with permanent mentalizing impairments after surgery, both at the cortical and at the subcortical level, and thus warrants special attention in the operating room. It is worthing of note that, in this study, trackwise analyses were performed on the amount of residual infiltrations of white matter tracts, not on the volume of resection of these tracts. As a result, it was unknown whether the surgical resection itself of these tracts may be also associated with a behavioral impairment. To tackle this issue, the authors planned a second large-scale neuropsychological study in which it was shown that the volume of resection of the right AF was a strong predictor of a permanent decline in low-level mentalizing abilities [43].

In another work, Herbet et al. [42] provided a neuropsychological study that aimed to assess the functional consequences of structural disconnection on subjective empathy. More specifically, subjective empathy was assessed with the "empathy quotient" [56] in 107 patients in whom a surgical removal for a diffuse low-grade glioma had been performed. This self-report has been constructed to estimate dispositional, long-lasting traits of empathy, especially in pathological populations such as autism spectrum disorders. Of interest, three subscales can be derived from the empathy quotient total score [57], in particular the cognitive empathy index, the emotional reactivity index, and the social skills index. The cognitive empathy and the emotional reactivity indices can be used as proxy indicators for the constructs of cognitive empathy and emotional empathy, respectively. As in Herbet et al. [52], voxelwise and tract-oriented lesion-symptom analyses were conducted. While the first type of anatomo-clinical analyses were inconclusive, meaning that empathy disturbances were hardly "localizable," multivariate models performed on disconnection data led to significant results. In particular, the amount of infiltration of the left cingulum was found to be a strong predictor of impaired cognitive empathy whereas the degree of lesion infiltration of the right IFOF was predictive of an increase of social skills. In brief, this study demonstrate that structural disconnections of distinct white matter tracts cause changes in the subjective experience of empathy.

In Nakajima et al. [51], a combination of voxelwise and trackwise lesion-symptom analyses were achieved on the mentalizing performance of 20 patients with a right-sided tumor (false-belief paradigm). The results from the first analysis demonstrated that resection of the orbito-frontal cortex caused persistent mentalizing difficulties while the second one showed that damage to both the SLF and the fronto-striatal tract was also associated with mentalizing impairments.

Finally, Campanella et al. [58] submitted basic emotion recognition and mentalizing performances acquired in 77 tumor patients presenting with a low-grade or a high-grade glioma, or a meningioma to both a lobe-based and a voxel-based lesion-symptom analysis. More specifically, the analyses were conducted on the behavioral difference between scores obtained usually the day before surgery and scores obtained a few days after surgery. Significant brain-behavior relationships were observed between disrupted emotion recognition abilities and both the right anterior temporal structures and the posterior insular cortex whereas impaired low-level mentalizing abilities were rather associated with the posteriormost portion of the superior temporal gyrus extending to the inferior parietal lobule, and the insulo-opercular cortex. As the analyses were not conducted with behavioral data obtained in the chronic postoperative period, it remained unestablished in this study whether the highlighted anatomo-functional correlations were permanent or just transitory. In a further study from the same research group [47], the authors processed again the data but added the results of the 4-month postoperative assessment. They found that deficits in recognizing basic facial emotions and in mentalizing were already present before the surgical procedure in high-grade glioma patients and that the surgery by itself did not induce a supplementary, negative effect on performances. Concerning patients with low-grade glioma, they were unimpaired on both tasks before surgery. However, the surgery did induce a significant decrease in performance just after surgery. Four months after surgery, the performances recovered significantly, but the behavior data were not displayed in the article so that it is unfortunately unknown whether patients fully recovered.

In Fig. 18.2, we provide an overview of the cortical and white matter structures known to be associated with long-lasting mentalizing deficits following surgery.

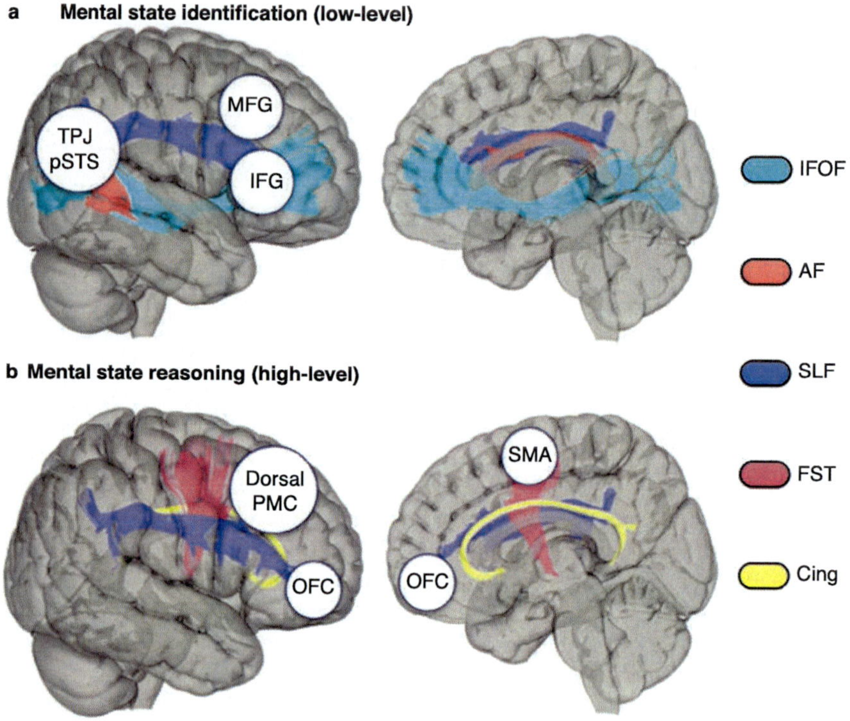

Fig. 18.2 Critical regions for social cognition as determined by lesion mapping or intraoperative brain mapping studies conducted with glioma patients. (**a**) Cortical and white matter structures associated with tasks assessing mental state identification (perceptive-based, low-level component of mentalizing). (**b**) Cortical and subcortical structures associated with tasks assessing mental state reasoning such as intention attribution or false-belief task (inference-based, high-level component of mentalizing). *IFG* inferior frontal gyrus, *MFG* middle frontal gyrus, *PMC* premotor cortex, *OFC* orbito-frontal cortex, *SMA* supplementary motor area

18.4 Review of the Different Tasks Newly Designed to Monitor Components of Social Cognition in the Operating Room Intraoperatively

18.4.1 Review of Studies

Earliest attempts to intraoperatively map aspects of social cognition was provided by Giussani et al. [59]. In this study, 18 patients with a right cerebral brain tumor (low-grade and high-grade glioma, metastases and meningioma) were required to recognize six basic emotions (anger, happiness, fear, surprise, disgust, and sadness) during cortical electrostimulation mapping. In total, five positive mapping sites were unmasked in five patients; they were located in the superior and middle temporal gyri and the supramarginal gyrus. None of the patients suffered from a permanent deficit in recognizing basic facial emotions after surgery. In the same vein, Papagno et al. [60] used the same kind of emotion tasks to ascertain the insular functional responsivity to facial expression of disgust in 13 patients with glioma. They did find that stimulating the left insula significantly impaired the ability in recognizing disgust, contrary to other basic emotions. Importantly, in this study, the insular structures were still removed for oncological reasons, and no long-lasting emotion recognition deficits were observed after surgery, suggesting ultra-fast recovery or compensation. The results obtained thus raise the question of the usefulness of using such a behavioral paradigm, at least in the context of insula removal. As developed in Mandonnet et al. [61], to decide whether or not a task must be included in the intraoperative mapping procedure, we need to assess the extent to which the surgery actually impacts the function under scrutiny. This is easily done by planning longitudinal behavioral studies (i.e., before, just after, late after surgery).

As developed above, Herbet et al. [49] provided a longitudinal study in which ten patients suffering from a low-grade glioma were behaviorally assessed with tasks tapping two aspects of mentalizing the day before, 4–5 days after, and 3 months after surgery. The authors found that high-level mentalizing quickly normalized after surgery contrary to low-level, perceptive-based mentalizing that did not fully recover 3 months after surgery, especially for patients with a glioma damaging the right inferior frontal gyrus—a key node of the mirror neuron network. These behavioral results prompt this clinical team to introduce a new task in the surgical theater in order to identify and spare structures involved in the lower aspect of mentalizing (see below for a complete description of the task). The results of this investigation have been published 2 years later [50]. Five cases of patients with a right frontal diffuse low-grade glioma were subjected to a precise mapping of the right inferior frontal gyrus. In agreement with Herbet et al. [49], and more generally with the supposed role of this structure in aspects of social cognition, six cortical sites were found to be associated with impaired performances during stimulation. They were mainly located in the lateral part of pars opercularis ($n = 4$), less frequently in the superiormost part of pars triangularis ($n = 2$). Importantly, two supplementary anatomical sites were unmasked deep in the white matter of the inferior frontal gyrus where cross the IFOF and the AF. These findings have had important implications, especially for the trans-opercular approach of insular gliomas which are the more frequent [62]. Three years later, the same research group reported another study using the same task, but it was conducted this time with a large group of 27 patients harboring a right-sided, diffuse low-grade glioma [45]. Contrary to the previous study, the mapping was performed without anatomical priors, at the whole-brain level. Cortically, the mapping results not only confirmed the involvement of the posterior part of inferior frontal gyrus, but also revealed a central role of the posterior dorsolateral prefrontal cortex as well as, to a lesser extent, of the superior temporal gyrus (posterior part). Critically, numerous sites were also identified in the white matter underneath the dorsolateral prefrontal cortex and the middle and superior temporal gyri. The disconnection analyses performed on the axonal stimulation dataset demonstrated that fibers of the IFOF and the SLF/AF had the highest probabilities of being disconnected during subcortical stimulation. Taken as a whole, the obtained results showed that the integrity of both the IFOF and SLF/AF is required for optimal tracking of mental states when inferred from the face. From a neurosurgical perspective, this shows how useful is the mentalizing task to find the functional margins in the event of right glioma.

In another study, Nakajima and associates [51] employed an alternative task to intraoperatively map the higher level aspect of mentalizing (see below for a complete description of the task). In particular, they assessed online mentalizing abilities in 20 patients presenting with a right cerebral glioma with a false-belief-like paradigm. They found mentalizing sites in four patients either in the inferior frontal gyrus or in the superior frontal gyrus, at the cortical or subcortical level.

18.4.2 Precise Description of Intraoperative Tasks

In Herbet et al. [50], Yordanova et al. [45], and Yordanova et al. [63], the "The read the Mind in the eyes" task, initially developed by the team of Baron-Cohen et al. [64] in an attempt to gauge social cognition difficulties in autism spectrum disorders, was adapted and used in the operating theater (see Fig. 18.3). This task has the advantage of being widely used and to be validated in numerous languages. In its standard version, 36 pictures of humans' eye region are presented to participants. The faces reflect either cognitive or affective mental states, and are mainly driven by the expression of eyes and/or by the motor configuration of the face. Four words describing different complex mental states are given, and the participant is required to select the one best describing what the person might think or feel. In the operating theater, the tasks are adapted to reach the surgical constraints and to increase task sensitivity. More specifically, on the basis of the preoperative assessment, only succeeded items are used. Moreover, only two words are selected instead of four. Note that "unstimulated" items are systematically performed before the mapping to ensure that the patient is able to perform the tasks without committing errors.

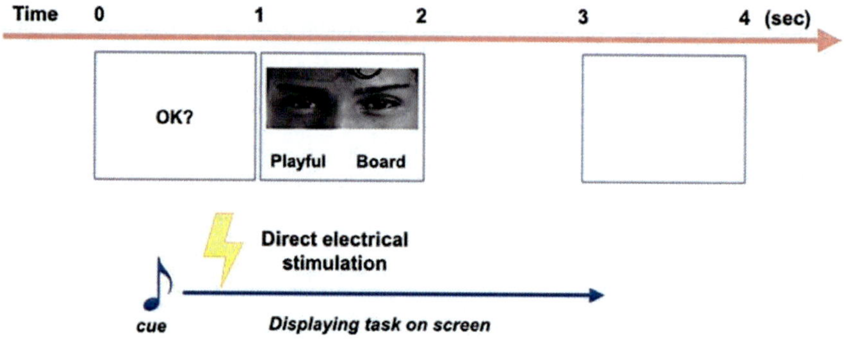

Fig. 18.3 Schematic illustration of the intraoperative procedure used to map and monitor mentalizing, especially the low-level aspect of this function (Reused with permission from [45])

Inappropriate word selection or a delayed response is accepted as a positive one. This task rather taps the perceptive, low-level aspect of mentalizing.

In Nakajima et al. [51], a standard picture-based false-belief paradigm was applied intraoperatively (Fig. 18.4). This behavioral task makes use of a stereotyped scenario in which a main character has left his/her asset unattended for a brief period of time. During that time, a second person removes the main character's asset. On return, the main character is surprised that his/her asset is missing. In the operating theater, the scenario is given to the patient in the format of four comic strips using a PowerPoint® slide show. The first three slides relate to the story course, while the fourth depicts two possible outcomes. The patient is instructed to select the option that would most logically conclude the scenario being seen. Stimulations, cortical or subcortical, are applied during the presentation of the second and third slides. An illogical selection or a delayed response is accepted as a positive mapping. This task rather assesses the inference-based, high-level aspect of mentalizing.

As a note of caution, neither of the two tasks should be considered as uniquely assessing the low-level versus the high-level aspect of mentalizing, but rather as preferentially gauging those aspects. Indeed, in the RME task, the patient is asked to overtly associate a complex mental state with a face. As such, this implies a reflective load. In the false-belief task, participants are needed to understand the story (basic intention decoding) and the main character's emotions; in this case, this

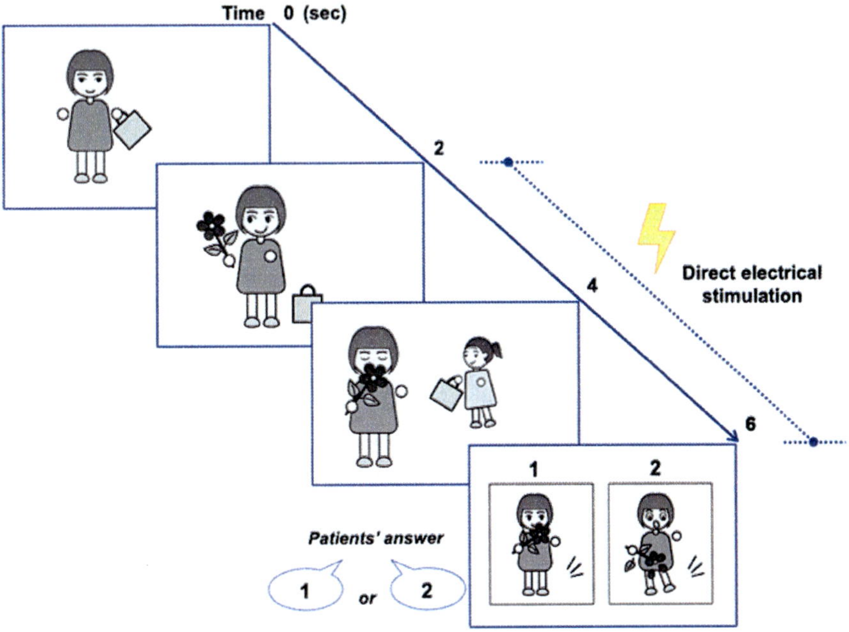

Fig. 18.4 Schematic illustration of the intraoperative procedure used to map and mentalizing with a false-belief task (Reused with permission from [73])

necessarily involves some of the low-level processes partly mediated by the mirror neuron or the emotion system.

18.5 Review of Studies Evidencing a Functional Improvement in Series of Patients Operated on with Versus Without Function Monitoring

To the best of our knowledge, only one paper directly comparing postoperative performances of patients having benefited or not from an intraoperative mapping of social cognition (in particular, mentalizing) has been published [51]. The results of this study suggest that intraoperative monitoring of mentalizing is useful. As a matter of fact, long-term scores of social cognition were significantly higher in the patient group exposed to intraoperative assessment compared with the group that was not. In another study, the same research group further investigated the functional outcomes of glioma patients who underwent awake surgery aiming at preserving a range of cognitive processes. Unfortunately, there were no direct comparisons between a group of patients with and without intraoperative monitoring. This longitudinal study showed that low- and high-level mentalizing performances were declined in the immediate postoperative phase, but recovered almost totally at 3 months postoperatively [65]. These findings indicate that wide-awake surgery aimed to decrease the probability of permanent social cognition disorders allows for good functional outcomes.

18.6 Which Additional Anatomo-Functional Knowledge Has Been Gained from Intraoperative Mapping Studies?

The use of direct electrostimulation for the study of mentalizing has allowed to gain fundamental insight into the network organization of this function, especially at the level of axonal pathways. Indeed, as electrostimulation remains to date the sole technique permitting direct interrogation of white matter pathways [66], it is a unique tool to study the role of fiber tracts in cognition and behavior. In general, the combination of network-lesion mapping [42, 43, 52] and axonal stimulation [45, 50] in glioma patients has been a pioneering approach in establishing the structural networks underlying mentalizing subprocesses. These efforts have led to the formulation of the triple-pathway model of mentalizing [10] (Fig. 18.5). This anatomo-functional model holds that mentalizing is performed through the solicitation of three subnetworks. The first one is underlain by the cingulum and supports high-level mentalistic inferences/attributions. The second one is underlain by the complex AF/SLF and rather supports the lower aspects of mentalizing, possibly through the white matter connections of the mirror neuron system. The third one is mediated by the IFOF and is possibly involved in the emotional aspects of mentalizing, through the analysis of visual cues (Fig. 18.5). These subsystems are thought to communicate in a context-sensitive manner, and to allow an optimal mapping of the

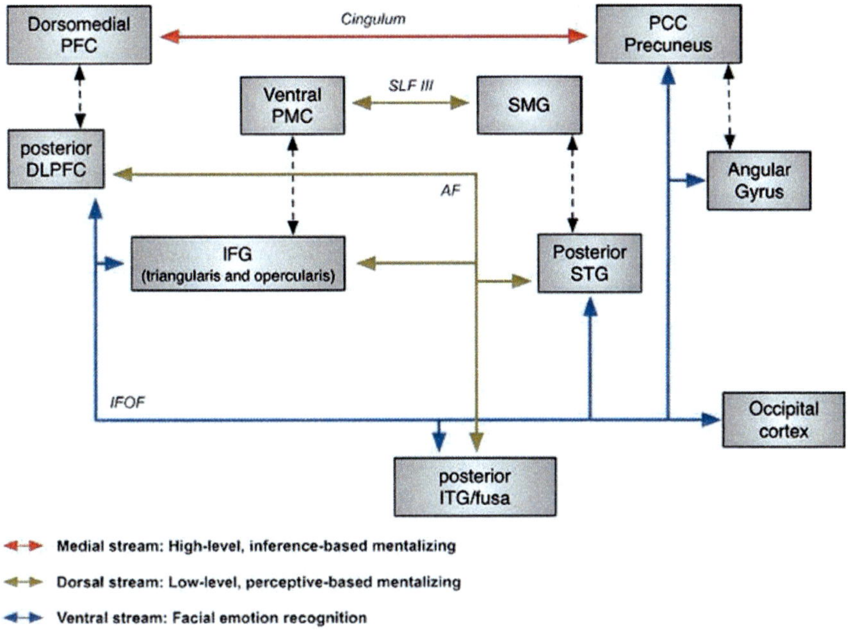

Fig. 18.5 The triple-stream model of mentalizing. *DLPFC* dorsolateral prefrontal cortex, *IFG* inferior frontal gyrus, *PFC* prefrontal cortex, *PMC* premotor cortex, *PCC* posterior cingulate gyrus, *SMG* supramarginal gyrus, *STG* Superior temporal gyrus (Reused with permission from [10])

surrounding social environment. It is a possibility that other tracts may have a significant contribution, in particular the FST that has been recently related to specific aspects of mentalizing [51].

Beyond these considerations, the combination of electrostimulation and neuroimaging methods, both structural and functional, has allowed to inaugurate a new way to map the human neurocognitive networks, with the advantage of transcending the limits inherent to each of the techniques. For example, in Yordanova et al. [63], fronto-cortical sites associated with a mentalistic impairment during direct stimulation were coupled with resting-state fMRI to identify the network of areas that might synchronize with the stimulated structures. Critically, the results showed that stimulation sites, located either in the posteriormost portion of the inferior frontal gyrus or in the dorsolateral prefrontal cortex, were functionally coupled with the dorsomedial prefrontal cortex, the temporo-parietal junction along with the posterior superior temporal sulcus and the posterior inferior temporal/fusiform gyrus; in other words, with the same network identified in activation fMRI studies using the same behavioral paradigm. This study not only confirmed that cortical sites unmasked with electrostimulation can be considered as gateways to the whole-brain network, but also demonstrated that combining resting-state fMRI and stimulation mapping is a powerful approach to identify functional networks in brain-damaged patients—as already suggested in a previous study concerning the motor and language domains [67].

In another work by Yordanova et al. [45], subcortical stimulations associated with mentalizing were combined with disconnection analyses to identify the white matter connections disrupted by electrical impulses. More specifically, based on a diffusion imaging-based white matter atlas [68], the method consists in visualizing the white matter fibers with the highest probabilities to be transitory "disconnected" by stimulation and thus in determining which tract is associated with the process under scrutiny. In this study, it was shown for the first time that the right IFOF may have a contributive role in mentalizing, a result that has been rapidly confirmed in another work using other types of methodological approaches in neurologically healthy subjects [40]. It is worthing of note that the method we described has been successfully applied to dissociate the motor-speech from the lexico-semantic system in the left frontal lobe [69] as well as to provide the white matter basis of the deafferentation model of verbal perseveration [69]—both studies had been conducted with the data from glioma patients.

To resume this part of the chapter, electrostimulation mapping datasets gained in glioma patients, coupled or uncoupled with other brain mapping methods, has permitted in recent years to provide first experimental evidence on the connectomics of the mentalistic system, especially regarding its white matter architecture.

18.7 Perspectives

18.7.1 The Need for Longitudinally Designed Studies

As mentioned in the first part of the chapter, social cognition has to be conceptualized as a mosaic of interactive processes, the efficient functioning of which allows individuals to navigate the social environment. If efforts have been made in the last 5 years to preserving social cognition in tumoral patients [43, 45, 50], the fact remains that such intraoperative mapping concerns only one aspect of social cognition, namely mentalizing. Whether or not should we introduce new tasks in the operating theater to assess "online" other components of social cognition is clinically unestablished. As developed recently [61] the only way to shed light scientifically on this issue is to determine if the vast range of sociocognitive abilities forming social cognition did not recover after surgery and to identify the physiopathological bases of this lack of recovery. In the latter case, it is important to keep in mind that limited recovery might not be related to the surgical procedure by itself but to other factors, clinical or sociodemographic, such as the amount of infiltration of white matter connectivity [70], age (i.e., older patients potentially have a reduced neuroplasticity potential), or education level (i.e., poorly educated patients may have a less resilient functional architecture) among others. This can be made by planning longitudinal studies designed to assess patients before surgery, immediately after surgery, and a few months after surgery using a variety of behavioral tasks. If permanent deficits are observed, this is a cue to reflect more deeply on the possibility of constructing new intraoperative paradigms. Such kind of studies may also offer the opportunity to assess the extent to which distinct social cognition impairments do impact patients' quality of life and daily life functioning.

18.7.2 Is There an Ideal Social Cognition Task to Be Used in the Operating Theater?

As the time devoted to the intraoperative mapping is limited for obvious reasons, an ideal social cognition task must be sensible, easy to perform, and appropriate to the temporal constraints of electrostimulation procedure (this is true for all intraoperative tasks). The mapping of low-level social cognition processes (i.e., basic emotion recognition, low-level mentalizing, and so on) is not really a problem since tasks tapping these processes are by very nature perceptual. The situation appears quite different for tasks measuring the higher level aspect of social cognition, as social inferences are mainly based on contextual information. For example, in comic strip-like tasks, patients are required to first analyze a scenario then to select the most logical end of this scenario (typically, between two or three alternatives). At what point of time exactly the neurosurgeon should stimulate, knowing that electrical impulses mustn't exceed 4 s? The response is not straightforward as mentalizing is solicited not only during the process of choosing the appropriate response, but also during the visualization of the scenario (i.e., the subject scan and rescan the visual scene to pick up all potential social cues). Moreover, current social cognition tasks are cognitively multi-determined. The "read the mind in the eye" task (the task used by the Montpellier neurosurgical team, France), albeit perceptual, necessitates to explicitly select (even if artificially) a mental state, and thus to make a conscious inference. On the other hand, a comic strip-like task (used notably by the Kanasawa neurosurgical team, Japan), beyond requiring the patient to infer the intention or belief of an acting agent, engages processes involved in action understanding and even in basic emotion recognition in the event of overtly expressed emotions. The bottom line is that the tasks we used in the operating theater have not a high degree of specificity—we acknowledge. The problem gains in importance when we consider what exactly a social interaction is. Currently, the main criticism in the field of social neuroscience is that the results obtained, most of the time with fMRI, are quite artificial because the tasks generally employed (usually, the same than used in clinical neuropsychology) are too reductionist and static to reflect the true functioning of the brain during interpersonal situations. Stated another way, the tasks very much lack ecological validity. This is the reason why a number of authors have strongly recommended the use of dynamic behavior paradigms able to replicate real-life demands on social cognition in general, and on mentalizing abilities in particular—the so-called second-person neurosciences [71]. In the context of neurosurgery, the question is indeed to know whether assessing social cognition with static pictorial items (a situation in which the patient is just a passive observer) is sufficient to maintain postoperatively efficient social abilities (situations in which the patient is in dynamic interactions with others). So, how to improve the validity of the tasks we used? Either we rework items in a way that we better target the sociocognitive process under scrutiny to increase specificity, at the expense of ecological validity, or we used dynamic items (e.g., short videos of interacting agents of 4 s in length) to increase ecological validity, but at the expense of specificity. In either case, this kind of development work has to be performed in the context of what has been stated in the preceding section (i.e., longitudinal studies). The key idea is to determine which tasks best predict lasting impairments in daily life social functioning and assess whether such tasks are feasible in a surgical context.

In connection with this, the choice of using a particular task among different alternatives must be made with the patient and its family. Awake surgery is by very nature a personalized medicine that needs be individually adjusted for each patient. For example, for obvious reasons, it is crucial to map and preserve different aspects of social cognition in a psychiatrist, while this need is less central in a handler.

18.7.3 Should We Map the Left Hemisphere?

Currently, only the right hemisphere is mapped in an attempt to avoid permanent mentalizing deficits in the chronic postoperative period. This choice appears to be constrained by several factors. First, even if it is highly questionable given the current literature, it is generally believed that the right hemisphere is dominant for social cognition. This view is largely influenced by studies showing that emotion recognition deficits are more severe in the event of right hemispheric lesions (for a review, [72]). Second, the tasks used for mapping the left hemisphere seem to be sufficient to identify most of the association or projection tracts, structures that have to be considered as building blocks for neurocognitive networks because refractory to functional compensation [62]. Third, social cognition tasks have often a language component, not allowing to be used for the left hemisphere. For example, if difficulties are induced on the "reading the mind in the eyes" task during electrostimulation of left structures, it is impossible to determine whether the deficit is due to mentalizing disturbances or semantic disturbances. Fourth, the handle of lesion-mapping studies performed in glioma patients have not found significant brain-behavior relationships with areas of the left hemisphere with the exception of Herbet et al. [42] in which subjective empathy changes were related to lesional infiltration of the left cingular bundle. However, in the two remaining studies, either patients with left-sided tumors were not included [43] or the number of included patients was limited for fully appropriate voxelwise lesion-symptom mapping analyses ($n = 63$) [52]. As a result, longitudinal studies with a large sample of patients and tasks may help deciding whether the left hemisphere should be the target of social cognition mapping.

References

1. Baron-Cohen S, Jolliffe T, Mortimore C, Robertson M. Another advanced test of theory of mind: evidence from very high functioning adults with autism or Asperger syndrome. J Child Psychol Psychiatry. 1997;38(7):813–22.
2. Brothers L. The social brain: a project for integrating primate behavior and neurophysiology in a new domain. Concepts Neurosci. 1990;1:27–61.
3. Baron-Cohen S, Ring HA, Bullmore ET, Wheelwright S, Ashwin C, Williams SC. The amygdala theory of autism. Neurosci Biobehav Rev. 2000;24(3):355–64. https://doi.org/10.1016/s0149-7634(00)00011-7.
4. Green MF, Horan WP, Lee J. Social cognition in schizophrenia. Nat Rev Neurosci. 2015;16(10):620–31. https://doi.org/10.1038/nrn4005.
5. Penn DL, Sanna LJ, Roberts DL. Social cognition in schizophrenia: an overview. Schizophr Bull. 2008;34(3):408–11. https://doi.org/10.1093/schbul/sbn014.
6. Adolphs R. The neurobiology of social cognition. Curr Opin Neurobiol. 2001;11(2):231–9. https://doi.org/10.1016/s0959-4388(00)00202-6.
7. Frith CD, Frith U. Mechanisms of social cognition. Annu Rev Psychol. 2012;63:287–313. https://doi.org/10.1146/annurev-psych-120710-100449.
8. Mar RA. The neural bases of social cognition and story comprehension. Annu Rev Psychol. 2011;62:103–34. https://doi.org/10.1146/annurev-psych-120709-145406.
9. Patterson K, Nestor PJ, Rogers TT. Where do you know what you know? The representation of semantic knowledge in the human brain. Nat Rev Neurosci. 2007;8(12):976–87. https://doi.org/10.1038/nrn2277.
10. Herbet G, Duffau H. Revisiting the functional anatomy of the human brain: toward a meta-networking theory of cerebral functions. Physiol Rev. 2020;100(3):1181–228. https://doi.org/10.1152/physrev.00033.2019.
11. Schaafsma SM, Pfaff DW, Spunt RP, Adolphs R. Deconstructing and reconstructing theory of mind. Trends Cogn Sci. 2015;19(2):65–72. https://doi.org/10.1016/j.tics.2014.11.007.
12. Keysers C, Gazzola V. Integrating simulation and theory of mind: from self to social cognition. Trends Cogn Sci. 2007;11(5):194–6. https://doi.org/10.1016/j.tics.2007.02.002.
13. Lieberman MD. Social cognitive neuroscience: a review of core processes. Annu Rev Psychol. 2007;58:259–89. https://doi.org/10.1146/annurev.psych.58.110405.085654.
14. Pan J, Zhan L, Hu C, Yang J, Wang C, Gu L, et al. Emotion regulation and complex brain networks: association between expressive suppression and efficiency in the fronto-parietal network and default-mode network. Front Hum Neurosci. 2018;12:70. https://doi.org/10.3389/fnhum.2018.00070.
15. Wang Y, Metoki A, Alm KH, Olson IR. White matter pathways and social cognition. Neurosci Biobehav Rev. 2018;90:350–70. https://doi.org/10.1016/j.neubiorev.2018.04.015.
16. Yang DY, Rosenblau G, Keifer C, Pelphrey KA. An integrative neural model of social perception, action observation, and theory of mind. Neurosci Biobehav Rev. 2015;51:263–75. https://doi.org/10.1016/j.neubiorev.2015.01.020.
17. Grill-Spector K, Weiner KS. The functional architecture of the ventral temporal cortex and its role in categorization. Nat Rev Neurosci. 2014;15(8):536–48. https://doi.org/10.1038/nrn3747.
18. Grill-Spector K, Weiner KS, Gomez J, Stigliani A, Natu VS. The functional neuroanatomy of face perception: from brain measurements to deep neural networks. Interface Focus. 2018;8(4):20180013. https://doi.org/10.1098/rsfs.2018.0013.
19. Grill-Spector K, Weiner KS, Kay K, Gomez J. The functional neuroanatomy of human face perception. Annu Rev Vis Sci. 2017;3:167–96. https://doi.org/10.1146/annurev-vision-102016-061214.
20. Haxby JV, Hoffman EA, Gobbini MI. Human neural systems for face recognition and social communication. Biol Psychiatry. 2002;51(1):59–67. https://doi.org/10.1016/s0006-3223(01)01330-0.

21. Weiner KS, Grill-Spector K. The evolution of face processing networks. Trends Cogn Sci. 2015;19(5):240–1. https://doi.org/10.1016/j.tics.2015.03.010.
22. Herbet G, Zemmoura I, Duffau H. Functional anatomy of the inferior longitudinal fasciculus: from historical reports to current hypotheses. Front Neuroanat. 2018;12:77. https://doi.org/10.3389/fnana.2018.00077.
23. Grossi D, Soricelli A, Ponari M, Salvatore E, Quarantelli M, Prinster A, et al. Structural connectivity in a single case of progressive prosopagnosia: the role of the right inferior longitudinal fasciculus. Cortex. 2014;56:111–20. https://doi.org/10.1016/j.cortex.2012.09.010.
24. Thomas C, Avidan G, Humphreys K, Jung KJ, Gao F, Behrmann M. Reduced structural connectivity in ventral visual cortex in congenital prosopagnosia. Nat Neurosci. 2009;12(1):29–31. https://doi.org/10.1038/nn.2224.
25. Rizzolatti G, Craighero L. The mirror-neuron system. Annu Rev Neurosci. 2004;27:169–92. https://doi.org/10.1146/annurev.neuro.27.070203.144230.
26. Rizzolatti G, Sinigaglia C. The functional role of the parieto-frontal mirror circuit: interpretations and misinterpretations. Nat Rev Neurosci. 2010;11(4):264–74. https://doi.org/10.1038/nrn2805.
27. Grossman ED, Battelli L, Pascual-Leone A. Repetitive TMS over posterior STS disrupts perception of biological motion. Vis Res. 2005;45(22):2847–53. https://doi.org/10.1016/j.visres.2005.05.027.
28. Thompson J, Parasuraman R. Attention, biological motion, and action recognition. Neuroimage. 2012;59(1):4–13. https://doi.org/10.1016/j.neuroimage.2011.05.044.
29. Bonini L. The extended mirror neuron network: anatomy, origin, and functions. Neuroscientist. 2017;23(1):56–67. https://doi.org/10.1177/1073858415626400.
30. Bufalari I, Aprile T, Avenanti A, Di Russo F, Aglioti SM. Empathy for pain and touch in the human somatosensory cortex. Cereb Cortex. 2007;17(11):2553–61. https://doi.org/10.1093/cercor/bhl161.
31. Singer T, Critchley HD, Preuschoff K. A common role of insula in feelings, empathy and uncertainty. Trends Cogn Sci. 2009;13(8):334–40. https://doi.org/10.1016/j.tics.2009.05.001.
32. Singer T, Frith C. The painful side of empathy. Nat Neurosci. 2005;8(7):845–6. https://doi.org/10.1038/nn0705-845.
33. Iacoboni M, Dapretto M. The mirror neuron system and the consequences of its dysfunction. Nat Rev Neurosci. 2006;7(12):942–51. https://doi.org/10.1038/nrn2024.
34. Premack D, Woodruff G. Does a chimpanzee have a theory of mind. Behav Brain Sci. 1978;1(4):515–26. https://doi.org/10.1017/S0140525X00076512.
35. Amodio DM, Frith CD. Meeting of minds: the medial frontal cortex and social cognition. Nat Rev Neurosci. 2006;7(4):268–77. https://doi.org/10.1038/nrn1884.
36. Carrington SJ, Bailey AJ. Are there theory of mind regions in the brain? A review of the neuroimaging literature. Hum Brain Mapp. 2009;30(8):2313–35. https://doi.org/10.1002/hbm.20671.
37. Schurz M, Radua J, Aichhorn M, Richlan F, Perner J. Fractionating theory of mind: a meta-analysis of functional brain imaging studies. Neurosci Biobehav Rev. 2014;42:9–34. https://doi.org/10.1016/j.neubiorev.2014.01.009.
38. Frith U, Frith CD. Development and neurophysiology of mentalizing. Philos Trans R Soc Lond Ser B Biol Sci. 2003;358(1431):459–73. https://doi.org/10.1098/rstb.2002.1218.
39. Van Overwalle F, Baetens K. Understanding others' actions and goals by mirror and mentalizing systems: a meta-analysis. Neuroimage. 2009;48(3):564–84. https://doi.org/10.1016/j.neuroimage.2009.06.009.
40. Grosse Wiesmann C, Schreiber J, Singer T, Steinbeis N, Friederici AD. White matter maturation is associated with the emergence of Theory of Mind in early childhood. Nat Commun. 2017;8:14692. https://doi.org/10.1038/ncomms14692.
41. Herbet G, Lafargue G, de Champfleur NM, Moritz-Gasser S, le Bars E, Bonnetblanc F, et al. Disrupting posterior cingulate connectivity disconnects consciousness from the external environment. Neuropsychologia. 2014b;56:239–44. https://doi.org/10.1016/j.neuropsychologia.2014.01.020.

42. Herbet G, Lafargue G, Moritz-Gasser S, Menjot de Champfleur N, Costi E, Bonnetblanc F, et al. A disconnection account of subjective empathy impairments in diffuse low-grade glioma patients. Neuropsychologia. 2015b;70:165–76. https://doi.org/10.1016/j.neuropsychologia.2015.02.015.
43. Nakajima R, Yordanova YN, Duffau H, Herbet G. Neuropsychological evidence for the crucial role of the right arcuate fasciculus in the face-based mentalizing network: a disconnection analysis. Neuropsychologia. 2018b;115:179–87. https://doi.org/10.1016/j.neuropsychologia.2018.01.024.
44. Wang Y, Olson IR. The original social network: white matter and social cognition. Trends Cogn Sci. 2018;22(6):504–16. https://doi.org/10.1016/j.tics.2018.03.005.
45. Yordanova YN, Duffau H, Herbet G. Neural pathways subserving face-based mentalizing. Brain Struct Funct. 2017;222(7):3087–105. https://doi.org/10.1007/s00429-017-1388-0.
46. Pertz M, Okoniewski A, Schlegel U, Thoma P. Impairment of sociocognitive functions in patients with brain tumours. Neurosci Biobehav Rev. 2020;108:370–92. https://doi.org/10.1016/j.neubiorev.2019.11.018.
47. Campanella F, Fabbro F, Ius T, Shallice T, Skrap M. Acute effects of surgery on emotion and personality of brain tumor patients: surgery impact, histological aspects, and recovery. Neuro Oncol. 2015;17(8):1121–31. https://doi.org/10.1093/neuonc/nov065.
48. Goebel S, Mehdorn HM, Wiesner CD. Social cognition in patients with intracranial tumors: do we forget something in the routine neuropsychological examination? J Neurooncol. 2018;140(3):687–96. https://doi.org/10.1007/s11060-018-3000-8.
49. Herbet G, Lafargue G, Bonnetblanc F, Moritz-Gasser S, Duffau H. Is the right frontal cortex really crucial in the mentalizing network? A longitudinal study in patients with a slow-growing lesion. Cortex. 2013;49(10):2711–27. https://doi.org/10.1016/j.cortex.2013.08.003.
50. Herbet G, Lafargue G, Moritz-Gasser S, Bonnetblanc F, Duffau H. Interfering with the neural activity of mirror-related frontal areas impairs mentalistic inferences. Brain Struct Funct. 2015a;220(4):2159–69. https://doi.org/10.1007/s00429-014-0777-x.
51. Nakajima R, Kinoshita M, Okita H, Yahata T, Matsui M, Nakada M. Neural networks mediating high-level mentalizing in patients with right cerebral hemispheric gliomas. Front Behav Neurosci. 2018a;12:33. https://doi.org/10.3389/fnbeh.2018.00033.
52. Herbet G, Lafargue G, Bonnetblanc F, Moritz-Gasser S, Menjot de Champfleur N, Duffau H. Inferring a dual-stream model of mentalizing from associative white matter fibres disconnection. Brain. 2014a;137(Pt 3):944–59. https://doi.org/10.1093/brain/awt370.
53. Abu-Akel A, Shamay-Tsoory S. Neuroanatomical and neurochemical bases of theory of mind. Neuropsychologia. 2011;49(11):2971–84.
54. Bates E, Wilson SM, Saygin AP, Dick F, Sereno MI, Knight RT, et al. Voxel-based lesion-symptom mapping. Nat Neurosci. 2003;6(5):448–50. https://doi.org/10.1038/nn1050.
55. Thiebaut de Schotten M, Urbanski M, Valabregue R, Bayle DJ, Volle E. Subdivision of the occipital lobes: an anatomical and functional MRI connectivity study. Cortex. 2014;56:121–37. https://doi.org/10.1016/j.cortex.2012.12.007.
56. Baron-Cohen S, Wheelwright S. The empathy quotient: an investigation of adults with Asperger syndrome or high functioning autism, and normal sex differences. J Autism Dev Disord. 2004;34(2):163–75. https://doi.org/10.1023/b:jadd.0000022607.19833.00.
57. Lawrence EJ, Shaw P, Baker D, Baron-Cohen S, David AS. Measuring empathy: reliability and validity of the Empathy Quotient. Psychol Med. 2004;34(5):911–9.
58. Campanella F, Shallice T, Ius T, Fabbro F, Skrap M. Impact of brain tumour location on emotion and personality: a voxel-based lesion-symptom mapping study on mentalization processes. Brain. 2014;137(Pt 9):2532–45. https://doi.org/10.1093/brain/awu183.
59. Giussani C, Pirillo D, Roux FE. Mirror of the soul: a cortical stimulation study on recognition of facial emotions. J Neurosurg. 2010;112(3):520–7. https://doi.org/10.3171/2009.5.JNS081522.
60. Papagno C, Pisoni A, Mattavelli G, Casarotti A, Comi A, Fumagalli F, et al. Specific disgust processing in the left insula: new evidence from direct electrical stimulation. Neuropsychologia. 2016;84:29–35. https://doi.org/10.1016/j.neuropsychologia.2016.01.036.

61. Mandonnet E, Herbet G, Duffau H. Letter: introducing new tasks for intraoperative mapping in awake glioma surgery: clearing the line between patient care and scientific research. Neurosurgery. 2020;86(2):E256–7. https://doi.org/10.1093/neuros/nyz447.
62. Herbet G, Maheu M, Costi E, Lafargue G, Duffau H. Mapping neuroplastic potential in brain-damaged patients. Brain. 2016;139(Pt 3):829–44. https://doi.org/10.1093/brain/awv394.
63. Yordanova YN, Cochereau J, Duffau H, Herbet G. Combining resting state functional MRI with intraoperative cortical stimulation to map the mentalizing network. Neuroimage. 2019;186:628–36. https://doi.org/10.1016/j.neuroimage.2018.11.046.
64. Baron-Cohen S, Wheelwright S, Hill J, Raste Y, Plumb I. The "Reading the Mind in the Eyes" Test revised version: a study with normal adults, and adults with Asperger syndrome or high-functioning autism. J Child Psychol Psychiatry. 2001;42(2):241–51.
65. Nakajima R, Kinoshita M, Okita H, Yahata T, Nakada M. Glioma surgery under awake condition can lead to good independence and functional outcome excluding deep sensation and visuospatial cognition. Neurooncol Pract. 2019;6(5):354–63. https://doi.org/10.1093/nop/npy054.
66. Duffau H. Stimulation mapping of white matter tracts to study brain functional connectivity. Nat Rev Neurol. 2015;11(5):255–65. https://doi.org/10.1038/nrneurol.2015.51.
67. Cochereau J, Deverdun J, Herbet G, Charroud C, Boyer A, Moritz-Gasser S, et al. Comparison between resting state fMRI networks and responsive cortical stimulations in glioma patients. Hum Brain Mapp. 2016;37(11):3721–32. https://doi.org/10.1002/hbm.23270.
68. Rojkova K, Volle E, Urbanski M, Humbert F, Dell'Acqua F, Thiebaut de Schotten M. Atlasing the frontal lobe connections and their variability due to age and education: a spherical deconvolution tractography study. Brain Struct Funct. 2016;221(3):1751–66. https://doi.org/10.1007/s00429-015-1001-3.
69. Mandonnet E, Herbet G, Moritz-Gasser S, Poisson I, Rheault F, Duffau H. Electrically induced verbal perseveration: a striatal deafferentation model. Neurology. 2019;92(6):e613–21. https://doi.org/10.1212/WNL.0000000000006880.
70. Almairac F, Herbet G, Moritz-Gasser S, de Champfleur NM, Duffau H. The left inferior fronto-occipital fasciculus subserves language semantics: a multilevel lesion study. Brain Struct Funct. 2015;220(4):1983–95. https://doi.org/10.1007/s00429-014-0773-1.
71. Schilbach L, Timmermans B, Reddy V, Costall A, Bente G, Schlicht T, et al. Toward a second-person neuroscience. Behav Brain Sci. 2013;36(4):393–414. https://doi.org/10.1017/S0140525X12000660.
72. Adolphs R. Recognizing emotion from facial expressions: psychological and neurological mechanisms. Behav Cogn Neurosci Rev. 2002;1(1):21–62. https://doi.org/10.1177/1534582302001001003.
73. Nakada M. The handbook of awake surgery. Tokyo: Chugai-igaku; 2019.

Multiple Tasks

19

Henry Colle, Barbara Tomasino, Erik Robert, Miran Skrap, and Tamara Ius

19.1 Introduction

Nowadays diffuse low-grade gliomas (DLGGs) surgery is based on the postulate that the maximal safe resection must be prosecuted [1–15]. To solve the classical dilemma between the oncological and functional issues, an individual cerebral mapping is mandatory in DLGGs surgery. Indeed, during their natural history, DLGGs induce cerebral reorganization which turns into considerable anatomo-functional variations among patients, representing a major issue in surgical management [16–19]. Intraoperative direct electrical stimulation (DES), especially in awake patients benefiting from a neuropsychological testing, is the best way to optimize the EOR while sparing eloquent neural networks [12, 14–16, 20–22]. Neuropsychological testing during AS should be customized "ad hoc" for each single patient, considering the high anatomo-functional variability due to patients' characteristics (age, education, job, cooperation degree, hemispherical dominance, preoperative cognitive assessment, daily activities) and tumor features (cortical and subcortical location, extension, tumor growth pattern, tumor lateralization, tumor development speed, individual plasticity reshaping in reaction to the tumor).

Although neuropsychological testing during AS is commonly used in DLGGs surgery, a standardized approved protocol has not yet been defined [14, 15, 23–25]. The main challenge in neuropsychological testing during AS is the patient collaboration and time limitation. A fundamental step in this approach is the choice of

H. Colle · E. Robert
Department of Neurosurgery, AZ Sint-Lucas, Ghent, Belgium
e-mail: Henry.Colle@AZSTLUCAS.BE; Erik.Robert@AZSTLUCAS.BE

B. Tomasino
IRCCS "E. Medea," Polo Regionale del FVG, San Vito al Tagliamento, Pordenone, Italy

M. Skrap · T. Ius (✉)
Neurosurgery Unit, Department of Neurosciences, Santa Maria della Misericordia University Hospital, Udine, Italy

E. Mandonnet, G. Herbet (eds.), *Intraoperative Mapping of Cognitive Networks*,
https://doi.org/10.1007/978-3-030-75071-8_19

neuropsychological testing, which should be tailored for the interested area. Considering the interindividual variability and the multifunctional areas, a combination of different specific tests is needed to obtain a useful feedback from the patient during surgery. In addition, most of the time DLGGs develop in multimodal areas requiring a multiple tasks approach.

In this chapter we summarize two different approaches for neuropsychological testing during AS:

1. Global Synthetical Multimodal Testing (GENTasks) based on global continuous multimodal testing elaborated to detect all the possible language functions that could be encountered in the peritumoral white matter. This is combined with an analytical sequential testing adapted to the operated area, in case an error appears at the G.E.N.T.
2. Real-Time Neuropsychological Testing (RTNT) is based on an intraoperative sequence of tasks to monitor several cognitive functions for the target area. The selected tasks for the target area are continuously repeated for immediate dysfunction detection. Even in case of negative mapping, this approach provides functional cognitive information, guiding the online decision to carry out or stop the resection.

19.2 Part I Multiple Tasks for Language Sub-functions Mapping

The ten chapters of part II dealing with language functions (Chaps. 5–14) demonstrated that relying intraoperatively on a sole picture naming test does not warrant to preserve language abilities in all its multifaceted aspects. Indeed, several studies indicated that some long-lasting deficits in some language subfunctions can be observed when testing picture naming only (see Table 19.1 for a summary, and Chaps. 5–14).

Hence the question arises how to optimize the selection of several language tasks and how to combine different specific language tasks sequentially or in a single more complex language task. We will deal in this chapter with two proposals regarding this issue:

- The global synthetical multimodal language testing (GSMLT), developed by the Gent team. It is an integrated new methodology of mapping; it is still under development and its interest should be demonstrated in a near future.
- The real-time neuropsychological testing (RTNT) developed by the Udine team. This method follows a slightly different philosophy, as it has been designed in the broader context of preserving both the language and other-than-language cognitive functions. Its use provided some promising results [32, 33].

Table 19.1 Literature review about long-term postoperative deficits in patients who did not benefit from intraoperative monitoring of the function

Function	Study	Test	Outcome at follow-up assessment
Verbal short-term memory [26]	Teixidor P, Gatignol P, Leroy M, Masuet-Aumatell C, Capelle L, Duffau H. (2007). Assessment of verbal working memory before and after surgery for low-grade glioma. J Neurooncol	Awake Surgery It is worth noting that WM was not mapped intraoperatively, because it was never demonstrated previously that this function was altered before and after DLGG surgery	Impaired At 3 months 8 examined 5 recovered surgery induced a transient vWM worsening, which nevertheless recovers within 3 months
Reading [27]	Mandonnet, E., Gatignol, P., & Duffau, H. (2009). Evidence for an occipito-temporal tract underlying visual recognition in picture naming. *Clinical neurology and neurosurgery*	Awake surgery Object naming	Recovery
Writing [28]	Scarone, P., Gatignol, P., Guillaume, S., Denvil, D., Capelle, L., & Duffau, H. (2009). Agraphia after awake surgery for brain tumor: new insights into the anatomo-functional network of writing. *Surgical neurology*, *72*(3), 223–241	Awake surgery the patient was asked to perform counting (regularly from 1 to 10 over and over) and picture naming	50% recovery among the patients, only those with lesions of the supplementary motor area did not recover from agraphia in the postoperative period (in 50% of cases)
Reading [29]	Gil-Robles, S., Carvallo, A., Jimenez, M., Gomez Caicoya, A., Martinez, R., Ruiz-Ocaña, C., & Duffau, H. (2013). Double dissociation between visual recognition and picture naming: a study of the visual language connectivity using tractography and brain stimulation. *Neurosurgery*	Awake surgery Intraoperative testing consisted of naming, reading, and recognition of symbols	Letter-by-Letter reading
Syntactic ability [30]	Teichmann, M., Rosso, C., Martini, J. B., Bloch, I., Brugières, P., Duffau, H., Lehéricy, S., & Bachoud-Lévi, A. C. (2015). A cortical-subcortical syntax pathway linking Broca's area and the striatum. *Human brain mapping*	Awake surgery Object naming tested	Impaired

(continued)

Table 19.1 (continued)

Function	Study	Test	Outcome at follow-up assessment
Proper name retrieval [31]	Papagno, C., Casarotti, A., Comi, A., Pisoni, A., Lucchelli, F., Bizzi, A., Riva, M., & Bello, L. (2016). Long-term proper name anomia after removal of the uncinate fasciculus. *Brain structure & function*	Not reported if awake, not tested intra-surgery	Impaired
Repetition [25]	Sierpowska, J., Gabarrós, A., Fernandez-Coello, A., Camins, À., Castañer, S., Juncadella, M., Morís, J., & Rodríguez-Fornells, A. (2017). Words are not enough: nonword repetition as an indicator of arcuate fasciculus integrity during brain tumor resection. *Journal of neurosurgery*	Real word repetition (WR) and nonword repetition (NWR) tasks as complements to standard picture naming	Still impaired

19.2.1 Global Synthetical Multimodal Testing (GSMLT)

19.2.1.1 Cortical Stimulation

Usually, once the stimulation threshold has been determined by testing motor and automatic speech like counting, an object naming (ON) task is first proposed. By accurate on-the-fly analysis of the error typology, a lot of information can be accessed about which language subfunction network has been disturbed [34]. However, some sites can be negative for ON, while they would be positive for other tasks, for example, a verb generation task or a syntactic task. This means that other tasks should be executed in a sequential way, and that the set of tasks should be adapted to the anatomical area at hand. We proposed to rely on the well-established anatomo-functional parcellation proposed by Corina [35] (see Fig. 19.1).

We tried to associate each parcel to some language subfunction(s), and to select specific tasks for each parcel. To this end, we recycled the Dutch Linguistic Intraoperative Protocol (DuLIP) [36]. From the ten basic tasks with 4 s time frame, we retained the six most useful tasks (Object Naming ON, Repetition RP, Semantic Odd Word Out SW, Semantic Odd Picture Out SP, Sentence Completion SC, Verb Generation VG), excluding the tasks with possible double use (Reading Phonological Odd Word Out, Action Naming, Semantic Association, Diadochokinesis). The resulting Parcel Adapted Specific Task (P.A.S.T.) is given in Fig. 19.2.

First, Object Naming is tested 3 times on each site; then parcel-specific tasks are proposed. Theoretically, at each stimulation point, each of the three selected tasks

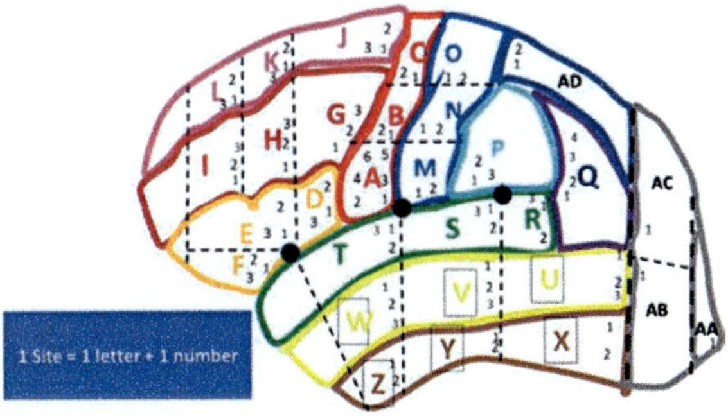

Fig. 19.1 Anatomo-functional parcellation for language, developed by Corina et al. Each parcel is named by a letter, and within a parcel, 1 cm^2 areas of stimulation are numbered

Cortical Stimulation: PARCEL (A-Z) / TASK (DuLIP 1-7)

DuLIP 1-7	A	B	C	D	E	F	G	H	I	J	K	L	M	N	O	P	Q	T	S	T	U	V	W	X	Y	Z
1 Object Naming	ON	ON	ON	ON	ON	ON	ON	ON	ON	ON	ON	ON	ON	ON	ON	ON	ON	ON	ON	ON	ON	ON	ON	ON	ON	ON
2 Verb Generation	VG	VG	VG	VG	VG	VG	VG	VG	VG	VG	VG	VG	VG	VG	VG											
3 Repetition	RP			RP									RP			RP	RP	RP	RP							
4 Semantic odd Picture out		SP			SP	SP	SP	SP	SP					SP		SP	SP	SP	SP	SP	SP	SP	SP	SP	SP	SP
5 Sentence Completion			SC							SC	SC	SC			SC			SC	SC	SC	SC	SC	SC	SC	SC	SC
6 Semantic odd Word out																SW	SW			SW	SW	SW	SW	SW	SW	SW
7 Action Naming	AN	AN	AN	AN	AN	AN	AN	AN	AN	AN	AN	AN	AN	AN	AN											

Fig. 19.2 Parcel Adapted Specific Tasks. For each parcel, no more than three specific tasks among six possible were selected (see Fig. 19.1 for the precise delineation of each cortical parcel)

should be tested three times. However, for a cortical exposition of, e.g., 6 × 6 cm = 36 cm^2, at the rate of 5 s per task, and with 1 stimulation point each square cm, the total duration would be 36 × 5 × 3 × 3 = 1620 s (27 min). This would be abusively too long, while the maximum of time should be kept for subcortical stimulation and resection. To overcome this issue, we hypothesized that because the tasks have been adapted to the parcel at hand, testing only once each of the three tasks would be already more sensitive than testing ON alone. Hence, at each stimulation point, three different tasks are performed, and the whole specific mapping lasts 9 min.

The selection of appropriate tasks is greatly facilitated by the preoperative definition of the stimulation points during the navigational planning ("functional planning"), with labeling with letter and number (A1 → Z9), see Fig. 19.3.

All the stimulation sites are reported in an Excel grid, personalized to each patient (see Fig. 19.4). The speech therapist will present successively the different tasks and tell to the surgeon which parcels should be stimulated for each task. Since the points are preselected, the sequence of stimulation can follow the sequence of the personalized grid (A1, B1, D1, E1, G1; A2, B2, D2, E2, G2; A3, B3….). This avoids successive stimulation of adjacent areas and limits the risk of seizures. For instance, when point A1 will be stimulated, the corresponding Excel cell is activated by clicking on it; if the patient's answer is correct (= negative = green), a click on (−) will change the color of the cell from white to light green, then cyan; if incorrect

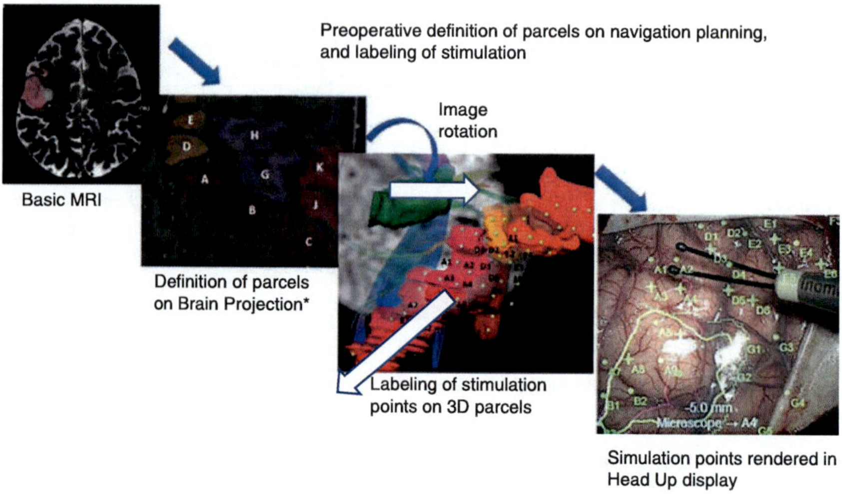

Fig. 19.3 Neuronavigated definition of stimulation sites. In the preplanning, the Corina parcels are manually segmented and labeled, and the 1 cm^2 stimulation sites are defined and labeled. Intraoperatively, the position of the stimulation sites is projected on the brain surface, through injection in the binocular microscope

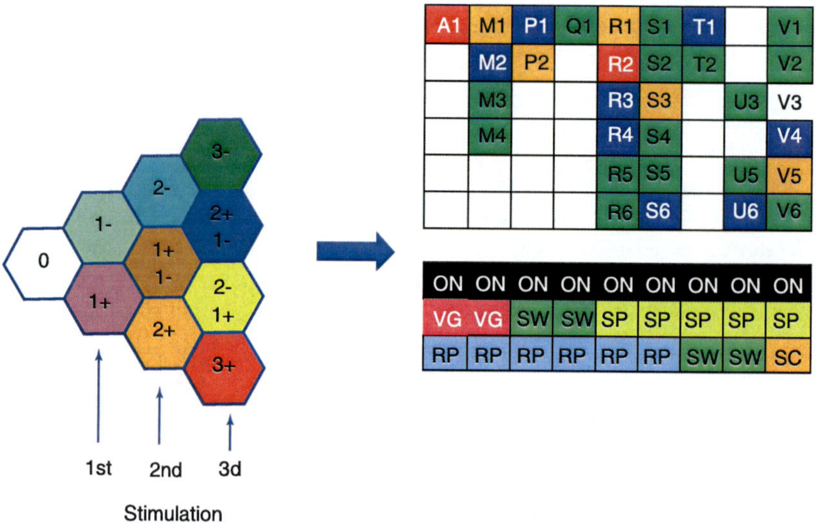

Fig. 19.4 Intraoperative results of cortical mapping. In excel files, parcels (letter labeled) are put in column, and within a parcel, stimulation sites are put in lines (letter-number labeled). The color of the cells indicates the results of the three stimulations

(=positive = red), a click on (+,) moves it to pink then yellow, and further to green (3× negative), red (3× positive), blue (+ − −), or orange (+ + −). So the color of the cell, universally understandable, immediately indicates the degree of positivity.

Subcortical Stimulation

The method explained above for cortical mapping was made possible thanks to our current knowledge of cortical anatomo-functional parcellation of language subfunctions. Despite considerable recent advances in our understanding of the anatomo-functional segregation of the subcortical pathways of language [37], such parcellation is not available for white matter.

For this reason, we developed a conceptually different approach when mapping white matter. We reasoned that a two-step procedure would optimize both the sensitivity and the specificity of mapping the white matter eloquent for language:

- First, a single task, called Global Evoked Naming Tasks (G.E.N.T.), is continuously monitored. This task taps all aspects of language and requires also a high cognitive load, in particular regarding executive functions. In other words, it is highly sensitive. The purpose of the G.E.N.T. (see Fig. 19.5) is to form a short sentence (the most obvious grammatical structures of which being Subject, Verb,

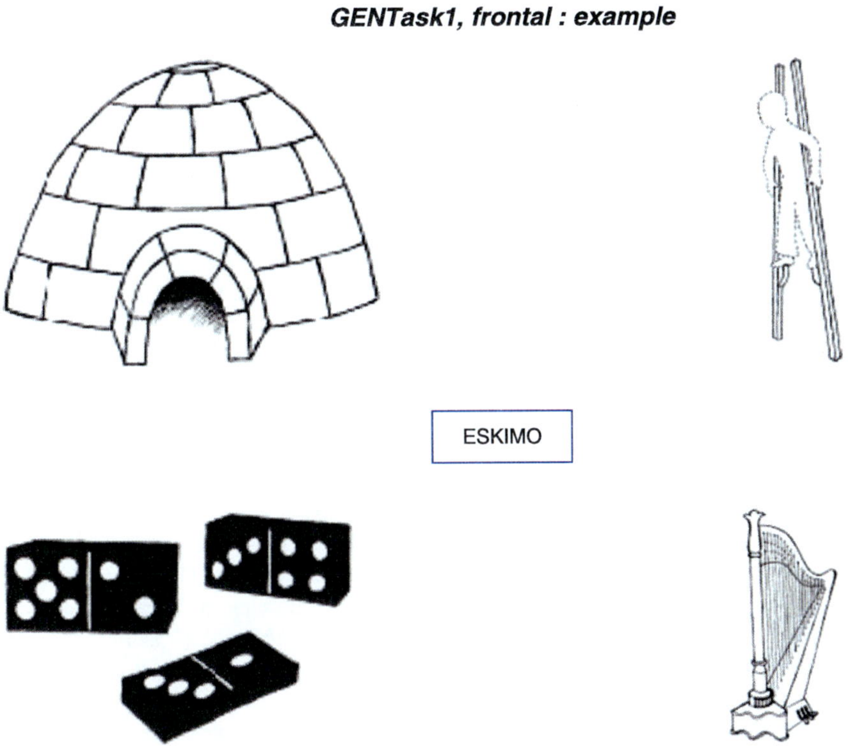

Fig. 19.5 The GENT task. The patient is asked to formulate a full relevant sentence that will make use of the written word at the center and of one of the four images at the corners. The task offers a high flexibility and versatility: the written word can be replaced by replaying an auditory recording, or the written word can be a verb, …

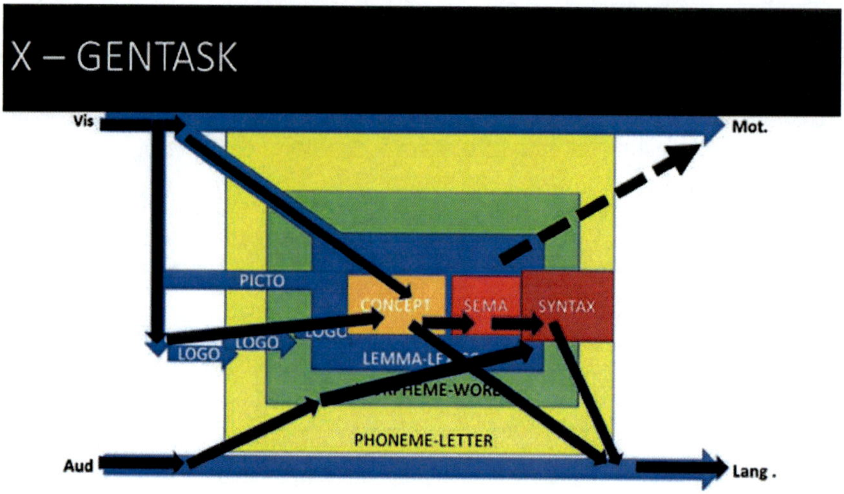

Fig. 19.6 The different language subfunctions explored by the GENT task

Object), where different elements are proposed via different inputs (e.g., visual + reading, auditive + visual,…): in this way, phonological, semantic, syntaxic, and articulatory functions as well must cooperate simultaneously (Fig. 19.6), and interface appropriately with executive functions. Usually, on the patient's screen, a *subject* is proposed written at the center of the slide, with the four Objects at the periphery, or a *verb* at the center and four *subjects* in the corners; instead of writing at the center, the word can also be "spoken" by the slide (interesting in analphabetic or "other-alphabetic" people), or combination of written *subject*, spoken *verb* and drawn *objects*. Attention should be paid to propose the "correct" *object* in the quadrant opposite to the lesion, particularly for parietal or temporal lesions (see Chap. 2). Moreover, the patient can be asked to indicate with the index finger the correct object: this allows to monitor the motor function and to register the motor response time, a measure which is particularly accurate when the cortical stimulation and the task presentation are started synchronously.

– Second, if an error is made by the patient in one trial of the GENT, then, depending on the approximate anatomical location in the white matter, three more specific tasks are selected and tested (Fascicle Adapted Sequential Testing: F.A.S.T.). The FAST has been built based on the DULIP, following the same rationale as for the PAST (see Fig. 19.7). Moreover, many additional, local specific tasks can be proposed, e.g., memory tasks at anterior temporal level, visuospatial tasks in right parietal areas, Lexical Semantic Judgment at temporoparietal level (Presentation of Subject + cannot + 3 Verbs), calculus in Angular Gyrus area, and Visual fields in temporo-parieto-occipital regions (Cf. Chap. 2).

This approach is greatly facilitated by the use of intermittent or continuous subcortical stimulation provided by CUSA-tip in monopolar or CUSA-and suction tip

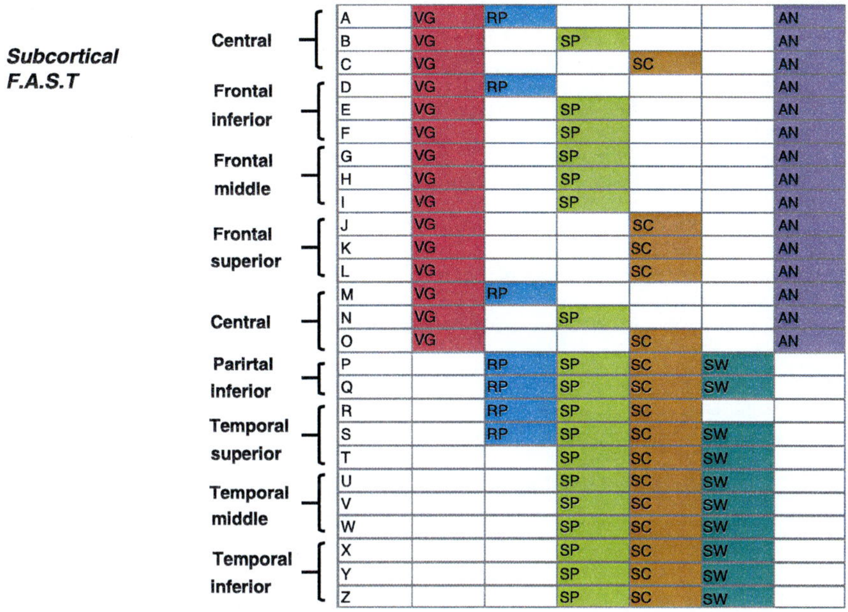

Fig. 19.7 Fascicle Adapted Sequential Testing (FAST). As for the PAST, three specific tasks are selected for each white matter location

in bipolar mode: no time gap occurs, neither by change of instruments, nor by omission of evaluation of a function during testing of other functions. Of note, there might be some periods of time during which task monitoring is not necessary. We take advantage of such periods to assess *spontaneous speech*, an important aspect of language for daily life. Indeed, dissociation between stimulus-induced language tasks and spontaneous auto-generated speech has been observed (see Chap. 6). Moreover, such conversation makes the patient feeling at ease, with possibility of relaxation between the exhausting tasking periods.

19.2.1.2 Real-Time Neuropsychological Testing (RTNT) Applied to Language Functions

RTNT Rational and Strategy

Since 2011, a new neuropsychological method called real-time neuropsychological testing (RTNT) has been adopted, in addition to direct electrical stimulation, at our Department in Udine [32]. The RTNT has been developed to respond to the surgeon's clinical need to have a simple, accurate, reliable, and fast testing of patient's cognitive status. In case of negative mapping, which could be related to an inappropriate task selection, RTNT provides a continuous functional feedback considering that it includes a wider task battery. Specifically, RTNT allows the immediate detection of neuropsychological dysfunction while resection occurs, thus providing a constant functional feedback to the surgeon, even between two consecutive DES

Table 19.2 Intraoperative RTNT performance of patient SR with a lesion to the left insular cortex

RTNT	1 run of RTNT	2 run of RTNT	3 run of RTNT	4 run of RTNT	5 run of RTNT	6 run of RTNT	7 run of RTNT
Naming nouns [1]	10/10	10/10	10/10	10/10	10/10	9/10	9/10
Reading words [38]	10/10	10/10	10/10	10/10	10/10	10/10	10/10
Repetition words [38]	10/10	10/10	9/10	10/10	10/10	10/10	10/10
Auditory grammar comprehension [39]	5/5	5/5	5/5	5/5	5/5[a]	5/5	5/5
Reading pseudowords [38]	10/10	10/10	10/10	10/10	10/10	10/10	10/10[a]
Repetition pseudowords [38]	10/10	10/10	10/10	10/10	10/10	10/10	10/10
Phonological discrimin [40]	16/16	15/15	16/16	15/15	15/15	15/15	15/15
Digit Span Forward [41]	6	5	6	5	5[a]	5	5
Naming verbs [1]	10/10	10/10	10/10	10/10	10/10	9/10	9/10
Token (revised)	10/10	10/10	10/10	10/10	10/10	10/10	
Production of narratives	3/3	3/3	3/3	3/3	3/3	3/3[a]	

[a]Tiredness

phases. A specific and precise panel of tasks can be selected for the RTNT according to the preoperative neuropsychological examination, tumor location and preoperative fMRI and DTI data (see Tables 19.2, 19.4, and 19.6 and a dedicated paragraph below).

The task sequence follows a fixed order and sequence of tasks was repeated (presenting a different stimuli list for each sequence) continuously until the end of the resection. Each task had a duration of about 30 s/1 min. In this way, task assessment and task switching were quick and dynamic for immediate dysfunction detection. This protocol not only prevents a problem of mismatch between task and anatomical point, but it also allows to reduce the mapping time.

Our experience on AS indeed taught us that achieving resection in the shortest time is of utmost importance. The time lapse in which RTNT was administered in our series ranged from 30 to 90 min.

The RTNT recalls the IONM concept. It is a *monitoring* technique that is applied *continuously* during resection, providing a continuous feedback of neuropsychological information [32, 33]., even when no specific sites can be identified with DES (negative mapping) (Fig. 19.8).

The RTNT was developed to obey four essential surgeon's queries on a neuropsychological monitoring: (1) constancy, (2) reliability, (3) immediacy, and (4) accuracy:

1. ***Constancy:*** to be administered and repeated several times through all the resection
2. ***Reliability:*** to guide the surgeon in the functional resection strategy based on repeated measures of patient's performance

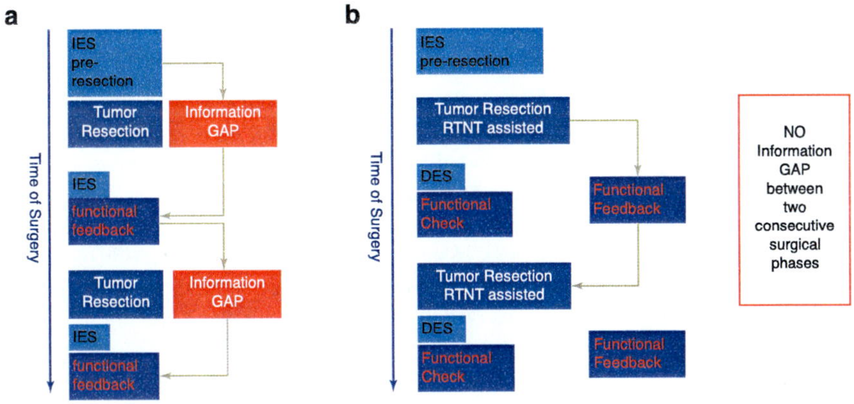

Fig. 19.8 A schematic representation of Surgical Time setting (**a**) DES assisted; (**b**) DES and RTNT assisted

3. ***Immediacy:*** to be applied in an intraoperative setting, the feedback on the patient's cognitive status should be quick; the patient's potential anxiety should be minimized by involving her/him continuously in solving tasks
4. ***Accuracy:*** to include tasks that could give unambiguous and precise measure of cognitive performance and to test the different functions of the area undergoing surgery.

The limit used to stop surgery temporarily or definitively coincides with a decrease in performance to 70% of baseline levels. As soon as the patient exhibits a decrement, the neurosurgeon is immediately informed and moves to another part of the surgical field. If the patient recovers the function, the surgical removal restarts in the previous critical site. When the RTNT shows a decrease in a test, the preordered task sequence is interrupted, and the neuropsychologist follows the principles of differential diagnosis [32, 33]. For example, if a patient manifests a decrease in nonword repetition, word repetition and speech comprehension are assessed to understand the nature of the decrease in performance. In this clinical setting, with selective nonword repetition decrease, the resection continues until the next RTNT run; otherwise if word repetition and speech comprehension are similarly decreased, the resection is stopped and the SLF (Superior Longitudinal Fasciculus) function is verified by using DES.

Intraoperative Tasks Selection

RTNT allows to monitor many neuropsychological functions. Ten/fifteen items are presented for each single test (for instance, 15 pictures for naming, 10 words for reading, 10 pseudowords for repetition) for about 30 s for each task, in a rotating manner, as previously described [32]. RTNT for surgery involving the *language-related* network is based on the use of both object and verb naming tasks (B.A.D.A.) [47]. Stimuli have to be tailored to patients' pre-surgery ability, as some patients may exhibit selective nouns or verb naming difficulties already in the pre-surgery testing [32, 33, 48]. The same stimuli are included in the pre-surgical fMRI naming tasks. The fMRI maps are used for planning and neuronavigation during surgery.

In few minutes the RTNT allows assessing object naming, word reading, pseudoword repetition, and so on. Repetition tasks for words, pseudowords, and sentences (B.A.D.A.) [47] are included as post-surgery patients may exhibit conduction aphasia [49]. Reading tasks of words and pseudowords (B.A.D.A.) [47] are also included, as such deficit could be very selective due to the circumscribed nature of some lesions [49]. In particular, reading is very useful for resection in the temporo-occipital areas and the white matter beneath such as the inferior fronto-occipital fasciculus (IFOF) [50] (see dedicated Chap. 7). In order to monitor comprehension and phonological input processing, RTNT protocols include phonemic discriminations (B.A.D.A.) [47], auditory object comprehensions (B.A.D.A.) [47], lexical decisions (B.A.D.A.) [47], sentence comprehension (B.A.D.A.) [47], and the Token test [51] tapping verbal comprehension. Ten stimuli for each task are continuously rotated and presented to the patient. Task rotation involves also task tapping semantic associations (Pyramids and Palm Trees Test) [52] and phonological fluency (1 min) [53]. In case of surgeries for bilingual patients, RTNT involves testing L1 and L2 as task switching phenomena could be observed intraoperatively [54].

Example of RTNT During a Left Anterior Temporo-Insular DLGG Resection
We report, as an example, a single case of a patient undergoing a left insular DLGG resection who performed AS assisted by RTNT (Table 19.2). SR is a 38-year-old, right-handed, primary-school teacher, with 13 years of schooling. In a period of well-being, she suffered for a series of four episodes characterized by *absence seizures* and déjà vu. She was hospitalized for a left DLGG (55 cm^3) involving the left insular cortex (Fig. 19.9a, b). The fMRI examination revealed an activation related to object naming close to the tumor in the region around Broca's area, and DTI showed that IFOF and SLF were tracked just close to the internal-anterior portion and just above the superior limit of the glioma, respectively (Fig. 19.9c, d).

Prior to starting resection, cortical DES during counting and object naming tasks revealed positive site in putative Broca's area, in agreement with the preoperative fMRI activation related to object naming (last axial slide in Fig. 19.9c). RTNT initiated when the resection started.

This patient performed the RTNT and maintained a normal level of accuracy in all the tasks (Table 19.2). At subcortical level, approaching the IFOF, DES phases were constantly confirmed as negative. At the end of resection, the cortical DES confirmed the positive sites related to object naming, the patient only reported tiredness in the second half of the resection. The resection lasted 1 h and 4 min: during this time lapse the patient performed 8 RTNT runs, each including 11 tasks. The EOR was 100% on T2-postoperative MRI weighted images. Figure 19.10 shows that activation in the area related to object naming close to the tumor in the region around Broca's area persisted, that a contralateral activation emerged, and that the

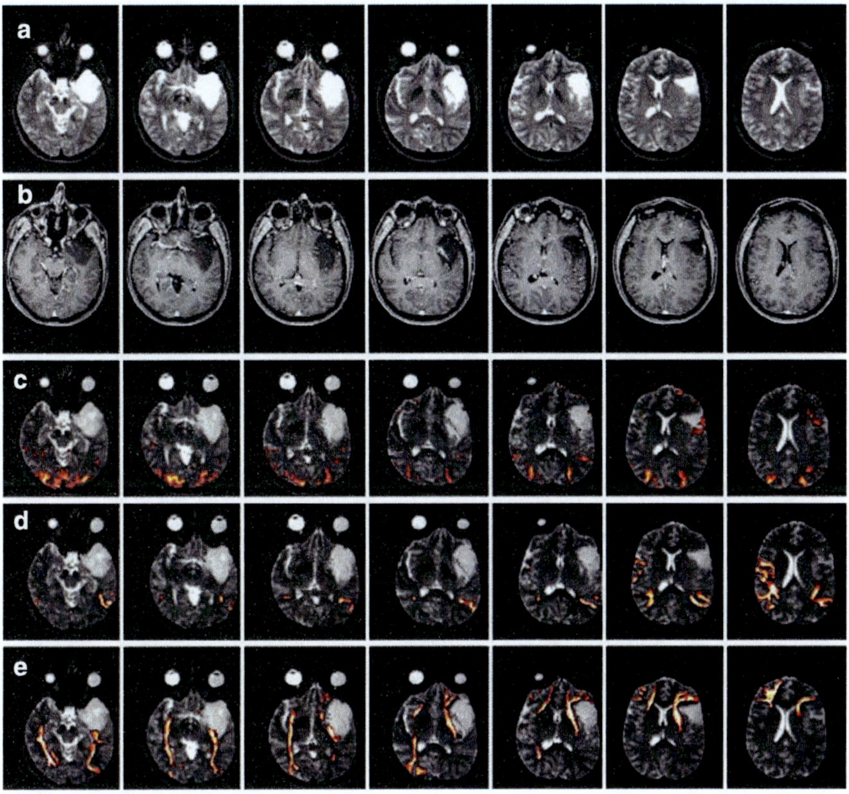

Fig. 19.9 Pre-surgery MRI images (T2 weighted and T1 weighted in **a** and **b**, respectively), the activation related to object naming (**c**), and the DTI tracking of the SLF and IFOF (**d** and **e**, respectively) are shown

IFOF and the SLF remained intact with respect to pre-surgery. When the patient was re-evaluated, her neuropsychological profile at the immediate post-surgery (at 1 week) and at follow-up (4 months after surgery) remained as at 1 week before surgery (Table 19.3).

Example of RTNT During a Left Posterior Temporal DLGG Resection

We present a second case with a DLGG in language area. This case illustrates intraoperative RTNT decrease and transient postoperative deficits. This example is part of a group of patients in which reading abilities have been studied preoperatively, intraoperatively, and in the postoperative follow-up [55]. We report, as an example, a single case of a patient undergoing a left posterior temporal resection who performed the RTNT (Table 19.4). AS is a 38-year-old, right-handed, men, with 18 years of schooling. In a period of well-being, he suffered of speech difficulties and fever. He was hospitalized for a left low-grade glioma (28 cm^3) involving the

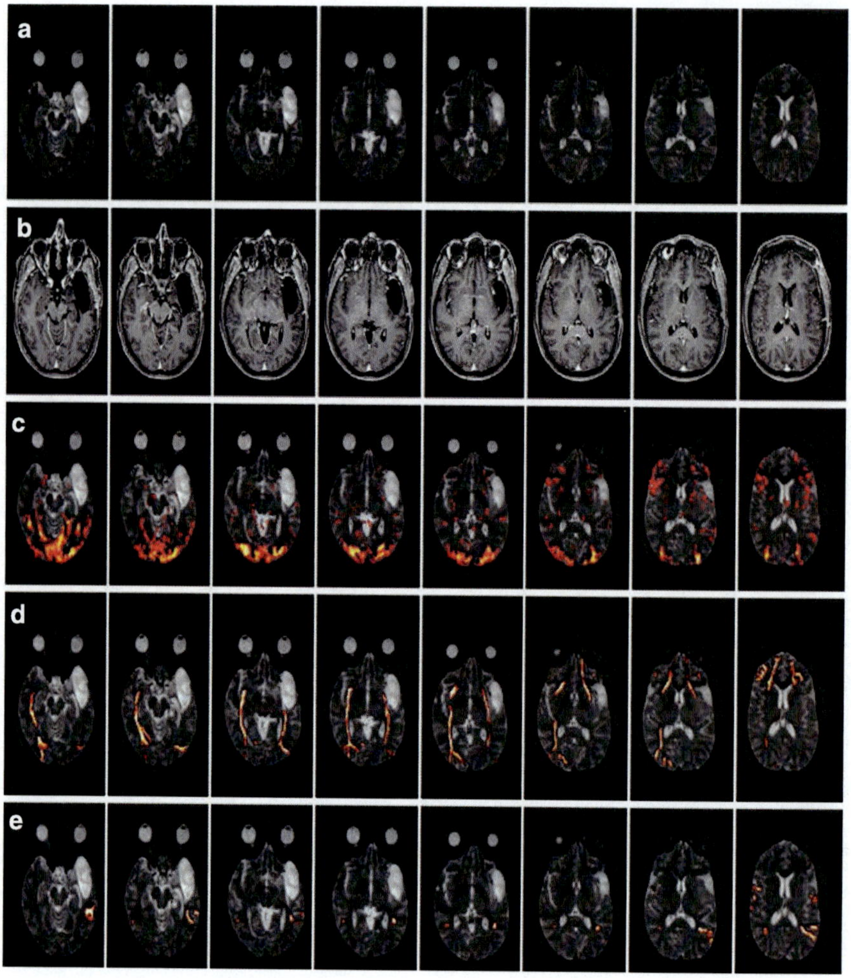

Fig. 19.10 Follow-up MRI images (T2 weighted and T1 weighted in **a** and **b**, respectively), the activation related to object naming (**c**), and the DTI tracking of the IFOF and SLF (**d** and **e**, respectively) are shown

left posterior temporal lobe (Fig. 19.11a). The fMRI examination revealed an activation related to reading close to the tumor. Pre-resective cortical DES was negative. This patient performed the RTNT and maintained a normal level of accuracy in all the tasks except for reading and naming in the final RTNT run. We verified the site with DES in the medial part of the surgical cavity. DES was positive and resection was stopped. The EOR was 82% on T2-postoperative MRI weighted images.

Table 19.3 Pre, immediate post, and follow-up performance of patient SR with a lesion to the left insular cortex

Neuropsychological test	Before surgery (Raw data)	+/–	1 week after surgery	+/–	Follow-up (4 months)	+/–
Raven coloured matrices	36/36	+	–		36/36	+
Digit Span forward	6	+	6	+	6	+
Digit span backward	3	+	4	+	4	+
Orofacial apraxia	20/20	+	20/20	+	20/20	+
Ideomotor apraxia	72/72	+	72/72	+	72/72	+
Letter fluency (3 min)	57	+	56	+	60	+
Category fluency (3 min)	60	+	59	+	61	+
Naming nouns	30/30	+	30/30	+	29/30	+
Naming verbs	28/28	+	28/28	+	28/28	+
Reading words	92/92	+	92/92	+	92/92	+
Reading pseudowords	45/45	+	45/45	+	45/45	+
Reading sentences	6/6	+	6/6	+	6/6	+
Repetition words	45/45	+	45/45	+	45/45	+
Repetition pseudowords	35/35	+	35/35	+	35/35	+
Repetition sentences	14/14	+	14/14	+	14/14	+
Writing words	46/46	+	46/46	+	46/46	+
Writing pseudowords	25/25	+	25/25	+	25/25	+
Auditory lexical decision	80/80	+	80/80	+	78/80	+
Visually lexical decision	80/80	+	80/80	+	78/80	+
Phonological discrimination	80/80	+	80/80	+	78/80	+
Token test	36/36	+	36/36	+	36/36	+
Nouns comprehension	40/40	+	40/40	+	40/40	+
Verbs comprehension	20/20	+	20/20	+	20/20	+
Palm and pyramid test	52/52	+	52/52		51/52	+
Rey auditory verbal learning test (immediate)	11		9		11	
Rey auditory verbal learning test (recall)	9/15	+	6/15	–	9/15	+

Table 19.4 Intraoperative RTNT performance of patient AS with a lesion to the left posterior temporal lobe

RTNT	1 run of RTNT	2 run of RTNT	3 run of RTNT	4 run of RTNT	5 run of RTNT
Naming nouns [1]	10/10	10/10	9/10	7/10	6/10
Reading words [38]	10/10	9/10	7/10	6/10	
Repetition words [38]	10/10	10/10	9/10	10/10	
Auditory grammar comprehension [39]	5/5	5/5	5/5	5/5	
Reading pseudowords [38]	10/10	10/10	8/10	7/10	
Repetition pseudowords [38]	10/10	10/10	9/10	10/10	
Phonological discrimin [40].	16/16	15/15	16/16	15/15	
Digit span forward [41]	5	5	5	4	
Token (revised)	10/10	10/10	10/10	10/10	

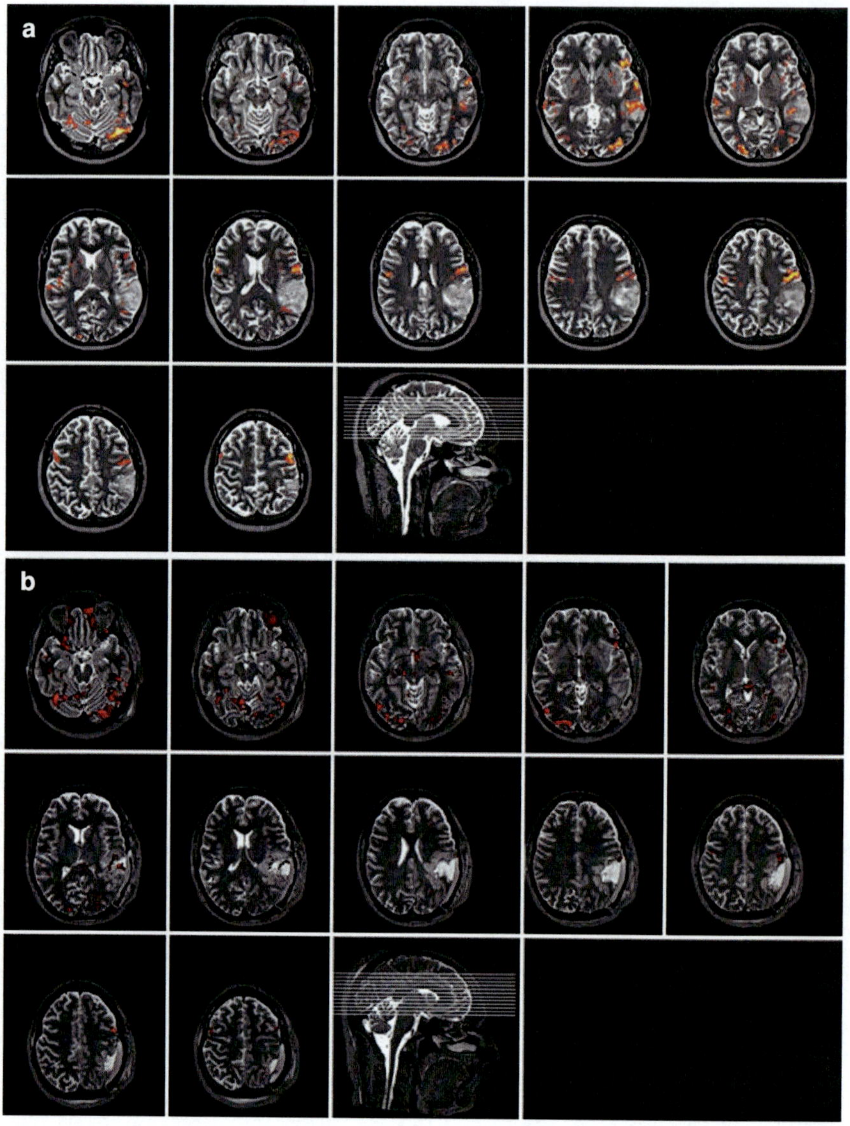

Fig. 19.11 Pre- (**a**) and post-surgery (**b**) MRI images of a DLGG in the left posterior temporal area with a non-total resection. The activation related to reading task is in close proximity to the glioma

Figure 19.11b shows that postoperative activation to reading were still detectable. When the patient was re-evaluated, her neuropsychological profile at the immediate post-surgery (at 1 week) showed an impaired naming and reading which recovered at follow-up (4 months after surgery) (see Table 19.5).

Table 19.5 Pre, immediate post, and follow-up performance of patient AS with a lesion to the left posterior temporal lobe

Neuropsychological test	Before surgery (Raw data)	+/–	1 week after surgery	+/–	Follow-up (4 months)	+/–
Raven coloured matrices	34/36	+	–		34/36	+
Digit span forward	5	+	4	+	4	+
Digit span backward	4	+	3	+	4	+
Orofacial apraxia	20/20	+	20/20	+	20/20	+
Ideomotor apraxia	72/72	+	72/72	+	72/72	+
Letter fluency (3 min)	32	+	28	+	28	+
Naming nouns	30/30	+	20/30	–	27/30	+
Naming verbs	24/28	–	23/28	–	23/28	–
Token test	36/36	+	35/36	+	33/36	+
Nouns comprehension	40/40	+	39/40	+	40/40	+
Verbs comprehension	20/20	+	20/20	+	20/20	+
Reading words	92/92	+	83/92	–	92/92	+
Reading pseudowords	45/45	+	31/45	–	44/45	+
Palm and pyramid test	51/52	+	50/52	+	50/52	+
Repetition words	45/45	+	45/45	+	45/45	+
Repetition pseudowords	35/35	+	35/35	+	35/35	+

19.2.2 Part II Multiple Tasks for Multiple Cognitive Function Mapping

The effect of surgery on cognitive performance is not so well investigated [56–59] and reliable data remains scarce. DES of cognitive functions by using specific cognitive test tapping other components than language is a potential promising tool to improve functional outcome [58]. In this perspective, the R.T.N.T approach does not only apply to the monitoring of language functions, but can also be used to monitor extra-language functions. The idea behind R.T.N.T. originates from the concept of the so-called negative mapping, that is, observing no DES effects. Negative mapping is not so frequently reported in DES literature, but it is instead frequently encountered during AS, especially while testing cognitive functions (for language mapping, effects such as speech arrest are easily evocable) [32, 60]. Despite negative DES mapping, often, cognitive deficits are reported in the postoperative testing. In this setting, uncontrolled resection of white matter connectivity, in which DES may result negative for inappropriate task selection or function complexity, could lead to permanent deficits. Hence, a better matching between intraoperative and postoperative tasks could contribute to avoid the resection of white matter supporting the cognitive function [57].

Thus, R.T.N.T. has been introduced, as a complementary approach, being aware that the ideal surgical need would be to have a continuous feedback on the patient's cognitive status. Moreover, stimulation does not allow to determine whether the responding area is essential so to stop the resection, or whether the function could have recovered in case the area would have been nevertheless resected. We argue that by using RTNT we obtain a gradual worsening of the patient's performance, and we have quantified, from the first preliminary case series, a possible percentage of acceptable decrease in performance, with good level of long-term recovery [32]. By using R.T.N.T. we observe fluctuations in performance, that is, observing a decrease and, after a brief period of resting, an improvement. Similar effects are observed, in the motor domain, when resecting areas close to the cortico-spinal tract [61] or during intramedullary surgery [62] and applying a wait-and-see approach. We argued [32] that the mechanical manipulation of the tissue can transiently disrupt the implicated function.

19.2.2.1 Intraoperative Tasks Selection

Ten/fifteen items are presented from each single test for about 30 s for each task, in a rotating manner, as previously described [32]. Short-term memory and working memory are assessed through Digit Span Forward [39] and Digit Span Backward [39], respectively. Executive functions assessment involves the administration of the Stroop Task [43], phonological and semantic fluency [63]. To control for information processing speed which can be influenced by sustained attention and selective attention we included also the oral version of the Symbol Digit Modalities Test [2]. In addition, for surgeries involving the frontal lobe or the temporo-insular region, RTNT involves also tasks tapping social cognition such as the Theory of Mind task [64], and task evoking emotions upon visual presentation of pictures (International Affective Picture Stimuli) [46] and asking the patient to rate valence and arousal to monitor their emotional experience. For a detailed description of RTNT in insular region, see Tomasino, Marin, Ius, & Skrap, 2018 [33] where we extensively describe the RTNT insular protocol.

For surgeries involving the right hemisphere, the RTNT protocols were devised for right frontal, right premotor, right temporo-insular, and right parietal areas. Visuo-spatial processing is assessed by using the landmark task [42], a visual scanning task requiring reading a list of words and of sentences (B.A.D.A.) [47] appearing in different positions and different quadrants on the PC screen, and a picture description task [65] in which patients are asked to detect all the relevant target stimuli appearing in different positions and different quadrants on the PC screen. Visual processing is tested by using an object decision task in which patients decide whether a stimulus is a real object or a chimera [66], while the ability to create and manipulate mental visual images is tested through an imagery 0' clock Test [44]. The patient is asked to imagine a pair of clock faces indicating different times, proposed verbally and to indicate where the clock hands appear. This task is useful also to monitor neglect. For surgeries involving the temporal areas, RTNT includes also a face recognition task [67]. The ability to comprehend figurative language is assessed by using a Metaphor comprehension [68].

For patients involving the parietal cortex, we use tasks requiring calculation [64].

For resections in both the left and the right hemisphere, sensorimotor tasks involve handedness decisions [69] since patients may exhibit an inability to predict and simulate action plans and hand/arm movements [70, 71]. The RTNT includes

Table 19.6 Intraoperative RTNT performance of patient DI with a lesion to the right temporal lobe

RTNT	1 run of RTNT	2 run of RTNT	3 run of RTNT	4 run of RTNT	5 run of RTNT
Milner landmark test [42]	13/14	14/14	14/14	13/14	14/14
Visual scanning: reading words [37]	10/10	10/10	10/10	10/10	10/10
Picture description [43]	+	+	+	+	+
Clock test [44]	10/10	10/10	10/10	10/10	9/10
Picture reality decision [33]	10/10	10/10	10/10	10/10	10/10
Theory of mind (emotion recognition) [45]	10/10	8/10	10/10	10/10	
Emotion processing [46]	10/10	10/10	10/10	10/10	

also the Florida praxis imagery test [53], Kissing and Dancing test [72], and a task assessing finger agnosia [41], oral apraxia [73], and ideomotor apraxia [74].

19.2.2.2 Example of RTNT During a Right Temporal DLGG Resection

The list of tasks we use for patients with a right temporal DLGG involves the tasks included in Table 19.6. We report, as an example, a single case of a patient undergoing a right temporal resection who performed the RTNT. DI is a 34-year-old, right-handed, men, with 18 years of schooling.

In a period of well-being, he had a car accident, followed by a seizure with loss of consciousness.

He was hospitalized for a right low-grade glioma (12 cm^3) involving the right temporal lobe (Fig. 19.12a). The fMRI examination revealed an activation related to sound listening close to the tumor. Pre-resective cortical DES was negative. This patient performed the RTNT and maintained a normal level of accuracy in all the tasks. The EOR was 100% on T2-postoperative MRI weighted images. Figure 19.12b shows that postoperative activation to sound listening persisted. When the patient was re-evaluated, her neuropsychological profile at the immediate post-surgery (at 1 week) and at follow-up (4 months after surgery) remained as at 1 week before surgery (see Table 19.7).

19.2.3 Discussion

Maximal resection is currently the first therapeutic option for DLGGs to prolong overall survival and to delay malignant transformation [1–6, 9–15, 22, 75, 76]. Given the tendency of DLGGs to infiltrate eloquent cortical areas and subcortical functional pathways, DES is the golden standard technique in awake patients to optimize the EOR while sparing the functional networks [12, 14, 15, 20–22, 75, 77, 78]. AS allows to map and to monitor not only basic motor and language functions but also the higher order cognitive and emotional functions, such as complex movement (e.g. bimanual coordination), visuospatial cognition and attention processing,

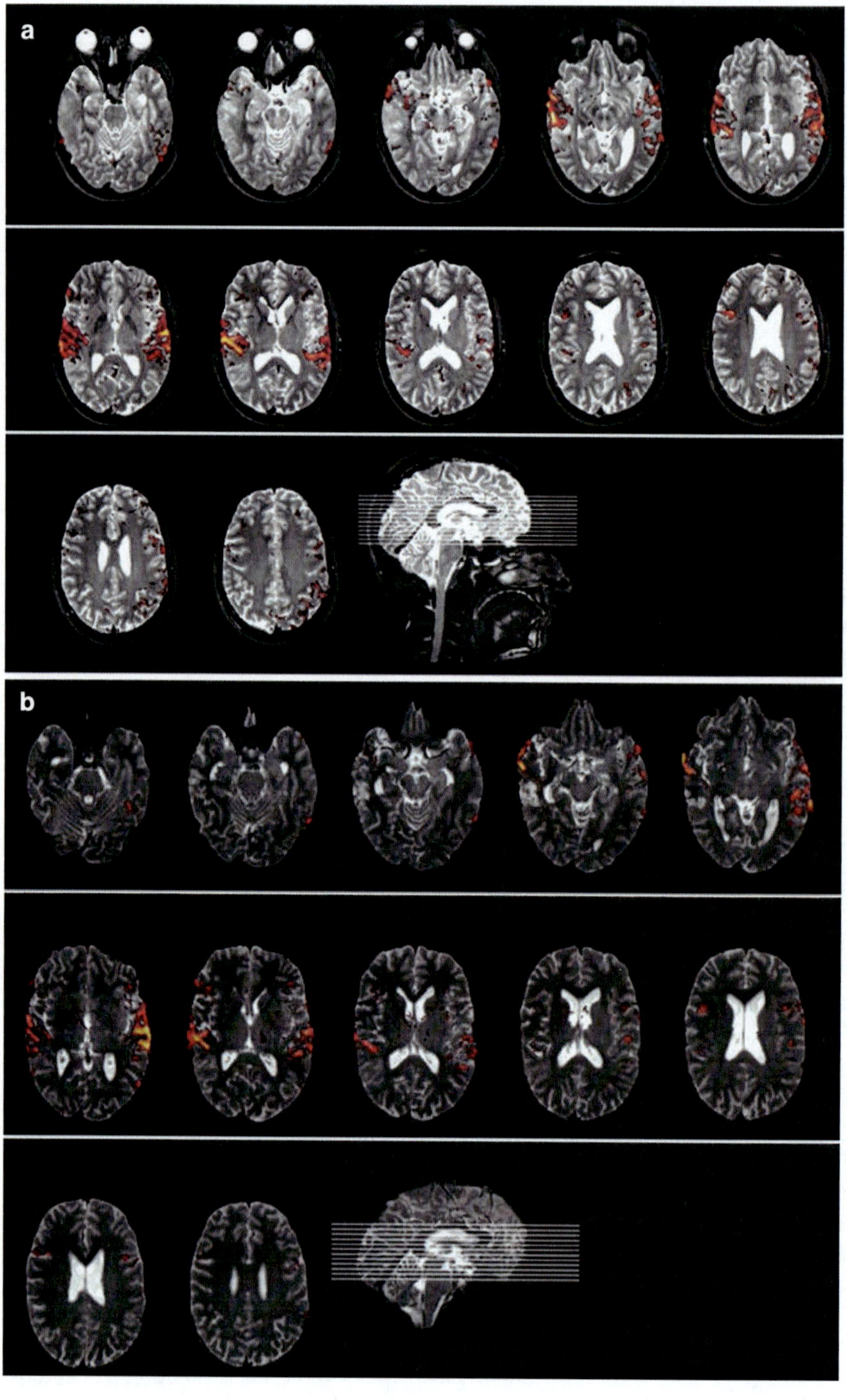

Fig. 19.12 Pre- (**a**) and post-surgery (**b**) MRI images of a DLGG in the right temporal lobe. The activation related to sound listening is in close proximity to the glioma

Table 19.7 Pre, immediate post, and follow-up performance of patient DI with a lesion to the right temporal lobe

Neuropsychological test	Before surgery (Raw data)	+/–	1 week after surgery	+/–	Follow-up (4 months)	+/–
Raven coloured matrices	34/36	+	–		34/36	+
Spatial span forward	6	+	6	+	6	+
Spatial span backward	5	+	5	+	5	+
Constructional praxis	14	+	14	+	14	+
Clock test	9.5/10	+	9.5/10	+	9.5/10	+
Star cancellation	54	+	54	+	54	+
Design fluency	30	+	34	+	29	+
TMT a	27	+	20	+	21	+
TMT b	56	+	47	+	46	+
TMT b-a	29	+	27	+	25	+
Mental rotation	21	+	21	+	21	+
Phonologic discrimination	60	+	60	+	60	+

calculation and reading, verbal and nonverbal semantics, working memory, judgment and even mentalizing (theory of mind) or metacognition [16, 18].

AS assisted by intraoperative neuropsychological monitoring is currently considered as a valid option for real-time optimization of EOR and clinical outcome ratio in DLGG surgery [32, 33]. Nowadays intraoperative neuropsychological testing during AS is increasingly being adopted, although a standardized and internationally approved battery for cognitive intraoperative monitoring has not yet been defined [14, 15, 23, 78–81]. Neuropsychological testing during AS permits monitoring of complex cognitive functions that rely on large functional network system with greater individual variability. When a deficit occurs in extra-language functions, the probability of functional recovery is greater than for motor or language functions.

In this chapter two methodologically different intraoperative neuropsychological monitoring strategies have been described.

GENTask and RTNT have been developed to meet the clinical need of providing a continuous monitoring of intraoperative cognitive network during AS, thus filling the functional information gap between two contiguous DES phases, especially at subcortical levels [32]. Both strategies attempt to provide simultaneously more information from the same anatomical spot to avoid the risk of mismatching the neuropsychological tests both at cortical and subcortical levels. The principle of having a more guaranteed feedback of the cognitive functions in a singular anatomical spot is the same in both approaches; however, the methodology is different between GENTtask and RTNT.

GENTtask relay on both a synthetical method and an analytical quick alternating monitoring. It combines the sensitivity and speed of a global approach with the specificity of an analytical sequential testing, which informs the surgeon which function is disturbed.

Specifically this method proposes a combination of analytical testing during cortical stimulation, with tasks dedicated to specific areas based on anatomo-functional parcellar distribution (**P**arcel **A**dapted **S**elected **T**asks-DuLIP), followed at subcortical level by global synthetical multimodal testing (GENTasks), covering different expected functions; if an error appears, immediate switching to analytical "plurimodal" testing (**F**ascicle **A**dapted **S**equential **T**asks) is indicated to determine the underlying fascicle. A maximum of information can be provided in a minimal time span, with a high level of accuracy considering the possibility of near constant stimulation and broad functional scan. The downside of the GENT task is that it is poorly informative in itself: the task is so complex and so cognitively demanding that a failure cannot be easily interpreted in terms of cognitive subfunctions. For example, it can happen that the GENT task would be positive, while none of the three FAST tasks would be positive. In such a situation, it remains speculative to decide whether the resection should be stopped, as there are no data that would demonstrate the long-term cognitive impact of resecting further.

Real-Time Neuropsychological Testing (RTNT) is a complementary method to DES. It is based on the continuous neuropsychological testing whose feedback is represented by the analysis of performance of the patient made intraoperatively by the neuropsychologist. The task sequence follows a fixed order and is continuously repeated throughout the entire resection. Continuously delivering neuropsychological information during brain tissue removal makes possible to closely monitor the single effects of resection in a step-by-step manner. In this way, task assessment and task switching are quick and dynamic to reduce the risk of mismatching the test.

RTNT is a reliable monitoring technique because it adds useful information, especially when DES produces a "negative mapping," i.e., when DES has no effect. Indeed, negative mapping does not necessarily imply that the area under stimulation is not involved in a certain function: such negative mapping might be caused by an inadequacy between the selected task and the location of the stimulated point.

The downside of the RTNT approach is that switching to a different task every 30 s/1 min comes in itself with a cognitive cost for the patient. There is no guarantee that a performance decrease would not be caused by this switching cost or by the cognitive fatigue, induced by the high level of flexibility required to shift every ten items from one task to another. Nonetheless, this drawback can be overcome by letting the patient rest a while and coming back later to the area where the performance decrease was observed.

In summary, the comparison of both methods shows that:

1. The GENTask approach consists of a combination of two types of tasks: a global one, which covers a wide spectrum of functions, which alternate with an analytical one, quite compact in number (max 3 tasks). The selected tasks are mainly linguistic in this approach.
2. RTNT relay on a continuous alternation of a broad spectrum of selected tasks (10–25) with fine tuning of neuropsychological, as well as neurolinguistics, functions. In case of negative language mapping, it provides functional cognitive information to decide to carry out or stop the resection.

Both methods offer the advantage of limitation of time gaps, with "scanning" of many different functions, more superficial and less complex for the GENTtask approach, more deepened and thorough for the RTNT approach.

In closing, in light of the distinctive features of each approach, RTNT strategy could be easily adopted in centers with an extensive dedicated team of neuropsychologists, while GENTask method is more suitable in smaller centers with limited, predominantly neurolinguistic staff.

19.2.4 Conclusions

GENTask and RTNT represent two efficient, valid, and reliable methods of intraoperative multitasking mapping to assist awake surgery for lesions in or close eloquent areas. Brain mapping in AS is the gold standard localization technique. GENTask and RTNT, although methodologically different, both represent valid intraoperative monitoring strategies capable of providing continuous and real-time information on the cognitive network status assisting AS.

By presenting two completely different approaches to subcortical testing, we not only demonstrate the complexity of (non) linguistic mapping, but also highlight the major challenge of awake neurosurgery. Moreover, the approaches play a fundamental role in uncovering an undiscovered gold vein within the linguistic subcortical connectivity.

A common and integrated standardized intraoperative protocol for cognitive intraoperative monitoring could be strategically developed in future studies to compare data from different centers and simplify the new trials design.

Disclosures All authors have nothing to declare.

Conflict of Interest The authors declare no conflict of interest.

References

1. Claus EB, Horlacher A, Hsu L, Schwartz RB, Dello-Iacono D, Talos F, et al. Survival rates in patients with low-grade glioma after intraoperative magnetic resonance image guidance. Cancer. 2005;103:1227–33.
2. Crepaldi D, Aggujaro S, Arduino LS, Zonca G, Ghirardi G, Inzaghi MG, et al. Noun-verb dissociation in aphasia: the role of imageability and functional locus of the lesion. Neuropsychologia. 2006;44:73–89.
3. Smith JS, Chang EF, Lamborn KR, Chang SM, Prados MD, Cha S, et al. Role of extent of resection in the long-term outcome of low-grade hemispheric gliomas. J Clin Oncol. 2008;26:1338–45.
4. Sanai N, Chang S, Berger MS. Low-grade gliomas in adults. J Neurosurg. 2011;115:948–65.
5. Ius T, Isola M, Budai R, Pauletto G, Tomasino B, Fadiga L, et al. Low-grade glioma surgery in eloquent areas: volumetric analysis of extent of resection and its impact on overall survival. A single-institution experience in 190 patients: clinical article. J Neurosurg. 2012; 117:1039–52.

6. Skrap M, Mondani M, Tomasino B, Weis L, Budai R, Pauletto G, et al. Surgery of insular non-enhancing gliomas: volumetric analysis of tumoral resection, clinical outcome, and survival in a consecutive series of 66 cases. Neurosurgery. 2012;70:1081–93.
7. Capelle L, Fontaine D, Mandonnet E, Taillandier L, Golmard JL, Bauchet L, et al. Spontaneous and therapeutic prognostic factors in adult hemispheric World Health Organization Grade II gliomas: a series of 1097 cases: clinical article. J Neurosurg. 2013;118:1157–68.
8. Nitta M, Muragaki Y, Maruyama T, Ikuta S, Komori T, Maebayashi K, et al. Proposed therapeutic strategy for adult low-grade glioma based on aggressive tumor resection. Neurosurg Focus. 2015;38:E7.
9. Hervey-Jumper SL, Berger MS. Maximizing safe resection of low- and high-grade glioma. J Neurooncol. 2016;130:269–82.
10. Weller M, van den Bent M, Tonn JC, Stupp R, Preusser M, Cohen-Jonathan-Moyal E, et al. European Association for Neuro-Oncology (EANO) guideline on the diagnosis and treatment of adult astrocytic and oligodendroglial gliomas. Lancet Oncol. 2017;18:e315–29.
11. Ius T, Ciani Y, Ruaro ME, Isola M, Sorrentino M, Bulfoni M, et al. An NF-kappaB signature predicts low-grade glioma prognosis: a precision medicine approach based on patient-derived stem cells. Neuro Oncol. 2018;20:776–87.
12. Mandonnet E, Duffau H. An attempt to conceptualize the individual onco-functional balance: why a standardized treatment is an illusion for diffuse low-grade glioma patients. Crit Rev Oncol Hematol. 2018;122:83–91.
13. Clark VE, Cahill DP. Extent of resection versus molecular classification: what matters when? Neurosurg Clin N Am. 2019;30:95–101.
14. Rudá R, Angileri FF, Ius T, Silvani A, Sarubbo S, Solari A, et al. Italian consensus and recommendations on diagnosis and treatment of low-grade gliomas. An intersocieties (SINch/AINO/SIN) document. J Neurosurg Sci. 2020;64(4):313–34. https://doi.org/10.23736/S0390-5616.20.04982-6.
15. Lombardi G, Barresi V, Castellano A, Tabouret E, Pasqualetti F, Salvalaggio A, et al. Clinical management of diffuse low-grade gliomas. Cancers. 2020;12(10):E3008.
16. Duffau H. Stimulation mapping of white matter tracts to study brain functional connectivity. Nat Rev Neurol. 2015;11:255–65.
17. Duffau H. A two-level model of interindividual anatomo-functional variability of the brain and its implications for neurosurgery. Cortex. 2017;86:303–13.
18. Duffau H. Diffuse low-grade glioma, oncological outcome and quality of life: a surgical perspective. Curr Opin Oncol. 2018;30:383–9.
19. Duffau H. Is non-awake surgery for supratentorial adult low-grade glioma treatment still feasible? Neurosurg Rev. 2018;41:133–9.
20. Duffau H. Surgery of low-grade gliomas: towards a 'functional neurooncology'. Curr Opin Oncol. 2009;21:543–9.
21. Bello L, Castellano A, Fava E, Casaceli G, Riva M, Scotti G, et al. Intraoperative use of diffusion tensor imaging fiber tractography and subcortical mapping for resection of gliomas: technical considerations. Neurosurg Focus. 2010;28:E6.
22. Bucci M, Mandelli ML, Berman JI, Amirbekian B, Nguyen C, Berger MS, et al. Quantifying diffusion MRI tractography of the corticospinal tract in brain tumors with deterministic and probabilistic methods. Neuroimage Clin. 2013;3:361–8.
23. De Witte E, Satoer D, Colle H, Robert E, Visch-Brink E, Mariën P. Subcortical language and non-language mapping in awake brain surgery: the use of multimodal tests. Acta Neurochir. 2015;157:577–88.
24. Mandonnet E, Sarubbo S, Duffau H. Proposal of an optimized strategy for intraoperative testing of speech and language during awake mapping. Neurosurg Rev. 2016;40:29–35.
25. Sierpowska J, Gabarrós A, Fernandez-Coello A, Camins À, Castañer S, Juncadella M, et al. Words are not enough: nonword repetition as an indicator of arcuate fasciculus integrity during brain tumor resection. J Neurosurg. 2017;126(2):435–45.

26. Teixidor P, Gatignol P, Leroy M, Masuet-Aumatell C, Capelle L, Duffau H. Assessment of verbal working memory before and after surgery for low-grade glioma. J Neurooncol. 2007;81(3):305–13.
27. Mandonnet E, Gatignol P, Duffau H. Evidence for an occipito-temporal tract underlying visual recognition in picture naming. Clin Neurol Neurosurg. 2009;111(7):601–5.
28. Scarone P, Gatignol P, Guillaume S, Denvil D, Capelle L, Duffau H. Agraphia after awake surgery for brain tumor: new insights into the anatomo-functional network of writing. Surg Neurol. 2009;72(3):223–41.
29. Gil-Robles S, Carvallo A, Jimenez Mdel M, Gomez Caicoya A, Martinez R, Ruiz-Ocaña C, Duffau H. Double dissociation between visual recognition and picture naming: a study of the visual language connectivity using tractography and brain stimulation. Neurosurgery. 2013;72(4):678–86.
30. Teichmann M, Rosso C, Martini JB, Bloch I, Brugières P, Duffau H, et al. A cortical-subcortical syntax pathway linking Broca's area and the striatum. Hum Brain Mapp. 2015;36(6):2270–83.
31. Papagno C, Casarotti A, Comi A, Pisoni A, Lucchelli F, Bizzi A, Riva M, Bello L. Long-term proper name anomia after removal of the uncinate fasciculus. Brain Struct Funct. 2016;221(1):687–94.
32. Skrap M, Marin D, Ius T, Fabbro F, Tomasino B. Brain mapping: a novel intraoperative neuropsychological approach. J Neurosurg. 2016;125:877–87.
33. Tomasino B, Marin D, Ius T, Skrap M. Neuropsychology in insular lesions prior-during and after brain surgery. In: Turgut M, Yurtta C, Tubbs S, editors. Island of Reil (Insula) in the human brain: anatomical, functional, clinical and surgical aspects. Springer; 2018.
34. Mandonnet E. A surgical approach to the anatomo-functional structure of language. Neurochirurgie. 2017;63(3):122–8. PMID: 28506484.
35. Martin R, Corina D, et al. Anatomical parcellation of cortical language sites. Medinfo CD:1742. 2004.
36. De Witte E, Satoer D, Robert E, Colle H, Verheyen S, Visch-Brink E, et al. The Dutch linguistic intraoperative protocol: a valid linguistic approach to awake brain surgery. Brain Lang. 2015;140:35–48.
37. Duffau H, Moritz-Gasser S, Mandonnet E. A re-examination of neural basis of language processing: proposal of a dynamic hodotopical model from data provided by brain stimulation mapping during picture naming. Brain Lang. 2014;131:1–10. https://doi.org/10.1016/j.bandl.2013.05.011.
38. Ripamonti E, Aggujaro S, Molteni F, Zonca G, Frustaci M, Luzzatti C. The anatomical foundations of acquired reading disorders: a neuropsychological verification of the dual-route model of reading. Brain Lang. 2014;134:44–67.
39. Orsini A, Grossi D, Capitani E, Laiacona M, Papagno C, Vallar G. Verbal and spatial immediate memory span: normative data from 1355 adults and 1112 children. Ital J Neurol Sci. 1987;8:539–48.
40. Shallice T. Specific impairments of planning. Philos Trans R Soc Lond Ser B Biol Sci. 1982;298(1089):199–209.
41. Spinnler M, Tognoni G. Standardizzazione e taratura italiana di test neuropsicologici. Ital J Neurol Sci. 1987;6(Suppl 8):1–120.
42. Capitani E, Neppi-Modona M, Bisiach E. Verbal-response and manual-response versions of the Milner Landmark task: normative data. Cortex. 2000;36:593–600.
43. Barbarotto R, Laiacona M, Frosio R, Vecchio M, Farinato A, Capitani E. A normative study on visual reaction times and two Stroop colour-word tests. Ital J Neurol Sci. 1998;19:161–70.
44. Antonietti A, Bartolomeo P, Colombi A, Incorpora C, Olivieri S. Batteria immaginazione e percezione (BIP) per la valutazione della cognizione visuo-spaziale. Traduzione e adattamento italiano. Milano: ISU—Università Cattolica del Sacro Cuore; 2008.
45. Prior M, Marchi S, Sartori G. Cognizione sociale e comportamento-Volume I. Domeneghini Editore UPSEL; 2003.

46. Lang PJ, Bradley MM, Cuthbert BN. International affective picture system (IAPS): instruction manual and affective ratings. Technical Report A-8. The Center for Research in Psychophysiology, University of Florida. Gainesville; 2008.
47. Miceli G, Laudanna A, Burani C, Capasso R. Batteria per l'analisi dei deficit afasici: BADA [BADA: a battery for the assessment of aphasic disorders]. Roma: CEPSAG; 1994.
48. Tomasino B, Tronchin G, Marin D, Maieron M, Fabbro F, Cubelli R, et al. Noun–verb naming dissociation in neurosurgical patients. Aphasiology. 2018;33:1418–40.
49. Tomasino B, Marin D, Maieron M, D'Agostini S, Medeossi I, Fabbro F, et al. A multimodal mapping study of conduction aphasia with impaired repetition and spared reading aloud. Neuropsychologia. 2015;70:214–26.
50. Tomasino B, Marin D, Maieron M, D'Agostini S, Fabbro F, Skrap M, et al. Double-letter processing in surface dyslexia and dysgraphia following a left temporal lesion: a multimodal neuroimaging study. Cortex. 2015;73:112–30.
51. De Renzi E, Faglioni P. Normative data and screening power of a shortened version of the Token Test. Cortex. 1978;14:41–9.
52. Gamboz N, Coluccia E, Iavarone A, Brandimonte MA. Normative data for the Pyramids and Palm Trees Test in the elderly Italian population. Neurol Sci. 2009;30:453–8.
53. Ochipa C, Rapcsak SZ, Maher LM, Rothi LJG, Bowers D, Heilman KM. Selective deficit of praxis imagery in ideomotor apraxia. Neurology. 1997;49:474–80.
54. Tomasino B, Marin D, Canderan C, Maieron M, Budai R, Fabbro F, et al. Involuntary switching into the native language induced by electrocortical stimulation of the superior temporal gyrus: a multimodal mapping study. Neuropsychologia. 2014;62:87–100.
55. Tomasino B, Ius T, Skrap M, Luzzatti C. Phonological and surface dyslexia in individuals with brain tumors: performance pre-, intra-, immediately post-surgery and at follow-up. Hum Brain Mapp. 2020;41(17):5015–31. https://doi.org/10.1002/hbm.25176. Epub 2020 Aug 28. PMID: 32857483.
56. Ille S, Engel L, Meyer B, Krieg S. Cortical functional reorganization of language function in glioma patients as measured by nrTMS. Abstracts/Brain Stimul. 2019;12:385–592.
57. Mandonnet E. Transopercular resection of IDH-mutated insular glioma: a critical appraisal of an initial experience. World Neurosurg. 2019;132:e563–76.
58. Puglisi G, Howells H, Sciortino T, Leonetti A, Rossi M, Conti Nibali M, et al. Frontal pathways in cognitive control: direct evidence from intraoperative stimulation and diffusion tractography. Brain. 2019;142(8):2451–65.
59. Rijnen SJM, Kaya G, Gehring K, Verheul JB, Wallis OC, Sitskoorn MM, et al. Cognitive functioning in patients with low-grade glioma: effects of hemispheric tumor location and surgical procedure. J Neurosurg. 2019;15:1–12.
60. Sanai N, Mirzadeh Z, Berger MS. Functional outcome after language mapping for glioma resection. N Engl J Med. 2008;358:18–27.
61. Skrap M, Vescovi MC, Pauletto G, Maieron M, Tomasino B, Bagatto D, Tuniz F. Supratentorial cavernous malformations involving the corticospinal tract and sensory motor cortex: treatment strategies, surgical considerations, and outcomes. Oper Neurosurg (Hagerstown). 2018;15(5):483–97.
62. Sala F, Bricolo A, Faccioli F, Lanteri P, Gerosa M. Surgery for intramedullary spinal cord tumors: the role of intraoperative (neurophysiological) monitoring. Eur Spine J. 2007;16(Suppl 2):S130–9.
63. Novelli G, Papagno C, Capitani E, Laiacona M, Vallar G, Cappa SF. Tre test clinici di ricerca e produzione lessicale. Taratura su soggetti normali. Arch Psicol Neurol Psichiatr. 1996;47:477–505.
64. Delazer M, Girelli L, Granà A, Domahs F. Number processing and calculation-normative dta from healthy adults. Clin Neuropsychol. 2003;17:331–50.
65. Paradis M. Bilingual aphasia test (Italian version). Bologna: EMS; 1986.
66. Rusconi ML. Test delle figure chimeriche nella valutazione dell'eminegligenza spaziale. Arch Psicol Neurol Psichiatr. 1998;LIX(6):810–23.

67. Bizzozero I, Ferrari F, Pozzoli S, Saetti MC, Spinnler H. Who is who: Italian norms for visual recognition and identification of celebrities. Neurol Sci. 2005;26:95–107.
68. Papagno C, Cappa SF, Forelli A, Garavaglia G, Laiacona M, Capitani E. Non-literal language comprehension: standardization of a metaphors and idiom comprehension test. Arch Psicol Neurol Psichiatr. 1995;56:402–20.
69. Tomasino B, Toraldo A, Rumiati RI. Dissociation between the mental rotation of visual images and motor images in unilateral brain-damaged patients. Brain Cogn. 2003;51:368–71.
70. Tomasino B, Vorano L, Skrap M, Gigli G, Rumiati RI. Effects of strategies of mental rotation performed by unilateral brain damaged patients. Cortex. 2004;40:197–9.
71. Tomasino B, Skrap M, Rumiati RI. Causal role of the sensorimotor cortex in action simulation: neuropsychological evidence. J Cogn Neurosci. 2011;23:2068–78.
72. Bak T, Hodges JR. Kissing and dancing—a test to distinguish the lexical and conceptual contributions to noun/verb and action/object dissociation. Preliminary results in patients with frontotemporal dementia. J Neurolinguistics. 2003;16:169–81.
73. De Renzi E, Piezcuro A, Vignolo LA. Oral apraxia and aphasia. Cortex. 1966;2:50–73.
74. De Renzi E, Motti F, Nichelli P. Imitating gestures. A quantitative approach to ideomotor apraxia. Arch Neurol. 1980;37:6–10.
75. Ius T, Turella L, Pauletto G, Isola M, Maieron M, Sciacca G, et al. Quantitative diffusion tensor imaging analysis of low-grade gliomas: from preclinical application to patient care. World Neurosurg. 2017;97:333–43.
76. Sanai N, Berger MS. Surgical oncology for gliomas: the state of the art. Nat Rev Clin Oncol. 2018;15:112–25.
77. Lang FF, Gilbert MR. Diffusely infiltrative low-grade gliomas in adults. J Clin Oncol. 2006;24:1236–45.
78. Hansmeyer L, Kruegert TB. Synchronized presentation of a language task to the electrical stimulation of cortical regions during speech mapping in an awake surgery. Curr Direct Biomed Eng. 2018;4:547–50.
79. De Witt Hamer PC, Robles SG, Zwinderman AH, Duffau H, Berger MS. Impact of intraoperative stimulation brain mapping on glioma surgery outcome: a meta-analysis. J Clin Oncol. 2012;30:2559–65.
80. Rofes A, Mandonnet E, Godden J, Baron MH, Colle H, Darlix A, et al. Survey on current cognitive practices within the European Low-Grade Glioma Network: towards a European assessment protocol. Acta Neurochir (Wien). 2017;159:1167–78.
81. Lu VM, Phan K, Rovin RA. Comparison of operative outcomes of eloquent glioma resection performed under awake versus general anesthesia: a systematic review and meta-analysis. Clin Neurol Neurosurg. 2018;169:121–7.

Part IV

Prospects

Creativity

20

Théophile Bieth, Alizée Lopez-Persem,
Marcela Ovando-Tellez, Marika Urbanski,
and Emmanuelle Volle

20.1 Introduction

The development of high-level cognitive functions in humans allows us to plan for future long-term goals, to adapt quickly to a changing environment, to innovate, and to create artwork. Among these functions, creativity is a cornerstone to our ability to cope with change and solve novel problems. Creativity is at the heart of many domains of human activity, including arts, sciences, education, or economy, and leads to innovation and discoveries. However, creative thinking is not restricted to extraordinary achievements or specific domains of expression (e.g. art). Finding original solutions to problems, achieving something novel, thinking away from pre-established ideas, and even coping with negative emotions [1, 2] are all creative requirements that also take place in everyday life. All human activities can involve creative thinking, as soon as we have to produce something new (e.g. an idea, a product, or a solution) to appropriately face situations with no established solution. Besides, in addition to the value of what we produce, creativity is also essential for well-being, as more creative people appear to be happier and more satisfied with their lives [3, 4]. Despite the importance of creativity in everyday life and society, the consequences of brain diseases on creative abilities are poorly known. As difficulties in creative thinking or creative problem-solving are not classically assessed in clinical practice, their impact on the daily life of patients with various brain diseases or damage is not understood [5–8].

T. Bieth
Sorbonne University, Paris Brain Institute (ICM), INSERM, CNRS, Paris, France

Neurology Department, Pitié-Salpêtrière Hospital, AP-HP, Paris, France

A. Lopez-Persem · M. Ovando-Tellez · E. Volle (✉)
Sorbonne University, Paris Brain Institute (ICM), INSERM, CNRS, Paris, France

M. Urbanski
Neurology Department, CHU Poitiers, Poitiers, France

E. Mandonnet, G. Herbet (eds.), *Intraoperative Mapping of Cognitive Networks*,
https://doi.org/10.1007/978-3-030-75071-8_20

To date, only a few studies have explored creativity in patients. Converging evidence indicates that damage to several brain regions or networks impact creative thinking, suggesting that patients with brain lesions requiring surgery may also have their creative abilities impaired. To our knowledge, creative abilities are not currently assessed as part of the perioperative planning of brain surgery, and no published study examined creative abilities intraoperatively (but see [9]). Unique case reports described intraoperative testing of particular artistic skills (mostly musical) that were critical for the patient (for instance, playing the violin, the flute, or the guitar; see [10–13]) but did not specifically assess creative abilities.

In this chapter, we first present some bases of creative cognition. Second, we review the recent neuroimaging literature in healthy subjects that revealed a set of brain regions involved in creativity tasks or related to creative abilities, and how they are organised into structured brain networks. Third, we present the few patient studies that explored the consequences of brain lesions on creative abilities. Although these studies were not conducted in neurosurgical patients specifically, they allow some predictions about the lesion locations at risk of long-term deficits. The improved knowledge of the creativity brain networks may hence be useful for planning and monitoring brain surgery in slow-growing lesions like glioma or malformations. However, as we discuss in the last part, the precise brain areas which integrity is necessary to preserve creative thinking and improve functional or mental outcomes of patients remain to be examined in neurosurgical patients specifically. As creativity has not been empirically tested in patients undergoing awake surgery, intraoperative mapping is unknown. Designing creativity tasks complying with the constraints of intraoperative mapping appears quite challenging. We finally suggest some avenues for future research and discuss how creativity tasks could be adapted for this purpose.

20.2 Creative Cognition

Creativity is usually defined as the ability to produce a work that is both original (unusual, novel, unexpected) and appropriate (useful, adaptive, valuable). From a neuroscience perspective, this capacity results from a set of mental operations that are normally found in all humans and can be studied experimentally. Several frameworks have been developed to explore creative abilities and the underlying cognitive and brain mechanisms: divergent thinking (DT), insight problem-solving, and associative combination.

The DT approach relies on the hypothesis that creativity depends on the ability to generate multiple solutions to an open-ended problem that does not have a right or wrong answer, and to search in different directions [14]. In completing DT tasks, participants should explore various options, think remotely, and generate unusual ideas. For instance, a typical DT task is the Alternate Uses Task (AUT, Fig. 20.1). The psychometric approach of DT provides a procedure for scoring creativity.

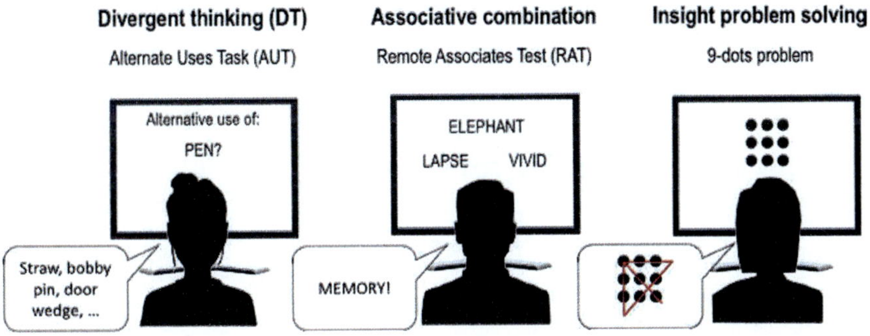

Fig. 20.1 Schematic representation of three main tasks used to assess creative abilities. The Alternate Uses Task (AUT) consists of asking participants to provide as many alternative and original uses as possible that one can make with a familiar object, such as a pen, with a time limit. The Remote Associates Test (RAT) consists, from three proposed words which have no apparent link between them (for example, "elephant", "lapse", and "vivid"), of finding a fourth word which is related to each of these words (in the previous example, "memory"). In the "9-dots problem" all nine points must be joined with only four continuous line segments

Typically, DT tasks responses are scored for fluency (quantity of relevant productions) and originality (quality of the productions in terms of originality, estimated either by a subjective consensual assessment or statistically by measuring the rarity of each response), as well as flexibility (number of different categories of productions), and elaboration (the degree of enrichment of productions).

A second approach, supported by Mednick [15], relies on the idea that creativity is the ability to connect things in new ways. It emphasises the role of semantic associations in creativity. Mednick defined creativity as the forming of associative elements into new combinations, which meet specified requirements. The more mutually remote the elements of the new combination, the more creative the process. The classical experimental task of this approach is the Remote Associates Test (RAT, Fig. 20.1).

The third approach to explore creativity is insight problem-solving. Insight problems can be visual, verbal, or mathematical. In insight problems, the solution can typically be found with the phenomenon of "Aha!" or "Eurêka". The "Eurêka" describes a subjective experience that arises when the solution to a given problem comes to mind suddenly, without being able to report the mental steps leading to this solution (as opposed to analytic solving). A feeling of pleasure and confidence often accompanies it. Insight problems usually include in their statements implicit constraints that one needs to overcome to find the solution. Hence, solving an insight problem implies a reorganisation of the problem representation. For example, in the visuospatial "nine-dots problem" (see [16], Fig. 20.1), the test-takers tend to stay inside a virtual square delimited by the dots, while the solution can only be found by drawing lines beyond the limits of the square. The RAT (described above) is, in fact, a particular type of verbal insight problem and is probably the most frequently used task to study insight problem-solving processes. Insight problems and RAT are usually viewed as convergent thinking tasks, where idea generation should converge to one correct solution.

In the cognitive neuroscience of creativity, the use of these approaches provides broad evidence in favour of the involvement of cognitive control functions that depend on the prefrontal cortex (PFC). Cognitive control functions that are important for creative abilities include inhibition (of inappropriate ideas or obvious non-creative ideas), working memory and attentional control (allowing to form and manipulate mental representations), response selection, and controlled retrieval in memory (to orient the search in memory) [17–22].

Besides deliberate cognitive control, creative cognition also involves another type of processes called associative processes [15]. Associative processes allow to spontaneously activate associated knowledge in memory [23, 24]. Psychological studies have shown that more creative people have more flexible semantic associations (i.e. related elements in their semantic memory), allowing them to connect more distant concepts or words. Researchers in the field now consider that creative abilities or performance result from an interaction, or a balance, between associative and controlled processes [18, 25]. Associative processes allow to spontaneously activate associations of ideas depending on the organisation of these associations in memory. Controlled processes allow controlling the way ideas are generated using a set of cognitive control functions. How these processes interact remains an open question.

In addition to this spontaneous versus controlled distinction, theories on creativity separate generative processes and evaluative processes of creative thinking [26]. Once a candidate idea is generated, it is evaluated for its originality and appropriateness before being selected (or rejected).

20.3 Brain Correlates of Creativity in Healthy Subjects

The cognitive frameworks mentioned above have been used to study the cerebral bases of creativity in neuroimaging, in particular in recent years in functional MRI. Consistent with the involvement of cognitive control processes in creative cognition, the PFC is one of the regions the most consistently associated with creativity tasks in functional imaging. Yet, different parts of the PFC have been reported, and the role of each subregion is still debated. Multiple other brain regions are also involved, in particular, parietal and temporal areas [27]. Recent research suggests that creativity involves interactions of large-scale brain systems—networks—rather than isolated brain regions [28]. With the development of network neuroscience based on functional connectivity, the neuroimaging of creative cognition in healthy subjects have started to clarify the multiple brain systems involved in creative processes. The main identified networks, i.e. sets of regions functionally interconnected, are the Default Mode Network (DMN), the Executive Control Network (ECN), and the Salience Network (SN) (Fig. 20.2).

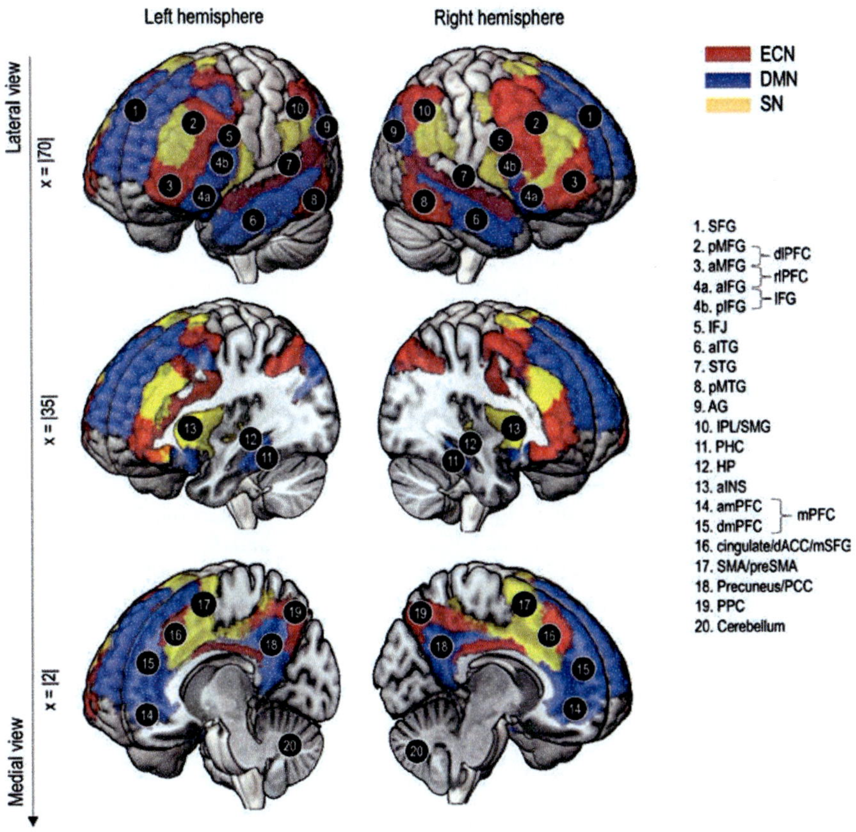

Fig. 20.2 Brain areas involved in creativity. Schematic representation of the main long-range brain networks and the main regions associated with creativity in neuroimaging studies are overlaid on a brain rendering. Brain networks are extracted from Yeo et al. [33]. *SFG* Superior frontal gyrus, *pMFG* posterior middle frontal gyrus, *aMFG* anterior middle frontal gyrus, *dlPFC* dorsolateral prefrontal cortex, *aIFG* anterior inferior frontal gyrus, *rlPFC* rostrolateral frontal gyrus, *pIFG* posterior frontal gyrus, *IFG* inferior frontal gyrus, *IFJ* inferior frontal junction, *aITG* anterior inferior temporal gyrus, *STG* superior temporal gyrus, *pMTG* posterior middle temporal gyrus, *AG* angular gyrus, *IPL* Inferior parietal lobule, *PHC* parahippocampal cortex, *HP* hippocampus, *aINS* anterior insula, *amPFC* anterior medial prefrontal cortex, *dmPFC* dorsomedial prefrontal cortex, *mPFC* medial prefrontal cortex, *dACC* dorsal anterior cingulate cortex, *mSFG* medial part of the SFG, *SMA* supplementary motor area, *PCC* posterior cingulate cortex, *PPC* posterior parietal cortex

20.3.1 Brain Networks Involved in Creativity

The DMN typically consists of three components: a core system, composed of the anterior medial PFC and the precuneus; a medial temporal subsystem, that comprises the ventromedial PFC, the hippocampus, and the parahippocampal cortex; and a dorsomedial subsystem, including the middle temporal gyrus, angular gyrus, and the dorsomedial PFC [29]. Regions of the core system appear to qualify as functional hubs interacting with the two subsystems. The DMN has been shown to support processes of self-generated thought and spontaneous cognition, but its role remains to be fully understood [30]. During creativity tasks, the DMN is assumed to process spontaneous idea generation, through unconstrained associative thinking [31]. The ECN is mainly composed of the dorsolateral PFC, especially its rostral and posterior parts, the dorsal anterior cingulate cortex, the superior parietal cortex, the dorsal part of the inferior parietal lobule, and the posterior part of the temporal lobe including the temporoparietal junction [32, 33]. It is classically associated with controlled processes such as working memory, inhibition, attentional control, memory retrieval, planning, and flexibility.

In cognitive neuroscience, the ECN and DMN are usually considered as having opposing activity patterns, as the former tend to be involved during active demanding tasks and the latter during rest or mind-wandering [30]. However, analyses of functional connectivity between those networks have shown that they interact during creativity tasks [28]. Based on those findings, Beaty et al. [28] have proposed that the two networks cooperate to balance associative and controlled processes for the generation and evaluation of ideas and that the SN network might mediate this cooperation. The central regions of SN are the bilateral anterior insula and dorsal anterior cingulate cortex; it also includes several subcortical and limbic structures, and possibly prefrontal/premotor areas. This network has been associated with attentional switching, detection of salient external or internal stimuli (especially via its insular node), and conflict monitoring (especially via its cingulate node). It may allow switching between associative processes (allowing idea generation) supported by the DMN and controlled processes (participating in idea evaluation and selection) supported by the ECN, according to the goal of the creativity task [34–36].

Recent functional connectivity studies also demonstrated that the way brain regions are connected within and between the DMN and ECN is predictive of individuals' creativity [37], assessed by DT tasks. Hence, functional connectivity patterns are a brain measurement highly relevant to investigation of the neural bases of creativity and should be taken into account.

20.3.2 The Specificity of Regions for Creativity Domains and Processes

Functional interactions between the DMN and ECN regions have typically been observed in verbal DT tasks, but also in various artistic performances, such as musical improvisation, poetry, visual art, and literature [28, 38]. Previous meta-analyses of neuroimaging studies on creativity also highlighted particular regions within the DMN, SN, or ECN that were associated with distinct creativity domains or tasks while others were more general, suggesting that both domain-general and domain-specific or task-specific regions co-exist within creativity networks [27, 39]. Both meta-analyses reported several regions that were recruited by different tasks and creativity domains across studies, including regions within the lateral PFC, medial PFC, and posterior parietal cortex, in particular in the left inferior frontal gyrus, inferior frontal junction, and left angular gyrus [27]. Boccia et al. [39] compared the brain correlates of musical, verbal, and visuospatial creativity and found that all three domains involved the dorsolateral PFC. As the dorsolateral PFC plays a role in mental effort, focused attention, working memory, and selection processes, this finding is consistent with its contribution to domain-general control processes for creativity. When examining creativity domains separately, the left inferior and middle frontal gyri were consistently involved in verbal creativity, together with the posterior part of the left temporal cortex [27], the left middle and superior temporal gyri, inferior parietal lobule, post-central and supramarginal gyri, right lingual gyrus, anterior insula, and cerebellum [39]. In the visuospatial domain, the typical brain regions observed in neuroimaging studies are the right inferior and middle frontal gyri, bilateral thalamus, and left precentral gyrus. In musical creativity, the most common regions that have been observed are the bilateral medial PFC (including premotor areas) and cingulate gyrus, the left middle frontal gyrus, left inferior parietal lobule, right fusiform gyrus, and cerebellum [39]. Additionally, the pre-supplementary motor area and dorsal premotor cortex seem to play a role in creativity [28, 40].

Gonen-Yaacovi et al. [27] also reported process-oriented regions. In this study, rostral regions of the lateral PFC were specialised for idea combination, and posterior prefrontal regions for idea generation. Idea combination recruited the left anterior inferior frontal gyrus (BA10/47 and 46) and left posterior middle temporal gyrus (BA 37/21) together with the right inferior frontal gyri (BA 44/45), while idea generation recruited the left dorsolateral PFC (BA 45/46), left supramarginal gyrus (BA 40), and anteromedial PFC (BA 10) (see also [41]). Overall, these studies indicate that process-general and process-specific regions co-exist. However, the role of each subregion in the creativity networks, and the way their functional connectivity is reconfigured according to the task demand or domain, is not yet fully understood.

20.3.3 Hemispheric Lateralisation

The previous meta-analyses of functional imaging have described bilateral but predominantly left brain activation during creativity tasks [27, 41], especially for verbal tasks [39]. Whether left dominance is related to the verbal domain of the creativity tasks that were used in the included studies remains an open question. Hemispheric lateralisation in creativity is a debated topic. First, it is important to keep in mind that both hemispheres are involved during creativity tasks. Yet, some studies have found some domain-dependent dissociations. For instance, Chen et al. [42] found that participants with high visuospatial creativity had stronger segregation of functional connectivity within some SN and DMN regions of the right hemisphere, while participants with high verbal creativity exhibited a balanced inter-hemispheric functional connectivity, suggesting that both hemispheres are involved in the verbal domain, with no particular dominance. Thus, even though language processes are more likely to recruit regions in the left hemisphere, both hemispheres are engaged and exchange information during verbal creativity.

Hence, functional imaging studies have shown that creative cognition is supported by a large set of brain areas that are organised in interacting networks. The data discussed above are mainly correlational and thus do not inform us about the brain regions and networks that are necessary for creativity. Brain lesion studies can help to elucidate how creative abilities are affected in patients and to identify the regions or networks which integrity is critical for creativity (Fig. 20.2).

20.4 Creativity in Brain-Damaged Patients

Only a few lesion studies measuring creativity have been conducted (Fig. 20.3), and they mostly used a group approach comparing patients with different lesion locations at the regional level, but not at the network or node level. Hence, the conclusions that can be drawn regarding the systems or networks that are critical are mostly indirect, and regional precision in delineating the critical areas is often limited.

Nevertheless, one study by Bendetowicz et al. [43] used a voxel-based lesion-symptom approach, and directly tested the impact of lesions at the network level. Although this study only examined frontal lesions, the authors revealed critical prefrontal nodes within the DMN and the ECN for different processes of verbal creativity. First, damage to either DMN or left ECN impacted performance on the RAT. Second, damage to specific nodes and anatomical connections affected distinct creativity processes. On the one hand, damage to the right rostromedial PFC, within the DMN, led to a decreased creative performance on the RAT along with difficulties in generating spontaneous and remote semantic associations. The difficulties in generating remote ideas were associated with a disconnection affecting the right cingulate fasciculus. Remote thinking difficulties of these patients with DMN damage were interpreted as a lack of flexibility in semantic associations, which impacted the ability to find the remote solution on the RAT [15].

On the other hand, patients with damage to the left rostrolateral PFC, in the left ECN, or to several tracts connected to it (frontomarginal tract, anterior thalamic radiations, and frontostriatal projections), were impaired on the same creativity task (the RAT), but had preserved flexibility in semantic associations and remote thinking. Impaired creativity in these patients is thus likely due to difficulties in the combination step that integrates the generated associates to produce the solution. Overall, consistent with results from functional imaging studies in healthy subjects, the DMN and the left ECN, involving distinct areas of the PFC, were found critical for creative abilities. Low creative performance could be explained by rigidity in semantic associations in patients with a rostromedial PFC lesion and by difficulties in more controlled combination processes in patients with a left rostrolateral PFC lesion.

Other lesions studies also suggest that damage to regions of the DMN, ECN, or SN impacts creative abilities. The assessment of creativity in patients with focal brain damage to supposedly DMN-related regions is sparse. Shamay-Tsoory et al.

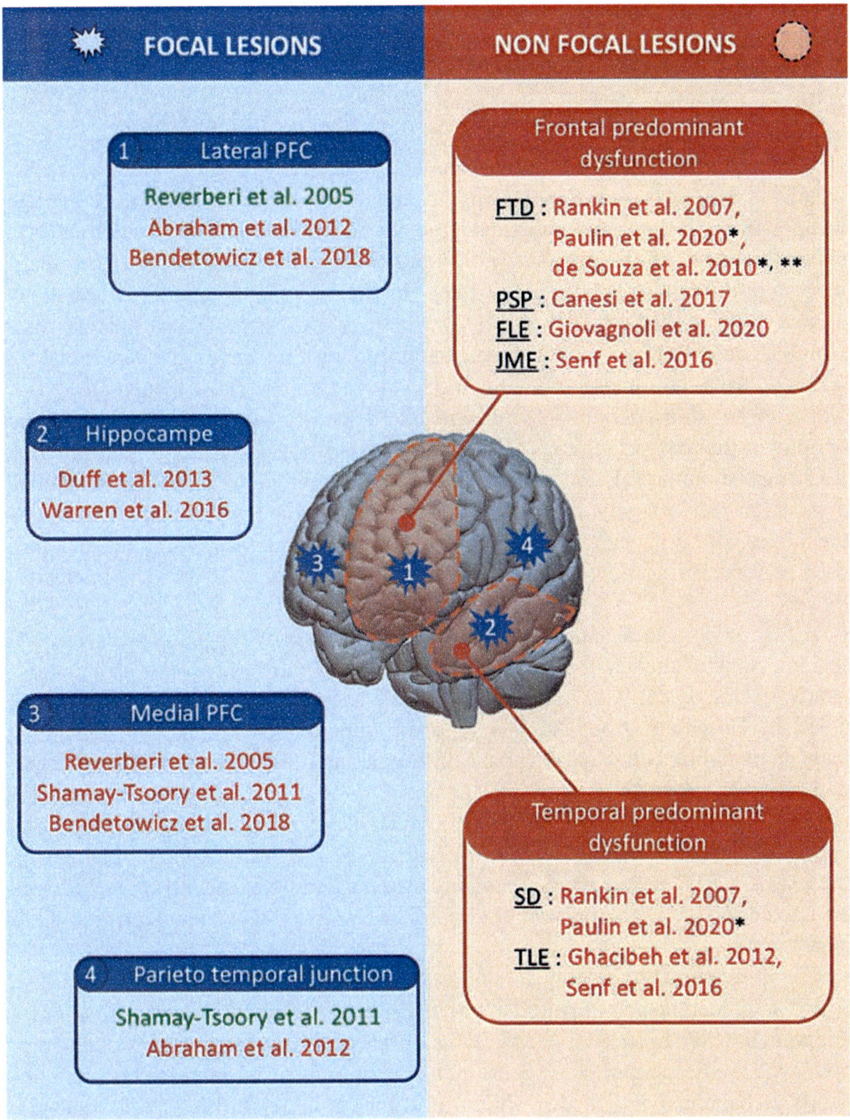

Fig. 20.3 Summary of studies in patients on creative cognition in adults. The figure includes patient studies that related creative abilities to focal anatomical lesions identified by neuroimaging methods (in blue, left side) and to more diffuse lesions based on disease-related brain dysfunctions (in orange, right side). References written in red indicate studies reporting creativity impairment related to lesion location. References written in green indicate studies reporting creativity enhancement related to lesion location. *: Indicates studies in patients suffering from a neurological illness which also used a neuroimaging approach. **: This study reports neuroimaging correlates of divergent thinking in parietal, temporal, and parieto-temporal regions in FTD patients. *PFC* Prefrontal cortex, *FTD* Frontotemporal dementia, *PSP* Progressive supranuclear palsy, *FLE* Frontal lobe epilepsy, *SD* Semantic dementia, *TLE* Temporal lobe epilepsy, *JME* Juvenile myoclonic epilepsy

[44] measured DT abilities in groups of patients with focal brain damage in the inferior frontal gyrus or the rostromedial PFC. The authors reported that patients with damage to the rostromedial PFC had difficulties in generating original ideas in DT tasks. Moreover, the larger the lesion in the right medial PFC was, the higher the impairment in creativity tasks. This result is consistent with Bendetowicz et al. [43]. However, another lesion study by Abraham et al. [45] did not observe creativity deficits after rostral prefrontal lesions, maybe due to differences in the nature and location of the lesions, and statistical approaches. Other studies focused on the hippocampus reported that patients with bilateral hippocampal damage had impairment in both DT task [46] and RAT [47]. Hippocampus is thought to participate in a subnetwork of the DMN [29, 48]. These findings suggest that, as for the rostromedial PFC, damage to the hippocampus impairs creative processes that are crucial for different tasks, presumably affecting associative thinking. These results are in line with a recent study in patients with semantic dementia with predominant bilateral atrophy in the anterior temporal lobe [49]. In this study, the patients had impaired performance on the DT task, and a voxel-based morphometry analysis revealed an association between grey matter volume in the left medial temporal lobe, centred on the left anterior hippocampus, and the DT scores. Overall, the few studies that have been performed in patients suggest that several DMN regions are critical to creativity tasks.

A few patient studies also highlight the critical role of supposedly ECN or SN regions. Several studies in patients with neurodegenerative diseases with predominantly frontal dysfunction support the importance of frontal control functions in creativity. Previous group studies reported impaired DT in neurodegenerative patients including behavioural variant of frontotemporal dementia (FTD), semantic dementia, or progressive supranuclear palsy [49–53]. De Souza et al. [51] first revealed that creativity scores correlated with a hypoperfusion in rostral prefrontal, lateral temporal and parietal regions in FTD patients, regions that may overlap with the ECN. In FTD and semantic dementia patients, Paulin et al. [49] recently found an association between grey matter atrophy in the left middle frontal gyrus and DT performance.

Creativity in other neurological diseases such as epilepsy has also been explored. A few studies indicated impaired creativity in epileptic patients with a frontal or a temporal lobe dysfunction [54, 55]. Some differences between frontal and temporal epilepsy have been reported, suggesting that temporal dysfunction affects predominantly verbal creativity [54, 55] while frontal lobe epilepsy mostly affects visuospatial creativity. No left-right difference in temporal lobe epilepsy patients regarding verbal creativity was observed [56]. Overall, these studies also support the hypothesis that both temporal and frontal lobes are critical for creativity. However, the studies mentioned above in neurodegenerative diseases and epilepsy do not allow definitive conclusions regarding which network is crucial.

Lesion studies of patients with more focal lesions affecting prefrontal and parietal regions that may belong to the ECN are scarce. Abraham et al. [45] showed that damage to frontolateral or temporoparietal regions affects several creativity tasks, including DT tasks. Conversely, it is interesting to note that a few lesion studies have suggested the possibility of a preserved or increased creative performance in patients with a left posterior parieto-temporal lesion or a lateral frontal lesion [44, 57]. Although these results remain to be replicated, they are consistent with a few brain stimulation studies (for a review see [58]). These findings may suggest that the organisation of the frontal and parietal regions for creativity is complex, with subregions possibly belonging to different functional systems, in turn playing distinct roles in creative cognition.

Overall, brain lesion studies converge with functional connectivity studies in healthy subjects and support the critical role of the DMN and ECN in different processes of creative thinking. Most studies highlight the critical role of the PFC either in its lateral or medial subregions. However, the PFC is a heterogeneous region with various connectivity patterns with the rest of the brain [59]. Understanding which network is impacted beyond the cortical lesion is thus essential to better understand the consequences of brain lesions on creativity [60].

20.5 Exploring Creativity in Patients Undergoing Brain Surgery

The patient studies presented above indicate that lesions affecting various brain areas in prefrontal, temporal, and parietal cortices impact creative thinking and problem-solving. These findings suggest that assessing creative abilities in patients suffering from neurological or neurosurgical diseases can be useful. However, problem-solving and creative abilities are not classically assessed in clinical practice.

Assessing creativity might be especially beneficial for patients with neurosurgical diseases such as gliomas or pharmaco-resistant epilepsy. Indeed, the brain regions or networks that were shown critical for creative thinking seem to overlap with some of the preferential locations of tumours or epileptogenic zones that require surgical intervention, e.g. frontoinsular, medial frontal, or temporal regions [61–63]. Hence, a proper assessment using creativity tasks before and after surgery would allow a more comprehensive understanding of the overall impact of the location of the lesion on cognition.

A few studies have assessed specific and personalised creativity-related skills, such as playing a musical instrument, before and during brain surgery [10–13], maximising the detection of a potential impact of a deficit on the patient's life. Nevertheless, when assessing the impact of the brain lesion or resection on the creative process, it is essential to distinguish the ability to think creatively as a domain-general process (tentatively captured by the creative tests described above) from specific creative domains or activities (for instance, playing music) that rely on domain-specific processes or skills. If brain lesions requiring brain surgery have an effect on creativity tests, affecting the patient's daily life, new tools to assess creativity during awake surgery may be developed. Similar approaches have been or are applied for more familiar cognitive functions such as language, unilateral spatial neglect, or executive functions and mentalizing [64–71].

Existing assessment tools of creative thinking and problem-solving could be adapted for clinical practice. The frameworks of DT and of insight problem-solving offer putative mechanisms and cognitive tasks that can be useful for this purpose, and the cerebral networks associated with these tasks have begun to be clarified [27, 28, 43]. Currently, several factors curb the assessment of creative processes during the perioperative planning of patients in clinical practice. Existing tools have not been yet normed and validated in clinical populations, and lack a pathological threshold. Besides, how impairment on creativity tasks relates to a detrimental change in functional outcomes, mental state, and quality of life remains to be measured, and may depend on the patient's profession, hobbies, or personality. As existing creativity assessments tap into nonspecific cognitive processes such as executive functions (inhibition, flexibility, working memory), semantic and episodic memory, functional consequences associated with poor creative abilities can be expected. However, the extent to which assessing creativity has an additional value will be important to examine. For instance, some DT tests were shown to discriminate dementia patients from control subjects more strongly than did classical fluency tests (category, phonemic; [72]). One can thus expect that creativity tasks are more complex and may be more sensitive to cognitive difficulties than more classical tests, and that they should reveal specific deficits that classical tests do not.

Regarding awake surgery, adding creativity tests to the toolbox of neurosurgeons for intraoperative monitoring may be worthy to be explored, especially if significant consequences are confirmed in their patients. There are strong constraints for intraoperative cognitive testing that may appear challenging regarding creativity tasks, including time constraints, repetition of many equivalent trials, and real-time evaluation of the patient responses as correct or not. Typical creativity tests usually do not satisfy these constraints, and adaptations are needed to make them suitable for functional intraoperative monitoring. For instance, the RAT or insight problem-solving tasks can be scored on a trial-by-trial basis, but response times are classically long (several seconds to several minutes). DT tasks have shorter response time, but determining the correctness of the response on a trial-by-trial basis is more difficult [73]. For DT tasks such as the AUT, automatic scoring methods have recently been developed and may allow an online scoring during surgery [74].

A task developed in our lab (Free Generation Associates Task; [43]) and others [75, 76] might offer an easier alternative. This task measures the ability to intentionally produce remote associations, with the instruction to think creatively. On each trial, a cue word is provided, and the participant is asked to generate a response word that is unusually associated with the cue word, with an original but existing link. The originality/singularity of responses at such task is positively correlated to the performance at creativity tests [75, 76], and depend on the integrity of the DMN, more especially the medial frontal pole [43] in brain-damaged patients.

In addition to the monitoring and planning of the surgery, the identification of deficits in creativity-related tasks can lead to proposing specific rehabilitation programs. Regarding creative abilities, cognitive training or stimulation programs have recently been developed and tested in healthy subjects [77–80]. Some studies suggest that engaging daily in creative activities is related to a better well-being and flourishing in individuals [3]. In patients, approaches based on creative activities (for instance, using art therapy) have shown beneficial effects in some neurological or psychiatric diseases [81–83]. To our knowledge, no specific training of creative processes has been tested in patients, and this is an avenue for future research.

20.6 Conclusions

The growing interest of the scientific community for creative thinking and its neural bases have allowed significant advances in the field. Neuroscientific studies have identified creativity-related brain regions, interconnected within and between mainly three long-range networks, the DMN, ECN, and SN. Although scarce, patient studies indicate that lesions affecting these networks impact creativity. These existing studies suggest that assessing creativity in a clinical context might be beneficial. However, to which extent slowly developing brain lesions damaging these networks requiring surgery affect creative abilities, creative processes, and the patients' everyday life remains to be quantified. In turn, such patient studies will have a scientific impact by offering new insights on creative cognition and on the plasticity that allows this function to recover.

References

1. Mastria S, Agnoli S, Zanon M, Lubart T, Corazza GE. Creative brain, creative mind, creative person. In: Kapoula Z, Volle E, Renoult J, Andreatta M, editors. Exploring transdisciplinarity in art and sciences. Heidelberg: Springer International Publishing; 2018. p. 3–29. https://doi.org/10.1007/978-3-319-76054-4_1.
2. Wu X, Guo T, Tan T, Zhang W, Qin S, Fan J, Luo J. Superior emotional regulating effects of creative cognitive reappraisal. Neuroimage. 2019;200:540–51. https://doi.org/10.1016/j.neuroimage.2019.06.061.
3. Conner T, Deyoung C, Silvia P. Everyday creative activity as a path to flourishing. J Posit Psychol. 2016;13(2):181–9. https://doi.org/10.1080/17439760.2016.1257049.
4. Shen W, Hua M, Wang M, Yuan Y. The mental welfare effect of creativity: how does creativity make people happy? Psychol Health Med. 2020:1–8. https://doi.org/10.1080/13548506.2020.1781910.
5. Abraham A. The neuropsychology of creativity. Curr Opin Behav Sci. 2019;27:71–6. https://doi.org/10.1016/j.cobeha.2018.09.011.
6. Ahmed FS, Miller LS. Adequate proverb interpretation is associated with performance on the independent living scales. Neuropsychol Dev Cogn B Aging Neuropsychol Cogn. 2015;22(3):376–87. https://doi.org/10.1080/13825585.2014.952613.
7. Bieth T, Ovando-Tellez M, Bernard M, Volle E. Contribution des études lésionnelles aux neurosciences de la créativité. Ann Méd-Psychol Rev Psychiatr. 2019;177(2):164–8.
8. Ovando-Tellez MP, Bieth T, Bernard M, Volle E. The contribution of the lesion approach to the neuroscience of creative cognition. Curr Opin Behav Sci. 2019;27:100–8. https://doi.org/10.1016/j.cobeha.2018.10.011.
9. Gonen T, Shofty B, Perry D, Levi R, Mayseless N, Korn A, Glikman A, Shamay-Tsoory S, Hendler T, Ram Z. Mapping original thinking by differential modulation of large-scale cortical networks: functional preservation of creativity in LGG patients. Brain Stimul Basic Transl Clin Res Neuromodul. 2017;10(2):369. https://doi.org/10.1016/j.brs.2017.01.087.

10. Piai V, Vos SH, Idelberger R, Gans P, Doorduin J, Ter Laan M. Awake surgery for a violin player: monitoring motor and music performance, a case report. Arch Clin Neuropsychol. 2019;34(1):132–7. https://doi.org/10.1093/arclin/acy009.
11. Riva M, Casarotti A, Comi A, Pessina F, Bello L. Brain and music: an intraoperative stimulation mapping study of a professional opera singer. World Neurosurg. 2016;93:486.e13–8. https://doi.org/10.1016/j.wneu.2016.06.130.
12. Scerrati A, Labanti S, Lofrese G, Mongardi L, Cavallo MA, Ricciardi L, De Bonis P. Artists playing music while undergoing brain surgery: a look into the scientific evidence and the social media perspective. Clin Neurol Neurosurg. 2020a;196:105911. https://doi.org/10.1016/j.clineuro.2020.105911.
13. Scerrati, A, Mongardi, L, Cavallo, MA, Labanti, S, Simioni, V, Ricciardi, L, De Bonis, P. Awake surgery for skills preservation during a sensory area tumor resection in a clarinet player. Acta Neurol Belg. 2020b;1-5. https://doi.org/10.1007/s13760-020-01368-5.
14. Guilford JP. Creativity. Am Psychol. 1950;5(9):444–54. https://doi.org/10.1037/h0063487.
15. Mednick SA. The associative basis of the creative process. Psychol Rev. 1962;69:220–32.
16. Patrick J, Ahmed A. Facilitating representation change in insight problems through training. J Exp Psychol Learn Mem Cogn. 2014;40(2):532–43. https://doi.org/10.1037/a0034304.
17. Beaty RE, Christensen AP, Benedek M, Silvia PJ, Schacter DL. Creative constraints: brain activity and network dynamics underlying semantic interference during idea production. NeuroImage. 2017;148:189–96. https://doi.org/10.1016/j.neuroimage.2017.01.012.
18. Benedek M, Jauk E. Spontaneous and controlled processes in creative cognition. In: The Oxford handbook of spontaneous thought. 2018. https://doi.org/10.1093/oxfordhb/9780190464745.013.22.
19. Cassotti M, Agogué M, Camarda A, Houdé O, Borst G. Inhibitory control as a core process of creative problem solving and idea generation from childhood to adulthood: inhibitory control as a core process of creative problem solving. New Dir Child Adolesc Dev. 2016;2016(151):61–72. https://doi.org/10.1002/cad.20153.
20. De Dreu CKW, Nijstad BA, Baas M, Wolsink I, Roskes M. Working memory benefits creative insight, musical improvisation, and original ideation through maintained task-focused attention. Personal Soc Psychol Bull. 2012;38(5):656–69. https://doi.org/10.1177/0146167211435795.
21. Edl S, Benedek M, Papousek I, Weiss EM, Fink A. Creativity and the Stroop interference effect. Personal Individ Differ. 2014;69:38–42. https://doi.org/10.1016/j.paid.2014.05.009.
22. Lee CS, Therriault DJ. The cognitive underpinnings of creative thought: a latent variable analysis exploring the roles of intelligence and working memory in three creative thinking processes. Intelligence. 2013;41(5):306–20. https://doi.org/10.1016/j.intell.2013.04.008.
23. Benedek M, Kenett YN, Umdasch C. How semantic memory structure and intelligence contribute to creative thought: a network science approach. Think Reason. 2017;23(2):158–83.
24. Kenett YN, Anaki D, Faust M. Investigating the structure of semantic networks in low and high creative persons. Front Hum Neurosci. 2014;8:407. https://doi.org/10.3389/fnhum.2014.00407.
25. Volle E. Associative and controlled cognition in divergent thinking: theoretical, experimental, neuroimaging evidence, and new directions. In: Jung RE, Vartanian O, editors. The Cambridge handbook of the neuroscience of creativity. New York: Cambridge University Press; 2017.
26. Ellamil M, Dobson C, Beeman M, Christoff K. Evaluative and generative modes of thought during the creative process. NeuroImage. 2012;59:1783–94. https://doi.org/10.1016/j.neuroimage.2011.08.008.
27. Gonen-Yaacovi G, de Souza LC, Levy R, Urbanski M, Josse G, Volle E. Rostral and caudal prefrontal contribution to creativity: a meta-analysis of functional imaging data. Front Hum Neurosci. 2013;7:465. https://doi.org/10.3389/fnhum.2013.00465.
28. Beaty RE, Benedek M, Silvia PJ, Schacter DL. Creative cognition and brain network dynamics. Trends Cogn Sci. 2016;20(2):87–95. https://doi.org/10.1016/j.tics.2015.10.004.
29. Andrews-Hanna JR, Reidler JS, Sepulcre J, Poulin R, Buckner RL. Functional-anatomic fractionation of the brain's default network. Neuron. 2010;65(4):550–62. https://doi.org/10.1016/j.neuron.2010.02.005.

30. Raichle ME. The restless brain: how intrinsic activity organizes brain function. Philos Trans R Soc Lond B Biol Sci. 2015;370(1668):20140172. Article 1668. https://doi.org/10.1098/rstb.2014.0172.
31. Marron TR, Lerner Y, Berant E, Kinreich S, Shapira-Lichter I, Hendler T, Faust M. Chain free association, creativity, and the default mode network. Neuropsychologia. 2018;118:40–58. https://doi.org/10.1016/j.neuropsychologia.2018.03.018.
32. Power JD, Petersen SE. Control-related systems in the human brain. Curr Opin Neurobiol. 2013;23(2):223–8. https://doi.org/10.1016/j.conb.2012.12.009.
33. Yeo BTT, Krienen FM, Sepulcre J, Sabuncu MR, Lashkari D, Hollinshead M, Roffman JL, Smoller JW, Zöllei L, Polimeni JR, Fischl B, Liu H, Buckner RL. The organization of the human cerebral cortex estimated by intrinsic functional connectivity. J Neurophysiol. 2011;106(3):1125–65. https://doi.org/10.1152/jn.00338.2011.
34. Adnan A, Beaty R, Silvia P, Spreng RN, Turner GR. Creative aging: functional brain networks associated with divergent thinking in older and younger adults. Neurobiol Aging. 2019;75:150–8. https://doi.org/10.1016/j.neurobiolaging.2018.11.004.
35. Jilka SR, Scott G, Ham T, Pickering A, Bonnelle V, Braga RM, Leech R, Sharp DJ. Damage to the salience network and interactions with the default mode network. J Neurosci. 2014;34(33):10798–807. https://doi.org/10.1523/JNEUROSCI.0518-14.2014.
36. Sridharan D, Levitin DJ, Menon V. A critical role for the right fronto-insular cortex in switching between central-executive and default-mode networks. Proc Natl Acad Sci. 2008;105(34):12569–74. https://doi.org/10.1073/pnas.0800005105.
37. Beaty RE, Kenett YN, Christensen AP, Rosenberg MD, Benedek M, Chen Q, Fink A, Qiu J, Kwapil TR, Kane MJ, Silvia PJ. Robust prediction of individual creative ability from brain functional connectivity. Proc Natl Acad Sci U S A. 2018;115(5):1087–92. https://doi.org/10.1073/pnas.1713532115.
38. Zhu W, Chen Q, Xia L, Beaty RE, Yang W, Tian F, Sun J, Cao G, Zhang Q, Chen X, Qiu J. Common and distinct brain networks underlying verbal and visual creativity: brain networks underlying verbal and visual creativity. Hum Brain Mapp. 2017;38(4):2094–111. https://doi.org/10.1002/hbm.23507.
39. Boccia M, Piccardi L, Palermo L, Nori R, Palmiero M. Where do bright ideas occur in our brain? Meta-analytic evidence from neuroimaging studies of domain-specific creativity. Front Psychol. 2015;6:1195. https://doi.org/10.3389/fpsyg.2015.01195.
40. Matheson HE, Kenett YN. The role of the motor system in generating creative thoughts. NeuroImage. 2020;213:116697. https://doi.org/10.1016/j.neuroimage.2020.116697.
41. Cogdell-Brooke LS, Sowden PT, Violante IR, Thompson HE. A meta-analysis of functional magnetic resonance imaging studies of divergent thinking using activation likelihood estimation. Hum Brain Mapp. 2020;41(17):5057–77. https://doi.org/10.1002/hbm.25170.
42. Chen Q, Beaty RE, Cui Z, Sun J, He H, Zhuang K, Ren Z, Liu G, Qiu J. Brain hemispheric involvement in visuospatial and verbal divergent thinking. Neuroimage. 2019;202:116065. https://doi.org/10.1016/j.neuroimage.2019.116065.
43. Bendetowicz D, Urbanski M, Garcin B, Foulon C, Levy R, Bréchemier M-L, Rosso C, Thiebaut de Schotten M, Volle E. Two critical brain networks for generation and combination of remote associations. Brain. 2018;141(1):217–33. https://doi.org/10.1093/brain/awx294.
44. Shamay-Tsoory SG, Adler N, Aharon-Peretz J, Perry D, Mayseless N. The origins of originality: the neural bases of creative thinking and originality. Neuropsychologia. 2011;49(2):178–85. https://doi.org/10.1016/j.neuropsychologia.2010.11.020.
45. Abraham A, Beudt S, Ott DVM, Yves von Cramon D. Creative cognition and the brain: dissociations between frontal, parietal–temporal and basal ganglia groups. Brain Res. 2012;1482:55–70. https://doi.org/10.1016/j.brainres.2012.09.007.
46. Duff MC, Kurczek J, Rubin R, Cohen NJ, Tranel D. Hippocampal amnesia disrupts creative thinking: creative thinking and the Hippocampus. Hippocampus. 2013;23(12):1143–9. https://doi.org/10.1002/hipo.22208.
47. Warren DE, Kurczek J, Duff MC. What relates newspaper, definite, and clothing? An article describing deficits in convergent problem solving and creativity following hippocampal

damage: hippocampal damage impairs convergent problem solving. Hippocampus. 2016;26(7):835–40. https://doi.org/10.1002/hipo.22591.
48. Alves PN, Foulon C, Karolis V, Bzdok D, Margulies DS, Volle E, Thiebaut de Schotten M. An improved neuroanatomical model of the default-mode network reconciles previous neuroimaging and neuropathological findings. Commun Biol. 2019;2:370. https://doi.org/10.1038/s42003-019-0611-3.
49. Paulin T, Roquet D, Kenett YN, Savage G, Irish M. The effect of semantic memory degeneration on creative thinking: a voxel-based morphometry analysis. NeuroImage. 2020;220:117073. https://doi.org/10.1016/j.neuroimage.2020.117073.
50. Canesi M, Rusconi ML, Cereda E, Ranghetti A, Cereda V, Moroni F, Pezzoli G. Divergent thinking in parkinsonism: a case–control study. Front Neurol. 2017;8:534. https://doi.org/10.3389/fneur.2017.00534.
51. de Souza LC, Volle E, Bertoux M, Czernecki V, Funkiewiez A, Allali G, Leroy B, Sarazin M, Habert M-O, Dubois B, Kas A, Levy R. Poor creativity in frontotemporal dementia: a window into the neural bases of the creative mind. Neuropsychologia. 2010;48(13):3733–42. https://doi.org/10.1016/j.neuropsychologia.2010.09.010.
52. Rankin KP, Liu AA, Howard S, Slama H, Hou CE, Shuster K, Miller BL. A case-controlled study of altered visual art production in Alzheimer's and FTLD. Cogn Behav Neurol. 2007;20(1):48–61. https://doi.org/10.1097/WNN.0b013e31803141dd.
53. Ruggiero F, Cortese F, Lavazza A, D'Urso G, Nuzzo CD, Marceglia S, Pravettoni G, Priori A, Ferrucci R. Do neurodegenerative diseases affect creativity? Divergent thinking in frontotemporal dementia and Parkinson's disease. Creat Res J. 2019;31(1):102–9. https://doi.org/10.1080/10400419.2019.1577667.
54. Giovagnoli AR. The contribution of the frontal lobe to creativity. Insights from epilepsy. Epilepsy Behav. 2020;111:107313. https://doi.org/10.1016/j.yebeh.2020.107313.
55. Senf P, Scheuren L, Holtkamp M. Is there a creative functional paradoxical facilitation in juvenile myoclonic epilepsy? Epilepsy Behav. 2016;62:285–90. https://doi.org/10.1016/j.yebeh.2016.07.023.
56. Ghacibeh GA, Heilman KM. Creative innovation with temporal lobe epilepsy and lobectomy. J Neurol Sci. 2013;324(1–2):45–8. https://doi.org/10.1016/j.jns.2012.09.029.
57. Reverberi C, Toraldo A, D'Agostini S, Skrap M. Better without (lateral) frontal cortex? Insight problems solved by frontal patients. Brain. 2005;128(12):2882–90. https://doi.org/10.1093/brain/awh577.
58. Weinberger AB, Green AE, Chrysikou EG. Using transcranial direct current stimulation to enhance creative cognition: interactions between task, polarity, and stimulation site. Front Hum Neurosci. 2017;11:246. https://doi.org/10.3389/fnhum.2017.00246.
59. Thiebaut de Schotten M, Urbanski M, Batrancourt B, Levy R, Dubois B, Cerliani L, Volle E. Rostro-caudal architecture of the frontal lobes in humans. Cereb Cortex. 2017;27(8):4033–47.
60. Foulon C, Cerliani L, Kinkingnéhun S, Levy R, Rosso C, Urbanski M, Volle E, Thiebaut de Schotten M. Advanced lesion symptom mapping analyses and implementation as BCBtoolkit. GigaScience. 2018;7(3). Article 3. https://doi.org/10.1093/gigascience/giy004.
61. Duffau H, Capelle L. Preferential brain locations of low-grade gliomas: comparison with glioblastomas and review of hypothesis. Cancer. 2004;100(12):2622–6. https://doi.org/10.1002/cncr.20297.
62. Mithani K, Boutet A, Germann J, Elias GJB, Weil AG, Shah A, Guillen M, Bernal B, Achua JK, Ragheb J, Donner E, Lozano AM, Widjaja E, Ibrahim GM. Lesion network localization of seizure freedom following MR-guided laser interstitial thermal ablation. Sci Rep. 2019;9(1):18598. https://doi.org/10.1038/s41598-019-55015-y.
63. Parisot S, Darlix A, Baumann C, Zouaoui S, Yordanova Y, Blonski M, Rigau V, Chemouny S, Taillandier L, Bauchet L, Duffau H, Paragios N. A probabilistic atlas of diffuse WHO Grade II glioma locations in the brain. PLoS One. 2016;11(1):e0144200. https://doi.org/10.1371/journal.pone.0144200.
64. Duffau H. Awake surgery for nonlanguage mapping. Neurosurgery. 2010;66:523–8.

65. Duffau H. Functional mapping before and after low-grade glioma surgery: a new way to decipher various spatiotemporal patterns of individual neuroplastic potential in brain tumor patients. Cancers. 2020;12(9):2611. Article 9. https://doi.org/10.3390/cancers12092611.
66. Mandonnet E, Cerliani L, Siuda-Krzywicka K, Poisson I, Zhi N, Volle E, Thiebaut de Schotten M. A network-level approach of cognitive flexibility impairment after surgery of a right temporo-parietal glioma. Neurochirurgie. 2017;63(4):308–13. https://doi.org/10.1016/j.neuchi.2017.03.003.
67. Mandonnet E, Vincent M, Valero-Cabré A, Facque V, Barberis M, Bonnetblanc F, Rheault F, Volle E, Descoteaux M, Margulies DS. Network-level causal analysis of set-shifting during trail making test part B: a multimodal analysis of a glioma surgery case. Cortex. 2020;132:238–49. https://doi.org/10.1016/j.cortex.2020.08.021.
68. Puglisi G, Sciortino T, Rossi M, Leonetti A, Fornia L, Conti Nibali M, Casarotti A, Pessina F, Riva M, Cerri G, Bello L. Preserving executive functions in nondominant frontal lobe glioma surgery: an intraoperative tool. J Neurosurg. 2018;131(2):474–80. https://doi.org/10.3171/2018.4.JNS18393.
69. Thiebaut de Schotten M, Urbanski M, Duffau H, Volle E, Levy R, Dubois B, Bartolomeo P. Direct evidence for a parietal-frontal pathway subserving spatial awareness in humans. Science. 2005;309(5744):2226–8. https://doi.org/10.1126/science.1116251.
70. Wager M, Du Boisgueheneuc F, Pluchon C, Bouyer C, Stal V, Bataille B, Guillevin CM, Gil R. Intraoperative monitoring of an aspect of executive functions: administration of the Stroop test in nine adult patients during awake surgery for resection of frontal glioma. Neurosurgery. 2013;72:ons169–80. https://doi.org/10.1227/NEU.0b013e31827bf1d6.
71. Yordanova YN, Cochereau J, Duffau H, Herbet G. Combining resting state functional MRI with intraoperative cortical stimulation to map the mentalizing network. Neuroimage. 2019;186:628–36. https://doi.org/10.1016/j.neuroimage.2018.11.046.
72. Hart RP, Wade JB. Divergent thinking in Alzheimer's and frontotemporal dementia. Aging Neuropsychol Cognit. 2006;13(3–4):281–90. https://doi.org/10.1080/13825580490904246.
73. Reiter-Palmon R, Murugavel V. The effect of problem construction on team process and creativity. Front Psychol. 2018;9:2098. https://doi.org/10.3389/fpsyg.2018.02098.
74. Beaty RE, Johnson DR. Automating creativity assessment with SemDis: an open platform for computing semantic distance. Behav Res Methods. 2021;53(2):757–80. https://doi.org/10.3758/s13428-020-01453-w.
75. Green AE, Cohen MS, Raab HA, Yedibalian CG, Gray JR. Frontopolar activity and connectivity support dynamic conscious augmentation of creative state: neuroimaging augmented state creativity. Hum Brain Mapp. 2015;36:923–34. https://doi.org/10.1002/hbm.22676.
76. Prabhakaran R, Green AE, Gray JR. Thin slices of creativity: using single-word utterances to assess creative cognition. Behav Res Methods. 2014;46:641–59. https://doi.org/10.3758/s13428-013-0401-7.
77. Fink A, Benedek M, Koschutnig K, Pirker E, Berger E, Meister S, Neubauer AC, Papousek I, Weiss EM. Training of verbal creativity modulates brain activity in regions associated with language- and memory-related demands: training of verbal creativity. Hum Brain Mapp. 2015;36(10):4104–15. https://doi.org/10.1002/hbm.22901.
78. Fink A, Grabner RH, Gebauer D, Reishofer G, Koschutnig K, Ebner F. Enhancing creativity by means of cognitive stimulation: evidence from an fMRI study. Neuroimage. 2010;52(4):1687–95. https://doi.org/10.1016/j.neuroimage.2010.05.072.
79. Fink A, Reim T, Benedek M, Grabner RH. The effects of a verbal and a figural creativity training on different facets of creative potential. J Creat Behav. 2020;54(3):676–85. https://doi.org/10.1002/jocb.402.
80. Sun M, Wang M, Wegerif R. Using computer-based cognitive mapping to improve students' divergent thinking for creativity development. Br J Educ Technol. 2019;50(5):2217–33. https://doi.org/10.1111/bjet.12825.
81. Forgeard MJC, Elstein JG. Advancing the clinical science of creativity. Front Psychol. 2014;5:613. https://doi.org/10.3389/fpsyg.2014.00613.

82. Silvia PJ, Beaty RE, Nusbaum EC, Eddington KM, Levin-Aspenson H, Kwapil TR. Everyday creativity in daily life: an experience-sampling study of "little c" creativity. Psychol Aesthet Creat Arts. 2014;8(2):183–8. https://doi.org/10.1037/a0035722.
83. Windle G, Gregory S, Howson-Griffiths T, Newman A, O'Brien D, Goulding A. Exploring the theoretical foundations of visual art programmes for people living with dementia. Dementia. 2018;17(6):702–27. https://doi.org/10.1177/1471301217726613.

21 Raising the Question of Personality Changes in Glioma Surgery

Anne-Laure Lemaitre, Gilles Lafargue, and Guillaume Herbet

21.1 Introduction

In recent years, the better understanding of both the natural history of low-grade glioma and the neuroplasticity dynamics deployed by the brain to functionally mitigate or even fully compensate the tumor-induced dysfunctions has jointly contributed to a proactive approach of the clinical management, the main goal of which is to maintain quality of life (QoL) as high as possible while performing a drastic cytoreduction of the tumor volume [1, 2]. As quality of life is indissociable from cognitive functioning (i.e., patients need to interact efficiently with their surrounding environment to continue assuming their daily-life activities), a central ambition of surgical oncology is to preserve functions, particularly through the intraoperative mapping and monitoring of various cognitive processes (beyond language and motor activities) in the operating theater [3], but also by means of a well-conducted neuropsychological care that includes perioperative and follow-up assessments and tailored cognitive rehabilitation. In this context, a great deal of studies has focused

A.-L. Lemaitre
Department of Neurosurgery, CHU Montpellier, Montpellier University Medical Center, Gui de Chauliac Hospital, Montpellier, France

Institute of Functional Genomics, INSERM, CNRS, INSERM U191, Montpellier, France
e-mail: al-lemaitre@chu-montpellier.fr

G. Lafargue (✉)
University of Reims Champagne Ardenne, C2S, EA 6291, Laboratoire Cognition, Santé, Socialisation, Reims, France
e-mail: gilles.lafargue@univ-reims.fr

G. Herbet
Department of Neurosurgery, Gui de Chauliac Hospital, Montpellier & Institute of Functional Genomics, University of Montpellier, INSERM, CNRS, Montpellier, France

E. Mandonnet, G. Herbet (eds.), *Intraoperative Mapping of Cognitive Networks*,
https://doi.org/10.1007/978-3-030-75071-8_21

on the cognitive status of patients before any neurosurgical treatments [4, 5] or longitudinally [4, 6–11], as considerably developed in the different chapters of this book. Contrary to patients with sudden diseases such as stroke or traumatic injuries, neuropsychological impairments are generally modest and aspecific in low-grade glioma patients despite large tumors and/or resections [12, 13]. As a matter of fact, previous neuropsychological works have suggested that surgical removal of the right inferior parietal cortex [14], the Broca's area [15], or the prefrontal cortex [16], even bilaterally [17, 18], did not necessarily cause, respectively, detectable abnormalities in the awareness of action, long-term expressive language impairment, or executive or metacognitive deficits. Taken as a whole, these clinical findings have provided compelling evidence that the brain has the potential to reshape dynamically its functional networks in reaction to lesion and resection. This is in line with the growing literature suggesting that cognitive activities and behavior are subserved by complex and distributed networks, not by static and isolated cortical structures.

Even if cognitive compensation and recovery in glioma patients have been well studied the last 10 years, the topic of personality and behavioral changes has received unfortunately little attention. This may sound quite paradoxical in the sense that it is generally conceded that personality is one of the fundamental components that make the uniqueness of our own behaviors. Broadly speaking, personality refers to the habitual modes of thoughts, feeling, and acting characterizing an individual [19, 20] and is often conceptualized as the base of inter-individual differences that explain various kind of behaviors [21–24]. As a consequence, lesion-related modifications of personality, even subtle, can alter the pattern of behaviors usually produced by an individual; stated another way, the acting self.

Behind empirical considerations/questions, there are the fundamental issues on what types of changes a given person can undergo while still being the same person and, in the clinical management, the questions raises how to anticipate these possible changes. Does a patient feel some modifications of his/her personality following surgery? Do the patient's relatives notice changes the patient remains unaware about? These questions should not be underappreciated as the medical or neuroscientific literature provides numerous cases of dramatic changes in personality following brain damage or following surgical interventions in the context of psychosurgery.

The first section of this chapter will explore the link between personality traits and the brain. In the second section, we will review the literature on personality changes after DLGG resection. Finally, in the third section, we will raise the question of personality in the clinical care of glioma patients.

21.2 Personality and the Brain

Raising the question of personality changes following brain damage is often associated with the depiction of clinical cases of patients displaying dramatic personality modifications like it is seen in acquired sociopathy [25–28]. One of the most famous depictions certainly remains the case of Phineas Gage whose personality modifications are summarizing in the sentence "*Gage was no longer Gage*" [27]. In the history of neuroscience, Phineas Gage has fueled many researches that attempted to precisely identify the lesioned structures, both cortical and subcortical, causally linked to the behavioral changes observed [29–34]. Today, we know that Gage had lesions spreading in the left frontal lobe, comprising the orbitofrontal and the dorsolateral prefrontal cortex as well as the temporopolar cortex [32] but also affecting the surrounding white matter connections [33, 34]. Other more recent clinical cases are also interesting to consider: for instance, patient E.V.R. who has undergone a surgery for a bilateral frontal tumor [26] and patient JZ operated on for a pituitary tumor for which the surgical approach damaged the left orbitofrontal cortex [28], like Phineas Gage.

Admittedly, the cases we described are unusual in terms of severity. However, the medical literature is filled with examples of patients experiencing less pronounced changes. Indeed, clinical symptoms such as irritability, apathy, emotional lability, and anxiety disorders are often described following neurological insult, including sudden and degenerative diseases [35–37]. In that respect, as neurosurgery is a voluntary act performed on the brain, any neurosurgeon should keep in mind that deep consequences on patient's personality can be caused. The history of neurosurgery itself calls for caution. For instance, we must remember that Egaz Moniz received the 1949 Nobel Prize for his pioneering use of prefrontal leucotomy to treat refractory cases of psychosis. How could it happen? How was it possible while this surgical treatment is now considered as one of the biggest scandals and "*the most spectacular failure*" in the history of medicine [38]? Indeed, prefrontal leucotomy and later prefrontal lobotomy [39] that consists in destroying the prefrontal white matter with a kitchen icepick-like instrument pushed into the brain through the skull bone behind the eyeball was later assimilated to a murder of the personality. This episode in the history of neurosurgery taught us that drastic changes in everyday life behaviors and personality can be masked by apparent benefits and are not easily accessible to an outside observer.

21.3 Personality and Diffuse Low-Grade Glioma

In the older literature personality changes in the context of brain tumor surgery were often investigated under the designation of "*mental symptoms.*" For instance, Bramwell [40] suggested that various and numerous mental symptoms were present in the majority of cases of intracranial tumors and those were sometimes so slight that only the individuals who were intimately acquainted with the patients were able to detect it [40]. In his review, Bramwell also presented a primary classification including on the one side the mental symptoms such as irritability, mania, or depression, and on the other side the cognitive symptoms. A couple of years later, Louis Minski [41] presented a compendium of 58 clinical observations of patients with brain tumors in which he described mental changes according to distinct classifications such as depression, excitement, anxiety, hysteria, and schizophrenic or obsessional states [41]. Based on these clinical observations, Minski argued that "*Mental symptoms in cerebral tumors do not appear to depend on localization, but rather on the rate of growth of the tumor and the previous personality of the patient*" [41]. This author further suggested a predominance of personality modifications in comparison to intellectual declines in the context of slow-growing brain tumors while rapidly growing tumors were associated with changes both in the intellectual and in the personality spheres.

Current research tends to support these pioneering clinical observations, as psychiatric symptoms have a reported incidence from 50 to 78%, in the context of brain tumors [42, 43]. In a recent meta-analysis, it was shown that 36% of patients with brain tumors suffered from mood disorders, 26% of patients had memory disturbances, and 22% psychotic symptoms [44]. In another study, Jenkins et al. [45] reported emotional and personality changes like apathy (for 21.21% of the patient's sample), irritability (33.33%), depression (42%), and moodiness (52%) following brain tumor resection [45]. Also, by investigating the Danish Psychiatric Central Register and the Danish Cancer Registry, Benros et al. [46] observed an increased incidence rate of brain tumors almost 19 times than expected during the first month of the psychiatric follow-up [46]. In this context psychiatric disorders could be one of the first manifestation of brain tumors [46, 47]. Nevertheless, most of these studies investigating personality changes included different tumor histologies such as meningioma, metastatic tumor, glioma, or glioblastoma. For example, in the meta-analysis by Madhusoodanan et al. [44] based on 148 previous published cases of patients, the proportion of patients with "glioma" (with no additional classification) was under-represented (5.1% of the cases).

To our best knowledge only three studies specifically explored possible changes in personality among patients with tagged diffuse low-grade glioma [48–50]. In the first study, Urgesi et al. [50] focused on one personality trait called self-transcendence, defined by Cloninger "*As the extent to which a person identifies the self as... an integral part of the universe as a whole*" ([51], p. 975)—in other words a sense of connection and movement beyond one's immediate self-boundaries [52, 53]. In this study, four groups of patients with different types of brain tumors, including DLGG, were assessed before and after surgical resection and their scores were analyzed separately. The main finding was that inferior parietal resections were associated with an increase in self-transcendence scores. In the two other studies, Campanella et al. [48, 49] used a personality questionnaire called Temperament and Character Inventory [54] and more specifically a derived measure called "self-maturity." Indeed, previous studies have demonstrated that individuals with low level of self-maturity tend to be at risk to develop personality disorders [55]. This time, three groups of patients with different types of brain tumor (high-grade glioma, low-grade glioma, and meningioma) were assessed before and after brain tumor resection and their scores were analyzed separately. In the first study using Voxel-Based Lesion–Symptom Mapping (VLSM), Campanella et al. [49] have highlighted an association between the inferolateral prefrontal cortex and lower self-maturity. In the second study [48], they statistically compared the self-maturity score of the different groups of patients before and after the surgical resections. They did not find significant differences in self-maturity scores of LGG patients, suggesting no personality changes following surgical resection [48]. These few researches showed an association between surgical resections in parietal or prefrontal cortex and changes in personality scale scores, suggesting that alteration of brain structures modulates personality. However, it must be noted that no major personality changes were identified.

The finding that resective surgery can lead to changes in personality traits is in accordance with a number of works demonstrating that psychological dysfunctions is related to aberrant functional connectivity in networks involving the frontal-striatal, frontal-parietal, and default mode networks [56–58]. Further, other findings tend to show modification of connectivity patterns in individual with pronounced personality traits. For example, functional connectivity of the insular cortex is increased in individuals with a high level of anxiety [59]. Our research group has also recently demonstrated that dysconnectivity of the left ventral fronto-temporal network (mainly supplied by the left uncinate fasciculus) was associated with heightened positive schizotypal traits [60]. In a third study, correlations were found between specific personality dimensions and distinct patterns of brain's functional connectivity [61]. Personality dimensions are thus encoded in the brain's intrinsic functional connectivity and may influence functional network efficiency. Therefore, a "large-scale" neural injury affecting the functional connectivity in one or more networks may lead to modifications of the premorbid personality.

Given possible changes in personality following surgery, it seems necessary to (1) exert some caution in the clinical management of glioma patients by adopting an individual and personalized clinical care, which will be the topic of the next section of this chapter, and (2) develop further researches aimed at assessing how DLGGs modulate patients' personality, ideally in longitudinally designed studies [62] in order to precisely gauge the impact of surgical resections.

21.4 Toward a *"Personalized"* Clinical Management of Glioma Patients

Investigating issues related to changes in personality and attitudes is essential to protect and preserve patients' quality of life and more generally to reflect on the most relevant and ethical management that patients have to receive. In this context, managing patients in a highly personalized manner appears to be the best option to capture the patient's personality dimensions and identify some of them that should require special attention such as, for example, anxiety or depressive traits. The medical team (including the neurosurgeon, speech therapist, neuropsychologist and anesthetist) must also clearly inform the patient about the standard care and the surgical procedure, to anticipate the psychological consequences of awake brain tumor surgery. Nevertheless, disregarding heightened personality traits like heightened anxiety or mood disorders (whatever their cause: preexisting intrinsic personality, reaction to the diagnosis of tumor, or connectivity changes induced by the tumor) may compromise the active participation and involvement of the patients to the awake procedure and the cognitive rehabilitation. Indeed, from our clinical experience, it seems that the immediate postoperative modifications are dictated by the premorbid personality, as if the psychological (or psychiatric) decompensation was an overexpression of the normal psychological characteristics or particular heightened personality characteristic (temperament, traits or characters) of the patients (Table 21.1). One could argue that the transitory modification of the personality of the patients may shift from a continuum that ranges from normal psychological characteristics and milder forms of personality traits (irritably, impulsivity, anxiety, etc.) to the overexpression of these traits and thus the emergence of psychiatric disorders (anxiety-depression disorders, violent behaviors, etc.).

Clinical interviews, made individually by the medical staff, are a valuable assistance to discuss about potential modifications of behaviors and personality of the patient with the patient himself and the patient's relative. In addition, psychological scales assessing distinct personality traits and behaviors can be used during the neuropsychological assessment like, for instance, anxiety (STAI, [63]), empathy [64], apathy [65], behavioral modifications [66, 67], and psychiatric disorders [68, 69]. This kind of self-evaluative questionnaires, and if possible hetero evaluation, can be useful for a longitudinal assessment in order to detect preoperatively patients with high risk of personality and behavioral decompensation and to adapt the clinical follow-up when detecting postoperative changes.

On the other hand, personality changes does not always lead to negative outcomes such as emotional liability, mood disorders, or irritability. In a recent study, King et al. [56] demonstrated positive changes in patients' personality and behaviors following neurological diseases, in particular stroke injury or benign brain tumor [56]. For instance, a decrease of irritability and distress and an improvement in executive functioning and social behavior were reported, while normal cognitive functioning was preserved; these favorable outcomes being associated with damage in the prefrontal cortex including frontopolar regions and the anterior part of the dorsolateral prefrontal cortex. Although counterintuitive, the idea that a brain lesion can in a few cases also be associated with rather positive changes in some aspects of the personality is in accordance with our clinical experience. Some of our patients, for example, told us that, following the resection, they had less depressive rumination or negative affects or they became less sad, irritable, or short-tempered. Other patients, or their relatives, report a slight disinhibition following the surgery, which was rather experienced as positive. While it is reasonable to think that certain personality traits could be amplified by tumor resection, it is also possible to consider that in certain cases rather negative premorbid tendencies could be reduced. It is not surprising that the resection of a structure in a dysfunctional network in patients with borderline traits can sometimes have positive consequences.

As emphasized by King et al. [56], considering the negative changes in behavioral functioning following a neurological disorder provides only a partial capture of the story. Further research should also investigate positive outcomes in order to identify the relevant factors leading sometimes to improvement in some personality and behavior characteristics.

Table 21.1 Example of patients with transitory changes in personality and behaviors

Patient 1: A case of transitory aggression
Patient 1 has undergone an awake neurosurgery for an incidental left prefrontal DLGG (with a preoperative volume around 20 cm^3). The surgical procedure was successfully achieved allowing a supratotal resection of tumor. This young man, aged 26 years, displayed no cognitive or behavioral impairments as determined by a comprehensive neuropsychological assessment. He was a high-level educational man enjoying a normal socio-professional life. Immediately after the surgery, the patient showed as expected transitory cognitive difficulties involving verbal fluency, most notably speech initiation problems, and executive functions
Few weeks later, the patient's mother called the neurosurgical team because her son developed some behavioral modifications. She explained that he becomes aggressive verbally and behaviorally. For example, following one comment about his disability, the patient had violent outburst. He broke the closet and other nearby objects, removing the surgical sutures and uttering insults. The patient and his mother came back to discuss with the neurosurgical team and to adapt the follow-up (including psychological follow up and an updating of the neurocognitive rehabilitation). The violent behaviors then decreased step by step until they disappeared a couple of weeks later. During the neuropsychological follow-up, 3 months after the surgery, the patient's relative indicated that it was not the first time that the patient developed aggressive behaviors. A few weeks before the surgery, the patient had already presented a first episode of "non-adaptive behaviors" that seemed to be linked to the diagnosis announce according to him. Thereafter, the patient was able to return to his previous socio-professional life and, according to him, never displayed again aggressive behaviors
Patient 2: A case of transitory irritability
Patient 2 is a 35-year-old businessman, married with a child. After a first inaugural seizure, a left operculo-insular glioma was discovered. The awake surgery allowed a subtotal resection. The preoperative neurocognitive assessment demonstrated executive difficulties (switching ability, working memory, and short-term memory) and the patient and his relatives mentioned subtle behavioral modifications such as irritability and occasionally perseverative ideas. Immediately after the surgery, the patient showed transitory language impairments and an intensification of the executive difficulties
Several days after homecoming, his wife reported an important increase of the behavioral modifications identified during the preoperative consultation, especially the development of a strong irritability (with a patient who get easily angry without legitime justifications, according to the patient's relative) and perseverative trouble were noticed by his acquaintance. As these behavioral changes were described preoperatively, the neurocognitive rehabilitation was already planned according to the patient's complaints before the neurosurgery. Therefore, an individually tailored rehabilitation program, dealing with mental flexibility, inhibitory control in addition to a reeducation of language process, was scheduled before the surgery. The heightened behavioral changes decreased progressively and returned to the same range than before the surgery
Patient 3: A case of transitory disinhibition
Patient 3 is a 50-year-old woman who suffers from chronic headaches since several years. In this context, an MRI was realized and a DLGG involving the right fronto-operculo-insular cortex was incidentally discovered (with a preoperative volume of 13 cm^3). A complete resection of the DLGG was performed under local anesthesia in accordance with the standard protocol of our institution. The neuropsychological assessment performed before the surgery demonstrated working memory impairment associated with attentional difficulties. As expected, these executive disorders increased immediately after the surgery, then a personalized cognitive rehabilitation program was prescribed

(continued)

Table 21.1 (continued)

Few days after the surgery, the patient subscribed to a dating site, met a young man, and finally had one sexual intercourse with him. The relationship with this young man deteriorated thereafter and the patient began to track this man and to wait for him in front of his own home. A harassment complaint against the patient was therefore lodged. Meanwhile, she wrote a love note intended to the neuropsychologist who performed the neurocognitive management of this patient. These harassment behaviors declined a few weeks after and the patient recovered quickly
Patient 4: A case of transitory nymphomania
Several weeks after the surgery, this 26-year-old patient who was operated on for a low-grade glioma infiltrating the right dorsomedial prefrontal cortex developed nymphomania symptoms. She had multiple sexual intercourses with distinct individuals (men and women). This risky behavior decreased progressively as the months passed
Patient 5: A case of transitory paranoid delusions
Patient 5 is a 48-year-old man with a high socio-educational level. He was married with several children. During the past years, he began to feel some negative changes in his cognitive functions, most notably lexical retrieval difficulty. He requested to perform an MRI and a right premotor DLGG (around 50 cm^3) was finally discovered. An awake neurosurgery was successfully performed with a complete resection of the tumor. The preoperative neuropsychological assessment indicated only episodic verbal memory deficits associated with subtle sustained attention difficulties. Three days after the surgery, the emergence of executive difficulties was observed during the immediate postoperative cognitive evaluation
Several weeks following surgery, the patient began progressively to present paranoia delusions with a strong jealousy (against his wife), a high level of stress leading to hypervigilance and insomnia, and rumination about ordinary details of the daily life. Progressively, these paranoiac symptoms decreased along with his cognitive recovery. Interestingly, the patient's spouse explained that his husband was disposed to jealousy before the surgery so that the behavioral modifications were regarded by her as an exaggeration of his premorbid temperament
Patient 6: A case of positive enhancement following brain neurosurgery
The patient 6 is a 43-year-old man enjoying normal socio-professional life. He is married with two children and works as a duty manager. The glioma, invading the right opercular frontal region, was incidentally discovered in a context of chronic headaches since several years. A complete resection of the DLGG (with a preoperative volume inferior to 5 cm^3) was performed under local anesthesia in accordance with the standard protocol of our institution
The preoperative neuropsychological examination did not objective cognitive impairment. After the surgery, the emergence of attentional and working memory difficulties was observed during the immediate postoperative cognitive evaluation for which a personalized cognitive rehabilitation program was indicated. In addition, behavioral modifications were noticed 3 days after the surgery. The patient was more talkative and seemed to be more outgoing, more joyful with the different individual he encountered (nurses, other patients in the hospitalization service for example). He was also more exhilarated but always in appropriate manner and never displayed non-adaptative behaviors or comments
Three months after the surgery, he explained that the surgery helped him to refocus on what seemed crucial for him (family life, children, wife) and reconsidered his priority. He felled more in agreement with himself and serene. On neuropsychological point of view, he recovered completely and was able to resume to his previous socio-professional life

21.5 Conclusion

If we throw a crystal to the floor, it breaks; but not into haphazard pieces. It comes apart along its lines of cleavage into fragments whose boundaries, though they were invisible, were predetermined by the crystal's structure [70].

The history of neuropsychology and neurosurgery is such that the neurosurgeon should always have in mind the question of personality changes, especially when the tumor to be resected is located in neural circuits that pass through the frontal and parietal structures. Therefore, since it is obvious that brain tumor surgery can have an impact on the personality characteristics of patients, it is important for the neurosurgeon to find, in the scientific literature, research data on the factors that could favor the occurrence personality changes. Unfortunately, to date, very few studies have addressed this problem in the context of a brain tumor and its resection (see the very recent study by Lemaitre et al. [71]). There are two main reasons for this lack of data. First, it is not possible to assess and map online during awake surgery the personality components of a human being. Second, even in retrospective studies, it is methodologically complex to objectify personality changes thanks to self-reports and reports by well-known family members or friends. Consequently, the only way to shed some lights on this matter is to plan longitudinally studies aimed at comprehensively assessing the different dimensions of personality before and after surgery. In this way, it would be theoretically possible to identify which personality dimensions are most likely to change, how these changes affect behaviors and social interactions, and which cerebral resections are the most likely to be associated with.

References

1. Duffau H. A new philosophy in surgery for diffuse low-grade glioma (DLGG): oncological and functional outcomes. Neurochirurgie. 2013;59:2–8. https://doi.org/10.1016/j.neuchi.2012.11.001.
2. Duffau H, Mandonnet E. The "onco-functional balance" in surgery for diffuse low-grade glioma: integrating the extent of resection with quality of life. Acta Neurochir. 2013;155:951–7.
3. Herbet G, Moritz-Gasser S. Beyond language: mapping cognition and emotion. Neurosurg Clin. 2019;30:75–83.
4. Tucha O, Smely C, Preier M, Lange KW. Cognitive deficits before treatment among patients with brain tumors. Neurosurgery. 2000;47:324–34.
5. van Kessel E, Baumfalk AE, van Zandvoort MJ, Robe PA, Snijders TJ. Tumor-related neurocognitive dysfunction in patients with diffuse glioma: a systematic review of neurocognitive functioning prior to anti-tumor treatment. J Neurooncol. 2017;134:9–18.
6. Herbet G, Lafargue G, Bonnetblanc F, Moritz-Gasser S, Duffau H. Is the right frontal cortex really crucial in the mentalizing network? A longitudinal study in patients with a slow-growing lesion. Cortex. 2013;49:2711–27. https://doi.org/10.1016/j.cortex.2013.08.003.
7. Talacchi A, Santini B, Savazzi S, Gerosa M. Cognitive effects of tumour and surgical treatment in glioma patients. J Neurooncol. 2011;103:541–9.
8. Taphoorn MJ, Klein M. Cognitive deficits in adult patients with brain tumours. Lancet Neurol. 2004;3:159–68.

9. van Kessel E, Snijders TJ, Baumfalk AE, Ruis C, van Baarsen KM, Broekman ML, van Zandvoort MJ, Robe PA. Neurocognitive changes after awake surgery in glioma patients: a retrospective cohort study. J Neurooncol. 2020;146:97–109.
10. Wu AS, Witgert ME, Lang FF, Xiao L, Bekele BN, Meyers CA, Ferson D, Wefel JS. Neurocognitive function before and after surgery for insular gliomas. J Neurosurg. 2011;115:1115–25.
11. Yoshii Y, Tominaga D, Sugimoto K, Tsuchida Y, Hyodo A, Yonaha H, Kushi S. Cognitive function of patients with brain tumor in pre-and postoperative stage. Surg Neurol. 2008;69:51–61.
12. Desmurget M, Bonnetblanc F, Duffau H. Contrasting acute and slow-growing lesions: a new door to brain plasticity. Brain. 2007;130:898–914. https://doi.org/10.1093/brain/awl300.
13. Duffau H, Capelle L, Denvil D, Sichez N, Gatignol P, Lopes M, Mitchell MC, Sichez JP, Van Effenterre R. Functional recovery after surgical resection of low grade gliomas in eloquent brain: hypothesis of brain compensation. J Neurol Neurosurg Psychiatry. 2003;74: 901–7.
14. Lafargue G, Duffau H. Awareness of intending to act following parietal cortex resection. Neuropsychologia. 2008;46:2662–7.
15. Plaza M, Gatignol P, Leroy M, Duffau H. Speaking without Broca's area after tumor resection. Neurocase. 2009;15:294–310.
16. Duffau H. The "frontal syndrome" revisited: lessons from electrostimulation mapping studies. Cortex. 2012;48:120–31.
17. Lemaitre A-L, Herbet G, Duffau H, Lafargue G. Preserved metacognitive ability despite unilateral or bilateral anterior prefrontal resection. Brain Cogn. 2018a;120:48–57. https://doi.org/10.1016/j.bandc.2017.10.004.
18. Plaza M, du Boullay V, Perrault A, Chaby L, Capelle L. A case of bilateral frontal tumors without "frontal syndrome". Neurocase. 2014;20:671–83. https://doi.org/10.1080/13554794.2013.826696.
19. Costa PT Jr, McCrae RR. Four ways five factors are basic. Personal Individ Differ. 1992;13:653–65.
20. Costa PT, McCrae RR, Kay GG. Persons, places, and personality: career assessment using the revised NEO personality inventory. J Career Assess. 1995;3:123–39. https://doi.org/10.1177/106907279500300202.
21. Allport GW. Personality and character. Psychol Bull. 1921;18:441–55. https://doi.org/10.1037/h0066265.
22. Kantor JR. Human personality and its pathology. J Philos Psychol Sci Methods. 1919;16:236–46. https://doi.org/10.2307/2940404.
23. Watson JB. Psychology: from the standpoint of a behaviorist. Philadelphia: Lippincott; 1919.
24. Weisberg YJ, DeYoung CG, Hirsh JB. Gender differences in personality across the ten aspects of the Big Five. Front Psychol. 2011;2:178.
25. Blair RJ, Cipolotti L. Impaired social response reversal: a case of 'acquired sociopathy'. Brain. 2000;123:1122–41.
26. Eslinger PJ, Damasio AR. Severe disturbance of higher cognition after bilateral frontal lobe ablation patient EVR. Neurology. 1985;35:1731.
27. Harlow JM. Passage of an iron rod through the head. Boston Med Surg J. 1948;39:389–93.
28. Meyers CA, Berman SA, Scheibel RS, Hayman A. Case report: acquired antisocial personality disorder associated with unilateral left orbital frontal lobe damage. J Psychiatry Neurosci. 1992;17:121.
29. Damasio AR, Anderson SW. The frontal lobes. Clin Neuropsychol. 1993;5:417–65.
30. Macmillan M. Phineas Gage: a case for all reasons. In: Classic cases in neuropsychology. 1996. p. 220–38.
31. Macmillan M. Restoring Phineas Gage: a 150th retrospective. J Hist Neurosci. 2000;9:46–66. https://doi.org/10.1076/0964-704X(200004)9:1;1-2;FT046.
32. Ratiu P, Talos I-F, Haker S, Lieberman D, Everett P. The tale of Phineas Gage, digitally remastered. J Neurotrauma. 2004;21:637–43.

33. Thiebaut de Schotten M, Dell'Acqua F, Ratiu P, Leslie A, Howells H, Cabanis E, Iba-Zizen MT, Plaisant O, Simmons A, Dronkers NF, Corkin S, Catani M. From Phineas Gage and Monsieur Leborgne to H.M.: revisiting disconnection syndromes. Cereb Cortex. 2015;25:4812–27. https://doi.org/10.1093/cercor/bhv173.
34. Van Horn JD, Irimia A, Torgerson CM, Chambers MC, Kikinis R, Toga AW. Mapping connectivity damage in the case of Phineas Gage. PLoS One. 2012;7:e37454.
35. Prigatano GP. Personality disturbances associated with traumatic brain injury. J Consult Clin Psychol. 1992;60:360.
36. Williams C, Wood RL, Howe H. Alexithymia is associated with aggressive tendencies following traumatic brain injury. Brain Inj. 2019;33:69–77.
37. Yeates GN, Gracey F, Mcgrath JC. A biopsychosocial deconstruction of "personality change" following acquired brain injury. Neuropsychol Rehabil. 2008;18:566–89.
38. Johnson J. A dark history: memories of lobotomy in the new era of psychosurgery. Med Stud. 2009;1:367–78.
39. Freeman W, Watts JW, Hunt TC. Psychosurgery: intelligence, emotion, and social behavior following prefrontal lobotomy for mental disorders. Arch Intern Med (Chic). 1942;70(1):179.
40. Bramwell B. Intracranial tumours. Edinburgh: Pentland; 1888.
41. Minski L. The mental symptoms associated with 58 cases of cerebral tumour. J Neurol Psychopathol. 1933;13:330.
42. Madhusoodanan S, Danan D, Brenner R, Bogunovic O. Brain tumor and psychiatric manifestations: a case report and brief review. Ann Clin Psychiatry. 2004;16:111–3.
43. Uribe VM. Psychiatric symptoms and brain tumor. Am Fam Physician. 1986;34:95–8.
44. Madhusoodanan S, Opler MG, Moise D, Gordon J, Danan DM, Sinha A, Babu RP. Brain tumor location and psychiatric symptoms: is there any association? A meta-analysis of published case studies. Expert Rev Neurother. 2010;10:1529–36.
45. Jenkins LM, Drummond KJ, Andrewes DG. Emotional and personality changes following brain tumour resection. J Clin Neurosci. 2016;29:128–32.
46. Benros ME, Laursen TM, Dalton SO, Mortensen PB. Psychiatric disorder as a first manifestation of cancer: a 10-year population-based study. Int J Cancer. 2009;124:2917–22.
47. Bunevicius A, Deltuva VP, Deltuviene D, Tamasauskas A, Bunevicius R. Brain lesions manifesting as psychiatric disorders: eight cases. CNS Spectr. 2008;13:950–8.
48. Campanella F, Fabbro F, Ius T, Shallice T, Skrap M. Acute effects of surgery on emotion and personality of brain tumor patients: surgery impact, histological aspects, and recovery. Neuro Oncol. 2015;17:1121–31. https://doi.org/10.1093/neuonc/nov065.
49. Campanella F, Shallice T, Ius T, Fabbro F, Skrap M. Impact of brain tumour location on emotion and personality: a voxel-based lesion–symptom mapping study on mentalization processes. Brain. 2014;137:2532–45.
50. Urgesi C, Aglioti SM, Skrap M, Fabbro F. The spiritual brain: selective cortical lesions modulate human self-transcendence. Neuron. 2010;65:309–19.
51. Cloninger CR, Svrakic DM, Przybeck TR. A psychobiological model of temperament and character. Arch Gen Psychiatry. 1993;50:975–90.
52. Garcia-Romeu A. Self-transcendence as a measurable transpersonal construct. J Transpers Psychol. 2010;42:26.
53. Levenson MR, Jennings PA, Aldwin CM, Shiraishi RW. Self-transcendence: conceptualization and measurement. Int J Aging Hum Dev. 2005;60:127–43.
54. Cloninger CR. Temperament and personality. Curr Opin Neurobiol. 1994;4:266–73.
55. Cloninger CR, Przybeck TR, Svrakic DM, Wetzel RD. The temperament and character inventory (TCI): A guide to its development and use. St-Louis, MO: Washington University. 1994.
56. King ML, Manzel K, Bruss J, Tranel D. Neural correlates of improvements in personality and behavior following a neurological event. Neuropsychologia. 2020;145:106579.
57. Liao W, Chen H, Feng Y, Mantini D, Gentili C, Pan Z, Ding J, Duan X, Qiu C, Lui S. Selective aberrant functional connectivity of resting state networks in social anxiety disorder. Neuroimage. 2010;52:1549–58.

58. Sheline YI, Price JL, Yan Z, Mintun MA. Resting-state functional MRI in depression unmasks increased connectivity between networks via the dorsal nexus. Proc Natl Acad Sci. 2010;107:11020–5.
59. Markett S, Weber B, Voigt G, Montag C, Felten A, Elger C, Reuter M. Intrinsic connectivity networks and personality: the temperament dimension harm avoidance moderates functional connectivity in the resting brain. Neuroscience. 2013;240:98–105.
60. Lemaitre A-L, Lafargue G, Duffau H, Herbet G. Damage to the left uncinate fasciculus is associated with heightened schizotypal traits: a multimodal lesion-mapping study. Schizophr Res. 2018b;197:240–8. https://doi.org/10.1016/j.schres.2018.02.027.
61. Adelstein JS, Shehzad Z, Mennes M, DeYoung CG, Zuo X-N, Kelly C, Margulies DS, Bloomfield A, Gray JR, Castellanos FX. Personality is reflected in the brain's intrinsic functional architecture. PLoS One. 2011;6:e27633.
62. Mandonnet E, Herbet G, Duffau H. Letter: Introducing new tasks for intraoperative mapping in awake glioma surgery: clearing the line between patient care and scientific research. Neurosurgery. 2020;86(2):E256–57.
63. Spielberger CD. Manual for the State-Trait Anxiety Inventory: STAI (Form Y). Palo Alto, CA: Consulting Psychologists Press. 1983.
64. Baron-Cohen S, Wheelwright S. The empathy quotient: an investigation of adults with Asperger syndrome or high functioning autism, and normal sex differences. J Autism Dev Disord. 2004;34:163–75.
65. Sockeel P, Dujardin K, Devos D, Deneve C, Destée A, Defebvre L. The Lille apathy rating scale (LARS), a new instrument for detecting and quantifying apathy: validation in Parkinson's disease. J Neurol Neurosurg Psychiatry. 2006;77:579–84.
66. Cummings JL, Mega M, Gray K, Rosenberg-Thompson S, Carusi DA, Gornbein J. The Neuropsychiatric Inventory: comprehensive assessment of psychopathology in dementia. Neurology. 1994;44:2308.
67. Godefroy O, Azouvi P, Robert P, Roussel M, LeGall D, Meulemans T, Behalf of the Groupe de Réflexion sur l'Evaluation des Fonctions Exécutives Study Group. Dysexecutive syndrome: diagnostic criteria and validation study. Ann Neurol. 2010;68:855–64. https://doi.org/10.1002/ana.22117.
68. Beck AT, Ward C, Mendelson M, Mock J, Erbaugh J. Beck depression inventory (BDI). Arch Gen Psychiatry. 1961;4:561–71.
69. Montgomery S, Åsberg M. A new depression scale designed to be sensitive to change. Acad. Department of Psychiatry, Guy's Hospital. 1977.
70. Freud S. New introductory lectures on psycho-analysis. In new introductory lectures on psycho-analysis and other works. The standard edition of the complete psychological works of sigmund freud, Hogarth Press, London. 1933;22.
71. Lemaitre AL, Herbet G, Duffau H, Lafargue G. Personality and behavioral changes after brain tumor resection: a lesion mapping study. Acta Neurochir. 2021;163(5):1257–67.

Patients with Barriers of Communication 22

Sandro M. Krieg, Sebastian Ille, and Matthieu Delion

22.1 Introduction

While awake surgery is more or less straightforward in regular LGG patients, specific language limitations—due to the functional impact of the tumor or to patients' characteristics like young age or language barrier—can make awake surgery and mapping considerably more challenging or even impossible. While in pediatric patients their general compliance and their global capability to perform the tasks (for example, regarding reading abilities) might require an adaption of the approach, adult patients can show completely different challenging situations. These can be marginally aphasic patients due to fast-growing or recurrent tumors, language barrier, deaf or mute people, and patients with severe myopia.

22.2 Pediatric Patients

Childhood brain cancer is an area still in need of advances. Currently, central nervous system tumors are the second most common childhood malignancy and the first cause of cancer-related death in childhood. The mean annual incidence rate is 39 per million according to the French National Registry of Childhood Solid Tumor [1]. Among these, only 30–40% are supratentorial, 40% of which are situated on the midline. Furthermore, supratentorial tumors are more frequent in the two first years of life. This low incidence of supratentorial tumors in children probably makes the

S. M. Krieg · S. Ille
Department of Neurosurgery, Klinikum rechts der Isar, Technische Universität München School of Medicine, Munich, Germany
e-mail: Sandro.Krieg@tum.de

M. Delion (✉)
Department of Neurosurgery, University Hospital of Angers, Angers Cedex, France
e-mail: Matthieu.Delion@chu-angers.fr

E. Mandonnet, G. Herbet (eds.), *Intraoperative Mapping of Cognitive Networks*,
https://doi.org/10.1007/978-3-030-75071-8_22

validation of any surgical technique in pediatric patients very challenging. However, it has been clearly demonstrated that the child's survival increases with the quality of the tumor resection. Therefore, given the vicinity of eloquent areas in a non-negligible number of supratentorial cases, awake craniotomy in these children could provide the best chances to obtain a gross total resection while preserving their functional status [2, 3]. One of the other reasons that explains the lack of validation of this method in children is the "famous" notion of brain plasticity. It could be that this "overvalued" brain plasticity of child might have limited the development of the technique. Until recently it was admitted by most neurosurgeons that a child can recover from a neurological deficit much more easily than an adult. But many recent publications demonstrated that brain tumor surgery in childhood might impact negatively the functional outcome. Even if children probably recover more easily than adults from a motor point of view, the neuropsychological side effect of surgery is difficult to avoid, causing real neurocognitive deficits [4–7]. According to the literature, it appears that young children can relocate language to the opposite hemisphere, but only during the first 5 years of life [8]. After 5 years, the reality is that the brain plasticity is not so different from the one observed in adults. On that basis, every resection-induced neurologic/cognitive impairment could become a long-lasting neurologic/cognitive sequelae. Hence, the respect of eloquent areas by awake craniotomy and cortico-subcortical mapping seems essential from the age of 5.

In our experience, as in the literature, awake surgery is feasible in children aged from 8 to 18 years old [2, 3, 9–12]. However, this procedure in children raises certain questions concerning ethics, psychological experience, brain plasticity, cortical language area organization, and intraoperative direct cortical stimulation in maturating brains.

We will review how the standard methodology of awake craniotomy in adults needs to be adapted in children, given the specificities encountered in this population.

22.2.1 Patient Selection and Preparation

Concerning patient selection, awake surgery is suitable for children suffering from brain lesions (tumors or cavernomas essentially) located in eloquent areas. A particular attention on the psychological evaluation and conditioning is necessary for these patients. In this way, every method expected to improve the psychological experience of this surgery should be applied.

At first, we suggest a psychiatric evaluation for each young patient before (and after) surgery. A psychiatric diagnosis based on DSM 4 or DSM 5 is carried out if necessary and eventually any contraindication to awake surgery identified. To date, the pediatric psychiatrist did not contraindicate any child for this procedure in our cohort. In our experience, as in the literature, the psychological experience of this surgery was good for each patient [11, 13].

Wherever possible we organize a meeting between the patient and his family and another child who had been operated on by awake craniotomy, in order to explain his psychological experience. We show the young patient and his family some pictures and a video describing the atmosphere of the operating theater and we offer the possibility to the child and his family to visit it and meet the surgical and anesthetic team before the surgery, allowing the child to get acquainted with the atmosphere.

We use hypnosis to improve the cooperation and the feelings of the children during anesthetic induction, intraoperative awakening, and periods without stimulation. The hypnosis conditioning is performed by the anesthetic team. The patient must be evaluated in hypnosis clinics 1–3 weeks before surgery by the same trained team to establish a confident relationship. The purpose of this meeting with the hypnotist is to collect some themes about pleasant places and pleasant sensations including visual, hearing, kinesthesia, smell, and taste. Above the analgesic effect, the aim of this management is to recreate during the induction and during the awakening a relaxing environment. In our experience this approach allows an induction and an awakening in very calm conditions. Hypnosis is also of major interest for the intraoperative periods without stimulation, like periods of tumor resection during which the cooperation of the child is not necessary, in creating a spatio-temporal distortion based on the pre-defined themes identified from the preoperative session. In focusing the attention of the child on pleasing situations, the psychological experience and the course of the operation are facilitated. Even in an emergency situation for a patient suffering from increased intracranial pressure, hypnosis proved to be a useful adjunct. This patient was examined by the hypnotist just before the surgery and was also sensitive to hypnosis during the anesthetic induction and the woken period, as well as the others. One of the best examples of the efficiency of hypnosis was seen in a 12-year-old girl. She had a very anxious personality and the psychiatrist's assessment suggested slight depression. Thanks to hypnosis, we obtained good cooperation and the atmosphere was very relaxed.

Concerning the analgesic effect, obviously, hypnosis is not sufficient. As a good cooperation and psychological experience require a total absence of pain, we add intravenous analgesic drugs. This is also achieved by the use of an efficient local anesthesia with nerve blocks of the entire scalp.

We recommend a functional MRI for children in the preoperative planning. The functional MRI in our experience contributes to shorten the duration of the intraoperative neuropsychological monitoring, by directly targeting the eloquent areas to be stimulated. However, care must be taken: the functional MRI does not replace the electrical cortical mapping and certainly not the subcortical mapping.

22.2.2 Test Selection and Limitations

A child language therapist evaluates the performances of each child before, during, and 3–6 months after the surgery. The pre- and postoperative evaluation is based on the BDAE (Boston Diagnosis Aphasia Examination) [14]. The intraoperative evaluation is based on the "object naming task" described in Ojemann's work on adults and children, corresponding to black line drawings of objects together with the carrier phrase "this is..." on a white slide [15, 16]. We use a French equivalent test based on the DO 80 [17]. There is ample evidence in the literature that this test is well suited for children older than 8 [2, 3, 9–12]. There is no data in the literature about child younger than 8. Between 5 and 8 years old, notably for a child who is not able to read, we can probably use the object naming task without the carrier phrase "this is" or we can directly present some real objects to the child, as described in extra-operative mapping for epilepsy surgery.

There are some data in the literature suggesting that maturating brain would require higher current intensities of stimulation, with a risk to exceed the after discharge threshold [18]. In our experience, we observed relevant cortical and subcortical mapping with involuntary stimulation-induced movement and stimulation-induced errors in naming, in all cases, whatever the level of brain maturation. This result could even be reproduced under general anesthesia for motor stimulation down to the age of 3. Whenever possible, the stimulation threshold should be determined on involuntary movements obtained by stimulating motor areas. The intensity used to obtain such cortical positive responses was not significantly different from the intensity used in adults. In the same way, even if differences in white matter myelination between pediatric and adult patients exist, it is not necessary in practice to increase stimulation intensities when stimulating subcortically.

According to Duchowny, the template of language organization is very similar in children and adults [8], but for Ojemann [16] and Berger [19]—as in adult patients—there is an important variability in language cortex localization among children. In practice, this cortical interindividual variability pleads for the use of language brain mapping in children.

22.2.3 Practical Aspects During Surgery

22.2.3.1 Anesthetic Technique

The children are put asleep by hypnosis in addition to intravenous remifentanil and propofol. The anesthetic team uses an adequately sized laryngeal airway mask. Indeed, in the literature, the use of laryngeal mask airway appeared extremely useful in the pediatric population undergoing awake craniotomy [1, 20]. The scalp incision, pin sites of the Mayfield head holder, scalp nerves, and dura are infiltrated with diluted 0.2% ropivacaine. The local nervous anesthetic block is done on the supratrochlear, auriculotemporal, retro auricular, and occipital nerve. They are woken and extubated after the completion of the bone flap and before opening the dura. After the tumor resection, in our experience, the patients are kept under conscious sedation until the end of the surgery. Some authors use the asleep-awake-asleep anesthetic technique [9].

22.2.3.2 Surgical Technique

The surgical technique is very similar to the adult. Patients are positioned in the supine or lateral position according to the location of the tumor. The skin incision, the bone flap, and the infiltration of the dura are done under general anesthesia. MR intraoperative neuronavigation based on preoperative images is used to assist in locating the brain lesion and to facilitate the gross total removal of the lesion.

After the awakening and the extubation of the child, and once he is able to clearly communicate with the neuropsychologist, we open the dura and start the electrical cortical mapping. For each patient we make a large bone flap with a large cortical exposure including, if possible, a motor area to clearly determine the stimulation threshold, which is defined by the lowest intensity producing a movement. This threshold is usually obtained around 3 mA and rarely above. In practice, a bipolar electrode delivering a biphasic current is applied to the cortex before the resection, starting with a 1 mA intensity and increasing with individual steps between 0.25 and 0.5 mA at a time. On a motor eloquent site, this electrical stimulation can induce an involuntary motor response. For the sites involved in language function, an object naming task is presented to the woken child during each stimulation, as described in the adult surgery [15]. We look for transient language disturbances (anomia, paraphasia, naming delay…). A speech therapist is present to interpret the exact kind of language impairments evoked. During surgical removal of a tumor, subcortical stimulation is also used to identify the white matter connections involved in language or motor activities. Subcortical stimulation is continuously alternated with ultrasonic aspiration in a back-and-forth fashion, as already described by some authors [21]. Additional tasks such as arithmetic processing, visuospatial functions, judgment, and others are applied, depending on the tumors' location and the patients' ability to complete the tasks [22–25].

22.2.4 Illustrative Case (Fig. 22.1)

We present the difficult situation of a right-handed 11-year-old boy suffering from a brain tumor of the left temporal lobe (Fig. 22.1a–c). This young man was already followed in our hospital for a medulloblastoma of the fourth ventricle treated 7 years before by chemotherapy and radiotherapy. We observed this infiltrative tumor on a control MRI without any change in its clinical presentation. He was at an adapted school for children with cognitive difficulties. His neuropsychological preoperative evaluation revealed a global lag of the cognitive abilities, essentially due to the first pathology, with notably visuoconstructive dyspraxia. The language examination revealed sometimes semantic paraphasias, anomia, and naming delay but the object naming task was perfectly realized for the majority of items. He presented also some behavioral disorders with restlessness crisis. Despite the uncertainty of cooperation of this child, we performed an awake surgery after an appropriate preparation of the child. The cooperation was good but for a short duration. We also decided to use for this surgery only object naming task and word repetition task according to the location of the tumor. We achieved a complete resection of the tumor without additional persisting alteration of his language abilities (Fig. 22.1d–f). The diagnosis was an anaplastic astrocytoma IDH wild type, probably induced by the radiation therapy. The young boy returned to school 3 months after the surgery.

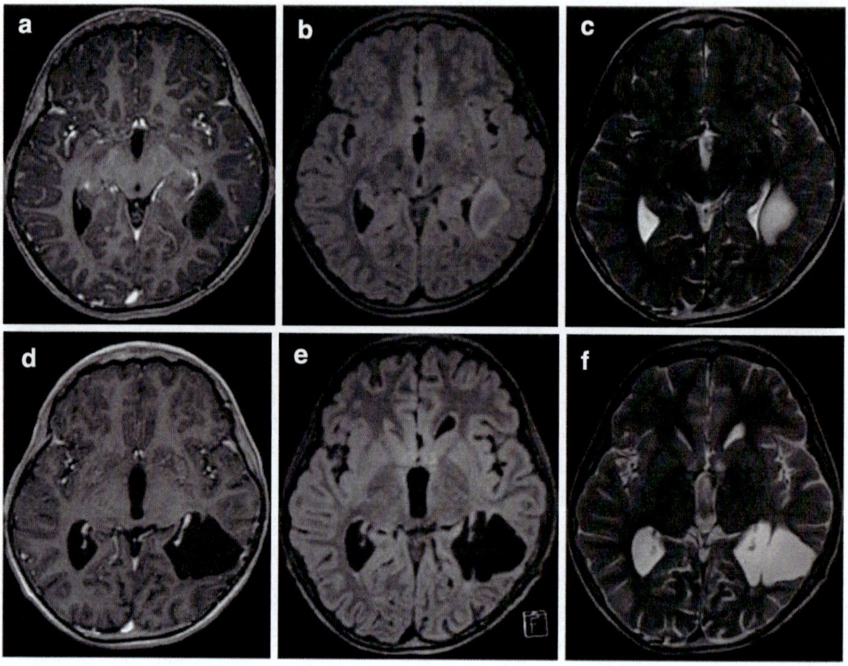

Fig. 22.1 Pediatric illustrative case. (**a–c**) Preoperative MRI scans showing an infiltrative left temporal anaplastic astrocytoma in an 11-year-old boy. (**d–f**) Postoperative MRI scans (2 months postoperative), showing the resection of the tumor

22.3 Adult Patients

22.3.1 Marginally Aphasic Patients

22.3.1.1 Patient Selection

Concerning patients with severe aphasia, pre- but also intraoperative testing might be nearly impossible in some cases. Moreover, data from studies which might help us to select our patients properly is missing. The only proper analysis tackling a number of issues is provided by a study of preoperative lesion-inducing mapping by navigated transcranial magnetic stimulation (nTMS). In this study the authors showed that the reliability of identifying language-involved cortical areas is severely impaired by aphasic symptoms [26]. In this large series, an object naming task was used and it was shown that an error rate of 28% for the baseline picture set could be regarded as a cutoff for reliable testing. From clinical experience, this value is quite comprehensible. For other testing than object naming, any of such data is missing. Yet, one series describes 55% of enrolled patients having a mild to severe aphasia while awake language testing was still feasible [27].

Moreover, it has been claimed that gross total resection of recurrent tumors might improve patients' survival [28]. Patients eligible for a redo surgery in this context commonly exhibit some degree of aphasia. Surgeons performing awake mapping need to accept that we have to deal also with such patients in whom reliability of testing is suboptimal, and not only with perfectly speaking, cognitively highly performing young patients.

22.3.1.2 Test Selection and Limitations

Marginally aphasic patients usually suffer from structural disconnection of white matter pathways of the language network. Keeping this in mind is crucial to properly understand the pathophysiological basis of their aphasia and how to properly select our test battery. In particular, the frequently used object-naming task can be impaired due to subcortical progressive disease [29]. Moreover, reduced language ability commonly comes along with severe cognitive disability due to subcortical impairment as a shared origin [30]. This also means that the selected tasks not only need to consider subcortical damage but also need to be easier than we are used to.

In particular, behavioral paradigms including assessment of semantic cognition or decision-making which can usually be very effective to identify language regions in non-aphasic patients can be challenging or even impossible in aphasic patients.

Several articles excellently provided an overview on currently used language tasks and their content does not need to be repeated here [31, 32]. However, when planning awake mapping in patients with borderline language function, the following needs to be considered, besides our usual standards when choosing the tasks:

- Consider subcortical damage and severe tract involvement
- Choose easier tasks
- Allow more time per item

22.3.1.3 Practical Aspects During Surgery

First, it is crucial to potentially optimize the patients' language abilities for surgery. Prior to surgery, this can be single or double dose of i.v. steroids in order to reduce white-matter compromising edema. Yet, despite this positive effect, we should not administer long-term steroids due to its proven negative effects in glioma patients [33, 34].

During surgery, this subgroup of patients shows much more language errors during testing than we are used to. Due to a natural rate of errors, it can be quite difficult to differentiate between real mapping-induced errors and background noise. First, removing from the intraoperative set all items misnamed at preoperative evaluation helps to reduce the baseline error rate during intraoperative mapping. Second, performing more trials per stimulation site is another way to improve reliability. Yet, surgeons have to admit that mapping results can still be less reliable in these patients, as compared to patients without tumor-induced deficits. Finally, it is crucial to tailor tasks and surgery in order to reduce as much as possible the total time of awake monitoring. As mentioned, those patients usually also suffer from additional cognitive impairment with reduced attention, and performances are declining with the awake time [35].

22.3.1.4 Illustrative Case (Fig. 22.2)

A 61-year-old male patient presented at our outpatient-clinic after non-conclusive stereotactic biopsy of a fast-growing left-hemispheric mass lesion at an external department. In suspicion of a contrast-enhancing, positron-emission-tomography-positive high-grade glioma, the neurooncological board decided for the resection of the mass lesion (Fig. 22.2a–d). However, preoperative language testing showed a severe tumor-induced combined aphasia (Aachener Aphasia Test grade 2AB) including a preoperative object naming score of 8 out of 80. After the application of a bolus of 40 mg dexamethasone, object naming was acceptable and fluent speaking especially improved; hence, we decided to perform an awake craniotomy.

Intraoperatively, the patient showed an adequate awakening and was able to perform a reduced version of simple object naming as defined preoperatively and particularly a continuous cortical and subcortical monitoring of language function under fluent conversation with our speech therapist. After initial resection based on the awake mapping and monitoring of language function, the patient was anesthetized and we performed an intraoperative MRI scan showing a cortical tumor residual (Fig. 22.2e). Due to the reliability of the adapted awake language mapping, we additionally resected the cortical tumor residual. The early postoperative MRI scan 1 day after resection showed a GTR (Fig. 22.2f).

Clinically, the patient showed a postoperative improvement of language function (Aachener Aphasia Test grade 1B), in keeping with the resection of the mass lesion and edema reduction. Histopathology showed a glioblastoma WHO grade IV (IDH wild type, no MGMT methylation). The neurooncological board decided for a combined adjuvant therapy, including radiation and chemotherapy with temozolomide. Late postoperative MRIs 1 month (Fig. 22.2g) and 3 months (Fig. 22.2h) still showed no tumor recurrence. Most importantly, the patient's language function was still only slightly impaired (Aachener Aphasia Test grade 1B), making daily communication feasible, and his quality of life was high with a Karnofsky Performance Scale of 90%.

22.3.2 Language Barriers

22.3.2.1 Patient Selection

Apart from medical tourism, we nowadays have an increasing number of patients who do not share any language with the surgical or neuropsychological team. In order to monitor patients' language function in their mother tongue, an interpreter is needed at each step of the process, rendering the whole procedure even more challenging.

22.3.2.2 Test Selection and Limitations

First, it is essential to find an interpreter who is able to do the job in the environment of an operating room (OR). The best solution is to make the interpreter and speech therapist (or neuropsychologist) work together hand in hand. If not possible, then the tests need to fulfill the following criteria:

- Execution is possible by a layperson in terms of neuropsychological testing.
- The resulting functional impairment can be detected by an untrained person.

Relying on videos showing language mapping and the induced errors can be very helpful to train the interpreter.

22.3.2.3 Practical Aspects During Surgery

The environment of an OR is not only new for the patients but can also be new for the interpreter. It is therefore helpful to get the interpreter used to the OR by attending another operation some days earlier.

In general, the feasibility of operating patients awake despite severe language barriers was shown in three recent articles [36–38]. Overall, these studies showed that the interpreter-mediated feedback implies a lower rate of gross total resection, longer duration of surgery, and unexpected tumor residuals. However, there was no difference concerning permanent surgery-related language deterioration.

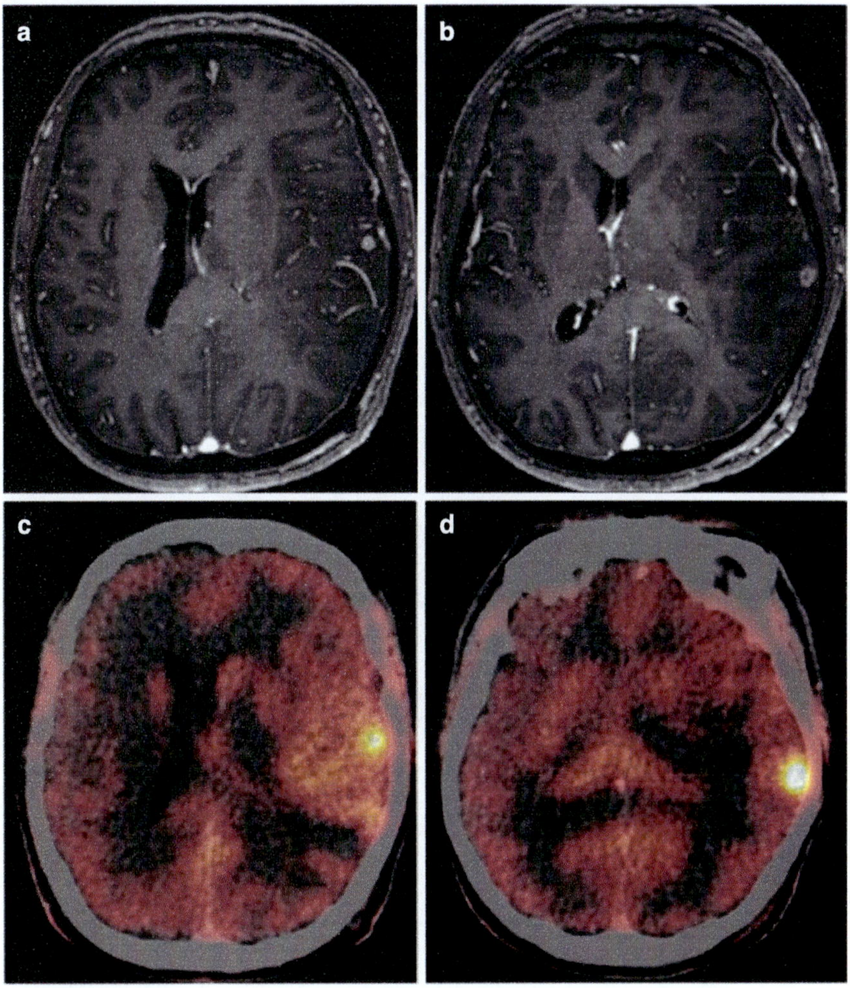

Fig. 22.2 Aphasic illustrative case. (**a**, **b**) Preoperative T1-MRI with gadolinium, showing a contrast-enhancing left temporal glioblastoma, in a 61-year-old patient. (**c**, **d**) Focus of positron-emission-tomography-positive. (**e**) Cortical residual tumor evidenced by the intraoperative MRI. (**f**) T1-MRI with gadolinium at postoperative day 1, demonstrating a gross total resection. (**g**) T1-MRI with gadolinium at 1 month postop. (**h**) T1-MRI with gadolinium at 3 months postop

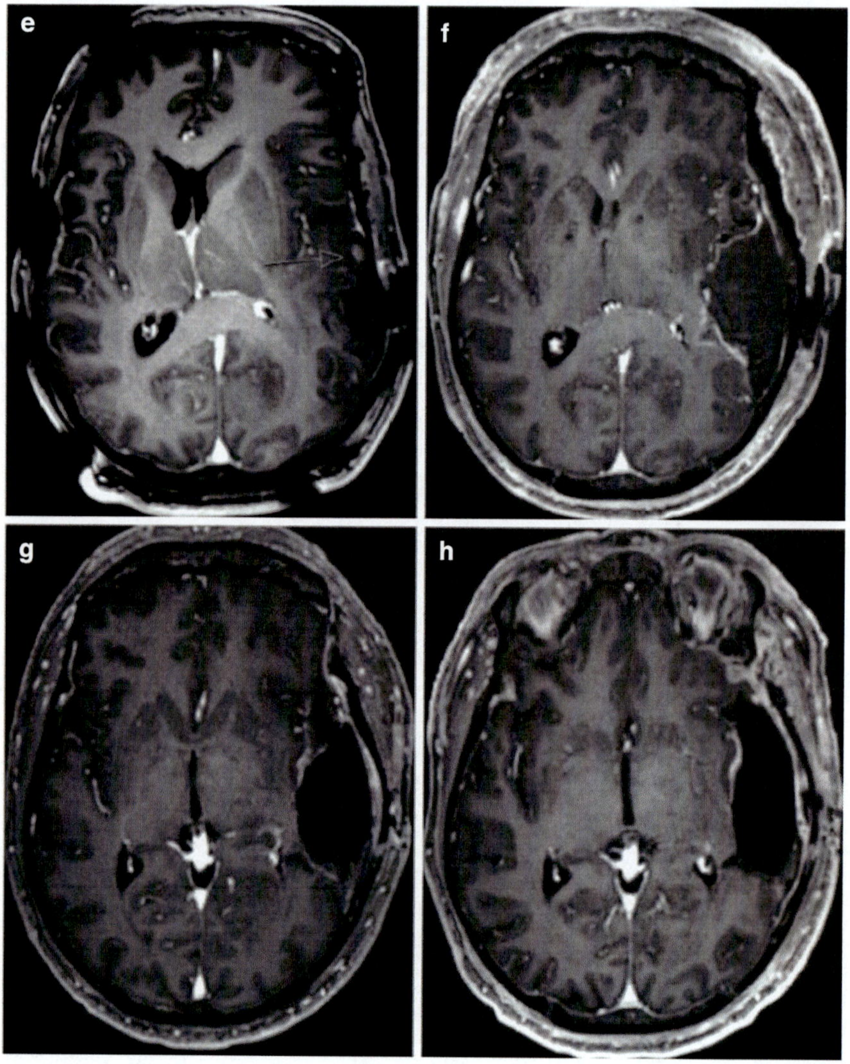

Fig. 22.2 (continued)

22.3.3 Deaf and Mute Patients

22.3.3.1 Patient Selection

Although literature is especially rare, awake surgery was proven to be feasible in deaf and mute people [39–41]. There is a huge number of articles investigating language perception and sign language conceptualization and their cortical representation. Irrespective from early deafness or postlinguistic deafness, cerebral reorganization seems to take place and conventional principles of language organization do not seem to apply anymore [42–44]. Thus, awake mapping of sign language communication in deaf and mute patients is mandatory when considering resective surgery. Particularly supplementary motor area but also other parts involved in sign language need to be preserved by all means [45–47].

Even within Broca's area and the supramarginal gyrus, direct electrical stimulation caused sign errors, indicating the importance of Broca's area even in mute patients [48].

22.3.3.2 Test Selection and Limitations

Theoretically, all tests from the current armamentarium can be adapted to patients communicating by signs or sign language [31, 32]. Published reports especially used object naming, text reading, and sign repetition tasks [39, 41].

22.3.3.3 Practical Aspects During Surgery

Since sign language is the only possibility of these patients to efficiently communicate with their environment, it is of even more importance to preserve their ability to communicate. A pattern of their language network is not as well established as it is for oral language; this fact requires consideration when it comes to indication, surgical planning, awake mapping, and resection itself [45].

Most importantly, this needs to be taken into account when resecting not only potentially language but also motor eloquent tumors [40].

Since deaf and mute patients also require an interpreter, all recommendations given in the paragraph above also adhere to this subgroup of patients.

22.3.4 Severe Myopia

22.3.4.1 Patient Selection

Severe myopia can be a challenge since glasses can be difficult to wear during awake surgery and myopia can interfere severely with most neuropsychological testing. Despite thorough literature search, no article was found on this issue; the authors therefore solely report on their own experience.

22.3.4.2 Test Selection and Limitations

Since myopia can interfere severely with most neuropsychological tests, it should be tried to put an emphasis on non-visual testing. Yet, as occipital projections are of major intraoperative relevance in many cases, this is only applicable in selected cases.

22.3.4.3 Practical Aspects During Surgery

There are four options in such patients, which need to be chosen depending on each particular case:

1. Increasing the screen size on which the tests are shown
2. Modifying the patients' glasses, e.g., by removing one temple or by providing suitable lenses via the ophthalmology department
3. Tailoring the test with some emphasis on non-visual tests if applicable.
4. Using contact lenses. This option, however, harbors some risk of dislocation of the contacts during the asleep phase and should preferably not be considered.

22.4 Conclusion

Performing awake surgery on patients with impaired communication abilities has to be thought thoroughly and requires an extra portion of patience, and experience, both in awake surgery and in neuropsychological testing. Concerning children, a particular attention on the psychological evaluation and conditioning is necessary for performing awake craniotomy. Only then, awake surgery and mapping may provide a benefit to the patient compared to asleep resection based on non-invasive mapping techniques.

References

1. Desandes E, Guissou S, Chastagner P, Lacour B. Incidence and survival of children with central nervous system primitive tumors in the French national registry of childhood solid tumors. Neuro-Oncol. 2014;16(7):975–83. https://doi.org/10.1093/neuonc/not309.
2. Balogun JA, Khan OH, Taylor M, Dirks P, Der T, Carter Snead Iii O, et al. Pediatric awake craniotomy and intra-operative stimulation mapping. J Clin Neurosci. 2014;21(11):1891–4. https://doi.org/10.1016/j.jocn.2014.07.013.
3. Lohkamp LN, Beuriat PA, Desmurget M, Cristofori I, Szathmari A, Huguet L, et al. Awake brain surgery in children-a single-center experience. Childs Nerv Syst. 2020;36(5):967–74. https://doi.org/10.1007/s00381-020-04522-9.
4. Grill J, Viguier D, Kieffer V, Bulteau C, Sainte-Rose C, Hartmann O, Kalifa C, Dellatolas G. Critical risk factors for intellectual impairment in children with posterior fossa tumors: the role of cerebellar damage. J Neurosurg. 2004;101(2 suppl):152–8. https://doi.org/10.3171/ped.2004.101.2.0152.
5. Konczak J, Schoch B, Dimitrova A, Gizewski E, Timmann D. Functional recovery of children and adolescents after cerebellar tumour resection. Brain JNeurol. 2005;128(Pt 6):1428–41. https://doi.org/10.1093/brain/awh385.
6. Nazemi KJ, Butler RW. Neuropsychological rehabilitation for survivors of childhood and adolescent brain tumors: a view of the past and a vision for a promising future. J Pediatr Rehabil Med. 2011;4(1):37–46. https://doi.org/10.3233/PRM-2011-0151.
7. Vago C, Bulgheroni S, Usilla A, Biassoni V, Serra A, Gentile S, Ajovalasit D, Leonardi M, Massimino M, Fidani P, Riva D. Adaptive functioning in children in the first six months after surgery for brain tumours. Disabil Rehabil. 2011;33(11):953–60. https://doi.org/10.3109/09638288.2010.520804.
8. Duchowny M, Jayakar P, Harvey AS, Resnick T, Alvarez L, Dean P, Levin B. Language cortex representation: effects of developmental versus acquired pathology. Ann Neurol. 1996;40(1):31–8. https://doi.org/10.1002/ana.410400108.
9. Alcaraz García-Tejedor G, Echániz G, Strantzas S, Jalloh I, Rutka J, Drake J, Der T. Feasibility of awake craniotomy in the pediatric population. Paediatr Anaesth. 2020;30(4):480–9. https://doi.org/10.1111/pan.13833. Epub 2020 Feb 13. PMID: 31997512.
10. Delion M, Terminassian A, Lehousse T, Aubin G, Malka J, N'Guyen S, Mercier P, Menei P. Specificities of Awake Craniotomy and Brain Mapping in children for resection of supratentorial tumors in the language area. World Neurosurgery. 2015;84(6):1645–52.
11. Riquin E, Dinomais M, Malka J, Lehousse T, Duverger P, Menei P, Delion M. Psychiatric and psychologic impact of surgery while awake in children for resection of brain tumors. World Neurosurg. 2017;
12. Talabaev M, Venegas K, Zabrodets G, Zmachinskaya V, Antonenko A, Naumenko D, Salauyeva H, Churyla N. Result of awake surgery for pediatric eloquent brain area tumors: single-center experience. Childs Nerv Syst. 2020; https://doi.org/10.1007/s00381-020-04666-8.
13. Huguet L, Lohkamp LN, Beuriat PA, Desmurget M, Bapteste L, Szathmari A, Mottolese C, Di Rocco F. Psychological aspects of awake brain surgery in children interests and risks. Childs Nerv Syst. 2020;36(2):273–9. https://doi.org/10.1007/s00381-019-04308-8.

14. Goodglass H, Kaplan E. The assessment of aphasia and related disorders. Lea & Febiger; 1972.
15. Ojemann G, Ojemann J, Lettich E, Berger M. Cortical language localization in left, dominant hemisphere. An electrical stimulation mapping investigation in 117 patients. J Neurosurg. 1989;71(3):316–26. https://doi.org/10.3171/jns.1989.71.3.0316.
16. Ojemann SG, Berger MS, Lettich E, Ojemann GA. Localization of language function in children: results of electrical stimulation mapping. J Neurosurg. 2003;98(3):465–70. https://doi.org/10.3171/jns.2003.98.3.0465.
17. Deloche G, Hannequin D: Test de dénomination orale d'images: DO 80. Éd. duCentre de psychologie appliquée; 1997.
18. Jayakar P, Alvarez LA, Duchowny MS, Resnick TJ. A safe and effective paradigm to functionally map the cortex in childhood. J Clin Neurophysiol Off Publ Am Electroencephalogr Soc. 1992;9(2):288–93.
19. Berger MS, Kincaid J, Ojemann GA, Lettich E. Brain mapping techniques tomaximize resection, safety, and seizure control in children with brain tumors. Neurosurgery. 1989;25(5):786–92.
20. Hagberg CA, Gollas A, Berry JM. The laryngeal mask airway for awake craniotomy in the pediatric patient: report of three cases. J Clin Anesth. 2004;16(1):43–7. https://doi.org/10.1016/j.jclinane.2003.02.011.
21. Bello L, Gallucci M, Fava M, Carrabba G, Giussani C, Acerbi F, Baratta P, Songa V, Conte V, Branca V, Stocchetti N, Papagno C, Gaini SM. Intraoperative subcortical language tract mapping guides surgical removal of gliomas involving speech areas. Neurosurgery. 2007;60(1):67–80. https://doi.org/10.1227/01.NEU.0000249206.58601.DE.
22. Della Puppa A, De Pellegrin S, Rossetto M, Rustemi O, Saladini M, Munari M, Scienza R. Intraoperative functional mapping of calculation in parietal surgery. New insights and clinical implications. Acta Neurochir (Wien). 2015;157(6):971–977; discussion 977. https://doi.org/10.1007/s00701-015-2426-4.
23. Plaza M, Gatignol P, Cohen H, Berger B, Duffau H. A discrete area within the left dorsolateral prefrontal cortex involved in visual-verbal incongruence judgment. Cereb Cortex. 2008;18(6):1253–9. https://doi.org/10.1093/cercor/bhm169.
24. Roux FE, Boukhatem L, Draper L, Sacko O, Démonet JF. Cortical calculation localization using electrostimulation. J Neurosurg. 2009;110(6):1291–9. https://doi.org/10.3171/2008.8.Jns17649.
25. Thiebaut de Schotten M, Urbanski M, Duffau H, Volle E, Lévy R, Dubois B, Bartolomeo P. Direct evidence for a parietal-frontal pathway subserving spatial awareness in humans. Science. 2005;309(5744):2226–8. https://doi.org/10.1126/science.1116251.
26. Schwarzer V, Bahrend I, Rosenstock T, Dreyer FR, Vajkoczy P, Picht T. Aphasia and cognitive impairment decrease the reliability of rnTMS language mapping. Acta Neurochir (Wien). 2018;160(2):343–56. https://doi.org/10.1007/s00701-017-3397-4.
27. Bilotta F, Stazi E, Titi L, Lalli D, Delfini R, Santoro A, Rosa G. Diagnostic work up for language testing in patients undergoing awake craniotomy for brain lesions in language areas. Br J Neurosurg. 2014;28(3):363–7. https://doi.org/10.3109/02688697.2013.854313.
28. Ringel F, Pape H, Sabel M, Krex D, Bock HC, Misch M, et al. Clinical benefit from resection of recurrent glioblastomas: results of a multicenter study including 503 patients with recurrent glioblastomas undergoing surgical resection. Neuro Oncol. 2016;18(1):96–104. https://doi.org/10.1093/neuonc/nov145.
29. Papagno C, Gallucci M, Casarotti A, Castellano A, Falini A, Fava E, et al. Connectivity constraints on cortical reorganization of neural circuits involved in object naming. Neuroimage. 2011;55(3):1306–13. https://doi.org/10.1016/j.neuroimage.2011.01.005.
30. Wall KJ, Cumming TB, Copland DA. Determining the association between language and cognitive tests in poststroke aphasia. Front Neurol. 2017;8:149. https://doi.org/10.3389/fneur.2017.00149.
31. De Witte E, Satoer D, Robert E, Colle H, Verheyen S, Visch-Brink E, Marien P. The Dutch Linguistic Intraoperative Protocol: a valid linguistic approach to awake brain surgery. Brain Lang. 2015;140:35–48. https://doi.org/10.1016/j.bandl.2014.10.011.
32. Rofes A, Spena G, Miozzo A, Fontanella MM, Miceli G. Advantages and disadvantages of intraoperative language tasks in awake surgery: a three-task approach for prefrontal tumors. J Neurosurg Sci. 2015;59(4):337–49. https://www.ncbi.nlm.nih.gov/pubmed/26159550.

33. Hui CY, Rudra S, Ma S, Campian JL, Huang J. Impact of overall corticosteroid exposure during chemoradiotherapy on lymphopenia and survival of glioblastoma patients. J Neurooncol. 2019;143(1):129–36. https://doi.org/10.1007/s11060-019-03146-7.
34. Pitter KL, Tamagno I, Alikhanyan K, Hosni-Ahmed A, Pattwell SS, Donnola S, et al. Corticosteroids compromise survival in glioblastoma. Brain. 2016;139(Pt 5):1458–71. https://doi.org/10.1093/brain/aww046.
35. Meskelevicius D, Schafer A, Weber JK, Hegmann L, Haddad L, Kamp MA, et al. Determination of optimal time window for cortical mapping in awake craniotomy: assessment of intraoperative reaction speed. Neurosurg Rev. 2020;43(2):633–42. https://doi.org/10.1007/s10143-019-01094-4.
36. Aubrun S, Poisson I, Barberis M, Draou C, Toure M, Madadaki C, et al. The challenge of overcoming the language barrier for brain tumor awake surgery in migrants: a feasibility study in five patient cases. Acta Neurochir (Wien). 2020;162(2):389–95. https://doi.org/10.1007/s00701-019-04101-1.
37. Kelm A, Sollmann N, Ille S, Meyer B, Ringel F, Krieg SM. Resection of gliomas with and without neuropsychological support during awake craniotomy-effects on surgery and clinical outcome. Front Oncol. 2017;7:176. https://doi.org/10.3389/fonc.2017.00176.
38. Sellier A, Moritz-Gasser S, Lemaitre AL, Herbet G, Duffau H. Presence of a translator in the operating theater for awake mapping in foreign patients with low-grade glioma: a surgical experience based on 18 different native languages. J Neurosurg. 2020:1–9. https://doi.org/10.3171/2020.6.Jns201071.
39. Chen PA, Chen YC, Wei KC, Chen KT. Awake craniotomy for a left pan-hippocampal diffuse low-grade glioma in a deaf and mute patient using sign language. World Neurosurg. 2020;134:629–634.e1. https://doi.org/10.1016/j.wneu.2019.11.129.
40. Martino J, Velasquez C, Vazquez-Bourgon J, de Lucas EM, Gomez E. Cross-modal recruitment of auditory and orofacial areas during sign language in a deaf subject. World Neurosurg. 2017;105:1033.e1–5. https://doi.org/10.1016/j.wneu.2017.05.170.
41. Metellus P, Boussen S, Guye M, Trebuchon A. Successful insular glioma removal in a deaf signer patient during an awake craniotomy procedure. World Neurosurg. 2017;98:883.e1–5. https://doi.org/10.1016/j.wneu.2016.08.098.
42. Cardon G, Sharma A. Somatosensory cross-modal reorganization in adults with age-related, early-stage hearing loss. Front Hum Neurosci. 2018;12:172. https://doi.org/10.3389/fnhum.2018.00172.
43. Moreno A, Limousin F, Dehaene S, Pallier C. Brain correlates of constituent structure in sign language comprehension. Neuroimage. 2018;167:151–61. https://doi.org/10.1016/j.neuroimage.2017.11.040.
44. Trumpp NM, Kiefer M. Functional reorganization of the conceptual brain system after deafness in early childhood. PLoS One. 2018;13(7):e0198894. https://doi.org/10.1371/journal.pone.0198894.
45. Cardin V, Orfanidou E, Kastner L, Ronnberg J, Woll B, Capek CM, Rudner M. Monitoring different phonological parameters of sign language engages the same cortical language network but distinctive perceptual ones. J Cogn Neurosci. 2016;28(1):20–40. https://doi.org/10.1162/jocn_a_00872.
46. Simon M, Campbell E, Genest F, MacLean MW, Champoux F, Lepore F. The impact of early deafness on brain plasticity: a systematic review of the white and gray matter changes. Front Neurosci. 2020;14:206. https://doi.org/10.3389/fnins.2020.00206.
47. Stroh AL, Rosler F, Dormal G, Salden U, Skotara N, Hanel-Faulhaber B, Roder B. Neural correlates of semantic and syntactic processing in German Sign Language. Neuroimage. 2019;200:231–41. https://doi.org/10.1016/j.neuroimage.2019.06.025.
48. Corina DP, McBurney SL, Dodrill C, Hinshaw K, Brinkley J, Ojemann G. Functional roles of Broca's area and SMG: evidence from cortical stimulation mapping in a deaf signer. Neuroimage. 1999;10(5):570–81. https://doi.org/10.1006/nimg.1999.0499.

Inner Speech Brain Mapping. Is It Possible to Map What We Cannot Observe?

23

Antoni Rodriguez-Fornells, Patricia León-Cabrera,
Andreu Gabarros, and Joanna Sierpowska

A large part of language occurs internally, without overt expression, in most cases as the subjective experience of "that voice in our head"—formally known as inner speech (IS). Forms of inner speech probably range from very vague, fragmented, passive, elliptic realizations or pre-conceptualizations to phonologically encoded or

---

Converso con el hombre que siempre va conmigo
- quien habla solo espera hablar a Dios un día -;
mi soliloquio es plática con ese buen amigo
que me enseñó el secreto de la filantropía.
[I am in conversation with a friend who is always with me.
- Who talks alone can hope someday to talk with the Divine -
All my soliloquy amounts to talk with this companion
Who shared with me the secret key to loving humankind.]
Antonio Machado, "Retratos"

Voices inside my head
Echoes of things that you said
(The Police, Voices inside my head, from Zenyatta Mondatta 1980)

A. Rodriguez-Fornells (✉)
Cognition and Brain Plasticity Unit (CBPU), ICREA and Department of Cognition, Development and Education Psychology and IDIBELL (Campus de Bellvitge), University of Barcelona, Barcelona, Spain
e-mail: antoni.rodriguez@icrea.cat

P. León-Cabrera
Department of Cognition, Development and Educational Psychology, Barcelona, Spain

A. Gabarros
Department of Neurosurgery, University Hospital of Bellvitge, Barcelona, Spain
e-mail: agabarros@bellvitgehospital.cat

J. Sierpowska
Donders Institute for Brain, Cognition and Behaviour and Donders Centre for Medical Neuroscience, Department of Medical Psychology, Radboud University and Radboud University Medical Center, Nijmegen, The Netherlands
e-mail: j.sierpowska@donders.ru.nl

E. Mandonnet, G. Herbet (eds.), *Intraoperative Mapping of Cognitive Networks*,
https://doi.org/10.1007/978-3-030-75071-8_23

subvocalized formats. From simple words to an elaborated soliloquy. Because of its introspective nature, IS has been clearly left behind in the progress of language science. The advancement of new neuroimaging techniques and methodological strategies has facilitated understanding of this complex phenomenon during the last two decades. Considering the importance of IS in our daily life, being central to a variety of higher-level cognitive functions such as language, working memory, thought, and consciousness, it is worth investigating how to best monitor IS during intraoperative electrical stimulation mapping (ESM). ESM can help to avoid lesions that may affect the internal experience of a rich mental life. This chapter aims to provide an understanding of this broad cognitive phenomenon, discuss its possible neural correlates, and suggest several cognitive tasks that could be useful in the future to monitor IS intraoperatively via awake intraoperative electrical stimulation mapping (ESM).

23.1 What Is Inner Speech?

A quite accepted understanding of IS is that proposed by Alderson-Day and Fernyhough [1] who define it as "the subjective experience of language in the absence of overt and audible articulation.". One critical aspect of this definition that may lead to disagreement among researchers is the idea of "subjective experience" which puts a strong emphasis in introspection and first-person experience (see discussion in [2]). One might argue that, in certain situations, inner verbal thoughts might occur or run in our mind without being aware of or attentive to our subjective experience. Indeed, many of us have the introspective experience that, to a certain extent, part of our rich inner life is triggered unconsciously or unwillingly. There is a large amount of mental content that pops into our conscious realm that is experienced passively, without intention. In many cases, this information is reactivated or replayed from episodic and semantic memory, especially autobiographical memories. Indeed, sometimes it is difficult to stop or halt oneself from engaging in IS. In some cases, the overuse or dysfunctional use of IS can become problematic and even pathological, as in the case of rumination [3], that is, obsessive and recurrent thoughts recognized to be common symptoms of mood and anxiety disorders. In these studies, experience sampling and questionnaires showed that rumination involved increased frequency of verbal thoughts and more evaluative and dialogic forms of inner speech. In a recent study in which the content of inner speech was explored in a student sample, the most frequent content sampled was the experience of "negative emotions," highlighting the important role of IS in emotional regulation [4]. Dysfunctional IS has also been linked to the genesis of verbal hallucinations [5], a symptom usually present in schizophrenia and to a lesser degree in the healthy population [6] which appears without a sense of agency ("I am not the one originating this thought or action") [7–9]. Therefore, both aspects, sense of agency and awareness (i.e., conscious accessibility) are important factors to consider when characterizing IS.

To obtain a comprehensive understanding of this phenomenon, it is worth considering that IS can have different levels of information specification—from only conceptual-semantic representations, without specific phonological formulation and articulation (i.e., abstract/condensed IS), to full articulatory and phonological specifications (i.e., concrete/expanded IS) (see [5, 10–12]). Accordingly, we will use the term IS in this chapter to refer to the subjective experience of verbalizing in one's head independent from overt speech that can vary from a nonverbalized conceptual message (i.e., condensed IS, ISc) to an experience of a voice percept (i.e., expanded IS, ISe) [12, 13].

Beyond the realm of linguistics, IS has offered an opportunity to explore thinking and reasoning processes and the possibility to understand conceptual analysis. IS could be seen as the vehicle of what we experience as our internal stream of consciousness. In this view, one might suggest that IS needs to be formalized as a pre-verbal component of our mind that navigates between thinking processes and their materialization into an elaborative language frame (from condensed to expanded IS forms). Due to its relationship with thought-related processes, IS has ignited an intriguing and unresolved debate in cognitive science, namely, whether language and thought processes are functionally inseparable or not [14–16]. The "lingualism" theory suggests that there is no thought without language ([17–19], p. 196, see also [20]), whereas the "language of thought" view proposes that language is inessential to private thought (see [21] for a review; [22], see also [23]). According to the first theory, mental operations such as mental calculation are per se supported by IS [15, 22], whereas the later standpoint proposes that the brain may hold these processes separately [24, 25]. Although this debate is out of the scope of this chapter, it is worth noting that IS lies at crossroads between language and thought—laying between nonverbal thoughts and more formulated language sentences, soliloquies or even internal dialogues. Furthermore, conscious accessibility to these contents may be different. IS represents a point of intersection for other cognitive processes, such as working memory (i.e., covert verbal rehearsal), subvocalization, abstract thinking, executive control, counting, metacognition, self-regulation, theory of mind, and auditory imagery, among others. Many of these functions are associated with introspective IS, consciousness and self-reflection, and in particular with conscious processes involved in gaining access to self-relevant-related information [26].

Interestingly, some authors view language as an important cognitive achievement that evolved as a mechanism needed for communication [27]. From this view, IS could be considered a by-product of language, representing an internalized language form that is also able to improve and support symbolic thinking. As IS is flexible and malleable in its forms, it could provide substantial advantages for thinking as compared to more structured or formalized versions of language in which the message is fully assembled. For example, Vygotsky [28], emphasized the self-referential and predicative quality of IS, being predicative in the sense that the topic of the sentence is missing, whereas in external language the topic is normally well known in the speaker's mind (but see [29] for a critique). This economic, fragmented, and elliptical form of IS might represent an advantage when trying to decode and transform thoughts into language.

23.1.1 Development and Frequency of IS

An early and very influential proposal from Vygotsky [28] stated that IS develops progressively as overt self-directed speech becomes more covert during elementary school years, and is used by children to increase internal rehearsal, simulation-planning capacity, and self-regulatory functions. Therefore, Vygotsky's view considered IS as an internalized form of egocentric speech, which is shaped by social interaction during childhood. Interestingly, previous research showed that preschool 4-year-old children had poor awareness of their own IS and of the existence of IS in the mind of other adults [30]. For example, when 4-year-old children were asked if "*a person can tell himself things or talk to himself up in his head,*" only 45% of infants stated that this is possible (compared to 95% of 6- to 7-year-old children).

Moving from childhood to adulthood, an important question is how frequently IS takes place in the general adult population during daily life. Heavey and Hurlburt [31] used a *descriptive experience sampling method* which consisted of a random beeper in a device that participants carried throughout the day. When the beep sounded, participants were requested to pay attention to the subjective experience that was going on in their mind just immediately before the beep and to write it down. The authors defined IS to participants as "*speaking words in your own voice, usually with the same vocal characteristics as your own external speech, but with no external (real) sound or motion*" (p. 5, [31]). In this survey, participants reported IS experiences in approximately 26% of the sampled moments, with a large variability across participants ranging from 0 to 75% of the time. It is worth noticing that nearly 16% of the sample reported that they never experienced IS during the interrupted moments. Another category that the authors explored and that is relevant to our purpose here was *unsymbolized thinking*. The survey requested participants to report their mental states of thinking without words or any other symbols. This category was defined as "*thinking a particular, definitive thought without the awareness of that thought's being conveyed in words, images, or any other symbols.*" Nearly 22% of the times participants reported this mental state of "word void" (with a large variability across participants ranging from 0 to 90%). Of note, the frequency of these mental states correlated negatively with the frequency of IS. These results suggest substantial individual differences in the experience of IS that needs to be considered as well as the interrelation between both types of experiences.

Although these sampling methods inform about the quantitative aspects of IS, they do not tackle the specific mental contents. A recent study [4] investigated the qualitative aspect of naturally occurring IS in everyday life. In brief, the authors carried out a factor analysis of the different questionnaires and mental content categories sampled and showed that four factors explained most of the variance: self-reflection (i.e., ideas, who I am, motives, beliefs, and preferences), cognition (i.e., planning, problem-solving, critical thinking, and memory), IS accompanying activities (i.e., on transit, performing hygiene, and meetings), and self-management (i.e., finances, education, and errands). In addition, the authors administered the self-regulatory IS questionnaire (Self-Talk scale, [32]) which taps into several components including self-assessment, self-criticism, self-management, and self-reinforcement. A strong correlation was observed between this scale and the questionnaire pointing to the importance of the self-regulatory role of IS as previously proposed [28]. Interestingly, the abovementioned mental content factors of IS correlated negatively with mindfulness tendencies, a non-evaluative and non-elaborative mental state in which thoughts and emotions are simply noticed as they arise without elaboration and rumination.

23.1.2 IS and Forward Simulation Process

Another interesting issue to address is the extent to which IS might represent a mental simulation of speech, relevant to planning, prediction, and error monitoring functions during language production [33]. Several models have proposed that IS might co-occur simultaneously with overt language production [34]. This idea concurs with the existence of mechanisms allowing self-monitoring of one's own speech production [35–38]. Self-corrections of overt speech have been reported to occur in about 50% of all speech errors [39], being speech interrupted in order to covertly correct the error [36]. Crucially, it is unlikely that the monitoring of one's overt speech using only external feedback explains fast interruptions or covert repair phenomena. Therefore, a fast "inner monitoring loop" [36] in the form of IS [40] has been often assumed [41] to be in charge of error monitoring.

Error monitoring in language production might be an indirect proof of the existence of accurate internal representations (e.g., "the expected word or lexical output") that are needed to detect the mismatch between the internal covert production and the expected correct item (what is going to be uttered). These internal representations, known as *efference copies*, are the by-product of a forward simulation model that can predict if the issued action, word, or thought will be the expected one, as well as its consequences in the world (e.g., how it will sound). This forward mechanism is essential in motor control to adjust ongoing movements very rapidly introducing very fast unconscious error corrections [42]. For some authors, IS might be associated with this type of forward simulations. For example, Carruthers [43] clearly advocated for a definition of IS in terms of "attended" sensory forward models involved in mentally rehearsed actions. In this sense, several proposals explaining IS have used this rich framework from motor control to explain IS.

However, it is unclear to what extent feedforward models of error monitoring are required for successful IS specially for those unintended or unbidden thoughts ([44–46]; but see; [47]). For example, error awareness is possible without proper word retrieval, as it has been reported in *tip-of-tongue* states of language production. Besides, Oppenheim and Dell [48, 49] showed that when participants are encouraged to read tongue twisters using only internal speech, the type of errors that appear are more abstract in nature, comprising phonological features but not articulatory components. The tongue twister paradigm consists on reciting repetitively and in a fast pace word strings that are formed as combinations of similar phonemes or phoneme arrangements (e.g., *l*eap *n*ote *n*ap *l*ute), inducing frequently phonological errors in the speaker. One possibility is that forward modeling could issue multiple efference copies of internal information at different levels of representation (phonological, articulatory) (see Fig. 23.1) that could be sent to the comparator mechanisms (eliciting or not eliciting error signals and corrections). This is in agreement with prediction coding accounts [50–52].

It is worth noting that one of the most influential views explaining verbal auditory hallucinations relies on the use of forward models and comparison processes to understand the lack of agency (the feeling that certain thoughts are not originated by oneself, but instead that they have somehow been inserted) [7]. As forward models allow for the prediction of the consequences of actions, the comparison process between expected and external information allows to create a sense of agency, most

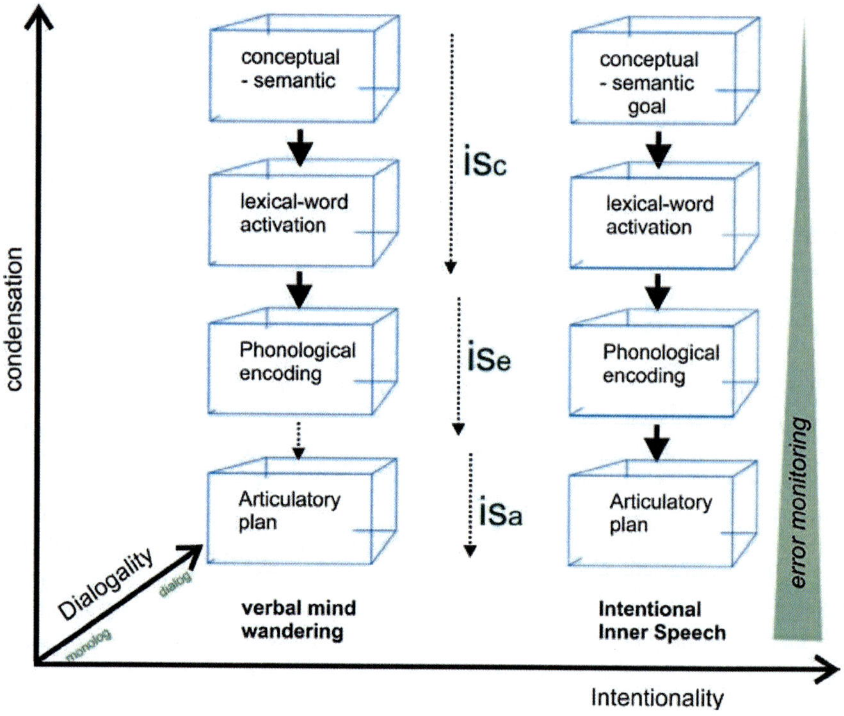

Fig. 23.1 Language production model for possible varieties of IS adapted from Grandchamp and colleagues [12]. The model is organized in three dimensions: level of condensation, from highest condensed forms IS (conceptual forms, ISc) to more expanded forms where phonological (ISe) or articulatory encoding is produced (ISa) and it is experienced as internal voices. The Intentionality dimension of the model seeks to address the issue of spontaneous or unbidden thoughts that range from producing verbal mind-wandering states to more stimulus-driven or goal-directed internal speech (intentional IS). Finally, the Dialogality dimension attempts to recognize the qualitative aspect of the inner voice conversation, ranging from a simple monologue to a conversation simulation. Notice that error monitoring is highlighted only in the intentional IS loop, as its participation is more questionable in the case of unintentional thoughts

probably feed-forwarding the information to sensory brain regions. Although these types of models seem to operate well in the realm of real actions, it is unknown if the same operations could be at play in our internal mental life. For instance, it seems that many thoughts and internal experiences are issued without clear intentions, or at least they seem to be spontaneously triggered instead of stimulus-driven thoughts. As these internal representations are not preceded by intentions, the forward simulation is not possible in this scenario, which opens a debate about the necessary implication of forward modeling in the production of IS (see [44] for further discussion). Fernyhough [5] suggested that having an accurate phonological and/or articulatory representation may not be a necessary condition for IS. This is even more relevant if we realize that, while overt speech might require *veto* or the implementation of inhibitory functions (i.e., preventing certain words in particular contexts), it is questionable if this *veto* is mandatory or even easy to apply for internal thoughts or certain forms of IS. To exemplify this point, in the model proposed by Grandchamp and colleagues [12], only expanded forms of IS might entail verbal monitoring through internal feedforward models (see Fig. 23.1). Thus, it remains a matter of current debate whether all forms of IS might involve error monitoring and the extent to which forward modeling is required.

23.2 How to Measure IS?

When thinking about IS and its measurement, it is worth considering language production models (see, for example, [12]; summarized and adapted at Fig. 23.1) and what happens in between the formulation of a message to be conveyed and its final articulatory or overt speech outcome. In most of these models, a distinction is made at least between the intention-conceptual plan (i.e., a non-linguistic form of knowledge) and two further lexical access processes that occur prior to articulation: (1) the activation of a lexical representation (i.e., an abstract word form level) and (2) the encoding of a phonological representation (i.e., auditory-phonological form) (see Fig. 23.1). Phonological encoding is followed by the activation of an articulatory plan [53–55] (see Fig. 23.1 for a scheme). These four language production stages are distinguished in most language production models and, simplifying it for the current purpose of this chapter, this division could be partially mapped onto the different forms observed in IS as follows (see Fig. 23.1): (1) **semantic level-IS** or condensed IS (**ISc**), representing IS without a clear auditory component and related to semantic-conceptual internal representations, (2) **auditory-phonological level** (IS expanded forms, **ISe**) in which IS comprises a subjective experience of talking to oneself activating auditory-phonological representations of speech but without uttering the sound, and (3) **motor articulatory level (ISa)** in which IS includes some sort of motor plan representations (ISa) (phonological representations pre-activate articulatory motor representations). This last level might range from less elaborated representations (i.e., motor articulatory imagery plans) to more developed ones producing the utterance (i.e., activation of real articulations, e.g., sub-articulation or subvocalization) [15]. Notice, however, that this mapping between language production stages and the three types of IS is not perfect as there is diffuse territory on how to classify IS forms when they represent internal thoughts or activation of abstract word form realizations without auditory-phonological representation (see discussion below).

Further, it is important to bear in mind that the different tasks used to measure IS could be classified considering if they are content-dependent or not, to the extent that they could provide information about the content of IS (i.e., what is the information that is being conveyed during the IS episode). Similarly, an important dimension to consider is the extent to which the measures employed tap on simple word productions or measure internal production of sentences, monologic or even dialogic forms.

A final important point to consider is that, in some cases, especially when using psycholinguistic tasks, the task at hand requires several cognitive processes besides the activation of representations associated with IS. For example, while judging if two words rhyme requires the internal activation of auditory-phonological representations, the participation of working memory (i.e., online manipulation of information) and executive control (i.e., monitoring) is also necessary to properly solve the task. Therefore, caution is needed when interpreting performance on these tasks as direct evidence of the absence of IS, as failures in other cognitive processes could result in impoverished behavioral observations. In most cases, these measures should be considered indirect proxies of preserved IS with relative ecological validity. In the light of these issues, it might be advisable to use an extensive battery of IS to observe convergent effects across different indexes.

23.2.1 Content-Independent Inner Speech Measures

23.2.1.1 Auditory-Phonological IS Level (ISe)

Several methods can be employed to measure IS auditory-phonological forms (i.e., auditory word forms) in a narrow sense without the evaluation of the semantic and articulatory components. For example, it is possible to focus on the evaluation of structural information regarding how words are internally encoded (e.g., dividing words into syllables, detecting homonyms or rhymes). These psycholinguistic tasks could provide a proxy of preserved IS or the internal representation of auditory word forms (i.e., ISe forms). Interesting systematized proposals for the evaluation of this type of IS in neuropsychological patients can be found in recent literature [56, 57]. Considering these proposals and other studies on this topic, we propose that several tasks could be employed to properly evaluate ISe.

1. *Rhyme detection task* (reading and picture naming). Participants are required to silently judge whether two written words that are spelled differently rhyme (e.g., "bear" and "chair"). To solve this task correctly, the activation of both phonological forms is necessary. The task also demands the participation of working memory processes [57]. If the two words are not the same orthographically, the participation of IS is necessary to make the correct judgment. The same task

could also be applied using pictures (see [57]) instead of words which diminishes the influence of single-word orthography as the task does not require reading.

2. *Homophone judgment tasks* (words). Participants are requested to silently judge if two written words that are orthographically dissimilar are homophones, that is, if the two words sound the same (e.g., "buy" and "bye"). Participants need to access the phonological forms of the words in order to solve this task correctly [58].
3. *Location of lexical stress.* In this task, participants are requested to identify where the stress is produced in written words [59, 60].
4. *Word syllable count.* A similar task is the one used by Levine and colleagues [61] in which participants silently count the number of syllables in a word.
5. *Phonological monitoring during picture naming.* Phonological monitoring tasks that require accessing the phonological representation of a pictured word exemplar may also be used as participants have to decide if the name of the picture begins with a consonant or a vowel, or if the picture name contains a particular letter (see [41]). Rodriguez-Fornells et al. [62] used a Go/noGo variant that could be practical in ESM settings as the task only requires an affirmative response (e.g., when the picture begins with a vowel). To the best of our knowledge, these tasks have not been used to monitor IS in patients.
6. *Repetition of tongue twisters.* The task used by Oppenheim and Dell [48] requests participants to repeat internally four word "tongue twisters" phrases and to report if they produced an internal error. Notice however that this task requires an introspective component of error detection as the participants need to monitor if their own inner production contains an error.
7. *Silent reading.* Reading could be accomplished via two different pathways (dual route model): (1) the "lexical route" which proceeds directly from orthography to lexical access, and (2) the "sublexical or letter-to-sound route" in which the orthographic form is converted to its phonological representation prior to lexical access, by applying a specific set of orthographic-phonological spelling rules [63]. When using this letter-to-sound route, IS is indeed being used as it is the case in low-proficient skill readers when reading difficult texts, under stress or with low attentional resources.
8. *Subjective experience during picture naming.* A very small number of studies in aphasia have been devoted to study the subjective experience of anomia (see [64, 65]). In an interesting recent study, Fama and colleagues [66] requested aphasic patients to report their internal experience of anomia. The goal of the study was to gather information about the experiences that anomic patients often present, especially when stating "*I know it but I can't say it.*" Two specific questions were asked to participants after presenting a picture: "*I can't say it out loud, but I can say the right word in my head*" and "*I can't say it out loud, but I know what it is in my head.*". Notice that the first question, which the authors refer to as successful IS (ISe in Fig. 23.1), refers to the correct activation of the auditory word form. In turn, the second might correspond to a semantic level of IS as the authors refer to it as an "*idea without the word,*" which might correspond to ISc forms in

Fig. 23.1. In this study, participants were requested to say yes/no to each question and during the presentation of each item, a pictured description of each question was also presented to support their understanding of the task instructions. Their findings provided important information about the preservation of IS in aphasic patients: 78% of the patients reported a positive experience regarding the first question addressing internal phonological representations, whereas 83% reported a positive experience regarding the second question addressing ideas without words. Furthermore, if self-report in patients is produced correctly regarding their IS experiences, this outcome should correlate with other psycholinguistic variables (e.g., word frequency, naming accuracy, likelihood of phonological errors, and even further success in re-learning these items) (see [65]). The convergence with self-report and overt language effects supports the reliability of the introspective information provided by patients regarding their IS.

It is worth considering that the main aim of these tasks is to provide indirect evidence of internal activation of auditory-verbal phonological information. In most of the cases, these tasks correspond to variations of phonological monitoring tasks [41]. However, a distinction seems important between tasks that require active manipulation of IS auditory-phonological information (e.g., rhyme or homophone judgments) and tasks that demand simple repetition and silent reading. In the latter, the act of repetition is not enough to demonstrate explicit activation and manipulation of phonological forms (no indirect behavioral evidence). Moreover, silent reading could be carried out through a pure lexical route without the use of the orthographic to phonological conversion mechanism (internally reading aloud), which is the mechanism supposedly targeted in these tasks. Fama and Turkeltaub [56] also emphasized the difference between tasks that request internal introspection about the quality of the performance (e.g., repetition of tongue twisters) and those in which introspection does not need to be assessed, thus being less affected by individual biases.

As mentioned above, it is important to bear in mind that the proposed tasks to assess ISe rely on several simultaneous cognitive processes and as such, their use carries the risk of detecting failures in specific tasks that may not be directly associated with impoverished IS. The use of picture naming instead of written words may facilitate the evaluation of IS in most cases, since it provides fewer confounding factors as compared to reading. Similarly, choosing simple phonological monitoring tasks may facilitate this evaluation, especially if these tasks rely less on working memory and executive control. In this regard, the study of Geva and Warburton [57] using several of these measures (i.e., picture and word rhyme judgment, word and non-word homophone judgment and lexical stress detection) showed that the educational level correlated positively with performance on some of the tasks (e.g., homophone judgments) in healthy adults. This finding suggests that in order to achieve proper monitoring of ISe in intraoperative awake monitoring contexts, tasks need to be moderately easy due to complex setting and assessment conditions. Interestingly, as expected, the IS tasks used by Geva and Warburton [57] were positively intercorrelated. However, the strength of the associations was not extremely high in adult healthy samples, suggesting that these tasks measure and capture different processes. This correlation pattern might change to a larger extent for patients with altered IS, as the impairment will affect performance on most tasks, increasing the shared variance of their performance across tasks. Overall, this result highlights the importance of employing multiple tasks to correctly map the IS construct. Finally, it is also important to underscore that these tasks evaluate single-word IS production for the most part, and do not encompass more elaborate forms as internal sentence production.

23.2.1.2 Motor Articulatory IS Level (ISa)

An interesting aspect to be assessed during ESM in brain tumor operated patients is subvocal speech, that is, the production of articulatory movements without sound production. Such experimental manipulations can indirectly assess preserved ISa [67, 68] and the possible implication of subvocalization or sub-articulation as well as the disruption of these processes as indirect measures of preserved IS.

1. *Electromyographic recordings.* Tongue and pharyngeal electromyogram (EMG) could be used for frequency estimations of inner speech production during completion of demanding cognitive tasks (e.g., calculating; [15]). These authors showed that the amplitude of the laryngeal EMG increased for difficult arithmetic problems, as for example solving the Raven matrices test or calculation tasks. Subvocal speech has been recorded electromyographically during mental calculations [69].
2. *Recording of lip movements.* For example, Frings and colleagues [70] evaluated the implication of the cerebellum in the generation of verbs using overt and IS conditions. To monitor IS, participants' lip movements were recorded using a camera inside the scanner. In an intraoperative context, this could be achieved by placing cameras in the operating room.
3. *Articulatory suppression tasks.* These tasks can provide a proxy of IS preservation causing its blocking since articulatory suppression and irrelevant speech have their effects by specifically blocking subvocal rehearsal and the phonological store. In the influential working memory model of Baddeley & Hitch [71], the phonological loop component is assumed to be related to inner speech, being important for manipulation and rehearsal functions [72]. Using articulatory suppression, participants are asked to produce a particular word or sound repeatedly in order to block rehearsal and storage, thus consequently preventing them from engaging in IS [73]. Articulatory suppression methods have been previously used to interfere with IS in children and adults [74, 75].
4. *Silent reading in difficult conditions.* It has been proposed that when reading difficulty increases (e.g., complex text) there is larger involvement of subvocal speech, which indeed could aid the comprehension of complex written material [76]. If subvocalization is disrupted, comprehension of the text becomes impaired. Similarly, this research adds to previous studies showing that vocalization helps learning and encoding verbal material.

5. *Disruption of primary motor regions for overt speech production*. Several studies have used navigated Transcranial Magnetic Stimulation (nTMS) mapping in order to cause disruptions of articulation and overt speech [77, 78]. For example, nTMS could be used to directly stimulate the ventral part of the precentral gyrus which is implicated in execution of motor speech [79] (see Fig. 23.2). Intraoperatively, direct electrical stimulation over this particular region produces speech arrests and language disruptions (see [81–84] for detailed analysis of sensorimotor activations associated to vocal production). Moreover, direct stimulation of the primary motor region for the laryngeal muscle produces language dysarthria [85–87]. With appropriate intraoperative neurophysiologic monitoring control conditions and careful ESM protocols as used in the awake patients reported by Deletis and colleagues [80], it might be possible to block specific articulatory aspects of language while selectively impairing certain forms of IS (see Fig. 23.2 for an example of intraoperative direct cortical brain mapping for language and neurophysiologic recording of the cricothyroid muscle activity after stimulation of IFG-ventral premotor cortex and motor laryngeal points).

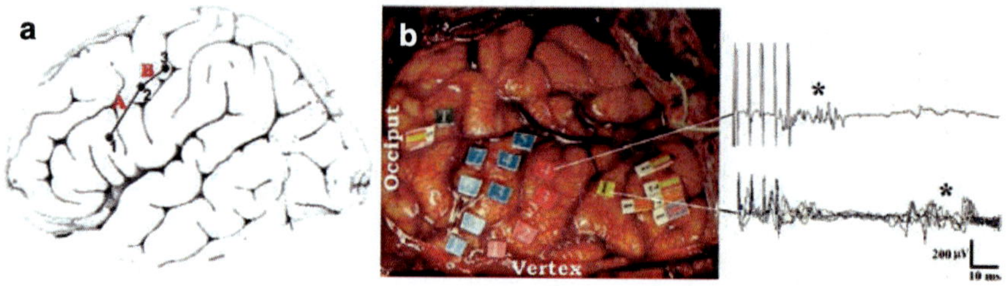

Fig. 23.2 (**a**) MR image obtained in a participant during a **navigated TMS** mapping procedure where the following stimulation points were measured: (3) M1 (primary motor) for abductor pollicis brevis (a control point of a muscle in the hand needed for thumb movement), (2) M1 for a laryngeal muscle, the cricothyroid muscles and (1) junction between inferior frontal sulcus and precentral gyrus (ventral premotor cortex) producing transient language disruptions. At the middle, Euclidean cortical distance between M1 for the abductor pollicis brevis muscle (3), M1 for the cricothyroid muscle (2), and ventral premotor cortical spot (1) (adapted from [79]). (**b**) **Intraoperative mapping during awake craniotomy** in a patient during a picture naming task (adapted from [80]). The neurophysiologic markers generated by primary motor and premotor cortex for laryngeal muscles, recorded from laryngeal muscle (short latency response and long latency response from cricothyroid muscle). Direct stimulation of the red spot 4 [M1 or primary motor region for the laryngeal muscles] elicited short latency responses (at about 20 ms) in the cricothyroid muscle, which is normally accompanied by dysarthria. Stimulation at the yellow spot 1 [located at the ventral premotor cortex in the caudal opercular part of inferior frontal gyrus] elicited long latency response at about 200 ms and generated speech arrest in patients. Notice that stimulating the other Flag points [English, Catalan, and Spanish flags = cortical spots for speech arrest for these languages] surrounding the yellow spot 1 did not show changes in the long latency response of the cricothyroid muscle. [T = tumor location; Blue markers 1–7 = somatosensory cortex; Red markers 1–4 = primary motor cortex]. Adapted with permission obtained from the authors

23.2.1.3 Semantic-Conceptual IS Level (ISc)

The evaluation of this level of analysis is more complex as it represents a form of IS that does not require proper activation of the auditory-phonological form (see Fig. 23.1). An interesting topic for research inquiry is whether ISc (at least at this level of analysis) is possible when overt language is lost in aphasia, or when the inability to put thoughts into words takes place. Is it possible to articulate thinking and reasoning without the capacity to convey such mental processes into meaningful language or words? If yes, how could these conditions be measured without language? Answers to these questions might be very relevant to the debate about how thought and language processes interact (see for a review on this issue [21, 88–90]).

In this regard, recent studies have contributed to this controversy with anatomo-functional observations. Results from voxel-lesion-symptom mapping studies with patients and functional magnetic resonance imaging (fMRI) studies using linguistic and non-linguistic tasks in healthy participants have provided partial evidence to support both views [10, 74, 91]. More interestingly, Varley and Siegal [92] described an aphasic patient with severe agrammatism due to a large lesion in left perisylvian regions encompassing the posterior prefrontal regions, inferior regions of the parietal lobe, and an extended lesion in the temporal lobe. Despite the profound deficit in grammar in this patient, his reasoning and theory of mind abilities (i.e., inferring the mental states of others) were fully preserved. This case provides evidence of the possible dissociation and independence between thought (and to certain extent preservation of ISc) and language processes (see also [93]). These findings further contradict previous views proposing that the processes involved in theory of mind require propositional language [94].

Moreover, it has been observed that individuals with milder forms of aphasia may preserve their IS despite failures in overt speech production [66, 95, 96]. For instance, aphasic patients with anomia often report that they can "*say or hear the correct words in their mind*" despite failing to produce them out loud [66]. Indeed, there is some evidence that IS and overt speech can dissociate in aphasia [10] indicating that the two are at least partially independent. Conversely, several studies have reported impaired IS with partially preserved language functions in frontal-aphasic patients [61]. Levine and collaborators [61] reported the case of a patient who, despite excellent albeit slow speech comprehension, reading, and writing skills, seemed incapable of internally eliciting the spoken word forms (e.g., failed completely on rhyme judgment tasks) (see also [97]). Loss of IS seems to occur to varying degrees in people with aphasia who also present corresponding outer speech deficits [10, 98].

Recently, we reported a single-case study that provided partial evidence of preserved ISc despite global aphasia occurring in the aftermath of brain tumor removal ([99]; see Fig. 23.3 for a lesion description affecting the left middle frontal gyrus and subjacent white matter, most probably affecting frontal lobe projections of the arcuate fasciculus). Patient TD presented global aphasia in the first few days after brain tumor removal but maintained a good level of performance on tasks that

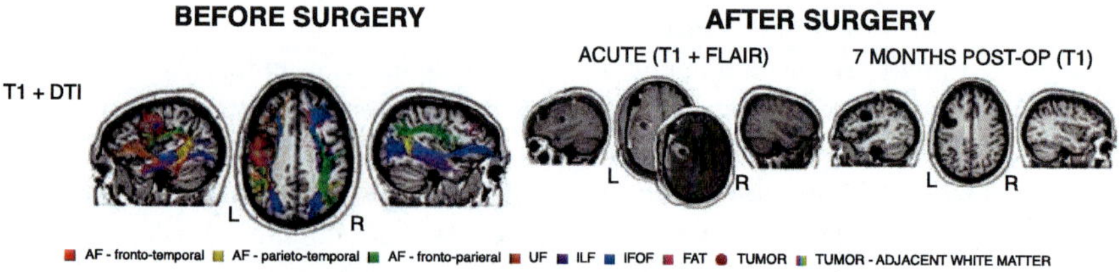

Fig. 23.3 Patient TD's t lesion described by Sierpowska and collaborators [99]. On the left side—tumor location and white matter, presurgical organization. Right side—postsurgical cavity anatomical location (both the acute and early recovery). Notice the left lateralization of white matter language-related tracts before surgery (left section) and the presence of the pericavitarian, subdural extra-axial blood collection in the acute stage of recovery (right section), *T1* T1-weighted structural image, *DTI* Diffusion Tensor Imaging, *FLAIR* Fluid-Attenuated Inversion Recovery Sequence, *AF* arcuate fasciculus, *UF* uncinate fasciculus, *ILF* inferior longitudinal fasciculus, *IFOF* inferior fronto-occipital fasciculus, *FAT* frontal aslant tract. Adapted with authors' permission (original figure published under CC-BY 4.0 license)

required conceptual analysis and nonverbal operations when these were possible to carry out by covert communication (e.g., indication of a correct semantic relationship). Reporting this case was critical given the scarce evidence on whether individuals with global aphasia preserve their IS ability [100] and the fact that global aphasia represents the most severe form of all aphasic syndromes affecting all facets of language production and comprehension. Moreover, the prognosis of language recovery is usually poor in these patients. The severe breakdown in language ability in TD made it impossible for her to communicate with her family, friends, and medical staff. Yet, she was actively reaching out—trying to communicate her thoughts and understand others' communicative intents. Severe aphasia does not occur often after brain tumor removal, but TD's case showed that this is indeed possible. The inability to communicate with TD by means of any of the numerous language and neuropsychological widely accessible assessment tools revealed that current postsurgical medical assistance needs to advance and include alternative ways to measure preserved abilities, as it is the case of IS, especially at the semantic level.

Once TD fully recovered during the first month after awake brain tumor surgery and her language production ability was restored, she reported on her subjective experience while dealing with global aphasia. She clearly explained being able to internally elaborate conceptual messages while being unable to utter them, which suggested that she had preserved ISc forms. Additionally, objective measures carried out during her global aphasia episode (see below) indicated good semantic matching performance. During her recovery process, TD also attempted responding to informal fill-the-gap exercises, the results of which again supported at least partial preservation of lexical access. Interestingly, she produced a series of phonological errors in formal testing in both writing and repetition. Preservation of word retrieval despite articulatory output impairments has been thought to underlie the preservation of IS in other aphasic patients [66]. Summing up, we consider that this evidence points to a partial preservation of language function during the global aphasia episode, probably through the partial involvement of IS. Although we acknowledge that inference based on subjective reports is not enough to unequivocally conclude in favor of preserved IS, this case study hints on the idea that it might not be enough to rely on overt language production tasks to predict actual functional status of individuals with severe aphasia -there may still be a silent, covert reality that is often left unassessed.

The tasks we used in this single-case study might be useful for assessing language ability at the conceptual level (e.g., ISc in ESM settings), without necessarily involving overt language production. Some of these tasks have been proven to be especially useful in cognitive assessment of semantic dementia patients. TD was remarkably successful in two crucial semantic matching tasks:

1. The *Pyramids and Palm Tress* (PPT, [101]). This task requires precise semantic judgments as patients are requested to find the best combination between a target image (e.g., *bottle*) and one of two other images (e.g., *cup* and *grass*).
2. The *Environmental Sound test* [102]. Participants indicate the best match between a target environmental sound and one of the six images presented at the computer screen.

Notice that to correctly solve these tasks, patients need to have detailed access to semantic information regarding each picture or sound, which will be necessary for the identification of the analogies between them, but no word production is mandatory. Besides, their implementation can be achieved by simply indicating the correct semantic match on the computer screen (see also Chap. 15 about verbal and nonverbal semantic cognition).

Other tasks could be used in addition to evaluate preserved semantic knowledge, as for example,

3. *Camel and Cactus Test* (CCT, [102]), which is a variation of the PPT, but including four response options (in color) instead of two (in black and white).
4. *Picture sorting task* [103]. This task is used to assess preserved semantic knowledge systematically in a nonverbal modality. Participants are required to sort 64 pictures at a superordinate level (living vs. manmade), then into basic categories (e.g., for living things: animals vs. birds vs. fruits), and finally at a subordinate level (e.g., for living things: native vs. foreign, larger than a man vs. smaller than a man, meat-eating vs. non-meat eating).
5. *Sound-to-picture matching* [103]. Participants are presented with 64 picture arrays, one for each item, with each array consisting of ten items from the same category (e.g., birds); the task is to point to the item named by the examiner.
6. *Gesture comprehension test* [104]. This task requires the evaluation of the meaning of a gesture. Patients are requested to match a specific videotaped pantomime to one of four presented images.

A recent study observed intraoperative electrical stimulation (ESM) in the vicinity of the ventral language white-matter tracks (i.e., the inferior longitudinal and inferior fronto-occipital fasciculi) involved in sound to meaning mapping, disturbed performance on several of these tasks ([105]; see also [106, 107]).

Overall, the previous aforementioned single-case study reported by our team [99] was an example of how to operationalize several forms of ISc. However, it is worth noting that the evaluation of this IS component is more challenging than the other levels (ISe and ISa) as it navigates between thought and language processes (at least the semantic-intentional stage and the first lexical access stage, *word level access without phonological realization*) (see Fig. 23.1). Thus, a priori, one might argue that any task that weights on thinking and reasoning, mentalizing, mental calculation, metacognition, etc., could be indirectly suggestive of partial preservation of ISc, at least in its more conceptual-semantic level. This IS level might be to some extent similar to the definition of Heavey and Hurlburt [31] of *unsymbolized thinking* (see above), a type of conceptual-semantic content of an inner speech act but without the presence of words. Furthermore, states like "tip-of-the-tongue" phenomena [108], defined as the failure to recall a word of which one has knowledge, could be a proxy measure of word-activation ISc. Considering language production models, a "tip-of-the-tongue" state might correspond to the failure to know *how a word sounds* (i.e., impaired phonological representation) despite successful access to its semantic and more abstract word form representations [109–111]. In convergence with this, the study reviewed above from Fama and colleagues [66] indeed included a question that could provide a distinction between ISe ("*I can say the right word in my head*") and ISc (as an "*idea without the word*"). In sum, further work is largely needed in this "fuzzy terrain" to understand condensed forms of IS and to define the extent to which preservation of these functions might be important to diminish postsurgical language impairments and their subsequent impact on internal mental life.

23.2.2 Content-Dependent Measures

As already mentioned (see first section), several measures developed to capture the mental content of IS are based on asking individuals to report their IS content using structured or open-ended interviews [112]. Multiple authors have reviewed this research and pointed to possible critiques to each one of these techniques (see [1]). However, despite the problems associated with the reliability of introspection [113], the techniques developed have accrued important information about the nature of the subjective experiences associated with IS and with self-referential activity. An example of such techniques is the one mentioned before, the Descriptive Experience Sampling [31]. Another self-report questionnaire is the Varieties of Inner Speech Questionnaire (VISQ, [114]), which measures important phenomenological qualities of IS, such as condensed and expanded IS forms and dialogality. On the other hand, other available questionnaires focus on the self-regulatory components of IS (The Self-Talk Scale, STS; [32]). The STS questionnaire includes 16 items across four scales that measure social assessment (e.g., "I talk to *myself when I'm imagining how other people respond to things I've said*"), self-criticism (e.g., "*.... when I'm really upset with myself*"), self-management (e.g., "*.... I need to figure out what*

I should say or do"), and self-reinforcement (e.g., ".... *when I'm proud of something I've done*").

Most of these questionnaires tap into a variety of constructs related to IS (which are nevertheless not largely correlated with one another) and, in most of the cases, the questions are related to one function of IS, as it is the case for the STS. Another aspect to take into account about these scales is that they do not report the inherent content of IS (i.e., what people say to themselves in daily life). A more recent study by Racy and colleagues [4] presented the General Inner Speech Questionnaire (GISQ), which aims to provide a more comprehensive and ecologically valid measure, including content-wise information of naturally occurring IS in everyday life.

23.3 Neuroanatomical Correlates of IS

The implication of the dorsal stream of language processing might be highly relevant considering the importance of internally activating phonological representations during IS (at least in some encapsulated forms). The dorsal stream is in charge of mapping sounds into their articulatory representations [115–117]. This stream involves the posterior superior temporal gyrus (STG) and supramarginal gyrus (SMG)—which operate as sensorimotor interfaces for phonological encoding—and the ventral motor and premotor cortices which are necessary for proper motor articulation [118–121]. In support of the crucial role of the white-matter fibers conveying information into these regions, a recent ESM study showed that disruption of the arcuate fasciculus affected non-word repetition, a process that requires the precise use of auditory-articulatory encoding [122]. More recently, Geva and Fernyhough [11] suggested a crucial relationship between the dorsal language stream and IS, based on the premise that IS emerges in early childhood in parallel with the maturation of dorsally located white-matter fascicles [123]. Geva and Fernyhough [11] also proposed that IS development might rely mostly on the fronto-temporal and frontoparietal white matter connectivity.

This idea is similar to early proposals from Wernicke, who suggested that, over the course of development, the systematic association between auditory and motor representations during speech production might form the basis of word-concept representations and be responsible of what we conceive as IS (see [124]). Wernicke also emphasized the importance of IS during phonological reading and comprehension or "sounding words out." Of note, self-monitoring and error correction functions attributed to a certain extent to IS are probably subserved by feedforward and feedback connections in the dorsal language stream [115, 125, 126], as it would be in charge of eliciting predicted speech output representations that need to be conveyed back to the auditory regions (see discussion in [127]).

The involvement of the dorsal language stream in IS has been supported, at least to some extent, by early neuroimaging studies [128–130]. However, the tasks used in these studies are rather diverse and range from simple, silent repetition of single words to more active requirements such as silent object definition, rhyme judgments, or syllable stress judgments, which complicate the interpretation of their results. A Positron Emission Tomography (PET) study by McGuire and colleagues [129] showed that, when participants were asked to recite sentences silently (i.e., without speaking and without subvocal articulatory movements), the left IFG as well as the superior temporal and middle cortices (STG/MTG) were activated. In fact, the activation of the left IFG during IS might be one of the most systematic results across studies. IS related to working memory and with the articulatory rehearsal phonological loop in particular has been shown to be associated with the posterior STG [131]. In a rhyme and homophone judgment task (ISe forms), Geva and collaborators [10] showed that IS was additionally associated with the inferior parietal lobe. Other fMRI studies have also reported activations in the SMG as well as IFG when participants were completing rhyme judgment tasks [132, 133].

Several studies have shown that overt and covert language production involve similar brain regions. However, other results point in a different direction as they have revealed that overt speech, when compared to covert speech, is associated with larger activations in sensorimotor and premotor as well as the auditory regions [134, 135]. As an example, Simmonds and colleagues [136] compared overt versus covert speech and reported a symmetrical, bilateral increase in both hemispheres of the medial premotor cortex (SMA), primary sensorimotor and auditory cortices, thalami, putamen, and cerebellum. No activation is usually observed for the reverse contrast comprising covert versus overt speech. Similarly, a recent study by Kell and colleagues [137] contrasted overt versus covert reading and showed increased activation at posterior and mid portions of the STS bilaterally, probably due to the presence of auditory feedback in the overt speech condition (Fig. 23.4d). Moreover, in that same study, two types of IS were evaluated, namely IS with no articulation (i.e., ISe, covert reading of sentences) and IS with articulation (i.e., ISa, covert reading with silent articulation). The crucial comparison between the two IS conditions showed somatosensory feedback processing during articulation at the inferior Rolandic cortex (activations in the sensorimotor cortex associated with articulation, the secondary somatosensory cortex, and the anterior supramarginal gyrus). In turn, the reverse contrast comprising covert reading versus silent articulation did not show increased activation.

It is important, however, to consider that IS, especially in its more condensed forms, is associated with semantic processing, and therefore the interplay between the ventral and the dorsal language streams should be carefully considered. As an example of this necessary interplay, Fama and colleagues [66] used a multivariate lesion-symptom mapping study to show that lesions in the dorsal stream involved in articulatory and motor speech output (left IFG, pars opercularis and ventral precentral gyrus) were associated with problems with "saying a word correctly in one's head" (i.e., proper phonological word form activation) (see Fig. 23.4c) (see also [10], Fig. 23.4a). These lesions correspond well with the lesions observed in TD patient ([99], see also Sect. 23.2.1.3. of this chapter). In contrast, in the study of Fama and colleagues [66] lesions in sites located more ventrally and associated with semantic retrieval (posterior middle temporal gyrus, MTG and angular gyrus) affected IS experiences related to having the idea of the word without proper reactivation of the phonological component (see Fig. 23.4c). Overall, proper semantic retrieval via the

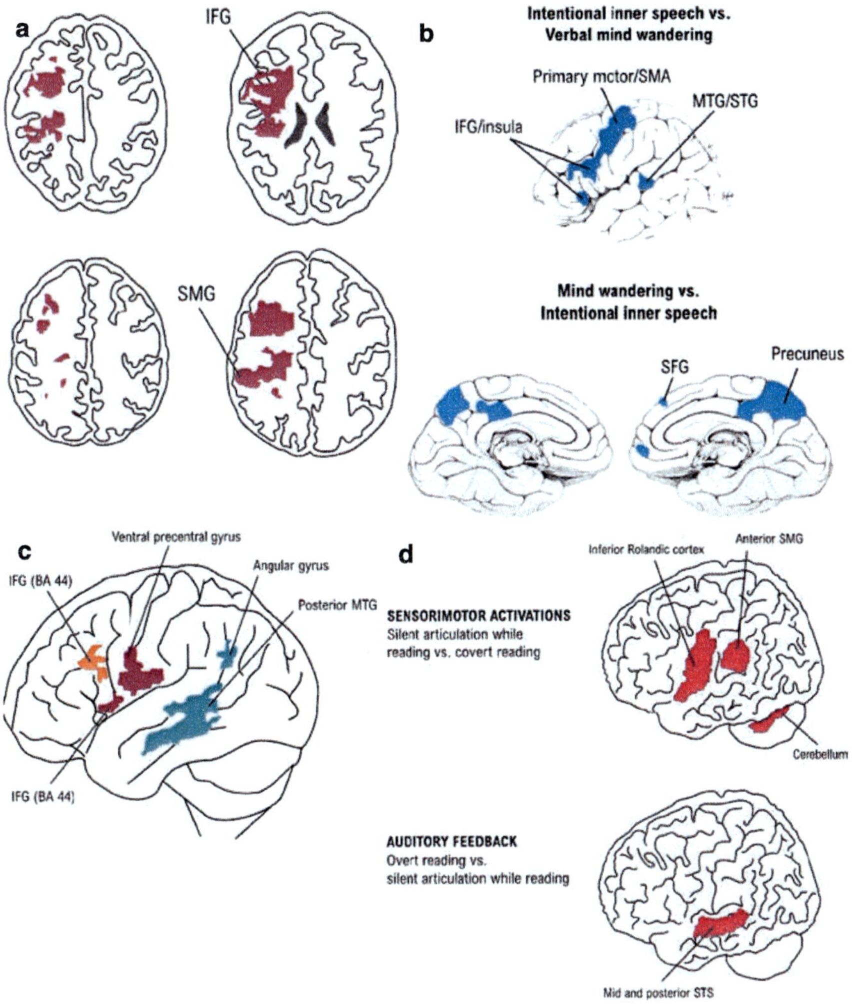

Fig. 23.4 (**a**) Voxel-based lesion-symptom mapping study showing the association between brain lesions and a rhyme judgment task, specially regions involving the dorsal language stream ($n = 18$ stroke patients) (adapted from [10]). (**b**) Comparison of intentional IS (mentally generating a definition of a specific object) and verbal mind wandering states. Notice the larger activation of the Default Model Network in the Mind wandering condition (adapted from [12]). (**c**) Results of the multivariate lesion-symptom mapping study from Fama and colleagues ([66]; $n = 37$ aphasic patients). Lesions associated to problems in producing the inner auditory representation of a word (during picture naming) are depicted in purple, whereas lesions associated to IS forms related to having the idea of but not activating the proper word (most probably a semantic form of IS) are shown in blue. Orange areas represent *tip-of-the-tongue* states during naming. (**d**) IS mapping using fMRI [137]. Two types of IS were assessed in this study: covert reading of sentences (IS with no articulation) and articulation while reading (IS with silent articulation). Notice the increased activation in the lower panel for the critical comparison between both IS conditions. The observed activation reflects somatosensory feedback processing during articulation at the inferior Rolandic cortex (sensorimotor cortex associated with articulation), the sensorimotor thalamus, bilateral cerebellum, and left secondary somatosensory cortex in the anterior portion of the supramarginal gyrus. The reverse contrast covert reading versus silent articulation did not show any increased activation. Figures have been adapted with permission obtained from the authors

ventral stream involved in accessing the meaning of words [138] may allow eliciting a clear concept of the word to be retrieved, but a lesion in the prefrontal branch of the dorsal stream might prevent the proper reactivation of its phonological form.

Finally, it is important to notice that mind-wandering states are also related to IS, and especially to its condensed or unintentional forms (see Fig. 23.1, left column). Increased mind-wandering and stimulus-independent thinking has been associated with the activation of the default mode network (DMN, [139]). Therefore, it is equally interesting to understand the cross-talk between regions activated during IS (i.e., specially IFG and perisylvian regions) and those involved in the DMN (i.e., medial prefrontal regions: posterior-cingulate/precuneus and bilateral insular cortices). A recent study by Grandchamp et al. [12] addressed this issue by evaluating unintended versus intended IS forms (see Fig. 23.4b). In this study, intentional IS was elicited by requesting participants to generate internal definitions of a presented object whereas unintentional use of IS was defined as using periods of verbal mind wandering that were self-reported by the participants. The authors assumed that expanded IS forms are present in intentional speech, whereas verbal mind wandering is usually characterized as being more condensed and probably blurred while at the same time being less susceptible to error monitoring processes [12]. The critical comparison between mind wandering and intentional speech showed activations in the classical DMN regions comprising the medial superior frontal gyrus, precuneus, posterior inferior parietal regions, and lateral temporal cortex (See Fig. 23.4b). The reverse contrast (intentional versus unintentional IS) showed larger activation in the left SMA, primary motor and left temporal regions (MTG/STG), as well as IFG, SMG, ACC, putamen, caudate, and bilateral premotor cortex. Here, reduced activation in left temporal regions in the mind-wandering condition speaks in favor of a reduced subjective quality and probably evanescence of IS in these periods (more condensed forms of IS).

Another source of relevant information is Electrocorticography (ECoG, intracranial recordings using intracranial EEG) used in service of localizing seizure onset prior to brain resection in patients with intractable epilepsy. The temporal implementation of electrode grids allows a unique opportunity to investigate human speech-related processes. This research is paving the way to the possibility of implementing neuroprosthetic and brain computer interfaces in the future. In this context, recent research using this approach revealed a large amount of similarity in the high-frequency (70–500 Hz) and low-frequency activity (theta, in between 4 and 8 Hz) recorded in speech-related areas when comparing inner and overt speech [140–143]. This resemblance sheds light upon the possibility of decoding neural activity into possible auditory features during inner speech (see [144, 145]). For example, recordings near the vicinity of the ventral sensorimotor cortex have been used to detect kinematic representations of laryngeal movements and decode speech features [146, 147]. In more recent research, the authors were able to decode speech units in real time and consider possible neuro-prosthetic designs for patients that are unable to communicate [145].

In summary, a large body of evidence supports the involvement of dorsal stream networks in the reactivation of auditory-phonological forms during IS. Yet, more research is needed to understand the cross-talk between the dorsal stream and the ventral stream involved in sound-to-meaning mapping and storage of semantic memory, as well as their interrelation with other important networks most probably involved in IS, as semantic controlled retrieval [148], memory replying of internal states [149] and the DMN in relation to mind wandering and unbidden internal thinking [150].

23.4 Conclusions

This chapter presents an overview of the recent and growing amount of research on IS from different fields including cognitive science, neuropsychology, neuroscience, and neuroimaging that contribute to our current understanding of a complex, multicomponent, and broad phenomenon that lies at the crossroad of several cognitive process such as language, thought, working memory, reading, consciousness, metacognition, and self-reflection (see [1, 2, 43, 88, 151]). In agreement with recent views [12], we highlight the existence of different forms of IS, discuss the experimental manipulations that may be better to address these different IS forms, and review currently available information regarding the neural underpinnings of IS. We further emphasize that comprehensive and fine-grained evaluations are needed to understand the extent to which IS and its different realizations are preserved in neurological patients, especially those undergoing awake brain mapping. Additionally, we propose that modern neuroscientific methods such as ESM, intraoperative ECoG, or Transcranial Magnetic Stimulation could be added in the near future to the existing set of neural IS blueprints providing new evidence for the neural mechanisms subserving IS. We conclude that the acknowledgment of IS as a complex cognitive phenomenon that interacts with multiple cognitive domains is necessary to understand it and to measure it in a reliable manner. Cross-talk efforts between different research fields have been truly fruitful in this sense for IS research, representing a model of interdisciplinary collaboration (see [1, 2, 88]). ESM has a great potential to add to this complex landscape by adding new evidence on covert language production from the neurosurgical theater.

References

1. Alderson-Day B, Fernyhough C. Inner speech: development, cognitive functions, phenomenology, and neurobiology. Psychol Bull. 2015;141(5):931. https://doi.org/10.1037/bul0000021.
2. Langland-Hassan P. Inner speech. Wiley Interdiscip Rev Cogn Sci. 2020;18:e1544. https://doi.org/10.1002/wcs.1544.
3. Moffatt J, Mitrenga KJ, Alderson-Day B, Moseley P, Fernyhough C. Inner experience differs in rumination and distraction without a change in electromyographical correlates of inner speech. PLoS One. 2020;15(9):e0238920. https://doi.org/10.1371/journal.pone.0238920.

4. Racy F, Morin A, Duhnych C. Using a thought listing procedure to construct the general inner speech questionnaire: an ecological approach. J Constr Psychol. 2020;33(4):385–405. https://doi.org/10.1080/10720537.2019.1633572.
5. Fernyhough C. Alien voices and inner dialogue: towards a developmental account of auditory verbal hallucinations. New Ideas Psychol. 2004;22(1):49–68. https://doi.org/10.1016/j.newideapsych.2004.09.001.
6. Barrett TR, Etheridge JB. Verbal hallucinations in normals, I: people who hear 'voices'. Appl Cogn Psychol. 1992;6(5):379–87. https://doi.org/10.1002/acp.2350060503.
7. Frith CD. The cognitive neuropsychology of schizophrenia. London: Psychology Press; 1992.
8. Gallagher S. How the body shapes the mind. New York, Clarendon Press; 2006. https://doi.org/10.1093/0199271941.001.0001.
9. Gould LN. Verbal hallucinations as automatic speech: the reactivation of dormant speech habit. Am J Psychiatry. 1950;107(2):110–9. https://doi.org/10.1176/ajp.107.2.110.
10. Geva S, Jones PS, Crinion JT, Price CJ, Baron JC, Warburton EA. The neural correlates of inner speech defined by voxel-based lesion-symptom mapping. Brain. 2011;134(10):3071–82. https://doi.org/10.1093/brain/awr232.
11. Geva S, Fernyhough C. A penny for your thoughts: children's inner speech and its neurodevelopment. Front Psychol. 2019;10:1708. https://doi.org/10.3389/fpsyg.2019.01708.
12. Grandchamp R, Rapin L, Perrone-Bertolotti M, Pichat C, Haldin C, Cousin E, Lachaux JP, Dohen M, Perrier P, Garnier M, Baciu M. The ConDialInt Model: condensation, dialogality and intentionality dimensions of inner speech within a hierarchical predictive control framework. Front Psychol. 2019;10:2019. https://doi.org/10.3389/fpsyg.2019.02019.
13. Lœvenbruck H, Grandchamp R, Rapin L, Nalborczyk L, Dohen M. A cognitive neuroscience view of inner language. In: Inner speech: new voices. 2018. p. 131. https://doi.org/10.1093/oso/9780198796640.003.0006.
14. Gleitman L, Papafragou A. Language and thought. In: Cambridge handbook of thinking and reasoning. 2005. p. 633–61.
15. Sokolov A. Inner speech and thought. Berlin: Springer Science & Business Media; 2012.
16. Vygotsky LS. Thinking and speech. In: The collected works of LS Vygotsky. Vol. 1. 1987. p. 39–285.
17. Sapir E. Language, culture, and personality: Essays in Memory of Edward Sapir. Linguistic Society of America. 1941;18(3):238–45. https://doi.org/10.2307/409560.
18. Whorf BL. In: Carroll JB, editor. Language, thought and reality: selected writings. Cambridge: Technology Press of Massachusetts Institute of Technology; 1956.
19. Wittgenstein L. Tractatus Logico-Philosophicus/Logisch-philosophische Abhandlung. London: Kegan Paul. Kevin Klement; 1922.
20. Vicente A, Martinez Manrique F. Inner speech: nature and functions. Philos Compass. 2011;6(3):209–19. https://doi.org/10.1111/j.1747-9991.2010.00369.x.
21. Fodor JA. The language of thought. Cambridge: Harvard University Press; 1975.
22. Hermer-Vazquez L, Spelke ES, Katsnelson AS. Sources of flexibility in human cognition: dual-task studies of space and language. Cogn Psychol. 1999;39(1):3–6. https://doi.org/10.1006/cogp.1998.0713.
23. Edwards S, Ellams J, Thompson J. Language and intelligence in dysphasia: are they related? Int J Lang Commun Disord. 1976;11(2):83–94. https://doi.org/10.3109/13682827609011295.
24. Basso A, De Renzi E, Faglioni P, Scotti G, Spinnler H. Neuropsychological evidence for the existence of cerebral areas critical to the performance of intelligence tasks. Brain. 1973;96(4):715–28. https://doi.org/10.1093/brain/96.4.715.
25. Hamsher KE. Intelligence and aphasia. In: Acquired aphasia. 1991. p. 339–72.
26. Morin A, Michaud J. Self-awareness and the left inferior frontal gyrus: inner speech use during self-related processing. Brain Res Bull. 2007;74(6):387–96. https://doi.org/10.1016/j.brainresbull.2007.06.013.
27. Pinker S, Jackendoff R. The faculty of language: what's special about it? Cognition. 2005;95(2):201–36. https://doi.org/10.1016/j.cognition.2004.08.004.

28. Vygotsky LS. Thought and language. Cambridge: MIT Press; 1962. https://doi.org/10.1037/11193-000.
29. Hurlburt RT, Heavey CL, Kelsey JM. Toward a phenomenology of inner speaking. Conscious Cogn. 2013;22(4):1477–94. https://doi.org/10.1016/j.concog.2013.10.003.
30. Flavell JH, Green FL, Flavell ER, Grossman JB. The development of children's knowledge about inner speech. Child Dev. 1997;68(1):39–47. https://doi.org/10.2307/1131923.
31. Heavey CL, Hurlburt RT. The phenomena of inner experience. Conscious Cogn. 2008;17(3):798–810. https://doi.org/10.1016/j.concog.2007.12.006.
32. Brinthaupt TM, Hein MB, Kramer TE. The self-talk scale: development, factor analysis, and validation. J Pers Assess. 2009;91(1):82–92. https://doi.org/10.1080/00223890802484498.
33. Perrone-Bertolotti M, Rapin L, Lachaux JP, Baciu M, Loevenbruck H. What is that little voice inside my head? Inner speech phenomenology, its role in cognitive performance, and its relation to self-monitoring. Behav Brain Res. 2014;261:220–39. https://doi.org/10.1016/j.bbr.2013.12.034.
34. Pickering MJ, Garrod S. An integrated theory of language production and comprehension. Behav Brain Sci. 2013;36(04):329–47. https://doi.org/10.1017/S0140525X12001495.
35. Dell GS. A spreading-activation theory of retrieval in sentence production. Psychol Rev. 1986;93(3):283. https://doi.org/10.1037/0033-295X.93.3.283.
36. Levelt WJ. Speaking: from intention to articulation. Cambridge: MIT Press; 1993. https://doi.org/10.7551/mitpress/6393.001.0001.
37. Motley MT, Baars BJ, Camden CT. Experimental verbal slip studies: a review and an editing model of language encoding. Commun Monogr. 1983;50(2):79–101. https://doi.org/10.1080/03637758309390156.
38. Postma A. Detection of errors during speech production: a review of speech monitoring models. Cognition. 2000;77(2):97–132. https://doi.org/10.1016/S0010-0277(00)00090-1.
39. Nooteboom SG. Speaking and unspeaking: detection and correction of phonological and lexical errors in spontaneous speech. In: Fromkin V, editor. Errors in linguistic performance: slips of the tongue, ear, pen and hand. London: Academic; 1980. p. 87–95.
40. Dell GS, Repka RJ. Errors in inner speech. In: Baars BJ, editor. Experimental slips and human error: exploring the architecture of volition. New York: Plenum Press; 1992. p. 237–62. https://doi.org/10.1007/978-1-4899-1164-3_10.
41. Wheeldon LR, Levelt WJM. Monitoring the time course of phonological encoding. J Mem Lang. 1995;34:311–34. https://doi.org/10.1006/jmla.1995.1014.
42. Rodriguez-Fornells A, Kurzbuch AR, Münte TF. Time course of error detection and correction in humans: neurophysiological evidence. J Neurosci. 2002;22(22):9990–6. https://doi.org/10.1523/JNEUROSCI.22-22-09990.2002.
43. Carruthers P. The causes and contents of inner speech. In: Langland-Hassan P, Vicente A, editors. Inner speech: new voices. Oxford: Oxford University Press; 2018. https://doi.org/10.1093/oso/9780198796640.003.0002.
44. Gallagher S. Neurocognitive models of schizophrenia: a neurophenomenological critique. Psychopathology. 2004;37(1):8–19. https://doi.org/10.1159/000077014.
45. Jones SR, Fernyhough C. Thought as action: inner speech, self-monitoring, and auditory verbal hallucinations. Conscious Cogn. 2007;16(2):391–9. https://doi.org/10.1016/j.concog.2005.12.003.
46. Möller J, Jansma BM, Rodriguez-Fornells A, Münte TF. What the brain does before the tongue slips. Cereb Cortex. 2007;17(5):1173–8. https://doi.org/10.1093/cercor/bhl028.
47. Whitford TJ, Jack BN, Pearson D, Griffiths O, Luque D, Harris AW, Spencer KM, Le Pelley ME. Neurophysiological evidence of efference copies to inner speech. Elife. 2017;6:e28197. https://doi.org/10.7554/eLife.28197.
48. Oppenheim GM, Dell GS. Inner speech slips exhibit lexical bias, but not the phonemic similarity effect. Cognition. 2008;106(1):528–37. https://doi.org/10.1016/j.cognition.2007.02.006.
49. Oppenheim GM, Dell GS. Motor movement matters: the flexible abstractness of inner speech. Mem Cogn. 2010;38(8):1147–60. https://doi.org/10.3758/MC.38.8.1147.

50. Clark A. Whatever next? Predictive brains, situated agents, and the future of cognitive science. Behav Brain Sci. 2013;36(3):181–204. https://doi.org/10.1017/S0140525X12000477.
51. Friston K. A theory of cortical responses. Philos Trans R Soc B Biol Sci. 2005;360(1456):815–36. https://doi.org/10.1098/rstb.2005.1622.
52. Rao RP, Ballard DH. Predictive coding in the visual cortex: a functional interpretation of some extra-classical receptive-field effects. Nat Neurosci. 1999;2(1):79–87. https://doi.org/10.1038/4580.
53. Dell GS, O'Seaghdha PG. Stages of lexical access in language production. Cognition. 1992;42(1–3):287–314. https://doi.org/10.1016/0010-0277(92)90046-K.
54. Garrett M. Levels of processing in sentence production. In: Butterworth B, editor. Language production. Vol. 1. Speech and talk. London: Academic; 1980. p. 177–220.
55. Levelt WJ, Schriefers H, Vorberg D, Meyer AS, Pechmann T, Havinga J. The time course of lexical access in speech production: a study of picture naming. Psychol Rev. 1991;98(1):122. https://doi.org/10.1037/0033-295X.98.1.122.
56. Fama ME, Turkeltaub PE. Inner speech in aphasia: current evidence, clinical implications, and future directions. Am J Speech Lang Pathol. 2020;29(1S):560–73. https://doi.org/10.1044/2019_AJSLP-CAC48-18-0212.
57. Geva S, Warburton EA. A test battery for inner speech functions. Arch Clin Neuropsychol. 2019;34(1):97–113. https://doi.org/10.1093/arclin/acy018.
58. Davis DF, Herr PM. From bye to buy: homophones as a phonological route to priming. J Consum Res. 2014;40(6):1063–77. https://doi.org/10.1086/673960.
59. Arciuli J, Monaghan P, Seva N. Learning to assign lexical stress during reading aloud: corpus, behavioral, and computational investigations. J Mem Lang. 2010;63(2):180–96. https://doi.org/10.1016/j.jml.2010.03.005.
60. Campbell R, Rosen S, Solis-Macias V, White T. Stress in silent reading: effects of concurrent articulation on the detection of syllabic stress patterns in written words in English speakers. Lang Cogn Process. 1991;6(1):29–47. https://doi.org/10.1080/01690969108406937.
61. Levine DN, Calvanio R, Popovics A. Language in the absence of inner speech. Neuropsychologia. 1982;20(4):391–409. https://doi.org/10.1016/0028-3932(82)90039-2.
62. Rodriguez-Fornells A, Lugt AV, Rotte M, Britti B, Heinze HJ, Münte TF. Second language interferes with word production in fluent bilinguals: brain potential and functional imaging evidence. J Cogn Neurosci. 2005;17(3):422–33. https://doi.org/10.1162/0898929053279559.
63. Coltheart M, Curtis B, Atkins P, Haller M. Models of reading aloud: dual-route and parallel-distributed-processing approaches. Psychol Rev. 1993;100(4):589. https://doi.org/10.1037/0033-295X.100.4.589.
64. Goodglass H, Kaplan E, Weintraub S, Ackerman N. The "tip-of-the-tongue" phenomenon in aphasia. Cortex. 1976;12(2):145–53. https://doi.org/10.1016/S0010-9452(76)80018-4.
65. Hayward W, Snider SF, Luta G, Friedman RB, Turkeltaub PE. Objective support for subjective reports of successful inner speech in two people with aphasia. Cogn Neuropsychol. 2016;33(5–6):299–314. https://doi.org/10.1080/02643294.2016.1192998.
66. Fama ME, Hayward W, Snider SF, Friedman RB, Turkeltaub PE. Subjective experience of inner speech in aphasia: preliminary behavioral relationships and neural correlates. Brain Lang. 2017;164:32–42. https://doi.org/10.1016/j.bandl.2016.09.009.
67. Atkinson JR. The perceptual characteristics of voice-hallucinations in deaf people: insights into the nature of subvocal thought and sensory feedback loops. Schizophr Bull. 2006;32:701–8. https://doi.org/10.1093/schbul/sbj063.
68. Smith JD, Reisberg D, Wilson M. In: Reisberg D, editor. Subvocalisation and auditory imagery: interactions between the inner ear and inner voice. New Jersey: Lawrence Erlbaum Associates; 1992. p. 95–119.
69. Aarons L. Subvocalization: aural and EMG feedback in reading. Percept Mot Skills. 1971;33(1):271–306. https://doi.org/10.2466/pms.1971.33.1.271.
70. Frings M, Dimitrova A, Schorn CF, Elles HG, Hein-Kropp C, Gizewski ER, Diener HC, Timmann D. Cerebellar involvement in verb generation: an fMRI study. Neurosci Lett. 2006;409(1):19–23. https://doi.org/10.1016/j.neulet.2006.08.058.

71. Baddeley A, Hitch G. Working memory. In: Psychology of learning and motivation. Vol. 8. Academic; 1974. p. 47–89. https://doi.org/10.1016/S0079-7421(08)60452-1.
72. Tullett AM, Inzlicht M. The voice of self-control: blocking the inner voice increases impulsive responding. Acta Psychol. 2010;135(2):252–6. https://doi.org/10.1016/j.actpsy.2010.07.008.
73. Baddeley A, Chincotta D, Adlam A. Working memory and the control of action: evidence from task switching. J Exp Psychol Gen. 2001;130(4):641. https://doi.org/10.1037/0096-3445.130.4.641.
74. Baldo JV, Dronkers NF, Wilkins D, Ludy C, Raskin P, Kim J. Is problem solving dependent on language? Brain Lang. 2005;92(3):240–50. https://doi.org/10.1016/j.bandl.2004.06.103.
75. Lidstone JS, Meins E, Fernyhough C. The roles of private speech and inner speech in planning during middle childhood: evidence from a dual task paradigm. J Exp Child Psychol. 2010;107(4):438–51. https://doi.org/10.1016/j.jecp.2010.06.002.
76. Hardyck CD, Petrinovich LF. Subvocal speech and comprehension level as a function of the difficulty level of reading material. J Verbal Learn Verbal Behav. 1970;9(6):647–52. https://doi.org/10.1016/S0022-5371(70)80027-5.
77. Picht T, Krieg SM, Sollmann N, Rösler J, Niraula B, Neuvonen T, Savolainen P, Lioumis P, Mäkelä JP, Deletis V, Meyer B. A comparison of language mapping by preoperative navigated transcranial magnetic stimulation and direct cortical stimulation during awake surgery. Neurosurgery. 2013;72(5):808–19. https://doi.org/10.1227/NEU.0b013e3182889e01.
78. Tarapore PE, Findlay AM, Honma SM, Mizuiri D, Houde JF, Berger MS, Nagarajan SS. Language mapping with navigated repetitive TMS: proof of technique and validation. Neuroimage. 2013;82:260–72. https://doi.org/10.1016/j.neuroimage.2013.05.018.
79. Rogic M, Deletis V, Fernández-Conejero I. Inducing transient language disruptions by mapping of Broca's area with modified patterned repetitive transcranial magnetic stimulation protocol. J Neurosurg. 2014;120(5):1033–41. https://doi.org/10.3171/2013.11.JNS13952.
80. Deletis V, Rogić M, Fernández-Conejero I, Gabarrós A, Jerončić A. Neurophysiologic markers in laryngeal muscles indicate functional anatomy of laryngeal primary motor cortex and premotor cortex in the caudal opercular part of inferior frontal gyrus. Clin Neurophysiol. 2014;125(9):1912–22. https://doi.org/10.1016/j.clinph.2014.01.023.
81. Bouchard KE, Mesgarani N, Johnson K, Chang EF. Functional organization of human sensorimotor cortex for speech articulation. Nature. 2013;495:327–32. https://doi.org/10.1038/nature11911.
82. Brown S, Ngan E, Liotti M. A larynx area in the human motor cortex. Cereb Cortex. 2008;18(4):837–45. https://doi.org/10.1093/cercor/bhm131.
83. Carey D, Krishnan S, Callaghan MF, Sereno MI, Dick F. Functional and quantitative MRI mapping of somatomotor representations of human supralaryngeal vocal tract. Cereb Cortex. 2017;27(1):265–78. https://doi.org/10.1093/cercor/bhw393.
84. Simonyan K, Horwitz B. Laryngeal motor cortex and control of speech in humans. Neuroscientist. 2011;17(2):197–208. https://doi.org/10.1177/1073858410386727.
85. Deletis V, Fernández-Conejero I, Ulkatan S, Rogić M, Carbó EL, Hiltzik D. Methodology for intra-operative recording of the corticobulbar motor evoked potentials from cricothyroid muscles. Clin Neurophysiol. 2011;122(9):1883–9. https://doi.org/10.1016/j.clinph.2011.02.018.
86. Espadaler J, Rogić M, Deletis V, Leon A, Quijada C, Conesa G. Representation of cricothyroid muscles at the primary motor cortex (M1) in healthy subjects, mapped by navigated transcranial magnetic stimulation (nTMS). Clin Neurophysiol. 2012;123(11):2205–11. https://doi.org/10.1016/j.clinph.2012.04.008.
87. Rogic M, Vidaković MR, Vujović I. Preoperative mapping of primary motor and Broca's area with transcranial magnetic stimulation (TMS)-case report. J Neurol Exp Neurosci. 2017;3(1):25. https://doi.org/10.17756/jnen.2017-023.
88. Langland-Hassan P, Vicente A. Introduction. In: Langland-Hassan P, Vicente A, editors. Inner speech: new voices. Oxford: Oxford University Press; 2018. https://doi.org/10.1093/oso/9780198796640.001.0001.

89. Martínez-Manrique F, Vicente A. 'What the…!' The role of inner speech in conscious thought. J Conscious Stud. 2010;17(9–10):141–67.
90. Pinker S. The language instinct: the new science of language and mind. The Penguin Press, London. 1994.
91. Fedorenko E, Varley R. Language and thought are not the same thing: evidence from neuroimaging and neurological patients. Ann N Y Acad Sci. 2016;1369(1):132. https://doi.org/10.1111/nyas.13046.
92. Varley R, Siegal M. Evidence for cognition without grammar from causal reasoning and 'theory of mind' in an agrammatic aphasic patient. Curr Biol. 2000;10(12):723–6. https://doi.org/10.1016/S0960-9822(00)00538-8.
93. Varley RA, Klessinger NJ, Romanowski CA, Siegal M. Agrammatic but numerate. Proc Natl Acad Sci. 2005;102(9):3519–24.
94. Carruthers P. Language, thought and consciousness: an essay in philosophical psychology. Cambridge: Cambridge University; 1996. https://doi.org/10.1017/CBO9780511583360.
95. Fama ME, Snider SF, Henderson MP, Hayward W, Friedman RB, Turkeltaub PE. The subjective experience of inner speech in aphasia is a meaningful reflection of lexical retrieval. J Speech Lang Hear Res. 2019a;62(1):106–22. https://doi.org/10.1044/2018_JSLHR-L-18-0222.
96. Fama ME, Henderson MP, Snider SF, Hayward W, Friedman RB, Turkeltaub PE. Self-reported inner speech relates to phonological retrieval ability in people with aphasia. Conscious Cogn. 2019b;71:18–29. https://doi.org/10.1016/j.concog.2019.03.005.
97. Verstichel P, Bourak C, Font V, Crochet G. Langage interieur apres lesion cerebrale gauche: etude de la reprisentation phonologique des mots chez des patients aphasiques et non aphasiques. Rev Neuropsychol. 1997;7(3):281–312.
98. Langland-Hassan P, Faries FR, Richardson MJ, Dietz A. Inner speech deficits in people with aphasia. Front Psychol. 2015;6:528. https://doi.org/10.3389/fpsyg.2015.00528.
99. Sierpowska J, León-Cabrera P, Camins À, Juncadella M, Gabarrós A, Rodríguez-Fornells A. The black box of global aphasia: neuroanatomical underpinnings of remission from acute global aphasia with preserved inner language function. Cortex. 2020;130:340–50. https://doi.org/10.1016/j.cortex.2020.06.009.
100. Bek J, Blades M, Siegal M, Varley R. Language and spatial reorientation: evidence from severe aphasia. J Exp Psychol Learn Mem Cogn. 2010;36(3):646. https://doi.org/10.1037/a0018281.
101. Howard D, Patterson K. The Pyramids and Palm Trees Test: a test of semantic access from words and pictures. Pearson Assessment; 1992.
102. Bozeat S, Ralph MA, Patterson K, Garrard P, Hodges JR. Non-verbal semantic impairment in semantic dementia. Neuropsychologia. 2000;38(9):1207–15. https://doi.org/10.1016/S0028-3932(00)00034-8.
103. Adlam AL, Patterson K, Bozeat S, Hodges JR. The Cambridge Semantic Memory Test Battery: detection of semantic deficits in semantic dementia and Alzheimer's disease. Neurocase. 2010;16(3):193–207. https://doi.org/10.1080/13554790903405693.
104. Rothi LJ, Heilman KM, Watson RT. Pantomime comprehension and ideomotor apraxia. J Neurol Neurosurg Psychiatry. 1985;48(3):207–10.
105. Sierpowska J, Gabarrós A, Fernández-Coello A, Camins À, Castañer S, Juncadella M, François C, Rodríguez-Fornells A. White-matter pathways and semantic processing: intrasurgical and lesion-symptom mapping evidence. NeuroImage Clin. 2019;22:101704. https://doi.org/10.1016/j.nicl.2019.101704.
106. Duffau H, Gatignol P, Mandonnet E, Peruzzi P, Tzourio-Mazoyer N, Capelle L. New insights into the anatomo-functional connectivity of the semantic system: a study using cortico-subcortical electrostimulations. Brain. 2005;128(4):797–810.
107. Mandonnet E, Nouet A, Gatignol P, Capelle L, Duffau H. Does the left inferior longitudinal fasciculus play a role in language? A brain stimulation study. Brain. 2007;130(3):623–9.
108. Brown AS. A review of the tip-of-the-tongue experience. Psychol Bull. 1991;109(2):204. https://doi.org/10.1037/0033-2909.109.2.204.

109. Burke DM, MacKay DG, Worthley JS, Wade E. On the tip of the tongue: what causes word finding failures in young and older adults? J Mem Lang. 1991;30(5):542–79. https://doi.org/10.1016/0749-596X(91)90026-G.
110. Dell GS, Schwartz MF, Martin N, Saffran EM, Gagnon DA. Lexical access in aphasic and nonaphasic speakers. Psychol Rev. 1997;104(4):801. https://doi.org/10.1037/0033-295X.104.4.801.
111. Meyer AS, Bock K. The tip-of-the-tongue phenomenon: blocking or partial activation? Mem Cogn. 1992;20(6):715–26. https://doi.org/10.3758/BF03202721.
112. Morin A. The self-reflective functions of inner speech: thirteen years later. In: Langland-Hassan P, Vicente A, editors. Inner speech: new voices. Oxford: Oxford University Press; 2018. https://doi.org/10.1093/oso/9780198796640.003.0012.
113. Nisbett RE, Wilson TD. Telling more than we can know: verbal reports on mental processes. Psychol Rev. 1977;84(3):231. https://doi.org/10.1037/0033-295X.84.3.231.
114. McCarthy-Jones S, Fernyhough C. The varieties of inner speech: links between quality of inner speech and psychopathological variables in a sample of young adults. Conscious Cogn. 2011;20(4):1586–93. https://doi.org/10.1016/j.concog.2011.08.005.
115. Hickok G, Poeppel D. The cortical organization of speech processing. Nat Rev Neurosci. 2007;8(5):393–402. https://doi.org/10.1038/nrn2113.
116. Rauschecker JP. Ventral and dorsal streams in the evolution of speech and language. Front Evol Neurosci. 2012;4:7. https://doi.org/10.3389/fnevo.2012.00007.
117. Saur D, Kreher BW, Schnell S, Kümmerer D, Kellmeyer P, Vry MS, Umarova R, Musso M, Glauche V, Abel S, Huber W. Ventral and dorsal pathways for language. Proc Natl Acad Sci. 2008;105(46):18035–40. https://doi.org/10.1073/pnas.0805234105.
118. Hickok G. The functional neuroanatomy of language. Phys Life Rev. 2009;6(3):121–43. https://doi.org/10.1016/j.plrev.2009.06.001.
119. Hickok G, Houde J, Rong F. Sensorimotor integration in speech processing: computational basis and neural organization. Neuron. 2011;69(3):407–22. https://doi.org/10.1016/j.neuron.2011.01.019.
120. Indefrey P, Levelt WJ. The spatial and temporal signatures of word production components. Cognition. 2004;92(1–2):101–44. https://doi.org/10.1016/j.cognition.2002.06.001.
121. Price CJ. A review and synthesis of the first 20 years of PET and fMRI studies of heard speech, spoken language and reading. Neuroimage. 2012;62(2):816–47. https://doi.org/10.1016/j.neuroimage.2012.04.062.
122. Sierpowska J, Gabarrós A, Fernandez-Coello A, Camins À, Castañer S, Juncadella M, Morís J, Rodríguez-Fornells A. Words are not enough: nonword repetition as an indicator of arcuate fasciculus integrity during brain tumor resection. J Neurosurg. 2017;126(2):435–45. https://doi.org/10.3171/2016.2.JNS151592.
123. Weiss-Croft LJ, Baldeweg T. Maturation of language networks in children: a systematic review of 22 years of functional MRI. Neuroimage. 2015;123:269–81. https://doi.org/10.1016/j.neuroimage.2015.07.046.
124. Eggert GH. Wernicke's works on aphasia. The Hague: Mouton; 1977.
125. Rauschecker JP, Scott SK. Maps and streams in the auditory cortex: nonhuman primates illuminate human speech processing. Nat Neurosci. 2009;12(6):718–24. https://doi.org/10.1038/nn.2331.
126. Wise RJ, Scott SK, Blank SC, Mummery CJ, Murphy K, Warburton EA. Separate neural subsystems within 'Wernicke's area'. Brain. 2001;124(1):83–95. https://doi.org/10.1093/brain/124.1.83.
127. DeWitt I, Rauschecker JP. Wernicke's area revisited: parallel streams and word processing. Brain Lang. 2013;127(2):181–91. https://doi.org/10.1016/j.bandl.2013.09.014.
128. Aleman A, Formisano E, Koppenhagen H, Hagoort P, De Haan EH, Kahn RS. The functional neuroanatomy of metrical stress evaluation of perceived and imagined spoken words. Cereb Cortex. 2005;15(2):221–8. https://doi.org/10.1093/cercor/bhh124.
129. McGuire PK, Silbersweig DA, Frith CD. Functional neuroanatomy of verbal self-monitoring. Brain. 1996;119(3):907–17. https://doi.org/10.1093/brain/119.3.907.

130. Shergill SS, Bullmore ET, Brammer MJ, Williams SC, Murray RM, McGuire PK. A functional study of auditory verbal imagery. Psychol Med. 2001;31(2):241. https://doi.org/10.1017/S003329170100335X.
131. Buchsbaum BR, Olsen RK, Koch P, Berman KF. Human dorsal and ventral auditory streams subserve rehearsal-based and echoic processes during verbal working memory. Neuron. 2005;48(4):687–97. https://doi.org/10.1016/j.neuron.2005.09.029.
132. Hoeft F, Ueno T, Reiss AL, Meyler A, Whitfield-Gabrieli S, Glover GH, Keller TA, Kobayashi N, Mazaika P, Jo B, Just MA. Prediction of children's reading skills using behavioral, functional, and structural neuroimaging measures. Behav Neurosci. 2007;121(3):602. https://doi.org/10.1037/0735-7044.121.3.602.
133. Lurito JT, Kareken DA, Lowe MJ, Chen SH, Mathews VP. Comparison of rhyming and word generation with FMRI. Hum Brain Mapp. 2000;10(3):99–106. https://doi.org/10.1002/1097-0193(200007)10:3<99::AID-HBM10>3.0.CO;2-Q.
134. Owen WJ, Borowsky R, Sarty GE. FMRI of two measures of phonological processing in visual word recognition: ecological validity matters. Brain Lang. 2004;90(1–3):40–6. https://doi.org/10.1016/S0093-934X(03)00418-8.
135. Shuster LI, Lemieux SK. An fMRI investigation of covertly and overtly produced mono- and multisyllabic words. Brain Lang. 2005;93(1):20–31. https://doi.org/10.1016/j.bandl.2004.07.007.
136. Simmonds AJ, Leech R, Collins C, Redjep O, Wise RJ. Sensory-motor integration during speech production localizes to both left and right plana temporale. J Neurosci. 2014;34(39):12963–72. https://doi.org/10.1523/JNEUROSCI.0336-14.2014.
137. Kell CA, Darquea M, Behrens M, Cordani L, Keller C, Fuchs S. Phonetic detail and lateralization of reading-related inner speech and of auditory and somatosensory feedback processing during overt reading. Hum Brain Mapp. 2017;38(1):493–508. https://doi.org/10.1002/hbm.23398.
138. Binder JR, Desai RH, Graves WW, Conant LL. Where is the semantic system? A critical review and meta-analysis of 120 functional neuroimaging studies. Cereb Cortex. 2009;19(12):2767–96. https://doi.org/10.1093/cercor/bhp055.
139. Mason MF, Norton MI, Van Horn JD, Wegner DM, Grafton ST, Macrae CN. Wandering minds: the default network and stimulus-independent thought. Science. 2007;315(5810):393–5. https://doi.org/10.1126/science.1131295.
140. Brumberg JS, Krusienski DJ, Chakrabarti S, Gunduz A, Brunner P, Ritaccio AL, Schalk G. Spatio-temporal progression of cortical activity related to continuous overt and covert speech production in a reading task. PLoS One. 2016;11(11):e0166872. https://doi.org/10.1371/journal.pone.0166872.
141. Hermes D, Miller KJ, Vansteensel MJ, Edwards E, Ferrier CH, Bleichner MG, van Rijen PC, Aarnoutse EJ, Ramsey NF. Cortical theta wanes for language. Neuroimage. 2014;85:738–48. https://doi.org/10.1016/j.neuroimage.2013.07.029.
142. Leuthardt E, Pei XM, Breshears J, Gaona C, Sharma M, Freudenburg Z, Barbour D, Schalk G. Temporal evolution of gamma activity in human cortex during an overt and covert word repetition task. Front Hum Neurosci. 2012;6:99. https://doi.org/10.3389/fnhum.2012.00099.
143. Pei X, Leuthardt EC, Gaona CM, Brunner P, Wolpaw JR, Schalk G. Spatiotemporal dynamics of electrocorticographic high gamma activity during overt and covert word repetition. Neuroimage. 2011;54(4):2960–72. https://doi.org/10.1016/j.neuroimage.2010.10.029.
144. Martin S, Iturrate I, Millán JD, Knight RT, Pasley BN. Decoding inner speech using electrocorticography: progress and challenges toward a speech prosthesis. Front Neurosci. 2018;12:422. https://doi.org/10.3389/fnins.2018.00422.
145. Moses DA, Leonard MK, Makin JG, Chang EF. Real-time decoding of question-and-answer speech dialogue using human cortical activity. Nat Commun. 2019;10(1):1–4. https://doi.org/10.1038/s41467-019-10994-4.
146. Chartier J, Anumanchipalli GK, Johnson K, Chang EF. Encoding of articulatory kinematic trajectories in human speech sensorimotor cortex. Neuron. 2018;98(5):1042–54. https://doi.org/10.1016/j.neuron.2018.04.031.

147. Dichter BK, Breshears JD, Leonard MK, Chang EF. The control of vocal pitch in human laryngeal motor cortex. Cell. 2018;174(1):21–31. https://doi.org/10.1016/j.cell.2018.05.016.
148. Wagner AD, Paré-Blagoev EJ, Clark J, Poldrack RA. Recovering meaning: left prefrontal cortex guides controlled semantic retrieval. Neuron. 2001;31(2):329–38. https://doi.org/10.1016/S0896-6273(01)00359-2.
149. Chen J, Leong YC, Honey CJ, Yong CH, Norman KA, Hasson U. Shared memories reveal shared structure in neural activity across individuals. Nat Neurosci. 2017;20(1):115–25. https://doi.org/10.1038/nn.4450.
150. Alderson-Day B, Weis S, McCarthy-Jones S, Moseley P, Smailes D, Fernyhough C. The brain's conversation with itself: neural substrates of dialogic inner speech. Soc Cogn Affect Neurosci. 2016;11(1):110–20. https://doi.org/10.1093/scan/nsv094.
151. Fernyhough, C. The Voices Within: The History and Science of How We Talk to Ourselves. Basic Books. 2016.

Beyond Task: When Experience Shapes Intuition

24

Hugues Duffau

"It is by logic that we prove, but by intuition that we discover"

Henri Poincaré

24.1 Introduction

The main goal in surgical neurooncology is to maximize the extent of tumor resection while optimizing the quality of life of patients. Indeed, overall survival is significantly greater when a complete or (if feasible) a supracomplete resection can be achieved, in low-grade gliomas [1, 2], high-grade gliomas [3, 4], and metastasis [5]. In this spirit mainly based upon oncological considerations, the vast majority of neurosurgeons decided to achieve image-guided resection [6], initially relying on structural MRI and progressively by incorporating functional neuroimaging (especially fMRI and tractography) in the surgical selection and planning. However, a few years afterwards, numerous limitations and drawbacks of neuroimaging were evidenced (1) from an oncological perspective, in diffuse gliomas, due to the invasive pattern of this neoplasm, the tumoral cells exist far beyond the anatomic and metabolic neuroimaging [7] and (2) from a functional perspective, fMRI and tractography are not reliable enough in order to identify the cortical hubs and white matter tracts critical for brain functions (for a recent review, see [8]).

H. Duffau (✉)
Department of Neurosurgery, Montpellier University Medical Center, Montpellier, France

Institute of Functional Genomics, INSERM U-1191, University of Montpellier, Montpellier, France

Department of Neurosurgery, Gui de Chauliac Hospital, CHU Montpellier, Montpellier, France
e-mail: h-duffau@chu-montpellier.fr

E. Mandonnet, G. Herbet (eds.), *Intraoperative Mapping of Cognitive Networks*,
https://doi.org/10.1007/978-3-030-75071-8_24

Therefore, in order to tend toward an optimal onco-functional balance, and taking account of a considerable interindividual anatomo-functional variability, a first paradigmatic shift was to evolve to a functional guided-surgical removal, performed up to the essential cerebral structures for each patient [9]. Of note, this principle can also be applied to surgery for non-neoplastic brain diseases, such as cavernomas [10] or epilepsy [11]. The purpose is to detect and spare the essential neural networks, at both the cortical and subcortical levels, by means of direct electrostimulation in awake patients. Such a philosophy has resulted in a significant improvement of survival and in a significant decrease of disabling permanent disorders after functional-based brain surgery, including in areas previously thought as unresectable [12].

Interestingly, this original concept in neuroocology, that consists in seeing the individual brain dynamics first (not the lesion) as well as in investigating the neural remodeling induced by the tumor progression at this moment in this given patient, was born of intuition—guided by the fact that patients with a low-grade glioma in "eloquent" sites had no or only mild neurological deficits [13]. Intuition can be defined as an instantaneous apprehension of coherence resulting from cognitive processes that operate outside awareness, i.e., the ability to apprehend an idea without explicit explanation [14]. In fact, our decisions can be guided by feelings that are not founded on analytic reasoning or explicit weighting of alternative options: these intuitive emotional evaluations may be activated during the judgment process, even though they are not consciously available at the moment of decision [15].

Here, the purpose is to explore how experience has contributed to shape intuition, and the role that intuition has played in the rise of "connectomal neurosurgery."

24.2 First Step: When Empirical Observation Shapes Experience

Even in a new functional approach of tumor surgery, the usual way to select tasks for intraoperative mapping is still based on the lobar location of the lesion, in a rigid localizationist account of brain organization assuming that the cerebral area invaded should correspond to a discrete function (one-to-one mapping). According to this simplistic model, motor function is usually tested for tumors near the central region (possibly using intraoperative neurophysiological monitoring under general anesthesia in many teams), speech for tumors involving the left frontal operculum, comprehension for tumors invading the left posterior temporal regions, and so forth [16]. Because of this reductionist view, the "new standard" in practical neurooncology, even if questionable [17], has become to awake patients bearing a lesion within the "left dominant hemisphere" while removing the tumor in asleep patients when located in the "right non-dominant side."

Yet, neurosurgeons must remind that the experience of a medical doctor is mainly built on the power of clinical observation, which regularly raises into question the official "a priori knowledge" learnt at university. Therefore, in order to be capable to see the real truth face of every patient and every brain, the first step is to collect information without bias or blinders, even if not in agreement with our preconceptions about functional anatomy. In this state of mind, numerous reports have evidenced the existence of a neurological recovery following surgical resections involving the so-called "eloquent sites" (deemed as "inoperable" for many decades), with nonetheless a return to an active life—e.g., after tumor removal in Broca's area, Wernicke's area, Rolandic area, or the insula [18, 19]. Such a functional compensation should not be possible in an inflexible localizationist framework. Thus, on the basis of these discrepancies between theory and the real facts observed in clinical practice, in a second step, our own brain is spontaneously capable to propose alternative theories built on the cumulated empirical experience, guided by feelings and common sense which challenge dogmas: as mentioned above, this non-conscious process can be called intuition.

24.3 Second Step: When Experience Shapes Intuition

Intuition may be conceived as the sudden, experience-based impression of coherence elicited by cues in the environment [15]. A seminal example of intuition is given by Geschwind (1965) [20] and then Mesulam (1990) [21] who anticipated, without the current technological facilities, that brain processes are not mediated by hyper-specialized and fixed cortical regions, as previously claimed, but rather by distributed and resilient neural circuits. In line with these pioneering works on neo-associationism, which opened the door to the concept of connectome, an alternative view of cerebral organization was recently proposed, that is, a meta-networking theory of brain functions [22]. This principle is founded on a perpetual succession of equilibrium states made possible thanks to interactions between delocalized large-scale neural circuits which subserve sensorimotor, visuo-spatial, language, cognitive, and emotional functions, allowing the brain to produce adapted and flexible behaviors. Such a dynamic architecture in complex networks explains the huge potential of neuroplasticity, both in physiology (e.g., learning) and in brain-damaged patients (leading to some degrees of postlesional functional compensation), in a flexible framework breaking with the classical dogma of a "unique brain" [22].

With respect to the clinical applications, this original concept paved the way of connectome-based surgical resection. According to this philosophy, in addition to the results of the preoperative objective neuropsychological assessment, the aim is to determine the needs of the patient and his/her family before surgery, based upon his/her lifestyle (e.g., job, hobbies) and his environment (e.g., language, culture), in order to select the appropriate tasks allowing a reliable intraoperative functional mapping and cognitive monitoring under local anesthesia [23, 24]. Indeed, the ultimate goal is not only to prevent hemiplegia or aphasia, but to enable the patient getting life back to normal. To this end, a new way of thinking emanating from intuition is to administrate functional testing to the patient in real-time throughout the resection by adapting to his/her own definition of health-related quality of life as well as to an improved knowledge of the functional connectivity of the human brain

[25]. In other words, the tests should be tailored to the proximity of both the cortical hubs (e.g., complex movement near the perirolandic system, especially bimanual coordination in a patient who would like to enjoy a high degree of dexterity, such as a pianist or surgeon [26]; or multimodal semantics close to the dorsolateral prefrontal cortex, since this region is a crossroad between the dorsal and ventral streams, in particular in a patient who would like to preserve a high level of conceptual elaboration [27]; etc.) as well as the subcortical pathways mediating the large-scale networks, regardless of the lobar localization of the tumor [28]. For example, (verbal or non-verbal) semantic processing should be mapped and monitored for frontal, insular, temporal, parietal, and occipital lesions, whatever the hemisphere, because the inferior fronto-occipital fasciculus will be encountered in all these locations, and must represent the deep functional boundary of the resection in all cases to preserve a higher level of comprehension indispensable to enjoy an active life—since this system plays a pivotal role in noetic consciousness (knowing of knowing, see below) [29, 30]. Thus, a strong bridge should be created between fundamental neurosciences and surgery of the central nervous system, which cannot be based anymore upon the traditional surgical anatomy that relies on the limited framework of localizationism. Indeed, a translational view founded on a multidisciplinary background will help each physician to elaborate original integrated theories by making the link between clinical observations and basic research, thanks to a holistic multimodal reasoning challenging dogmas.

24.4 Third Step: To Validate the Intuition

The third step should consist in the validation of the new concepts that emerged from intuition, such as a meta-networking model of neural functions; adaptation of the surgical strategy according to a distributed and dynamic organization of cerebral circuitry, by taking into account the functional connectivity and neuroplastic potential at the individual level; selection of intraoperative tasks allowing a connectomal-based resection; tailored postoperative cognitive rehabilitation; etc. The best way is to go back to reality of the facts, based on the feedback provided by the patient before, during, and after surgery. Indeed, the priority is to prove that the cognitive scores are similar on the pre- and postoperative neuropsychological evaluations [29, 31], and that the patient resumed a normal life, including working full-time [32]—although not at the expense of the extent of resection. It is nonetheless worth noting that a validation is not complete until it is reproduced by other teams. Interestingly, by comparing results between teams with a long or a short experience in functional-based surgery, it has been demonstrated that both neurological and oncological outcomes were similar, confirming that stimulation mapping is independent of surgical expertise and supporting wider implementation [33].

For this purpose, that is, to make these results even more reproducible worldwide, it is of utmost importance to better understand the mechanisms mediating cerebral reshaping, in particular by performing serial functional mappings. Longitudinal investigations are currently possible by means of noninvasive pre- and postsurgical fMRI, compared with intrasurgical neurophysiological mapping and with cognitive assessments before and after rehabilitation. For example, a series using perioperative resting-state fMRI has evidenced a transient decrease of the inter-hemispheric functional connectivity after surgery of tumors involving the supplementary motor area, correlated to the immediate postoperative worsening. Interestingly, this inter-hemispheric connectivity increased a few weeks later, simultaneously with neurological recovery [34]. Besides movement, plastic phenomena underpinning language have recently been studied in patients who underwent awake surgery for low-grade gliomas in the left side, with no permanent aphasia. Significant changes in the functional connectome have been observed before and after resection, using both activation-tasks [35] and resting-state fMRI [36]. Of note, neural reallocation was demonstrated not only within the lesional hemisphere and/or in the contralateral side but also at the level of the thalamus and the cerebellum [37]. Similar investigations start to be performed with regard to high-order cognitive functions, such as attention processing [38] or memory reorganization after epilepsy surgery [39]. In addition, these series were also able to explain why some patients did not completely recover following brain surgery, most of the time due to a disconnection syndrome related to injury of the white matter tracts [40–42]. Therefore, such a basic research in cognitive neurosciences has immediate implications in neurosurgery, with in return the clinical outcomes that allow to validate the theoretical model.

24.5 Fourth Step: From Model Shift to a Higher Level of Automation

The next step is to replace the old model by the original philosophy in the medical and scientific communities. To achieve such a paradigmatic shift, the key lies in educational changes, by introducing the new models in the teaching of clinical neurology and basic neurosciences [22]. Beside institutional academic considerations, it is also crucial to found a school based on tutoring as well as multidisciplinary networks able to disseminate, refine, and finally go beyond the core concept. A typical illustration was the creation of the European Low Grade Glioma Network, which gathered departments managing patients with diffuse low-grade gliomas, and permitted to conduct collaborative and translational studies thanks to the emulation of specialists involved in different fields, such as neurosurgeons, neurooncologists, radiation therapists, pathologists, oncomolecular biologists, neuroradiologists, anesthesiologists, speech therapists, neuropsychologists, and neuroscientists involved in brain function mapping [43]. In particular, from a neuropsychological perspective, this network proposed the development of a European assessment protocol regarding perioperative and intraoperative cognitive assessment [44].

An additional way to popularize “connectome-based surgery” is to elaborate new tools that can be used by the vast majority of physicians and researchers, such as probabilistic atlases of the human brain, at the level of both the cortex [45] and white matter tracts [46]. Recently, a unique combination of cortical and subcortical data gained from intraoperative electrostimulation mapping, including 1821 functional responses and 16 functional domains in a series of 256 awake patients, has been used for computation of probabilistic maps of structures critical for neural functions [47, 48]. This atlas can be helpful for planning the more appropriate neuro-cognitive monitoring as well as for driving the cortico-subcortical mapping strategy, in particular for teams not yet trained in the most recent advances in structural and functional anatomy. They could use this new tool to rapidly improve their knowledge regarding the brain connectome and then to optimize their clinical results. In the same mind, an atlas of neuroplasticity is also available, with the aim of teaching the dynamics of neural networks in brain-damaged patients, the potentials and limitations of functional compensation, in order to predict if neurological recovery is possible at the individual level—or not [49]. A better understanding of cerebral plasticity may also lead to propose new dynamic therapeutic strategies, as, for example, new programs of postoperative cognitive rehabilitation stimulating neural reallocation and then facilitating multistage surgical approaches, especially in slow-growing lesion as low-grade glioma. This original management resulted in an increase of the extent of resection at reoperation, while preserving the quality of life thanks to remapping in comparison with the first surgery [50]. Interestingly, such a provocative attitude discovered by intuition [51], and that was a matter of debate for many years, has recently been validated [52], including by other teams [53].

With these new ideas in mind, both medical doctors and researchers may tend toward a higher level of automation, freeing up time and energy to continue to observe and listen the central nervous system in order to elaborate, update, and improve models closer to reality. Indeed, embedded information can in fine take the form of prior knowledge held by the neuroscientist, such a tacit knowledge being conductive to intuitive judgment [14, 54].

24.6 Perspectives: When Intuition Makes the Bed of Creativity

Intuition relies on the unconscious spreading activation of semantic associates [15]. This complex function seems to be underpinned by a large network involving notably the right superior temporal cortex, which is considered as reflecting the role of the unconsciously activated information, as well as the bilateral inferior parietal cortex, which is related to the process of decision-making under uncertainty [55]. Interestingly, this experience-based process of intuition can affect meta-cognitive judgment, based on both nonanalytic and analytic, theory-based processes [56]. Such inter-system interaction is in agreement with the new meta-networking model of brain functions and could be helpful to understand the ways of thinking that make “experts” expert.

To this end, it is critical to investigate the neural bases underlying behavior from two different perspectives: (1) as neuroscientists, in order to continue to refine our knowledge concerning cerebral networks dynamics (that is, segregation and integration of circuits subserving conation, cognition and emotion) and then to discover new insights into intuition and metacognition—the "proper of man," i.e., the awareness of knowing and understanding the world and the self, the ability to be aware of such an awareness [29], and even currently the capacity to study the brain foundations mediating such an integrated process making the human being what he is; (2) as medical doctors, especially in the field of neurooncology (at the interface between cancer and brain), in order not only to increase the survival of patients while avoiding neurological disorders but also to preserve their personality.

In practice, a preliminary stage guided by experience-based intuition, namely, relying on the fact that brain tumor patients and their family felt changes in behavior (with subjective complaints regarding motivation, affect, mood, desire, belief, empathy, and so on), resulted in the introduction of new tasks allowing a more accurate examination. For example, by using the Schizotypal Personality Questionaire after surgery for diffuse low-grade glioma, heightened schizotypal traits was observed, associated with damage to the left uncinate fasciculus [57]. Regarding mentalistic processes, seminal data evidenced that low-level mentalizing (mirror-system) performances, evaluated using The Read The Mind in The Eyes (RME) test before and after glioma surgery, were significantly correlated with the volume of resection of the pars opercularis of the right inferior frontal gyrus [58], and that subjective empathy impairment was associated with white matter tracts disconnection [59]. Later, a pivotal role of the dorsal stream (underpinned by the superior longitudinal fasciculus/arcuate fasciculus complex) was demonstrated in perceptual-based mentalizing, in addition to the medial stream (mediated by the cingulum) in high-level inference-based mentalizing and to the ventral stream (subserved by the inferior fronto-occipital fasciculus) in face-based mentalizing, such as complex facial emotion recognition [60]. Therefore, to prevent long-lasting postsurgical social cognition disturbances, an adapted version of the RME task has been introduced into the operating theater, with the goal to preserve theory of mind following surgery [61]. Interestingly, these preliminary results have been reproduced by other teams, and even extended to the monitoring of high-level inference-based mentalizing processing [62]. Undoubtedly, in the near future, new intraoperative tasks will be proposed to evaluate more precisely the behavior of patients throughout the resection: however, it is worth noting that additional testing should be introduced into the operating theater primarily for patient care, and not for scientific research—even though the data collected during surgery could finally be analyzed off-line to improve our understanding of the connectome [63].

For this purpose, such a refinement of intraoperative functional mapping and monitoring which relies on more sophisticated tasks must be extensively explained to each patient and his/her relatives before surgery, in order to give him/her the choice according to his/her philosophy of life and his/her own weighting of the onco-functional balance [64]. In other words, because every patient (and every brain) is unique, the decision-making process should be achieved in a personalized-medicine concept, in agreement with the Hippocratic oath, making the protocols issued from evidence-based medicine questionable in this setting of surgical neurooncology [65]. Similarly, decisional algorithms emerging from the so-called "artificial intelligence" expose us to risk of deprivation of decision, disempowerment, then involution of neural networks which need perpetual problem-solving to find adapted strategies—with ultimately a threat for intuition, (meta)cognition, and behavior, i.e., with a debasement of the spirit, both for medical doctors and patients [66].

Therefore, to offer a wider range of therapeutic strategies tailored to each patient, medical doctors should continue to potentiate their own creative scientific work based upon amodal integration between cognition, conscious awareness, and tacit knowledge as a source of inspiration to stimulate intuition. In fact, a meta-networking account of brain functioning renders conceivable an infinity of spatiotemporal combinations between specialized and more integrated neural circuits, resulting in an infinity of behaviors. This dynamic organization explains how the brain may adapt to the environment and makes possible the emergence of new ideas and thus creative behaviors [22]. The ultimate aim of this unending virtuous spiral founded on observation-experience-intuition-knowledge-health care is to enable patients not only to live longer but also to be human beings able to dream and to innovate [67]. Free will is the common thread to sublimate relationship between physician and patient. On the basis of this unique link, the purpose is to give the opportunity for each patient to potentiate his/her own meta-networking brain thanks to the profound thoughts imposed by the tumoral disease about his/her wishes in life (active participation in the selection of tasks before surgery, in awake monitoring during resection, in postoperative cognitive rehabilitation, in resuming familial and socioprofessional activities), in order to use his/her self-confidence to reach a higher level of transcendence and to become more creative, which is the essence of man—neither in agreement nor against the world, but in perfect symbiosis with him(her)self.

Fundings The author reports no fundings.

Financial Disclosure Statement The author reports no disclosures.

References

1. Duffau H. Long-term outcomes after supratotal resection of diffuse low-grade gliomas: a consecutive series with 11-year follow-up. Acta Neurochir (Wien). 2016;158:51–8.
2. Rossi M, Ambrogi F, Gay L, Gallucci M, Conti Nibali M, Leonetti A, et al. Is supratotal resection achievable in low-grade gliomas? Feasibility, putative factors, safety, and functional outcome. J Neurosurg. 2019;132(6):1692–705. https://doi.org/10.3171/2019.2.JNS183408.
3. Li YM, Suki D, Hess K, Sawaya R. The influence of maximum safe resection of glioblastoma on survival in 1229 patients: can we do better than gross-total resection? J Neurosurg. 2016;124:977–88.
4. Molinaro AM, Hervey-Jumper S, Morshed RA, Young J, Han SJ, Chunduru P, et al. Association of maximal extent of resection of contrast-enhanced and non-contrast-enhanced tumor with survival within molecular subgroups of patients with newly diagnosed glioblastoma. JAMA Oncol. 2020;6(4):495–503. https://doi.org/10.1001/jamaoncol.2019.6143.

5. Kamp MA, Rapp M, Slotty PJ, Turowski B, Sadat H, Smuga M, et al. Incidence of local in-brain progression after supramarginal resection of cerebral metastases. Acta Neurochir (Wien). 2015;157:905–10.
6. Barone DG, Lawrie TA, Hart MG. Image guided surgery for the resection of brain tumours. Cochrane Database Syst Rev. 2014;(1):CD009685.
7. Zetterling M, Roodakker KR, Berntsson SG, Edqvist PH, Latini F, Landtblom AM, et al. Extension of diffuse low-grade gliomas beyond radiological borders as shown by the coregistration of histopathological and magnetic resonance imaging data. J Neurosurg. 2016;125(5):1155–66.
8. Azad TD, Duffau H. Limitations of functional neuroimaging for patient selection and surgical planning in glioma surgery. Neurosurg Focus. 2020;48(2):E12.
9. Duffau H. Mapping the connectome in awake surgery for gliomas: an update. J Neurosurg Sci. 2017;61:612–30.
10. Zanello M, Meyer B, Still M, Goodden JR, Colle H, Schichor C, et al. Surgical resection of cavernous angioma located within eloquent brain areas: international survey of the practical management among 19 specialized centers. Seizure. 2019;69:31–40.
11. Bourdillon P, Apra C, Guénot M, Duffau H. Similarities and differences in neuroplasticity mechanisms between brain gliomas and nonlesional epilepsy. Epilepsia. 2017;58(12):2038–47.
12. Duffau H. Lessons from brain mapping in surgery for low-grade glioma: insights into associations between tumour and brain plasticity. Lancet Neurol. 2005;4:476–86.
13. Duffau H. Diffuse low-grade glioma, oncological outcome and quality of life: a surgical perspective. Curr Opin Oncol. 2018;30:383–9.
14. Zhang Z, Lei Y, Li H. Approaching the distinction between intuition and insight. Front Psychol. 2016;7:1195.
15. Zander T, Horr NK, Bolte A, Volz KG. Intuitive decision making as a gradual process: investigating semantic intuition-based and priming-based decisions with fMRI. Brain Behav. 2015;6(1):e00420.
16. Duffau H. The error of Broca: from the traditional localizationist concept to a connectomal anatomy of human brain. J Chem Neuroanat. 2018;89:73–81.
17. Vilasboas T, Herbet G, Duffau H. Challenging the myth of right nondominant hemisphere: lessons from corticosubcortical stimulation mapping in awake surgery and surgical implications. World Neurosurg. 2017;103:449–56.
18. Desmurget M, Bonnetblanc F, Duffau H. Contrasting acute and slow-growing lesions: a new door to brain plasticity. Brain. 2007;130(Pt 4):898–914.
19. Duffau H. The huge plastic potential of adult brain and the role of connectomics: new insights provided by serial mappings in glioma surgery. Cortex. 2014;58:325–37.
20. Geschwind N. Disconnexion syndromes in animals and man. Brain. 1965;88(3):585.
21. Mesulam MM. Large-scale neurocognitive networks and distributed processing for attention, language, and memory. Ann Neurol. 1990;28(5):597–613.
22. Herbet G, Duffau H. Revisiting the functional anatomy of the human brain: toward a meta-networking theory of cerebral functions. Physiol Rev. 2020;100(3):1181–228. https://doi.org/10.1152/physrev.00033.2019.
23. Duffau H. Awake surgery for nonlanguage mapping. Neurosurgery. 2010;66:523–8.
24. Vanacôr C, Duffau H. Analysis of legal, cultural, and socioeconomic parameters in low-grade glioma management: variability across countries and implications for awake surgery. World Neurosurg. 2018;120:47–53.
25. Duffau H. Stimulation mapping of white matter tracts to study brain functional connectivity. Nat Rev Neurol. 2015;11:255–65.
26. Rech F, Herbet G, Moritz-Gasser S, Duffau H. Disruption of bimanual movement by unilateral subcortical electrostimulation. Hum Brain Mapp. 2014;35:3439–45.
27. Herbet G, Moritz-Gasser S, Duffau H. Electrical stimulation of the dorsolateral prefrontal cortex impairs semantic cognition. Neurology. 2018;90:e1077–84.
28. Fernández Coello A, Moritz-Gasser S, Martino J, Martinoni M, Matsuda R, Duffau H. Selection of intraoperative tasks for awake mapping based on relationships between tumor location and functional networks. J Neurosurg. 2013;119:1380–94.

29. Moritz-Gasser S, Herbet G, Duffau H. Mapping the connectivity underlying multimodal (verbal and non-verbal) semantic processing: a brain electrostimulation study. Neuropsychologia. 2013;51:1814–22.
30. Lemaitre AL, Herbet G, Duffau H, Lafargue G. Preserved metacognitive ability despite unilateral or bilateral anterior prefrontal resection. Brain Cogn. 2018;120:48–57.
31. Herbet G, Moritz-Gasser S, Duffau H. Direct evidence for the contributive role of the right inferior fronto-occipital fasciculus in non-verbal semantic cognition. Brain Struct Funct. 2017;222:1597–610.
32. Ng S, Herbet G, Moritz-Gasser S, Duffau H. Return to work following surgery for incidental diffuse low-grade glioma: a prospective series with 74 patients. Neurosurgery. 2020;87(4):720–9. https://doi.org/10.1093/neuros/nyz513. pii: nyz513.
33. De Witt Hamer PC, Hendriks EJ, Mandonnet E, Barkhof F, Zwinderman AH, Duffau H. Resection probability maps for quality assessment of glioma surgery without brain location bias. PLoS One. 2013;8(9):e73353.
34. Vassal M, Charroud C, Deverdun J, Le Bars E, Molino F, Bonnetblanc F, et al. Recovery of functional connectivity of the sensorimotor network after surgery for diffuse low-grade gliomas involving the supplementary motor area. J Neurosurg. 2017;126:1181–90.
35. Deverdun J, van Dokkum LEH, Le Bars E, Herbet G, Mura T, D'agata B, et al. Language reorganization after resection of low-grade gliomas: an fMRI task based connectivity study. Brain Imaging Behav. 2020;14(5):1779–91. https://doi.org/10.1007/s11682-019-00114-7.
36. van Dokkum LEH, Moritz Gasser S, Deverdun J, Herbet G, Mura T, D'Agata B, et al. Resting state network plasticity related to picture naming in low-grade glioma patients before and after resection. Neuroimage Clin. 2019;24:102010.
37. Boyer A, Deverdun J, Duffau H, Le Bars E, Molino F, Menjot de Champfleur N, et al. Longitudinal changes in cerebellar and thalamic spontaneous neuronal activity after wide-awake surgery of brain tumors: a resting-state fMRI study. Cerebellum. 2016;15(4):451–65.
38. Charras P, Herbet G, Deverdun J, de Champfleur NM, Duffau H, Bartolomeo P, et al. Functional reorganization of the attentional networks in low-grade glioma patients: a longitudinal study. Cortex. 2015;63:27–41.
39. Bonelli SB, Thompson PJ, Yogarajah M, Powell RH, Samson RS, McEvoy AW, et al. Memory reorganization following anterior temporal lobe resection: a longitudinal functional MRI study. Brain. 2013;136(Pt 6):1889–900.
40. Herbet G, Latorre JG, Duffau H. The role of cerebral disconnection in cognitive recovery after brain damage. Neurology. 2015;84(14):1390–1.
41. Herbet G, Moritz-Gasser S, Lemaitre AL, Almairac F, Duffau H. Functional compensation of the left inferior longitudinal fasciculus for picture naming. Cogn Neuropsychol. 2019;36(3–4):140–57.
42. Mandonnet E, Cerliani L, Siuda-Krzywicka K, Poisson I, Zhi N, Volle E, et al. A network-level approach of cognitive flexibility impairment after surgery of a right temporo-parietal glioma. Neurochirurgie. 2017;63:308–13.
43. Mandonnet E, Wager M, Almairac F, Baron MH, Blonski M, Freyschlag CF, et al. Survey on current practice within the European Low-Grade Glioma Network: where do we stand and what is the next step? Neurooncol Pract. 2017;4(4):241–7.
44. Rofes A, Mandonnet E, Godden J, Baron MH, Colle H, Darlix A, et al. Survey on current cognitive practices within the European Low-Grade Glioma Network: towards a European assessment protocol. Acta Neurochir (Wien). 2017;159(7):1167–78.
45. Tate MC, Herbet G, Moritz-Gasser S, Tate JE, Duffau H. Probabilistic map of critical functional regions of the human cerebral cortex: Broca's area revisited. Brain. 2014;137:2773–82.
46. Sarubbo S, De Benedictis A, Merler S, Mandonnet E, Balbi S, Granieri E, et al. Towards a functional atlas of human white matter. Hum Brain Mapp. 2015;36:3117–36.
47. Sarubbo S, Tate M, De Benedictis A, Merler S, Moritz-Gasser S, Herbet G, et al. Mapping critical cortical hubs and white matter pathways by direct electrical stimulation: an original functional atlas of the human brain. Neuroimage. 2020;205:116237.

48. Sarubbo S, Tate M, De Benedictis A, Merler S, Moritz-Gasser S, Herbet G, et al. A normalized dataset of 1821 cortical and subcortical functional responses collected during direct electrical stimulation in patients undergoing awake brain surgery. Data Brief. 2019;28:104892.
49. Herbet G, Maheu M, Costi E, Lafargue G, Duffau H. Mapping neuroplastic potential in brain-damaged patients. Brain. 2016;139:829–44.
50. Robles SG, Gatignol P, Lehéricy S, Duffau H. Long-term brain plasticity allowing a multi-stage surgical approach to World Health Organization Grade II gliomas in eloquent areas. J Neurosurg. 2008;109(4):615–24.
51. Duffau H, Denvil D, Capelle L. Long term reshaping of language, sensory, and motor maps after glioma resection: a new parameter to integrate in the surgical strategy. J Neurol Neurosurg Psychiatry. 2002;72(4):511–6.
52. Picart T, Herbet G, Moritz-Gasser S, Duffau H. Iterative surgical resections of diffuse glioma with awake mapping: how to deal with cortical plasticity and connectomal constraints? Neurosurgery. 2018;85:105–16.
53. Southwell DG, Hervey-Jumper SL, Perry DW, Berger MS. Intraoperative mapping during repeat awake craniotomy reveals the functional plasticity of adult cortex. J Neurosurg. 2016;124(5):1460–9.
54. Walker AM. Tacit knowledge. Eur J Epidemiol. 2017;32(4):261–7.
55. Ilg R, Vogeley K, Goschke T, Bolte A, Shah JN, Pöppel E, et al. Neural processes underlying intuitive coherence judgments as revealed by fMRI on a semantic judgment task. Neuroimage. 2007;38(1):228–38. Epub 2007 Jul 24.
56. Undorf M, Zander T. Intuition and metacognition: the effect of semantic coherence on judgments of learning. Psychon Bull Rev. 2017;24(4):1217–24.
57. Lemaitre AL, Lafargue G, Duffau H, Herbet G. Damage to the left uncinate fasciculus is associated with heightened schizotypal traits: a multimodal lesion-mapping study. Schizophr Res. 2018;197:240–8.
58. Herbet G, Lafargue G, Bonnetblanc F, Moritz-Gasser S, Duffau H. Is the right frontal cortex really crucial in the mentalizing network? A longitudinal study in patients with a slow-growing lesion. Cortex. 2013;49:2711–27.
59. Herbet G, Lafargue G, Moritz-Gasser S, Menjot de Champfleur N, Costi E, Bonnetblanc F, et al. A disconnection account of subjective empathy impairments in diffuse low-grade glioma patients. Neuropsychologia. 2015;70:165–76.
60. Herbet G, Duffau H. Awake craniotomy and bedside cognitive mapping in neurosurgery. In: Pearson CM, Ecklund-Johnson E, Gale SD, editors. Neurosurgical neuropsychology. Chennai: Academic; 2019. p. 113–38.
61. Herbet G, Lafargue G, Moritz-Gasser S, Bonnetblanc F, Duffau H. Interfering with the neural activity of mirror-related frontal areas impairs mentalistic inferences. Brain Struct Funct. 2015;220:2159–69.
62. Nakajima R, Kinoshita M, Okita H, Yahata T, Matsui M, Nakada M. Neural networks mediating high-level mentalizing in patients with right cerebral hemispheric gliomas. Front Behav Neurosci. 2018;12:33.
63. Mandonnet E, Herbet G, Duffau H. Introducing new tasks for intraoperative mapping in awake glioma surgery: clearing the line between patient care and scientific research. Neurosurgery. 2020;86(2):E256–7.
64. Mandonnet E, Duffau H. An attempt to conceptualize the individual onco-functional balance: why a standardized treatment is an illusion for diffuse low-grade glioma patients. Crit Rev Oncol Hematol. 2018;122:83–91.
65. Duffau H. Paradoxes of evidence-based medicine in lower-grade glioma: to treat the tumor or the patient? Neurology. 2018;91(14):657–62.
66. Duffau H. Antagonisme entre la plasticité cérébrale humaine, le poids des dogmes et l'explosion incontrôlée de l'intelligence artificielle. Futuribles. 2019;431.
67. Duffau H. Jazz improvisation, creativity, and brain plasticity. World Neurosurg. 2014;81(3–4):508–10.